AN ATLAS OF
NORMAL DEVELOPMENTAL
ROENTGEN ANATOMY

Second Edition

Other books by Theodore E. Keats:

An Atlas of Normal Roentgen Variants That May Simulate Disease,
Fourth Edition

Atlas of Roentgenographic Measurement,
Fifth Edition,
with Lee B. Lusted

Emergency Radiology

AN ATLAS OF
NORMAL DEVELOPMENTAL
ROENTGEN ANATOMY

SECOND EDITION

THEODORE E. KEATS, M.D.

Professor and Chairman
Department of Radiology
University of Virginia School of Medicine
Charlottesville, Virginia

THOMAS H. SMITH, M.D.

Clinical Associate Professor of Radiology
University of Texas Health Science Center at Dallas
Director of Radiology
Children's Medical Center
Dallas, Texas

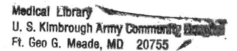

YEAR BOOK MEDICAL PUBLISHERS, INC.

Chicago • London • Boca Raton

1   2   3   4   5   6   7   8   9   0   KC   91   90   89   88   87

Library of Congress Cataloging-in-Publication Data

Keats, Theodore E. (Theodore Eliot), 1924-
An atlas of normal developmental roentgen anatomy.

  Includes bibliographies and index.
   1. Anatomy, Human—Atlases.   2. Radiography, Medical—
Atlases.   I. Smith, Thomas H. (Thomas Howard),
1938-   . II. Title. [DNLM: 1. Anatomy—atlases.
2. Radiography—atlases.   WN 17 K25a]
QM25.K4   1988   611′.0022′1   87-10667
ISBN 0-8151-5045-8

Sponsoring Editor: James D. Ryan, Jr.
Assistant Director, Manuscript Services: Frances M. Perveiler
Copyeditor: Julie DuSablon
Production Project Manager: Robert Allen Reedtz
Proofroom Supervisor: Shirley E. Taylor

To our Patricias

PREFACE TO THE FIRST EDITION

Decision making in diagnostic radiology is experience-dependent in that it requires a proper mental set for what is normal for the given anatomic part under observation at a particular age and for a particular sex. This is an enormous requirement that may take a lifetime to acquire if it is accomplished at all. The published atlases of skeletal development of the hand, knee, and foot have been very useful in this regard and are oriented largely to the determination of skeletal maturation, but the radiologist must rely on what resources he can muster for normal reference for the rest of the anatomy. This atlas of normal developmental roentgen anatomy is an effort to produce such ready source material for reference.

The atlas makes no attempt to duplicate the efforts of the published works on skeletal maturation and is not intended for this purpose, but rather to provide normal standards for relative size, proportion, density and configuration of the developing anatomy at various ages and for both sexes. The anatomic parts illustrated include the skeleton and those soft tissues that are obtainable by conventional radiography. The roentgenograms presented represent a composite individual at regular age intervals and include what was considered an average specimen from an accumulated series of normal individuals. The size of the sample of each part is variable and not all individuals are complete, despite several years of collection and searching of files, indicating some of the difficulty in finding normal roentgenograms on demand. The illustrated normal individual does not reflect the range of normal variation and is a reference guide to the normal only in a broad sense. The roentgenographic examples in this book should not be employed as determinants of skeletal maturation, since the sample size for any given part may not be adequate to provide statistically valid criteria for this kind of information. In short, this atlas is dedicated to answering the problems of the busy radiologist who requires that ever-elusive normal radiograph to compare with the case at hand for diagnosis.

We wish to express our special appreciation to Dr. Frederic N. Silverman of the Cincinnati Children's Hospital for permitting us to reproduce some of his material to complete entries where our own files were inadequate. His courtesy and willingness to help are much appreciated.

We wish also to thank the Division of Medical Photography of the University of Virginia School of Medicine for their dedication and cooperation in reproducing so large a volume of films; Patricia L. Hart, R.T., for her diligent assistance in critiquing, assembling, and mounting the illustrations for publication; and Dana Browne and Henry Matthews for their invaluable assistance in the collection of material.

THEODORE E. KEATS, M.D.

THOMAS H. SMITH, M.D.

PREFACE TO SECOND EDITION

In order to recognize pathology in radiologic diagnosis, one must have sound knowledge of the normal radiologic appearance of an anatomic part at any given age. Gaining this knowledge is an almost insurmountable task for most radiologists, particularly if they do not practice pediatric radiology exclusively. This atlas provides a ready reference source for this information. In our practices, the atlas has aided in innumerable decisions regarding radiographic appearances in growing individuals. These decisions often present problems of size, shape, and proportion that do not lend themselves to description in the texts on pediatric radiology.

To make the atlas more useful, we have replaced many of the illustrations with others of higher quality. The publishers have reproduced each of the figures individually rather than by composite page, as was done in the first edition. The greater clarity of these images should provide much more detail in each of the illustrations. In addition, we have provided maturation tables to assist in accurately determining skeletal maturation. We have also commented at the beginning of each chapter on the most important changes that are seen at each age. In reworking this edition, we discovered that there are no significant or even discernible radiographic changes in skeletal anatomy in the 20- to 25-year-old age group. Therefore, we have deleted the 21- to 25-year-olds from this edition in the interests of maintaining a manageable size and economy.

We believe that these modifications will enhance the value of this atlas.

THEODORE E. KEATS, M.D.

THOMAS H. SMITH, M.D.

CONTENTS

1

MATURATION STANDARDS

RADIOLOGIC ESTIMATION OF FETAL MATURITY

Technique

Central ray: Anteroposterior supine—to level of iliac crest on median plane.
Posteroanterior prone—to level of iliac crests on median plane.
Oblique posteroanterior—to symphysis pubis on median plane.
Positions: Anteroposterior supine abdomen.
Posteroanterior prone abdomen.
Oblique posteroanterior abdomen.
Target-film distance: Immaterial (36 inches used by Hartley).

Measurements

Figure 1–1:

10 wk. Ossification centers appear first in the transverse arches of the cervical vertebrae, subsequently appearing in the dorsal region and lumbar region.

Hartley believes that the centers are never dense enough to be identified before the end of the 10th week.

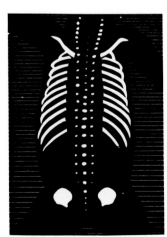

FIG 1–1 (left).
Radiologic estimation of fetal maturity.

FIG 1–2 (below).
Radiologic estimation of fetal maturity.

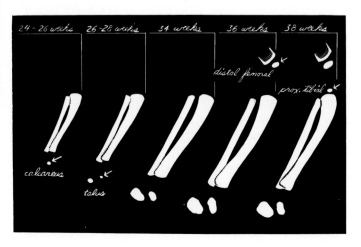

Figure 1–2:

- 10–24 wk. Size of skull is probably the best single index of fetal age. No carpal or tarsal centers are present, and no identifiable epiphyses have yet appeared.
- 24–26 wk. Calcaneous appears.
- 26–28 wk. Talus appears.
- 30–36 wk. Best guide is the study of developing foot ossification centers plus overall study of skull, vertebral bodies, femora, tibiae, and soft tissues.
- 36 wk. Distal femoral epiphysis appears.
- 38 wk. Proximal tibial epiphysis appears.

Source of Material

More than 10,000 cases from a large cross-section of the population in a large industrial center in Britain were studied.

MEASUREMENT OF THE NORMAL SKULL

Technique

Central ray: Posteroanterior—to glabella.

Lateral—to a point 1 inch anterior and 1 inch superior to external auditory meatus.

Positions: Posteroanterior.

Lateral.

Target-table distance: 91.4 cm (36 inches).

Table-film distance: 5.6 cm (enlargement factor of 16%).

Target-film distance: 97.0 cm (38 inches).

Measurements

Figure 1–3.

BR = greatest transverse diameter of skull in posteroanterior position.

L = greatest length of skull = distance from the glabella to the opisthocranion.

H = height of skull = total height from the basion to the vertex.

Note:

1. In roentgenograms the breadth averages from 4 to 8 mm less on the anteroposterior view than on the posteroanterior view.
2. Haas believes that it is best to measure breadth at the upper margin of the squamous suture, or slightly above it at the level of the stephanion, when the skull is wider there.

The modulus $M = \dfrac{L + H + Br}{3}$ is a better indicator of skull size than a single diameter. The computed modulus values conform to anthropologic data.

The cephalic index, $CI = Br_l \times 100$, is characteristic of skull shape.

Mesocephalic skull, CI = 75–84.

Brachycephalic skull, CI = 84 or greater.

Dolichocephalic skull, CI = 75 or less.

Skull size and measurements have diagnostic value. Deformity itself does not necessarily mean clinical pathology, but deviations in size call for detailed clinical and roentgenologic studies.

In Tables 1–1 through 1–5:

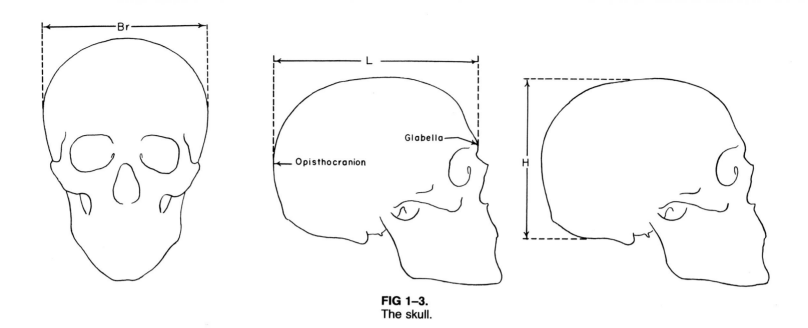

FIG 1–3.
The skull.

TABLE 1–1.

Breadth (cm) of Skull on Roentgenograms (Distortion: 16%)*

	MALE			FEMALE			TOTAL		
AGE	n	V_{min}-V_{max}	M	n	V_{min}-V_{max}	M	n	V_{min}-V_{max}	m†
–4 wk	2	11.1–11.6	11.3	3	10.0–12.0	10.8	5	10.0–12.0	11.0
2–6 mo	8	11.0–14.1	12.2	7	10.1–12.8	11.6	15	10.1–12.8	11.9
7–12 mo	14	12.7–15.6	13.9	12	12.0–15.0	13.2	26	12.0–15.6	13.6
13–18 mo	12	12.8–15.8	14.1	17	12.4–15.6	13.9	29	12.4–15.8	14.0
19–30 mo	22	14.0–16.7	15.1	9	13.2–16.0	14.4	31	13.2–16.7	14.9
3–5 yr	38	14.1–17.0	15.3	30	13.1–16.4	14.9	68	13.1–17.0	15.1
6–8 yr	32	14.1–17.2	15.9	27	13.6–16.6	15.3	59	13.6–17.2	15.6
9–11 yr	29	14.9–17.6	16.0	23	14.3–17.2	15.5	52	14.3–17.6	15.8
12–14 yr	29	15.2–17.3	16.2	23	14.7–17.0	15.7	52	14.7–17.3	16.0
15–17 yr	32	15.0–17.8	16.5	18	14.7–17.1	15.7	50	14.7–17.8	16.2
18–20 yr	31	14.7–18.9	16.5	24	15.5–17.2	16.1	55	14.7–18.9	16.3
21–	369	14.9–19.0	16.8	356	14.2–17.9	16.2	725	14.2–19.0	16.5
	$\sigma = -0.79 + 0.65$			$\sigma = -0.43 + 0.65$					
	$M \pm \sigma = 16.0 - 17.4 = 70.9\%$			$M \pm \sigma = 15.4 - 16.8 = 65.7\%$					
	$M \pm 2\sigma = 15.2 - 18.1 = 95.4\%$			$M \pm 2\sigma = 14.7 - 17.4 = 96.3\%$					
TOTAL	**618**			**549**			**1,167**		

*From Haas LL: *Am J Roentgenol* 1952; 67:197. Used by permission.
†m = Mean value.

TABLE 1–2.

Length Diameter (cm) of Racially Mixed Skulls on Roentgenograms (Distortion: 16%) of Various Age Groups of Both Sexes*

	MALE			FEMALE			TOTAL		
AGE	n	V_{min}-V_{max}	M	n	V_{min}-V_{max}	M	n	V_{min}-V_{max}	$m†$
–4 wk	2	13.7–14.2	13.9	3	12.6–14.0	13.2	5	12.6–14.2	13.5
2–6 mo	8	13.5–16.2	14.7	7	13.4–14.8	14.3	15	13.4–15.0	14.5
7–12 mo	14	14.0–17.8	16.4	12	14.5–16.9	15.8	26	14.0–17.6	16.1
13–18 mo	12	15.8–18.2	17.1	17	15.8–18.1	17.1	29	15.8–18.2	17.1
19–30 mo	22	16.1–19.8	18.1	12	15.7–19.5	17.7	34	15.7–19.8	17.9
3–5 yr	40	16.4–20.4	18.9	30	16.2–20.4	18.8	70	16.2–20.4	18.8
6–8 yr	33	17.1–20.8	19.4	29	16.0–20.7	19.0	62	16.0–20.8	19.2
9–11 yr	34	17.9–21.1	19.6	26	16.6–21.3	19.3	60	16.6–21.3	19.5
12–14 yr	32	18.3–21.8	20.3	26	17.9–21.0	19.7	58	17.9–21.8	20.0
15–17 yr	34	19.0–22.2	20.6	20	18.7–21.8	20.1	54	18.7–22.2	20.4
18–20 yr	33	19.6–22.6	20.8	29	19.2–21.0	20.1	62	19.2–22.6	20.5
21–	395	18.9–23.2	21.2	363	18.0–22.3	20.1	758	18.0–23.2	20.7
	$\sigma = -8.0 + 7.9$			$\sigma = -7.5 + 7.4$					
	M ± σ = 20.4–22.0 = 69.8%			M ± σ = 19.4–20.9 = 74.5%					
	M ± 2σ = 19.6–22.8 = 96.7%			M ± 2σ = 18.7–21.6 = 95.5%					
TOTAL	659			574			1,233		

*From Haas LL: *Am J Roentgenol* 1952; 67:197. Used by permission.
†m = Mean value.

TABLE 1–3.

Height (cm) of Skull on Roentgenograms (Roentgenologic Enlargement: 16%)*

	MALE			FEMALE			TOTAL		
AGE	n	V_{min}-V_{max}	M	n	V_{min}-V_{max}	M	n	V_{min}-V_{max}	$m†$
–4 wk	2	10.2–11.2	10.7	3	9.8–13.0	11.1	5	9.8–13.0	11.0
2–6 mo	8	10.5–13.7	11.7	7	10.8–13.5	11.8	15	10.5–13.7	11.7
7–12 mo	10	12.1–14.3	13.3	12	11.4–13.6	12.4	22	11.4–14.3	12.8
13–18 mo	9	12.6–15.0	14.0	17	12.1–15.5	13.6	26	12.1–15.5	13.8
19–30 mo	22	13.6–15.7	14.7	9	13.2–15.3	14.2	31	13.2–15.7	14.5
3–5 yr	40	13.5–16.3	14.9	26	13.5–16.0	14.6	66	13.5–16.3	14.7
6–8 yr	33	14.2–16.7	15.2	27	13.2–16.3	14.8	60	13.2–16.7	15.1
9–11 yr	34	14.0–17.0	15.3	25	13.8–15.8	14.8	59	13.8–17.0	15.1
12–14 yr	32	14.4–17.0	15.6	24	13.8–16.3	15.1	56	13.8–17.0	15.4
15–17 yr	32	14.5–17.1	15.7	19	13.8–15.7	15.0	51	13.8–17.1	15.4
18–20 yr	29	14.0–17.4	15.6	26	13.0–16.3	15.1	55	13.0–17.4	15.4
21–	379	13.4–17.7	15.6	353	13.4–17.1	15.1	732	13.4–17.7	15.3
	$\sigma = -0.72 + 0.68$			$\sigma = -0.64 + 0.64$					
	M ± σ = 14.9–16.3 = 75.7%			M ± σ = 14.5–15.8 = 70.0%					
	M ± 2σ = 14.1–16.9 = 95.0%			M ± 2σ = 13.8–16.4 = 95.3%					
TOTAL	630			548			1,178		

*From Haas LL: *Am J Roentgenol* 1952; 67:197. Used by permission.
†m = Mean value.

$$\text{Modulus } (M) = \frac{L + H + Br}{3} \qquad \text{Cephalic index } (CI) = \frac{Br}{L} \times 100$$

$$m = \text{mean value}$$

$V_{min} - V_{max}$ = variation range from minimum to maximum. Values outside this range are definitely abnormal.

Adults: $M \pm \sigma$ = range of variation for mesocephalic skull; σ (standard deviation) not computed for children.

TABLE 1–4.

Modulus (cm) of Skull on Roentgenograms*

AGE	MALE			FEMALE			TOTAL		
	n	V_{min}-V_{max}	M†	n	V_{min}-V_{max}	M	n	V_{min}-V_{max}	m†
–4 wk	2	11.6–12.3	12.0	3	10.8–12.8	11.6	5	10.8–12.3	11.8
2–6 mo	8	11.9–14.6	12.9	7	12.1–14.1	12.7	15	11.9–14.6	12.8
7–12 mo	11	13.0–15.3	14.9	12	12.9–15.0	13.8	23	12.9–15.3	14.2
13–18 mo	9	14.3–16.1	15.3	17	13.5–16.0	14.8	26	13.5–16.1	15.0
19–30 mo	23	14.5–16.8	15.9	12	13.6–16.6	15.1	35	13.6–16.8	15.7
3–5 yr	33	14.8–17.4	16.3	26	14.2–17.4	16.0	59	14.2–17.4	16.2
6–8 yr	29	15.5–17.7	16.8	27	14.3–17.5	16.3	56	14.3–17.7	16.6
9–11 yr	30	15.7–18.1	16.9	23	15.2–17.6	16.5	53	15.2–18.1	16.7
12–14 yr	30	16.4–18.5	17.4	23	16.0–17.6	16.7	53	16.0–18.5	17.1
15–17 yr	32	16.6–18.8	17.6	18	15.9–17.7	16.9	50	15.9–18.8	17.3
18–20 yr	30	16.3–19.2	17.7	22	16.3–17.8	17.1	52	16.3–19.2	17.5
21–	360	16.3–19.5	17.8	355	15.7–18.5	17.1	715	15.7–19.5	17.5
	$\sigma = -0.52 + 0.51$			$\sigma = -0.54 + 0.39$					
	M $\pm$ σ = 17.3–18.4 = 72.1%			M $\pm$ σ = 16.4–17.6 = 70.2%					
	M $\pm$ 2σ = 16.8–18.9 = 94.2%			M $\pm$ 2σ = 16.0–18.1 = 95.7%					
TOTAL	597			545			1,142		

*From Haas LL: *Am J Roentgenol* 1952; 67:197. Used by permission.
†M = modulus

TABLE 1–5.

Cephalic Index (Br $\times$ 100/L) on Roentgenograms*

AGE	MALE			FEMALE			TOTAL		
	n	V_{min}-V_{max}	M†	n	V_{min}-V_{max}	M	n	V_{min}-V_{max}	m
–4 wk	2	81.0–81.7	81.3	3	79.4–85.7	81.6	5	79.4–85.7	81.5
2–6 mo	11	73.5–88.1	81.7	12	72.7–87.7	80.8	23	72.7–87.7	81.4
7–12 mo	12	73.8–89.5	81.8	12	75.9–90.4	82.5	24	73.8–90.4	82.1
13–18 mo	11	78.3–90.3	82.3	11	73.7–87.9	81.5	22	73.7–90.3	81.8
19–30 mo	21	71.7–90.4	81.2	10	77.4–88.4	81.4	31	74.3–90.4	81.3
3–5 yr	35	72.4–90.0	81.2	26	72.7–91.1	81.0	61	72.4–91.1	81.1
6–8 yr	30	71.8–88.6	81.4	24	73.0–88.3	81.5	54	71.8–88.6	81.4
9–11 yr	30	72.0–89.8	81.1	22	74.9–88.5	80.3	52	72.0–89.8	80.8
12–14 yr	30	73.1–88.3	80.5	23	73.9–89.4	80.2	53	73.1–89.4	80.3
15–17 yr	35	72.8–87.7	80.6	17	72.0–83.4	79.6	52	72.8–87.7	80.0
18–20 yr	31	72.8–85.7	79.3	24	73.8–89.6	80.0	55	72.8–89.6	79.6
21–	351	71.3–89.4	79.5	354	71.0–90.4	80.0	705	71.0–90.4	79.8
	$\sigma = -3.66 + 3.87$			$\sigma = -3.87 + 3.33$					
	M $\pm$ σ = 75.9–83.4 = 65.7%			M $\pm$ σ = 76.1–84.2 = 66.2%					
	M $\pm$ 2σ = 72.2–87.3 = 96.5%			M $\pm$ 2 σ = 72.3–88.3 = 94.0%					
TOTAL	599			538			1,137		

*From Haas LL: *Am J Roentgenol* 1952; 67:197. Used by permission.
†M = modulus.

Values of *M* outside of *M* $\pm$ 2σ indicate hyperdolichocephaly, and in adults suggest previous pathology in childhood.

n = Number of individuals.

Source of Material

Studies were made of 1,300 racially mixed patients of various age groups and both sexes.

Frontal and Maxillary Sinuses

Technique

Central ray: perpendicular to table top.
Position: posteroanterior. Head on 23° board.
Target-film distance: 28 inches

Measurements

None

Source of Material

Figure 1–4 was made from tracings of roentgenograms of 100 children who were examined periodically from birth to maturity.

FIG 1–4.
A, changes in size and shape of the maxillary and frontal sinuses in one individual during infancy and childhood (*m*-month; *y*-year). **B,** postnatal growth of the sphenoid sinus from birth to maturity. (From Caffey J: *Pediatric X-Ray Diagnosis,* ed 3. Chicago, Year Book Medical Publishers, 1956, pp 93–101. Used by permission.)

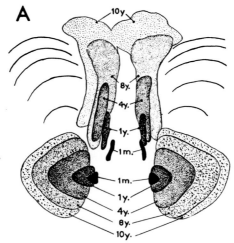
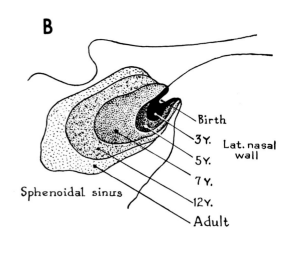

Sphenoid Sinus

Technique

Central ray: perpendicular to table top.
Position: true lateral.
Target-film distance: irrelevant.

Measurements

None

Source of Material

Maresh studied the frontal, ethmoid, and maxillary sinuses on routine anteroposterior roentgenograms of 100 children who were being examined from birth to maturity by the Child Research Council.

For studies on the sphenoid sinus, see the work of Schaeffer JP: *Pa Med J* 1936; 39:395. Schaeffer measured 3,000 sphenoid sinus specimens.

DEVELOPMENT OF THE TEETH (Table 1–6)

TABLE 1–6.

Approximate Periods of Eruption*
(see also Fig 1–5)

DECIDUOUS TEETH

TEETH	ERUPTION OCCURS	SHEDDING BEGINS
Medial incisors	6–8 mo	7th yr
Lateral incisors	7–12 mo	8th yr
First molars	14–15 mo	10th yr
Canines	18–19 mo	10th yr
Second molars	20–24 mo	11th–12th yr

*From Pendergrass EP, Schaeffer JP, Hodes P: *The Head and Neck in Roentgen Diagnosis*, (Springfield, Ill: Charles C Thomas, Publisher, 1956, vol I, p 442. Used by permission.

PERMANENT TEETH

TEETH	YEAR ERUPTION OCCURS	
	GIRLS	BOYS
First molars	6.0	6.5
Medial incisors	6.5	7.0
Lateral incisors	8.0	8.5
First premolars	9.0	10.0
Second premolars	10.0	11.0
Canines	11.0	11.5
Second molars	11.5	12.0
Third molars	17–25	17–25

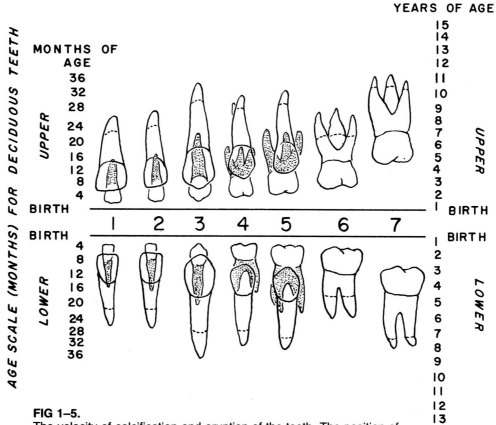

FIG 1–5.
The velocity of calcification and eruption of the teeth. The position of the biting edge of the crowns in the age scale indicates the age at which calcification of each tooth begins. *Dotted lines* on the roots signify the age at which each tooth erupts and its approximate size at that time. The position of the ends of the roots on the age scale measures the age at which calcification of each tooth is completed. The third permanent molar is not shown because of its great normal developmental variation. It usually begins to calcify between age 7 and 10, erupts between age 17 and 21, and completes calcification between age 18 and 25. Deciduous teeth are *shaded;* permanent teeth are *unshaded.* (Redrawn from Schour I, Poncher H: Development of Teeth. Copyright 1940 and 1945 by Mead Johnson & Company. Used by permission.)

SKELETAL MATURATION

Method of Sontag, Snell, and Anderson*

List of Centers (Total = 67)

Shoulder—Coracoid process
Humerus—Proximal medial epiphysis
      Proximal lateral epiphysis
      Capitellum
      Medial epicondyle
Radius—Proximal epiphysis
      Distal epiphysis
Hand—Capitatum
      Hamatum
      Triquetrum
      Lunate
      Navicula
      Greater multiangular bone
      Lesser multiangular bone
      5 distal phalangeal epiphyses
      4 middle phalangeal epiphyses
      5 proximal phalangeal epiphyses
      5 metacarpal epiphyses

Femur—Proximal epiphysis
      Greater trochanter
      Distal epiphysis
Knee—Patella
Tibia—Proximal epiphysis
      Distal epiphysis
Fibula—Proximal epiphysis
      Distal epiphysis
Foot—Cuboid
      First cuneiform
      Second cuneiform
      Third cuneiform
      Navicula
      Epiphysis of calcaneus
      5 distal phalangeal epiphyses
      4 middle phalangeal epiphyses
      5 proximal phalangeal epiphyses
      5 metatarsal epiphyses

TABLE 1–7.

Mean Total Number of Centers on the Left Side of Body Ossified at Given Age Levels*

AGE (MO)	BOYS		GIRLS	
	MEAN NO.	S.D.	MEAN NO.	SD.
1	4.11	1.41	4.58	1.76
3	6.63	1.86	7.78	2.16
6	9.61	1.95	11.44	2.53
9	11.88	2.66	15.36	4.92
12	13.96	3.96	22.40	6.93
18	19.27	6.61	34.10	8.44
24	29.21	8.10	43.44	6.65
30	37.59	7.40	48.91	6.50
36	43.42	5.34	52.73	5.48
42	47.06	5.26	56.61	3.98
48	51.24	4.59	57.94	3.91
54	53.94	4.35	59.89	3.36
60	56.24	4.07	61.52	2.69

*SD = Standard deviation.

Technique

Roentgenograms are taken of the following areas of the left side of the body: shoulder, elbow, wrist and hand, hip, knee (anteroposterior; lateral after 24 months), ankle and foot (anteroposterior; lateral after 48 months).

Measurements

The total number of ossification centers in the left half of the body is counted. A center is counted as soon as it casts a small shadow on the roentgenogram.

---

*Sontag LW, Snell D, Anderson M: *Am J Dis Child* 1939; 58:949.

Source of Material

These data have been taken from roentgenograms made at regular intervals of all the bones and joints of the left upper and lower extremities of 149 normal children during their first 5 years of life. The children came from the rural and metropolitan area near Yellow Springs, Ohio. There were 75 boys and 74 girls, and they represented a fair economic cross-section. Three black children (1 boy and 2 girls) were included.

Method of Girdany and Golden

Technique

Conventional technique for each body part.

Measurements

The numbers on Figures 1–6 and 1–7 indicate the range from the 10th to the 90th percentile in appearance time of centers of ossification, obtained from the studies on bone growth available in 1950. Statistically significant studies of the time of appearance of ossification centers have been made of relatively few portions of the skeleton after the 6th year of life. Figures followed by *m* indicate months; otherwise all numbers indicate years. Where two sets of numbers are given for one center of ossification, the *upper figures* refer to males and the *lower figures* refer to females. *Single figures* apply to both sexes. *AB* indicates that the ossification center is visible at birth. Figures in parentheses give approximate time of fusion.

Source of Material

The figures giving the range of time of appearance of the most important ossification centers have been taken from multiple sources, including:

Scammon RE, in Schaeffer JP (ed): *Morris' Human Anatomy*, ed. Philadelphia, Blakiston Company, 1953, p 11.

Vogt EC, Vickers VS: *Radiology* 1938; 31:441.

Milman DH, Bakwin H: *J Pediatr* 1950; 36:617.

Buehl CC, Pyle SI: *J Pediatr* 1942; 21:331.

Ruckensteiner E: *Die normale Entwicklung des Knochensystems im Roentgenbilg* Leipzig, Georg Thieme, 1931.

Bailey W: *Am J Roentgenol* 1939; 42:85.

Method of Graham

Technique

Central ray: Perpendicular to plane of film.
Position: Anteroposterior and lateral.
Target-film distance: Immaterial.

Measurements

The selected examinations that yield the most data at various ages are shown in Figure 1–8. The age-at-appearances for selected ossification center is shown in Table 1–8. Important "happenings" at various age levels are in *boldface* type. These data are based on a Caucasian population. American black and Hong Kong Chinese infants are relatively slightly advanced.

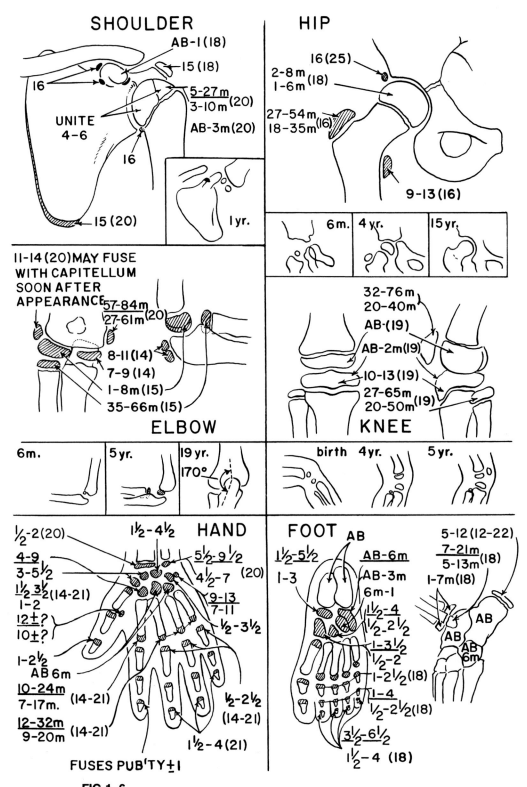

FIG 1–6.
Skeletal maturation—method of Girdany and Golden. (From Girdany BR, Golden R: *Am J Roentgenol* 1952; 68:922. Used by permission.)

VERTEBRA

OSSIFY FROM 3 PRIMARY CENTERS AND 9 SECONDARY CENTERS — ANY OF THESE SECONDARY CENTERS, EXCEPT FOR ANNULAR EPIPHYSES, MAY FAIL TO FUSE.

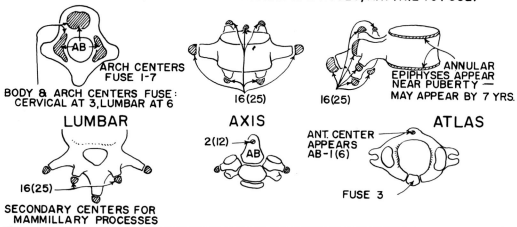

ARCH CENTERS FUSE 1-7

BODY & ARCH CENTERS FUSE: CERVICAL AT 3, LUMBAR AT 6

16(25)

16(25)

ANNULAR EPIPHYSES APPEAR NEAR PUBERTY — MAY APPEAR BY 7 YRS.

LUMBAR

16(25)

SECONDARY CENTERS FOR MAMMILLARY PROCESSES

AXIS

2(12) → AB

ATLAS

ANT. CENTER APPEARS AB-1(6)

FUSE 3

SACRUM & COCCYX

LOWER SACRAL BODIES FUSE AT 18 ··· ALL FUSE BY 30

INNOMINATE

PUBERTY ± 1

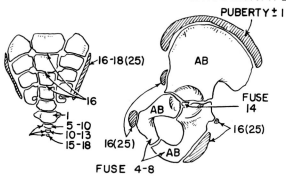

AB

16-18(25)

16

1
5-10
10-13
15-18

AB

FUSE 14

AB

16(25)

16(25)

AB

FUSE 4-8

PRIMARY CENTERS AB, SECONDARY CENTERS APPEAR NEAR PUBERTY, FUSE 16-30 YRS. — OCCASIONAL CENTERS AT PUBIC TUBERCLE, ANGLE, & CREST

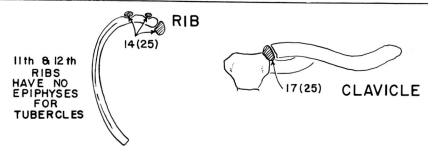

RIB

14(25)

11th & 12th RIBS HAVE NO EPIPHYSES FOR TUBERCLES

17(25)   CLAVICLE

FIG 1–7.
Skeletal maturation—method of Girdany and Golden. (From Girdany BR, Golden R: *Am J Roentgenol* 1952; 68:922. Used by permission.)

TABLE 1–8.

Age-at-Appearance (Years–Months) Percentiles for Selected Ossification Centers

CENTERS*	BOYS			GIRLS		
	5th	50th	95th	5th	50th	95th
1. Humerus, head	–	0–0	0–4	–	0–0	0–4
2. Tibia, proximal	–	0–0	0–1	–	0–0	0–0
3. Coracoid process of scapula	–	0–0	0–4	–	0–0	0–5
4. Cuboid	–	0–1	0–4	–	0–1	0–2
5. Capitate	**–**	**0–3**	**0–7**	**–**	**0–2**	**0–7**
6. Hamate	**0–0**	**0–4**	**0–10**	**–**	**0–2**	**0–7**
7. Capitellum of humerus	**0–1**	**0–4**	**1–1**	**0–1**	**0–3**	**0–9**
8. Femur, head	**0–1**	**0–4**	**0–8**	**0–0**	**0–4**	**0–7**
9. Cuneiform 3	**0–1**	**0–6**	**1–7**	**–**	**0–3**	**1–3**
10. Humerus, greater tuberosity	**0–3**	**0–10**	**2–4**	**0–2**	**0–6**	**1–2**
11. Toe phyalanx 5M	–	1–0	3–10	–	0–9	2–1
12. Radius, distal	0–6	1–1	2–4	0–5	0–10	1–8
13. Toe phalanx 1 D	0–9	1–3	2–1	0–5	0–9	1–8
14. Toe phalanx 4 M	0–5	1–3	2–11	0–5	0–11	3–0
15. Finger phalanx 3 P	0–9	1–4	2–2	0–5	0–10	1–7
16. Toe phalanx 3 M	0–5	1–5	4–3	0–3	1–0	2–6
17. Finger phalanx 2 P	0–9	1–5	2–2	0–5	0–10	1–8
18. Finger phalanx 4 P	0–10	1–6	2–5	0–5	0–11	1–8
19. Finger phalanx 1 D	0–9	1–6	2–8	0–5	1–0	1–9
20. Toe phalanx 3 P	0–11	1–7	2–6	0–6	1–1	1–11
21. Metacarpal 2	0–11	1–7	2–10	0–8	1–1	1–8
22. Toe phalanx 4 P	0–11	1–8	2–8	0–7	1–3	2–1
23. Toe phalanx 2 P	1–0	1–9	2–8	0–8	1–2	2–1
24. Metacarpal 3	0–11	1–9	3–0	0–8	1–2	1–11
25. Finger phalanx 5 P	1–0	1–10	2–10	0–8	1–2	2–1
26. Finger phalanx 3 M	1–0	2–0	3–4	0–8	1–3	2–4
27. Metacarpal 4	1–1	2–0	3–7	0–9	1–3	2–2
28. Toe phalanx 2 M	0–11	2–0	4–1	0–6	1–2	2–3
29. Finger phalanx 4 M	1–0	2–1	3–3	0–8	1–3	2–5
30. Metacarpal 5	1–3	2–2	3–10	0–10	1–4	2–4
31. Cuneiform 1	**0–11**	**2–2**	**3–9**	**0–6**	**1–5**	**2–10**
32. Metatarsal 1	1–5	2–2	3–1	1–0	1–7	2–3
33. Finger phalanx 2 M	1–4	2–2	3–4	0–8	1–4	2–6
34. Toe phalanx 1 P	1–5	2–4	3–4	0–11	1–7	2–6
35. Finger phalanx 3 D	1–4	2–5	3–9	0–9	1–6	2–8
36. Triquetrum	0–6	2–5	5–6	0–3	1–8	3–9
37. Finger phalanx 4 D	1–4	2–5	3–9	0–9	1–6	2–10
38. Toe phalanx 5 P	1–6	2–5	3–8	1–0	1–9	2–8
39. Metacarpal 1	1–5	2–7	4–4	0–11	1–7	2–8
40. Cuneiform 2	**1–2**	**2–8**	**4–3**	**0–10**	**1–10**	**3–0**
41. Metatarsal 2	1–11	2–10	4–4	1–3	2–2	3–5
42. Femur, greater trochanter	1–11	3–0	4–4	1–0	1–10	3–0
43. Finger phalanx 1 P	1–10	3–0	4–7	0–11	1–9	2–10
44. Navicular of foot	**1–1**	**3–0**	**5–5**	**0–9**	**1–11**	**3–7**
45. Finger phalanx 2 D	1–10	3–2	5–0	1–1	2–6	3–3
46. Finger phalanx 5 D	2–1	3–3	5–0	1–0	2–0	3–5
47. Finger phalanx 5 M	1–11	3–5	5–10	0–11	2–0	3–6
48. Fibula, proximal	**1–10**	**3–6**	**5–3**	**1–4**	**2–7**	**3–11**
49. Metatarsal 3	2–4	3–6	5–0	1–5	2–6	3–8
50. Toe phalanx 5 D	2–4	3–11	6–4	1–2	2–4	4–1
51. Patella	**2–7**	**4–0**	**6–0**	**1–6**	**2–6**	**4–0**
52. Metatarsal 4	2–11	4–0	5–9	1–9	2–10	4–1
53. Lunate	1–6	4–1	6–9	1–1	2–7	5–8
54. Toe phalanx 3 D	3–0	4–4	6–2	1–4	2–9	4–1
55. Metatarsal 5	3–1	4–4	6–4	2–1	3–3	4–11
56. Toe phalanx 4 D	2–11	4–5	6–5	1–4	2–7	4–1
57. Toe phalanx 2 D	3–3	4–8	6–9	1–6	2–11	4–6
58. Radius, head	**3–0**	**5–3**	**8–0**	**2–3**	**3–10**	**6–3**
59. Navicular of wrist	3–7	5–8	7–10	2–4	4–1	6–0
60. Greater multangular	3–6	5–10	9–0	1–11	4–1	6–4
61. Lesser multangular	3–1	6–3	8–6	2–5	4–2	6–0
62. Medial epicondyle of humerus	**4–3**	**6–3**	**8–5**	**2–1**	**3–5**	**5–1**
63. Ulna, distal	5–3	7–1	9–1	3–3	5–4	7–8
64. Calcaneal apophysis	**5–2**	**7–7**	**9–7**	**3–6**	**5–4**	**7–4**

(continued)

TABLE 1–8 (continued).

Age-at-Appearance (Years–Months) Percentiles for Selected Ossification Centers

	BOYS			GIRLS		
CENTERS*	5th	50th	95th	5th	50th	95th
65. Olecranon of ulna	7–9	9–8	11–11	5–7	8–0	9–11
66. Lateral epicondyle of humerus	9–3	11–3	13–8	7–2	9–3	11–3
67. Tibial tubercle	9–11	11–10	13–5	7–11	10–3	11–10
68. Adductor sesamoid of thumb	11–0	12–9	14–7	8–8	10–9	12–8
69. Os acetabulum	11–11	13–6	15–4	9–7	11–6	13–5
70. Acromion	12–2	13–9	15–6	10–4	11–11	13–9
71. Iliac crest	12–0	14–0	15–11	10–10	12–9	15–4
72. Coracoid apophysis	12–9	14–4	16–4	10–4	12–3	14–4
73. Ischial tuberosity	13–7	15–3	17–1	11–9	13–11	16–0

*P = proximal. M = middle. D = distal

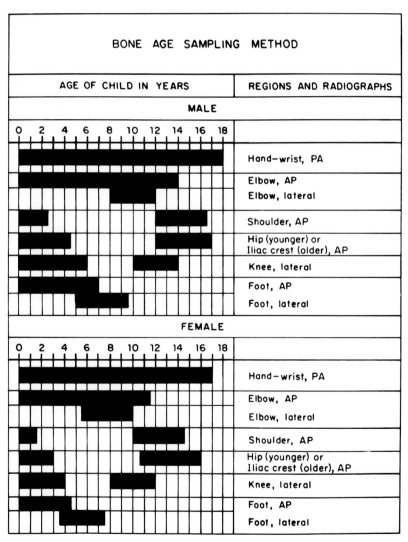

FIG 1–8.
Suggested films for determination of osseous maturation at various ages. (From Graham CB: *Radiol Clin North Am* 1972; 10:185. Used by permission.)

Data, derived by Garn et al.* in the Fels Research Institute Program of Human Development, were based on a study of 143 healthy, middle-class Ohio-born children of Northwestern European ancestry.

Method of Greulich-Pyle

Technique

Central ray: Perpendicular to plane of film and centered halfway between tips of fingers and distal end of radius.
Position: Posteroanterior.
Target-film distance. Immaterial.

Measurements

See Figures 1–9 through 1–13.
The patient's film is compared with the standard of the same sex and nearest chronologic age. It is next compared with adjacent standards, both older and younger than the one that is of the next chronologic age. Select, for a more detailed comparison, the standard that superficially appears to resemble the patient's film most closely.

Source of Material

Each of the standards was selected from 100 films of children of the same sex and age. The film chosen was selected as the most representative of the central tendency of the group. All children were white; all were born in the United States; almost all were of North European ancestry. The entire group included 1,000 children.

Note: Pyle, Waterhouse, and Greulich† have published a radiographic reference standard for the assessment of skeletal age from hand-wrist films of children and youths. The reference standard is based in part on the 1959 *Greulich and Pyle Atlas* that contains one series of reference films for males and another series for females. The new reference standard uses a single series of reference films. The osseous features indicating one and the same skeletal maturity level of each hand-wrist bone appear in the male and female at different chronologic ages. The films in the single film series are calibrated to show the natural chronologic differences between the appearance of the osseous features in males and females.

Studies of skeletal age assessments by research workers using left hand-wrist films and the bone-specific Greulich and Pyle method showed intra-observer differences ranging from 0.25 to 0.47 years. Observer training improves reliability of assessments. (Roche AF, et al: *Am J Roentgenol* 1970, 108:511; and Johnson GF, et al: *Am J Roentgenol* 1973; 118:320.

---

*Garn et al: *MCA Radiogr Photogr* 1967; 43:45.
†Pyle SI, Waterhouse Am, Greulich WW: *A Radiographic Standard of Reference for the Growing Hand and Wrist.* Cleveland, The Press of Case Western Reserve University, 1971.

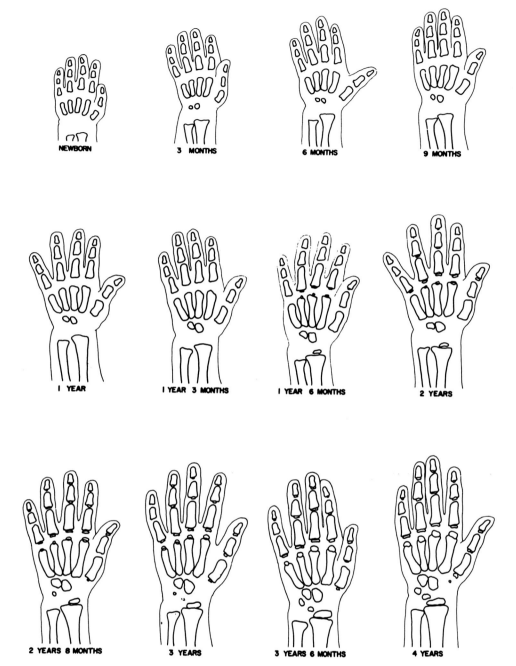

FIG 1–9.
Skeletal maturation—method of Greulich-Pyle. (Modified from Greulich WW, Pyle SI: *Radiographic Atlas of Skeletal Development of the Hand and Wrist,* ed 2. Stanford, Calif, Stanford University Press, 1959. Used by permission.)

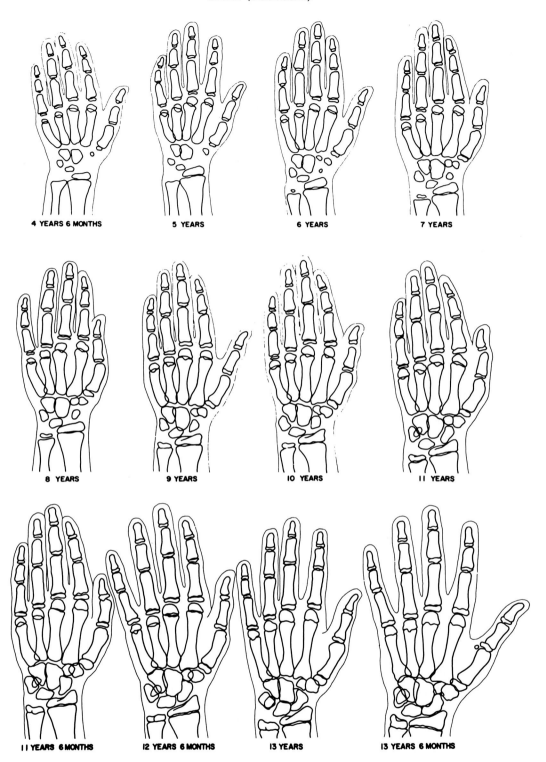

FIG 1–10.
Skeletal maturation—method of Greulich-Pyle. (Modified from Greulich WW, Pyle SI: *Radiographic Atlas of Skeletal Development of the Hand and Wrist,* ed 2. Stanford, Calif, Stanford University Press, 1959. Used by permission.)

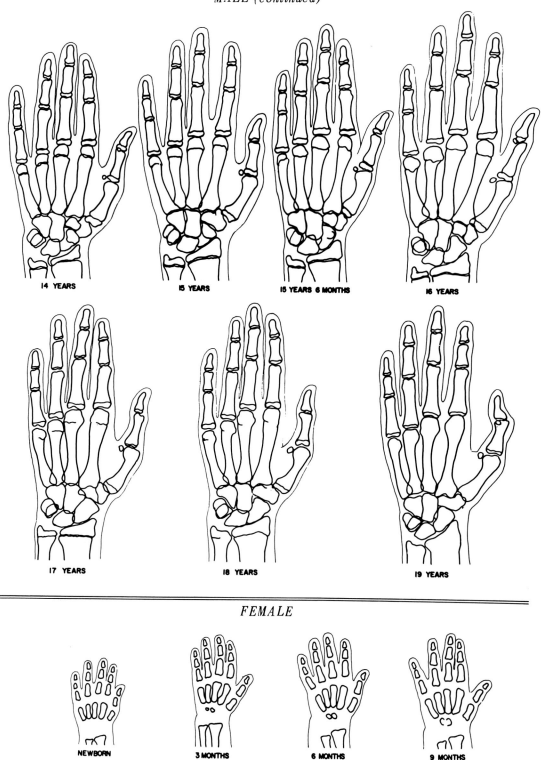

FIG 1–11.
Skeletal maturation—method of Greulich-Pyle. (Modified from Greulich WW, Pyle SI: *Radiographic Atlas of Skeletal Development of the Hand and Wrist,* ed 2. Stanford, Calif, Stanford University Press, 1959. Used by permission.)

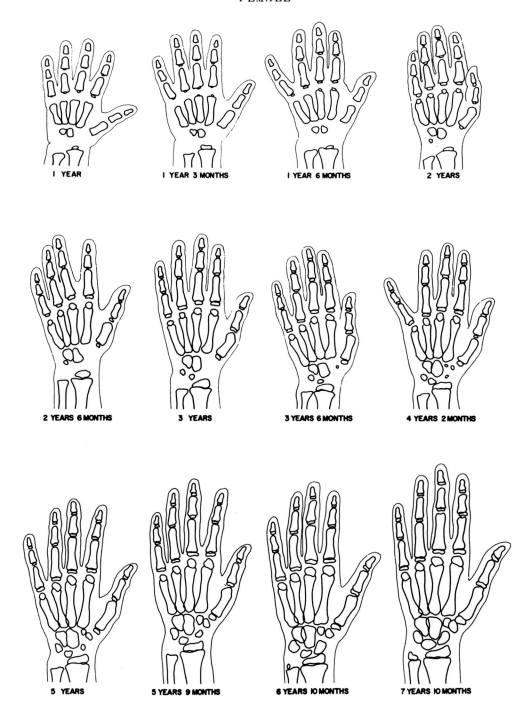

FIG 1–12.
Skeletal maturation—method of Greulich-Pyle. (Modified from Greulich WW, Pyle SI: *Radiographic Atlas of Skeletal Development of the Hand and Wrist,* ed 2. Stanford, Calif, Stanford University Press, 1959. Used by permission.)

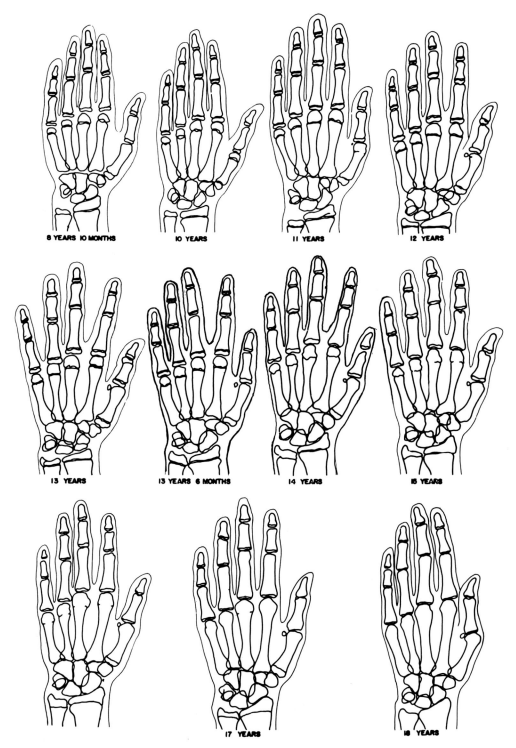

FIG 1–13.
Skeletal maturation—method of Greulich-Pyle. (Modified from Greulich WW, Pyle SI: *Radiographic Atlas of Skeletal Development of the Hand and Wrist,* ed 2. Stanford, Calif, Stanford University Press, 1959. Used by permission.)

2

NEWBORN

There is enormous variation in the configuration of the neonatal skull as a result of the molding of labor. An important observation is the ratio of skull to face size, which should be approximately 3 to 1. Sutural width is also extremely variable, but all the sutures should be visible. The orbits may be peaked superiorly.

The cervical spinal canal in children often appears disproportionately large. Measurements are available for determining the range of normal. The posterior elements are unfused. This is particularly clear in the lateral projection of the dorsal spine. The anterior and posterior surfaces of the dorsal and lumbar vertebrae are notched by vascular entry. The sacrum is poorly defined in the frontal plane.

In the pelvis, the degree of ossification of the ischia and pubes varies. The inner pelvic ring has a cup-like configuration. The capital femoral epiphyses are not evident as yet, but the distal femoral and proximal tibial epiphyses should be present.

The long bones are often quite dense, but this should not be mistaken for osteosclerosis. The ossification of the centers for the feet is highly variable. The relationship between the talus and calcaneus is important for determining deformity.

The proximal humeral ossification centers should be present. Normally, the acromioclavicular joints are wide. The appearance of the clavicle is extremely position-dependent and may appear bowed or twisted.

The organs of the chest and abdomen appear disproportionately large by adult criteria. The epiglottis should be visible. The size of the retropharyngeal soft tissues is respiration-dependent. Pulmonary vascularity is difficult to define. The ribs appear horizontal and gracile with bulbous ends.

Air bubbles may be seen in the stomach. It is difficult to differentiate the large from the small bowel. The pelvis may be gasless due to the filled bladder.

The esophagus should not exhibit any extrinsic impressions. The ligament of Treitz should lie at the level of the duodenal bulb. The small bowel is redundant. The cecum normally should overlap the ilium. The appendix is usually filled.

The renal cortical margins are difficult to define. The calyces should be sharp. The ureters are only partially filled. Bladder size is extremely variable.

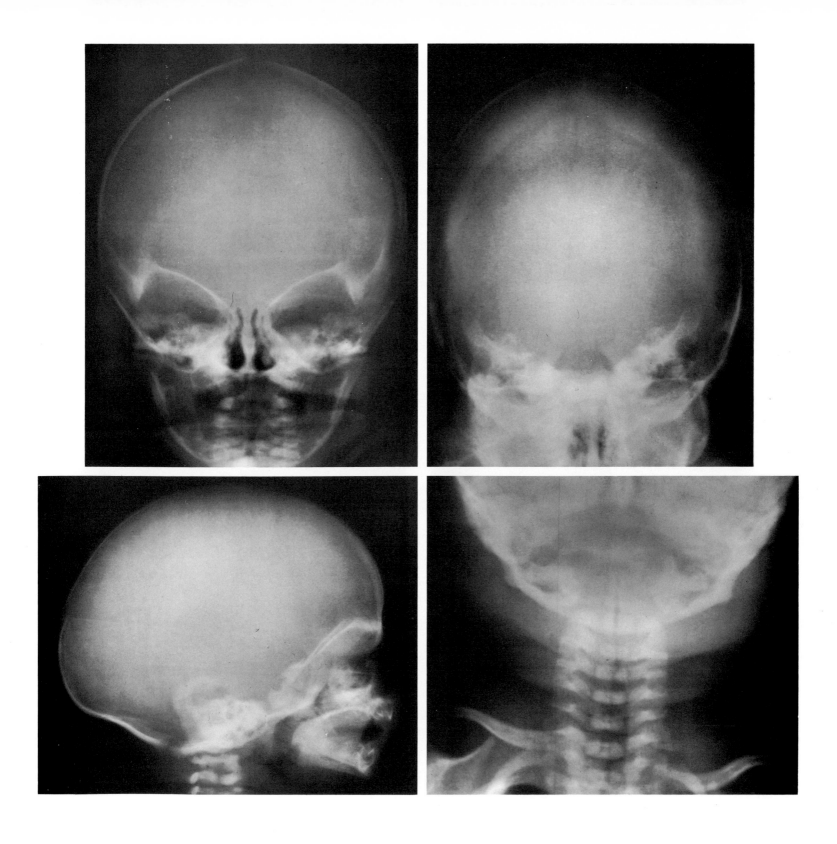

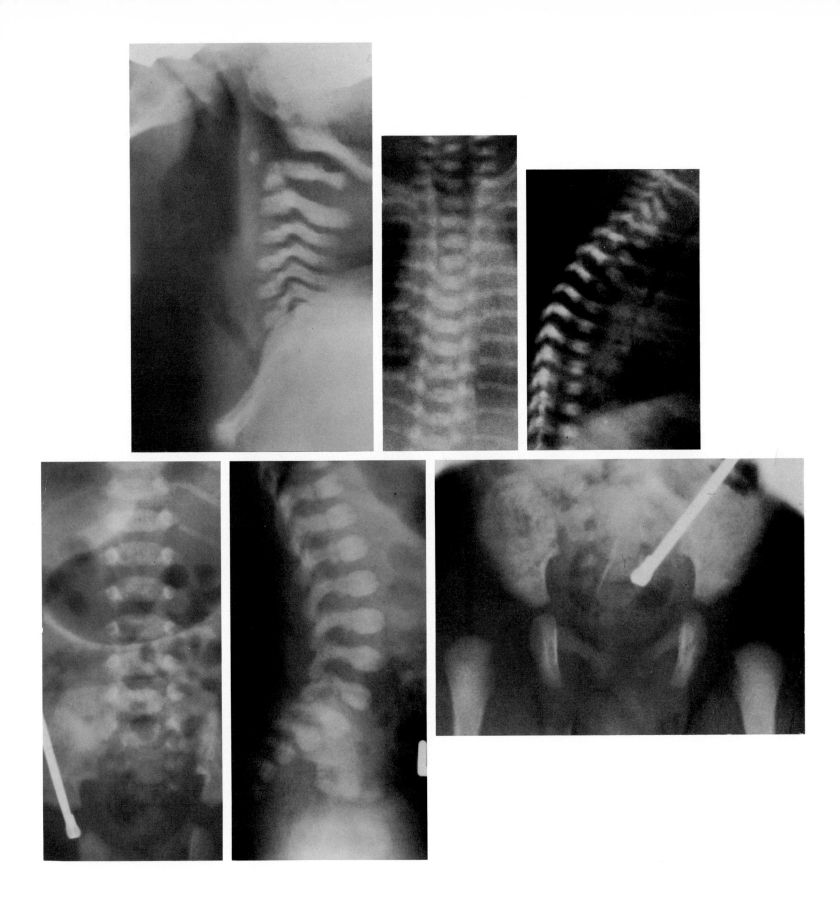

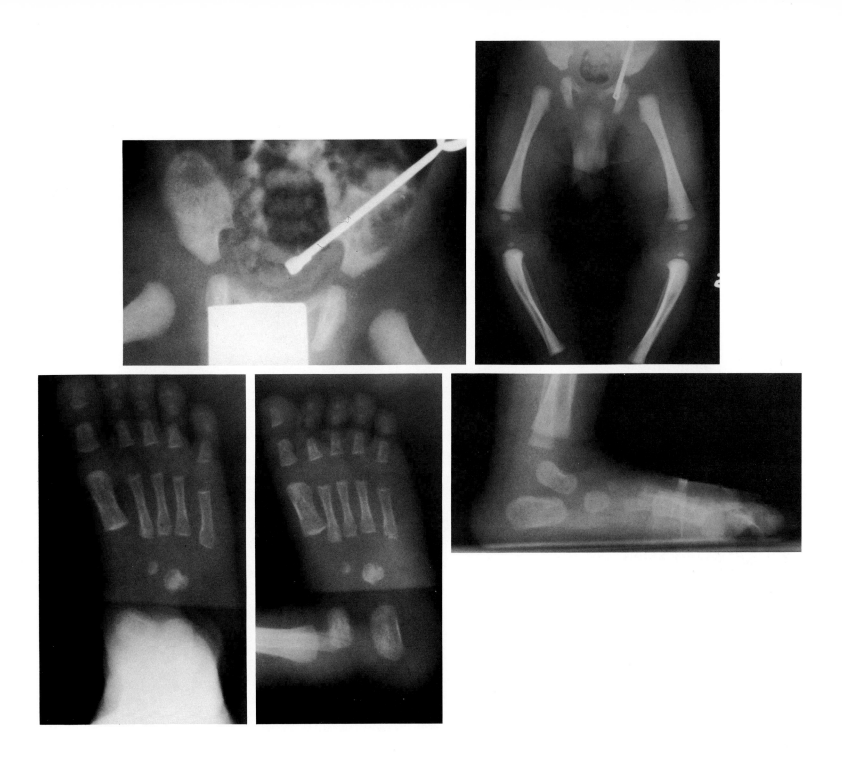

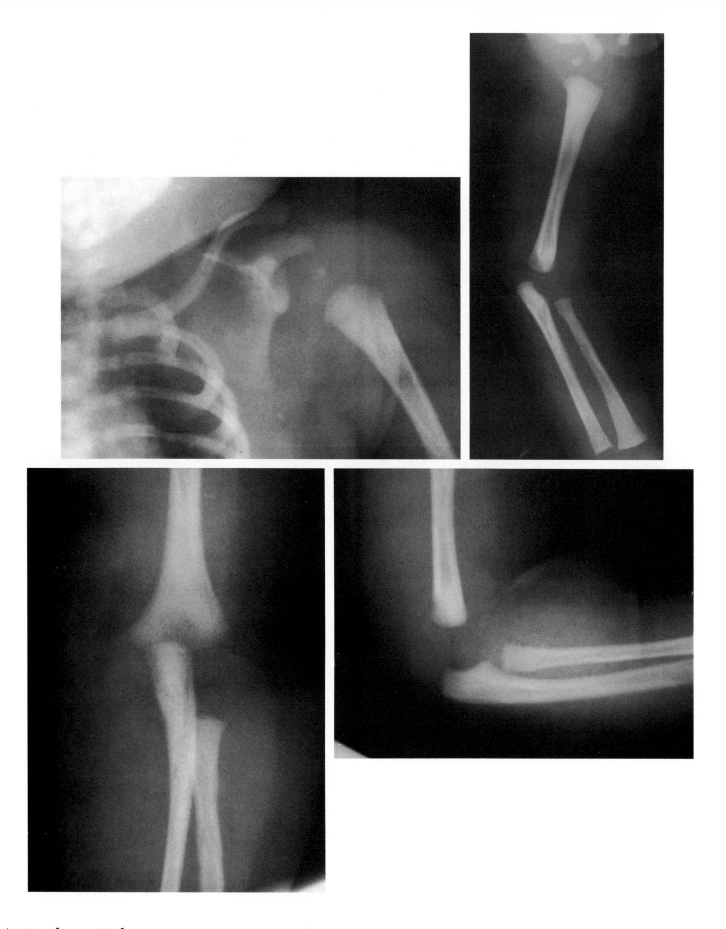

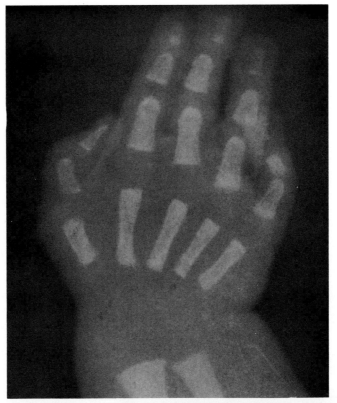

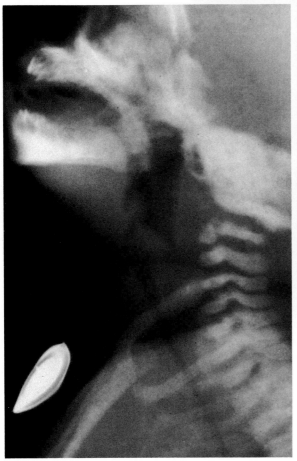

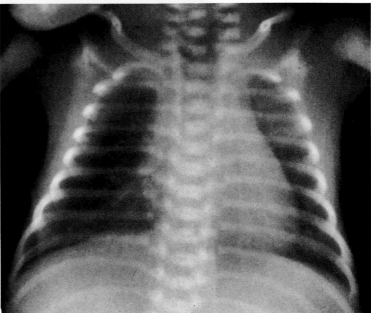

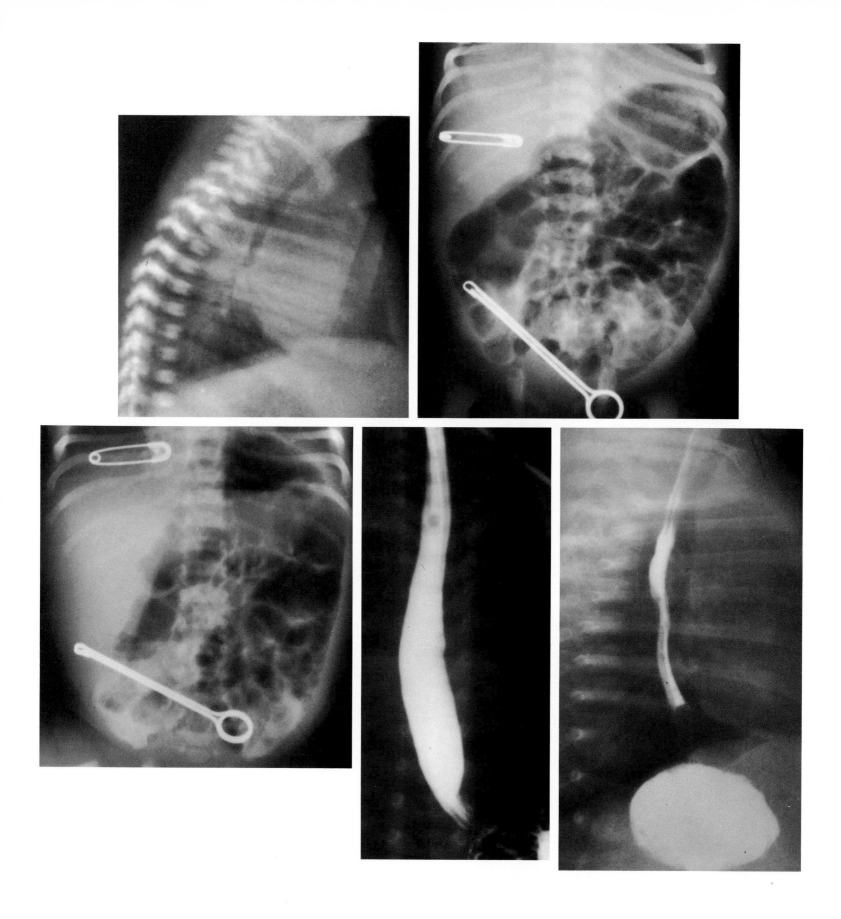

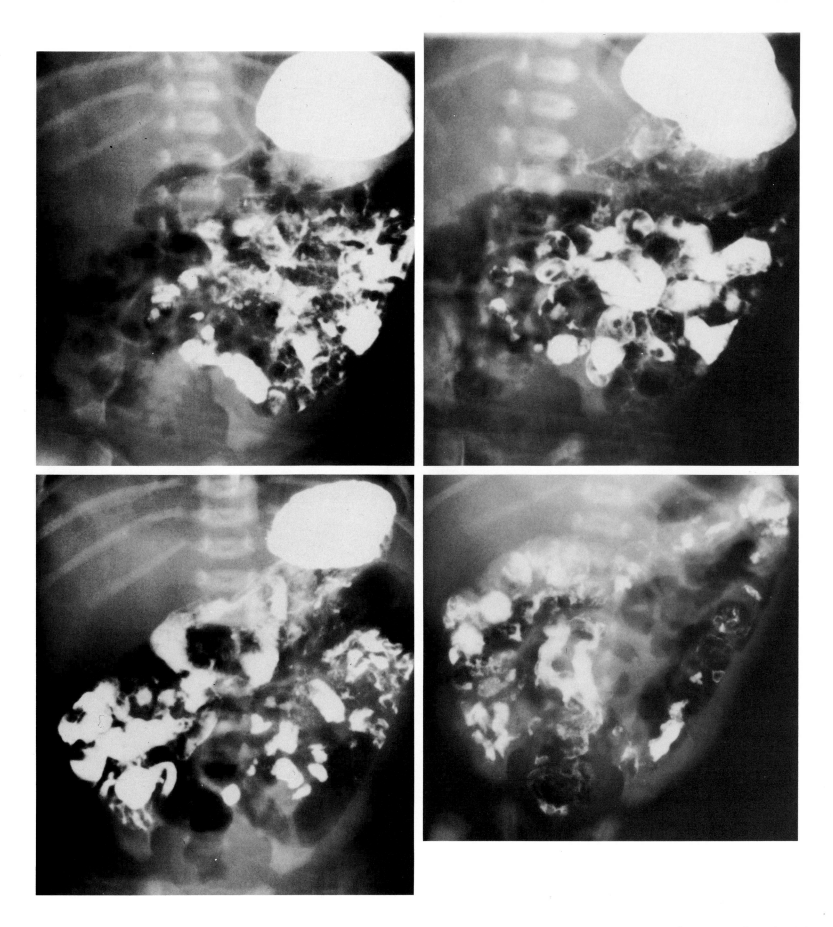

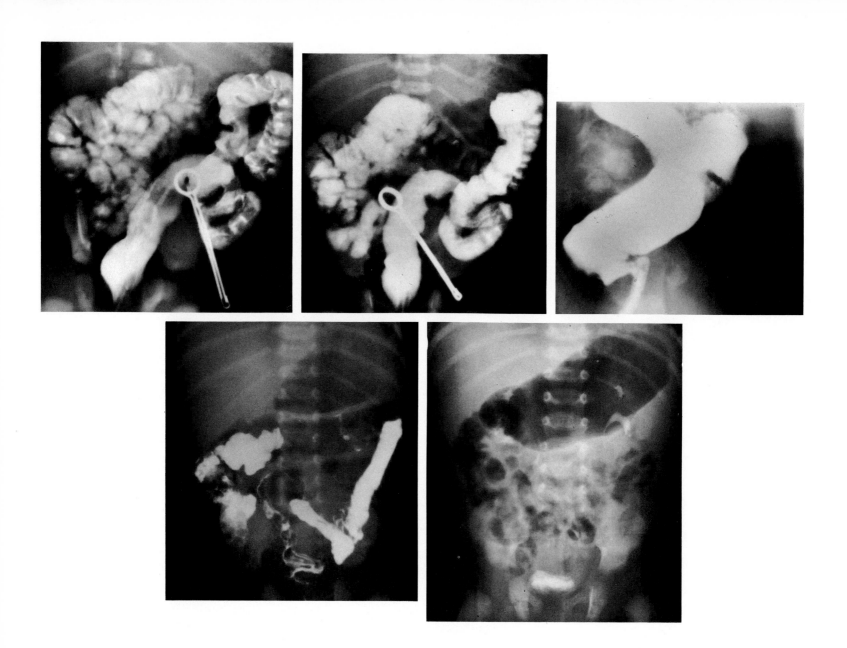

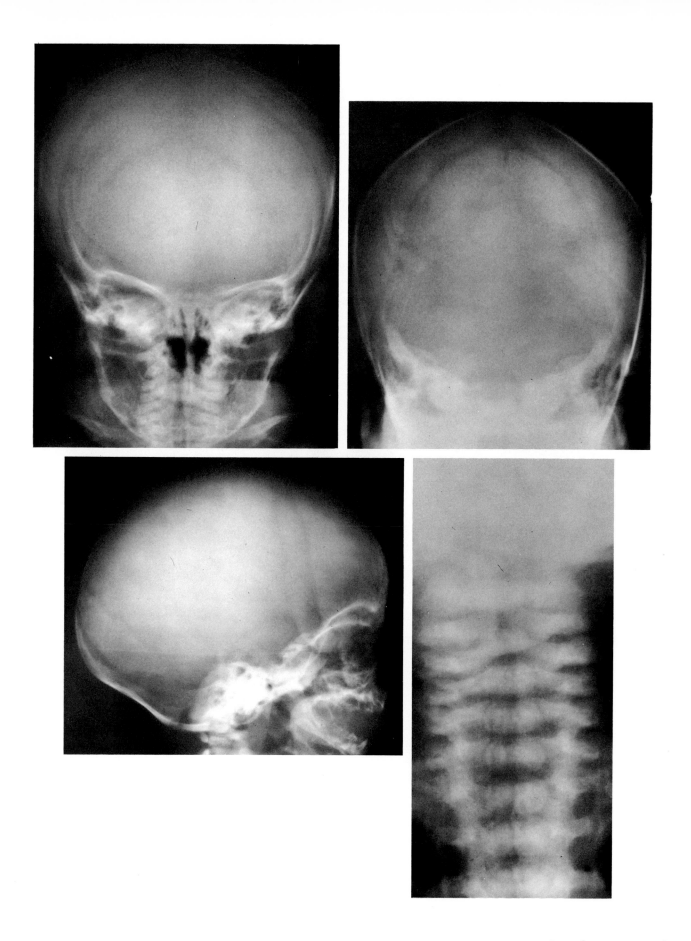

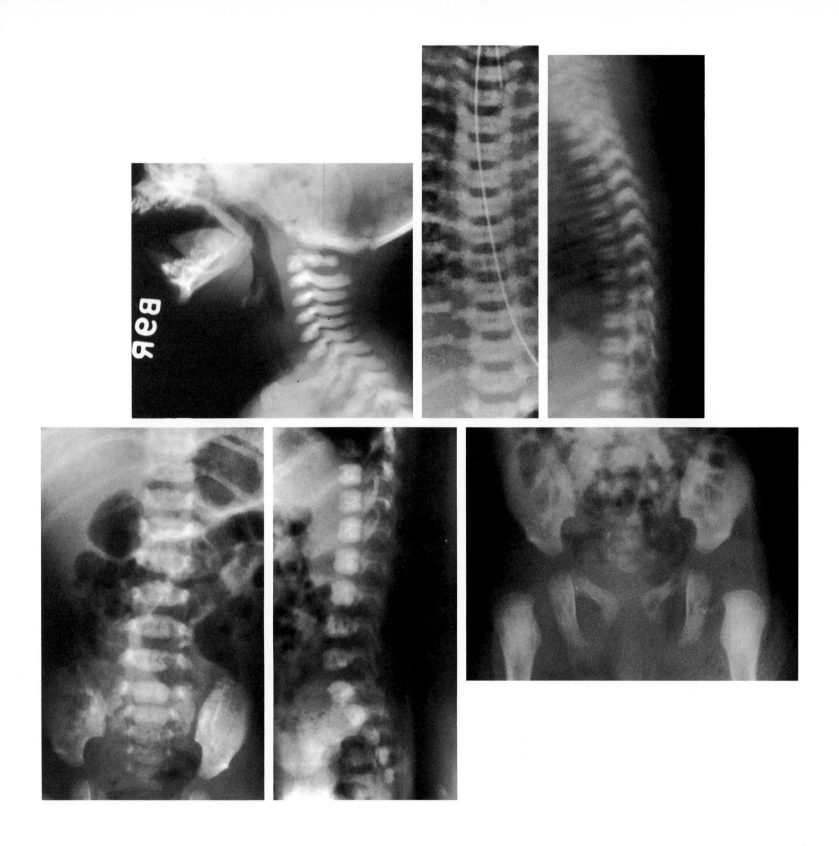

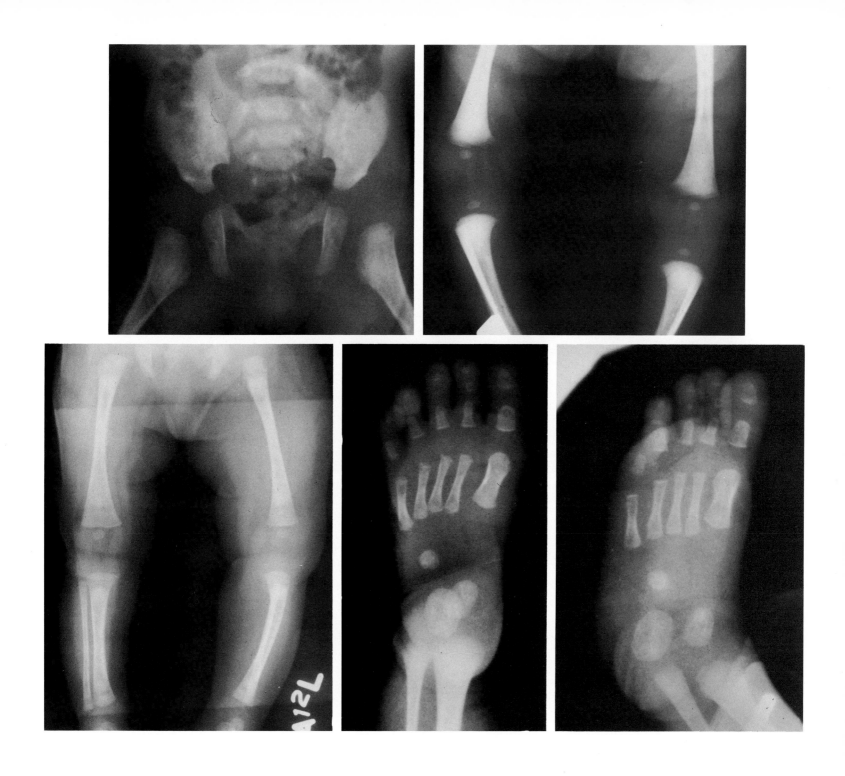

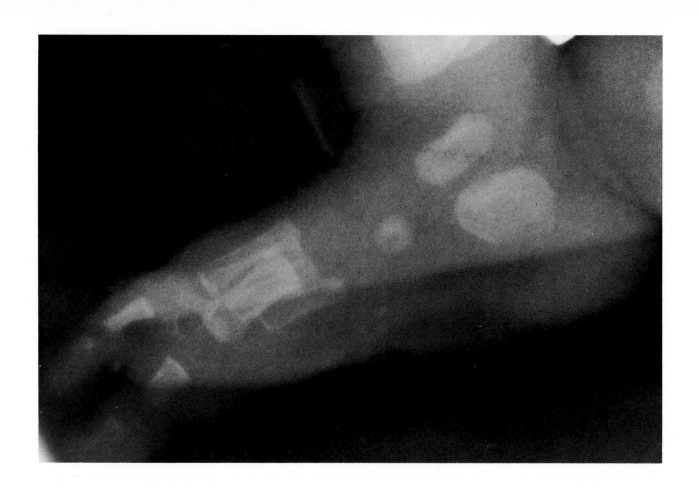

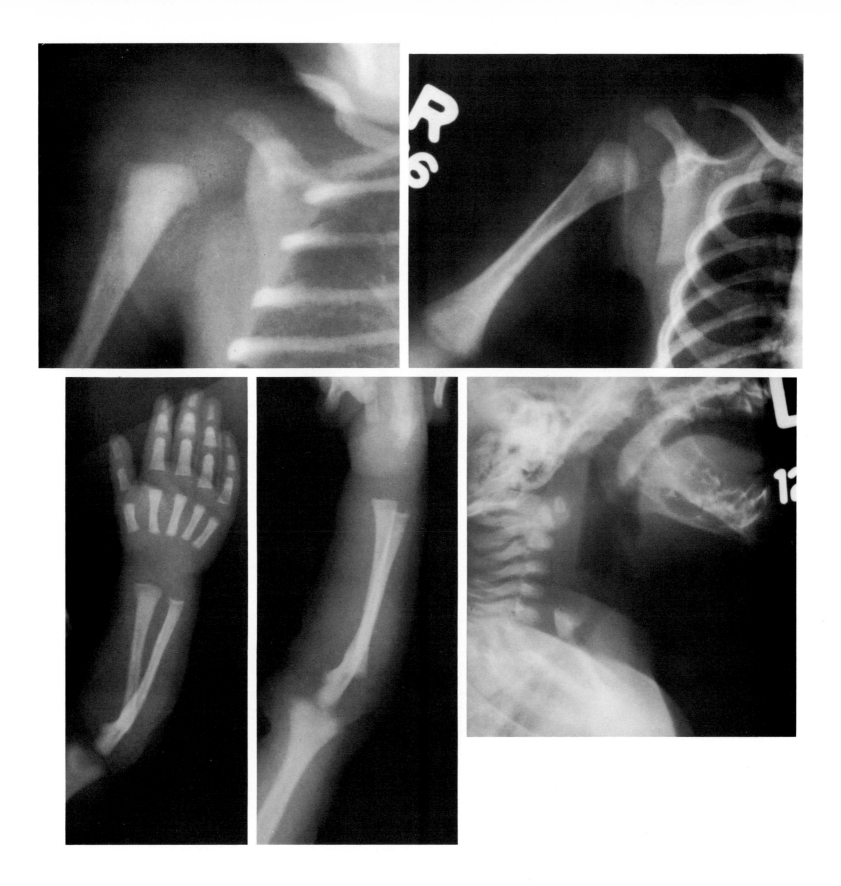

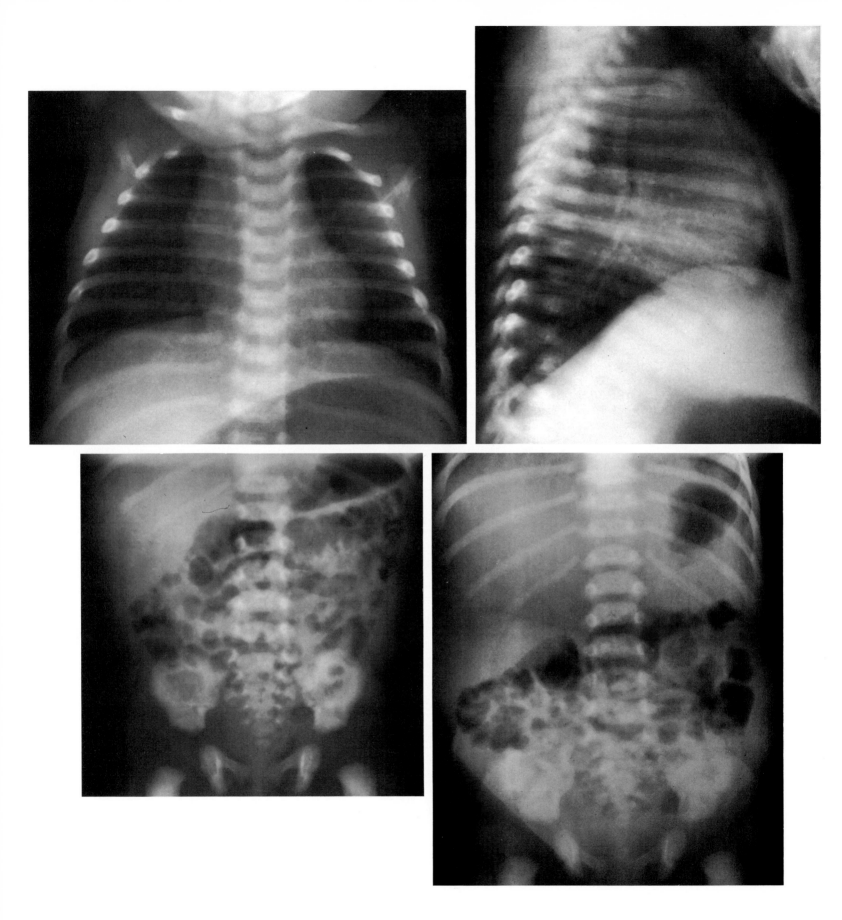

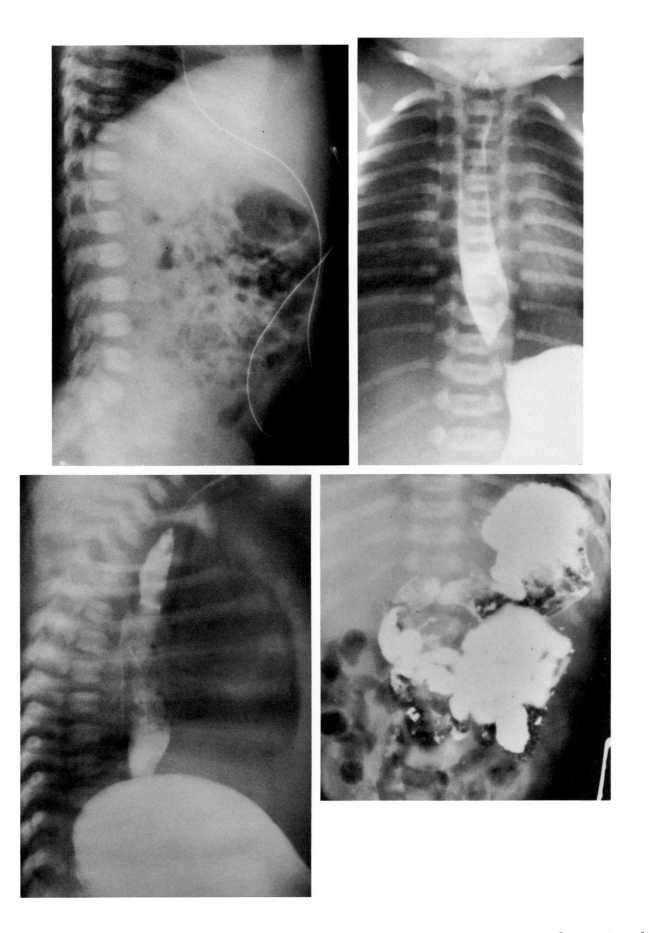

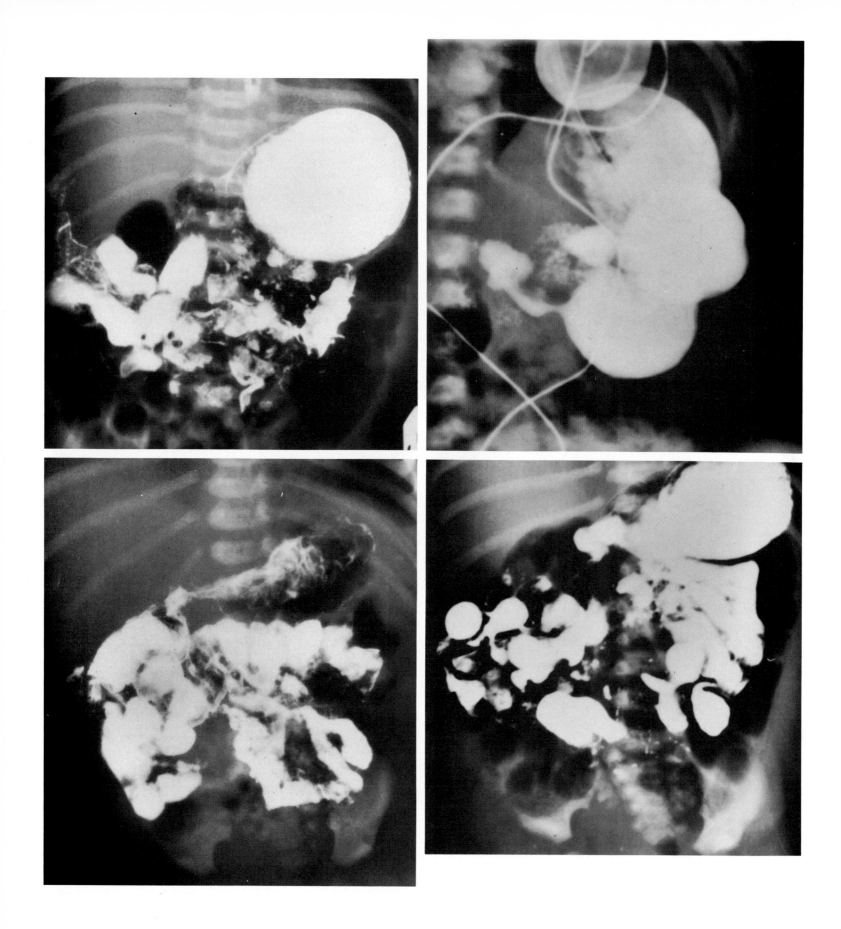

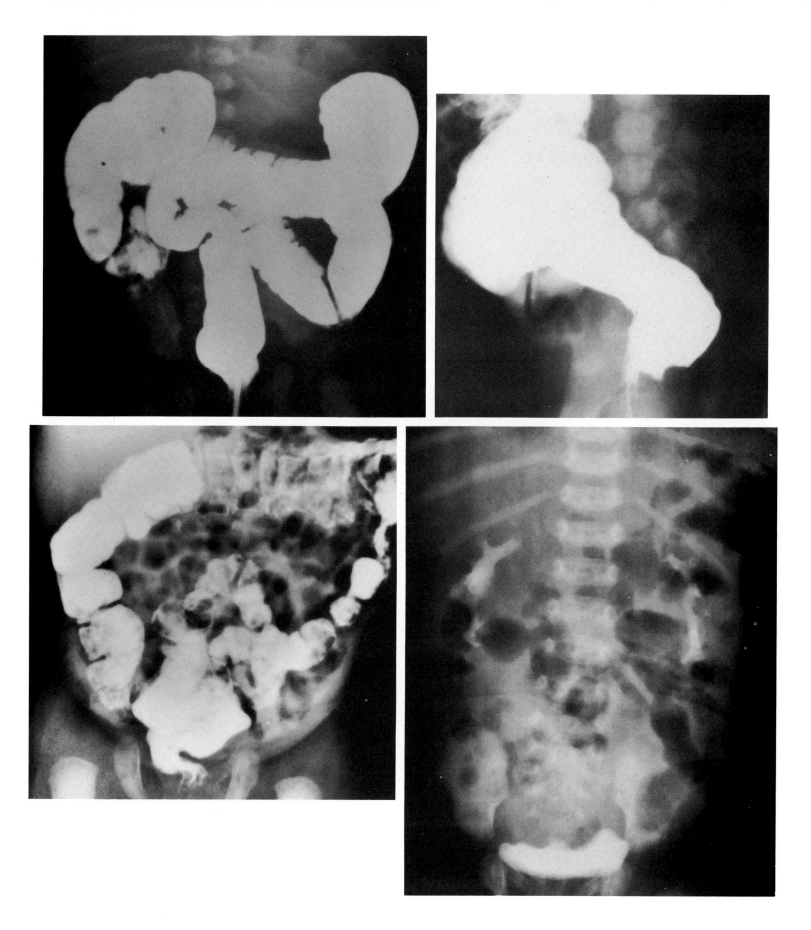

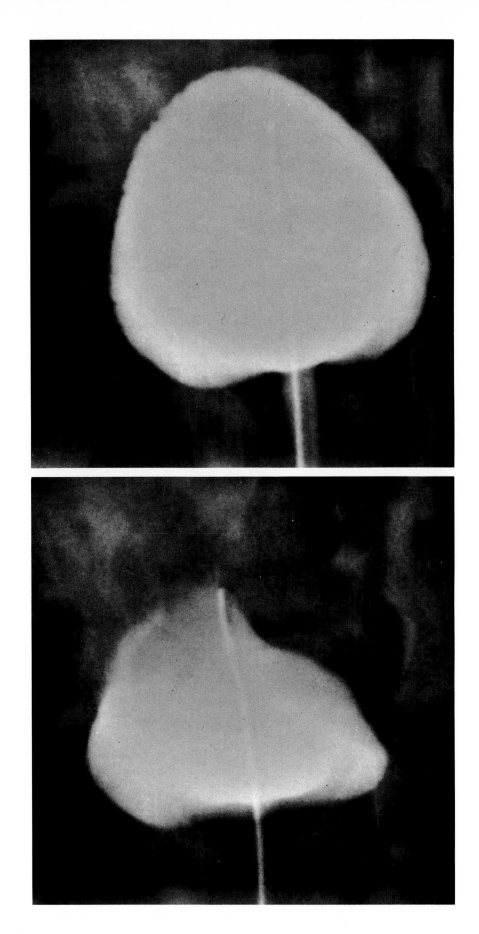

3

3 MONTHS

The effects of the molding of labor have disappeared. The sutures of the calvaria and the anterior fontanel are more clearly defined. Pneumatization of the mastoids is apparent. The cervical spinal canal still appears disproportionately large, and there is less separation of the fusing posterior elements. The capital humeral and the capital femoral epiphyses are present. The presence of the latter simplifies the diagnosis of congenital hip dislocation. The distal femoral and proximal epiphyses have grown larger. The distal tibial epiphysis appears. One or two ossificiation centers may be present in the tarsal and carpal areas. The long bones have lost their neonatal density.

The variable appearance of the thymus produces a spectrum of configurations of the mediastinum. The heart is relatively small in proportion to the chest. The ossification centers of the sternum appear as separate islands of bone.

The colon is more easily recognizable because of the presence of stool. The psoas and renal shadows are still not well defined.

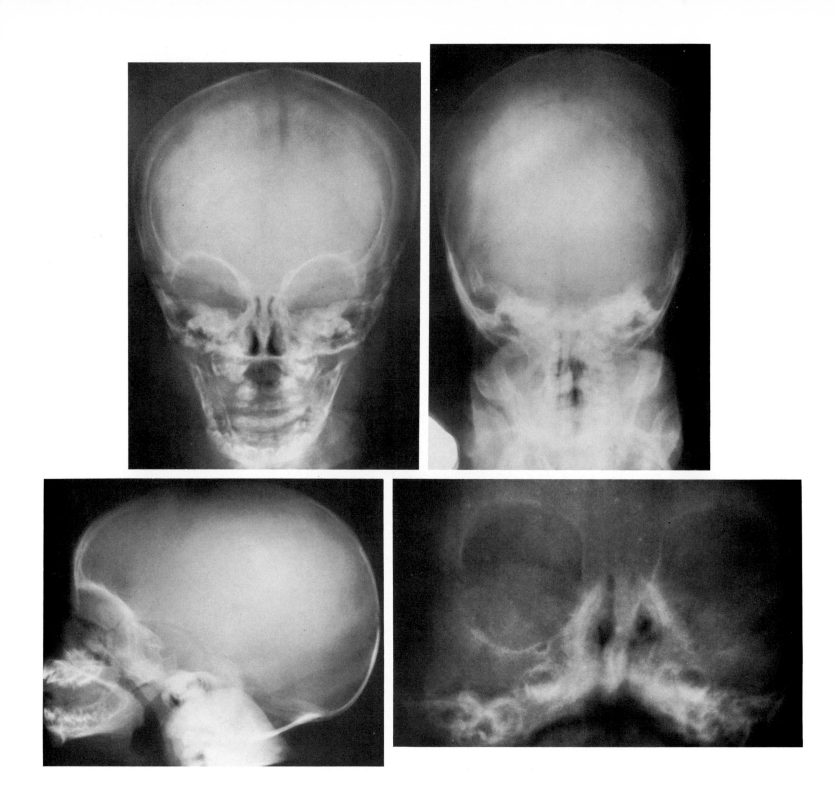

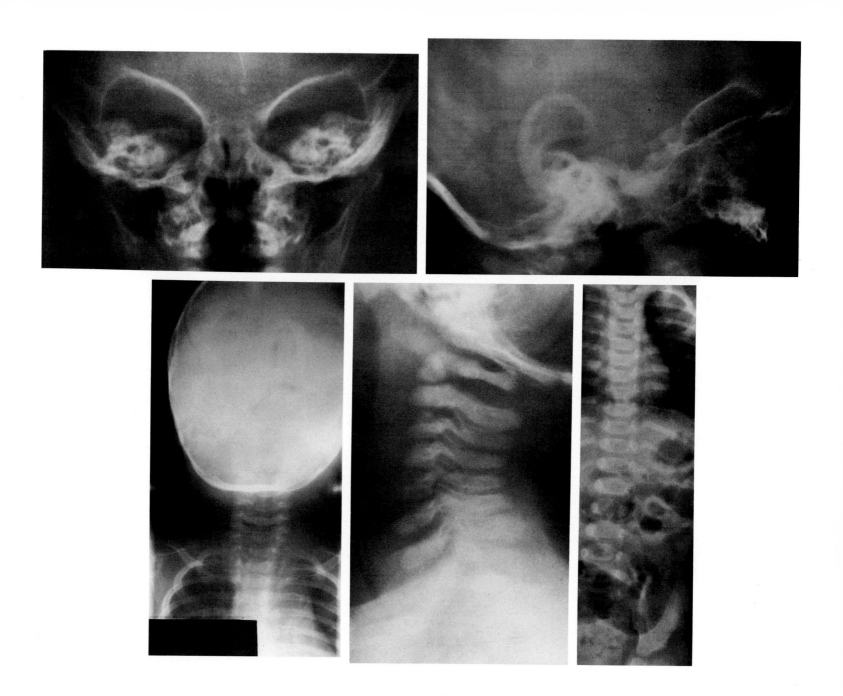

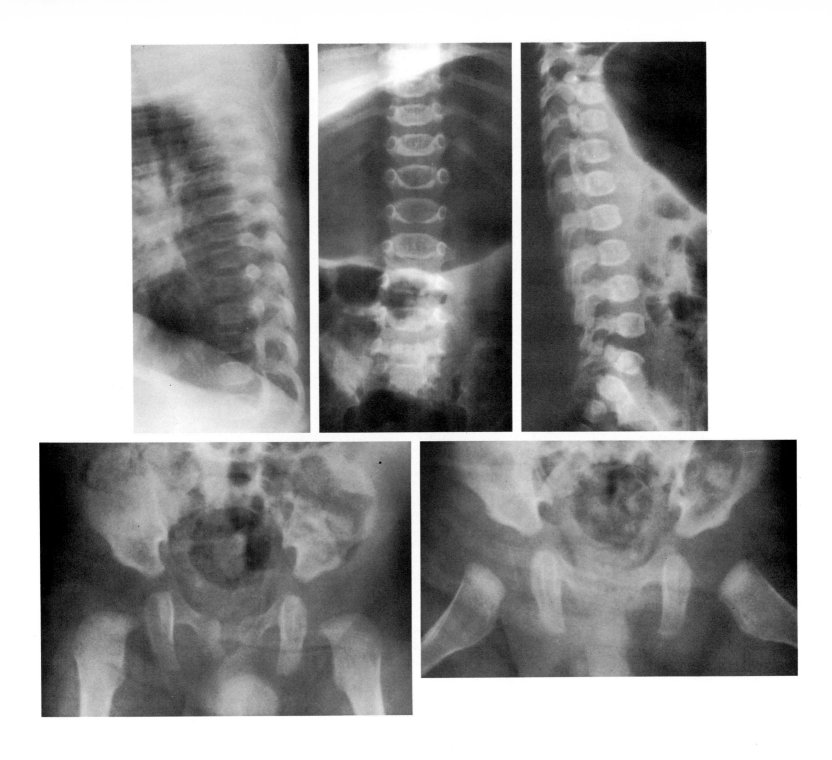

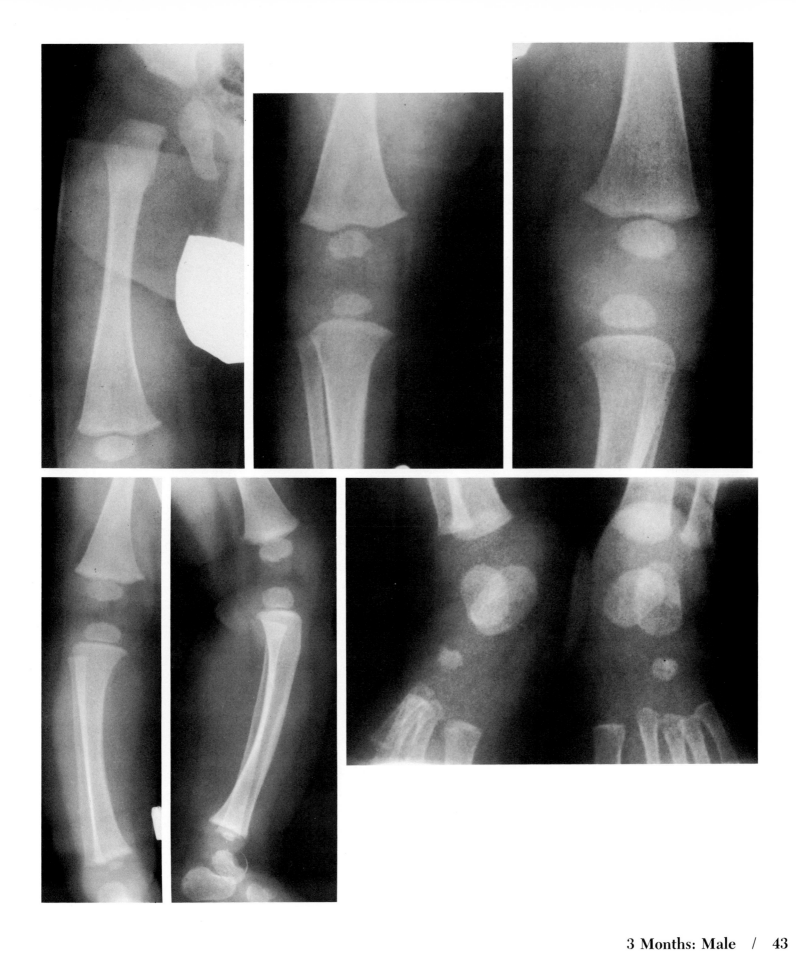

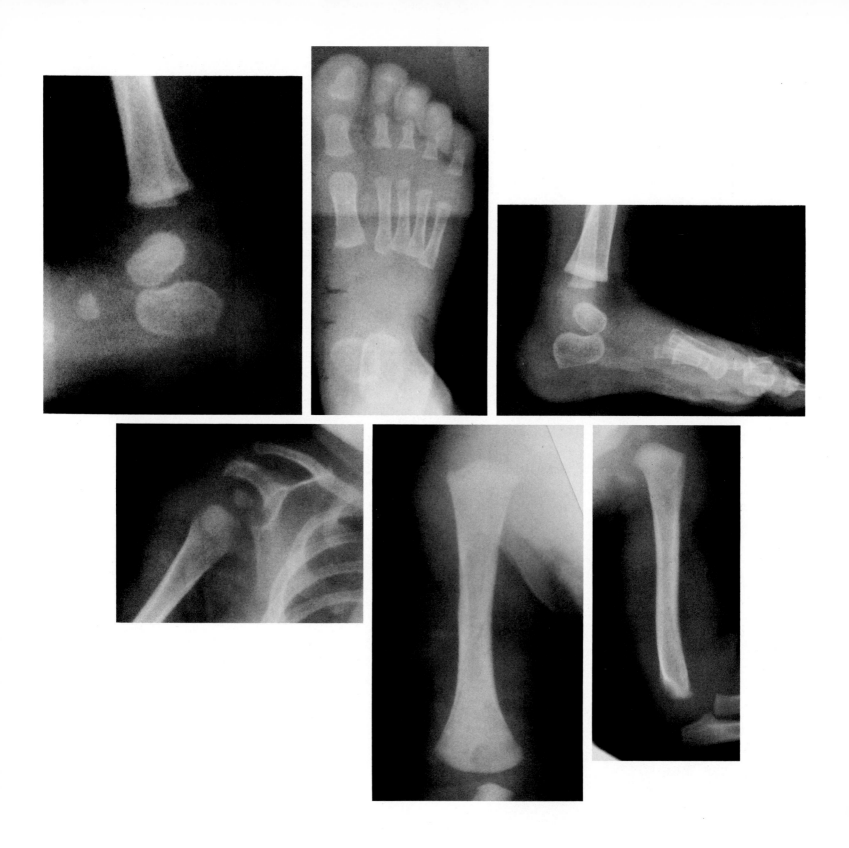

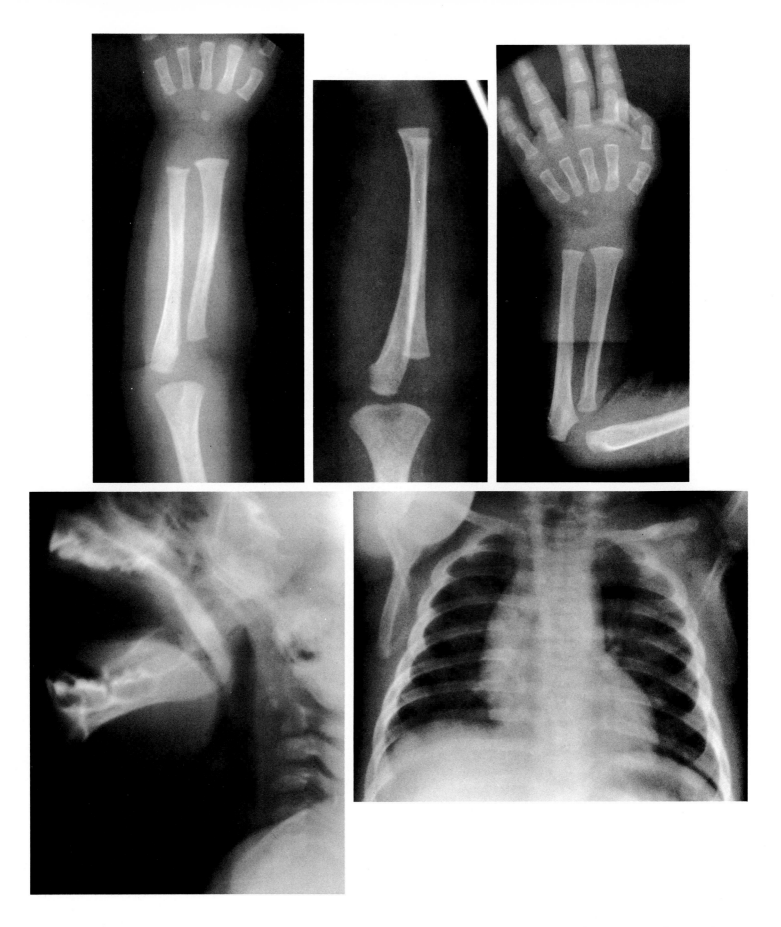

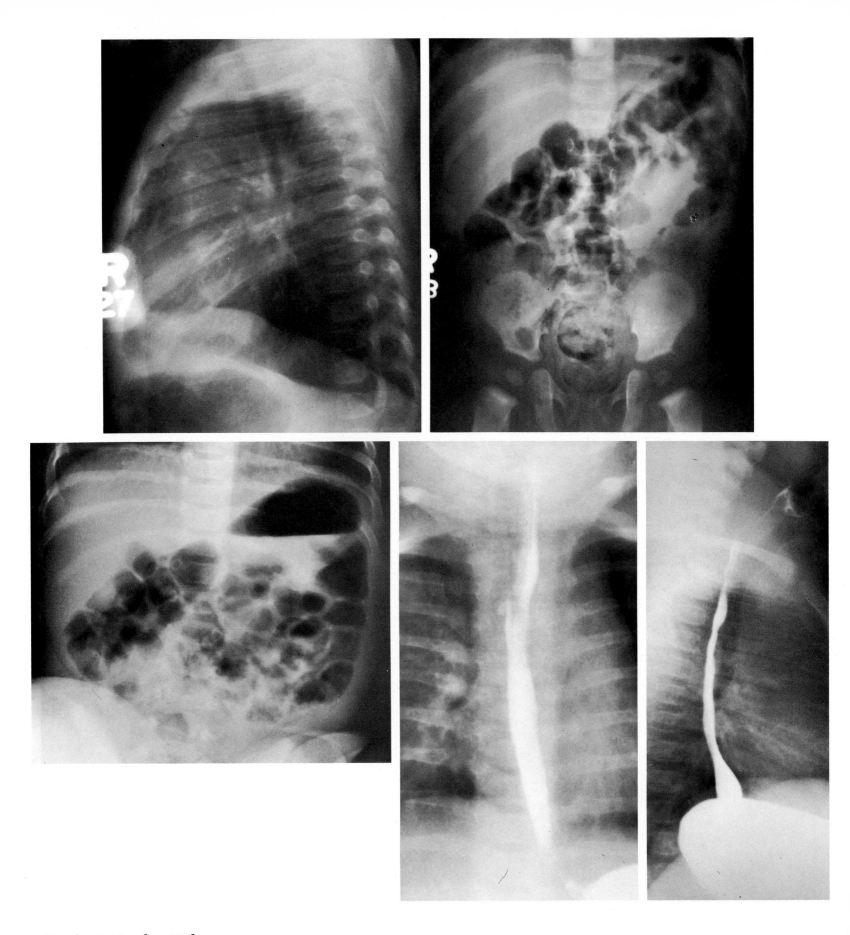

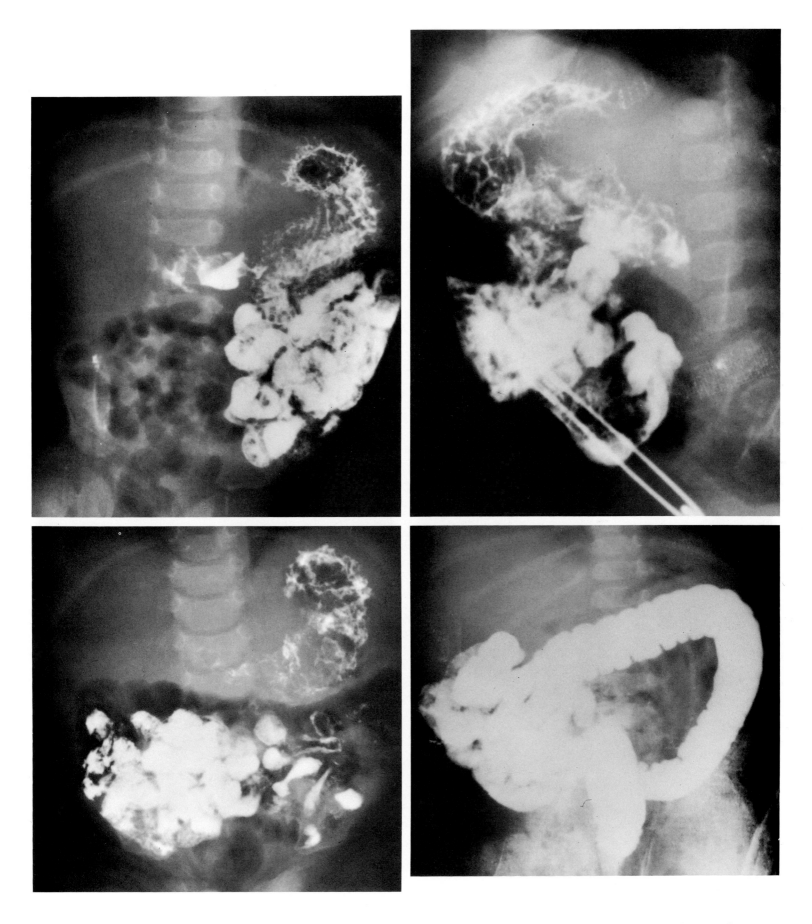

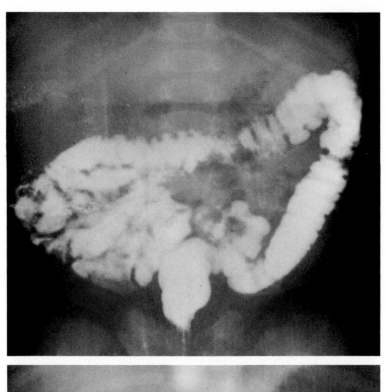

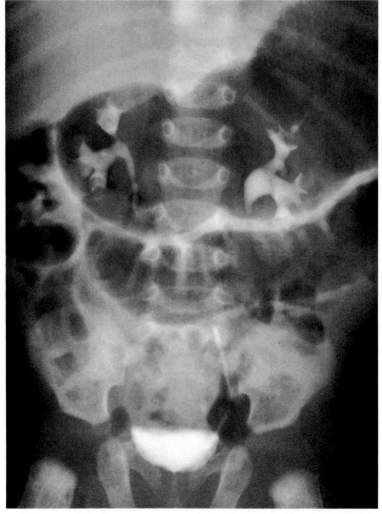

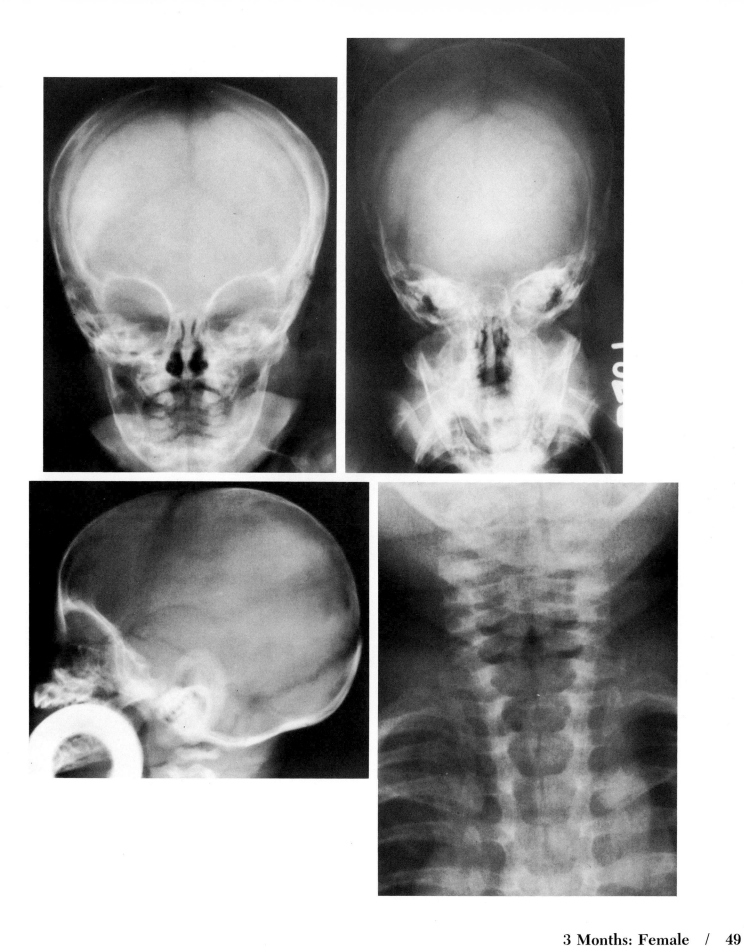

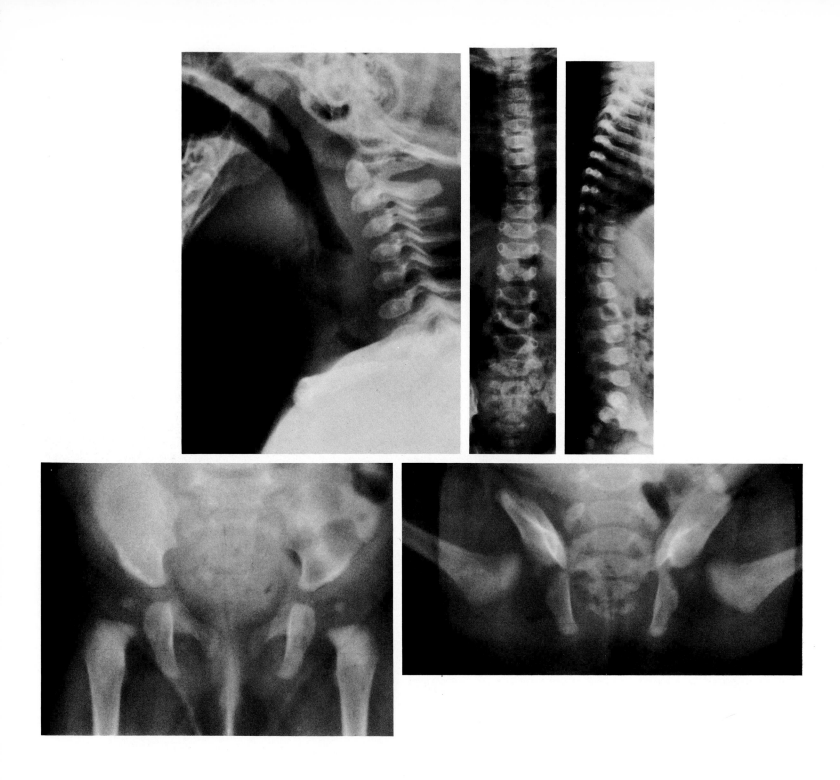

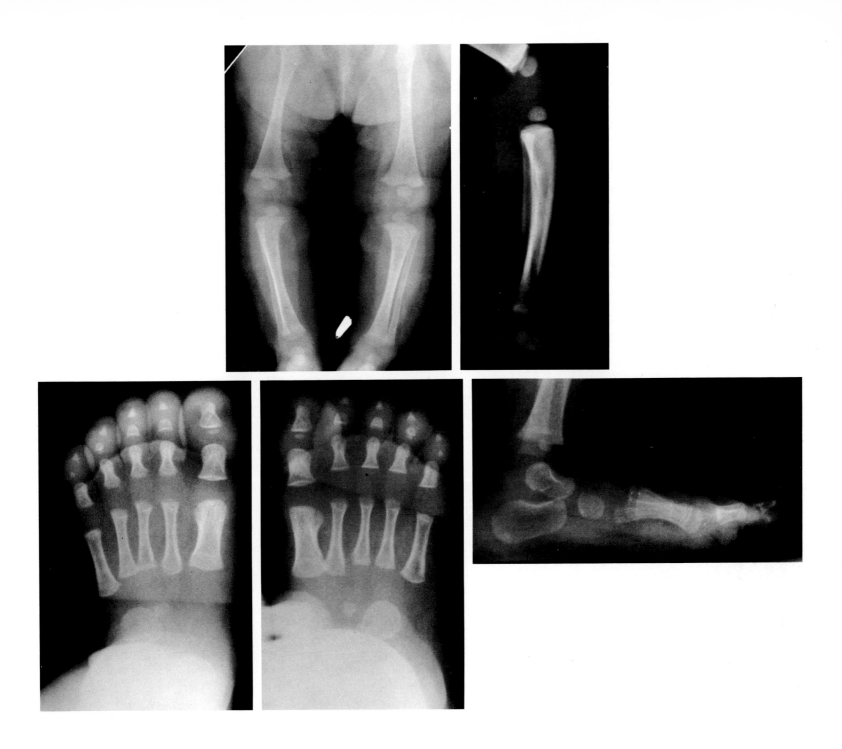

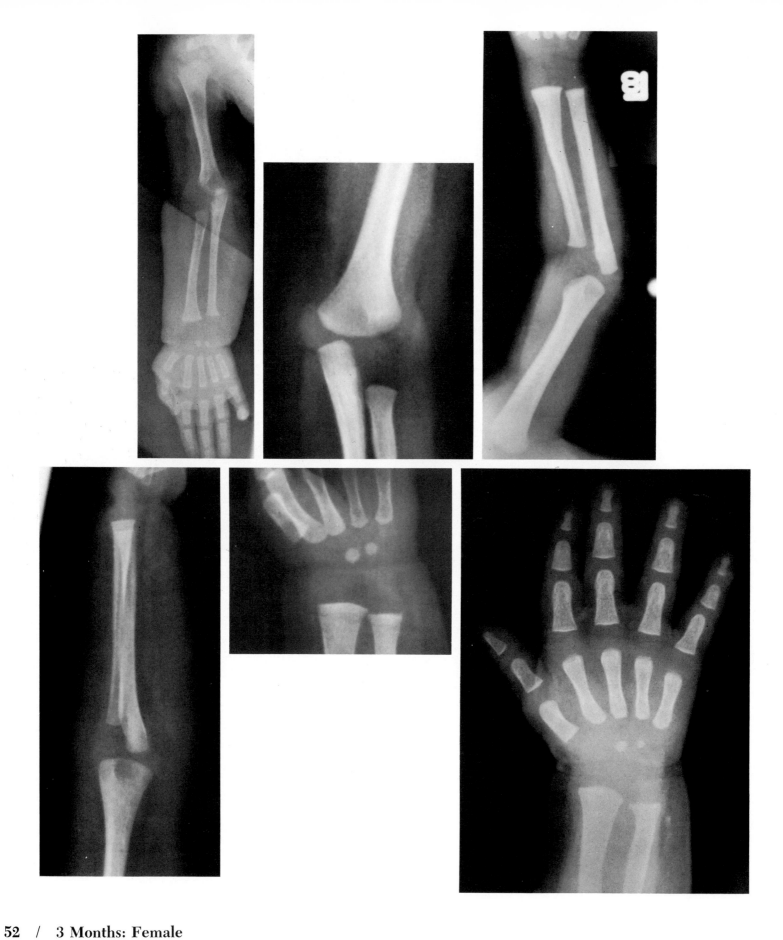

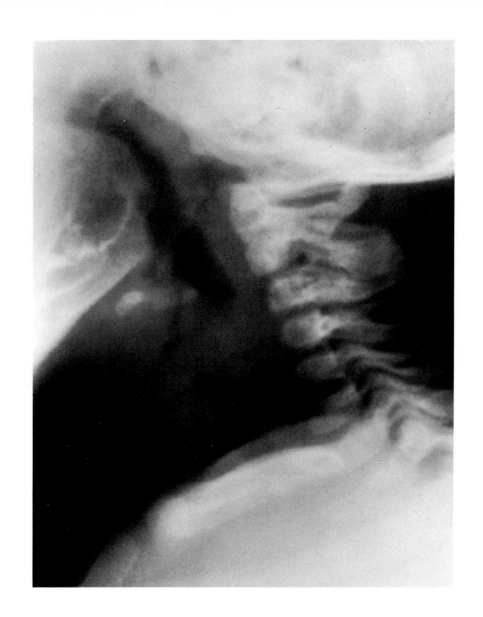

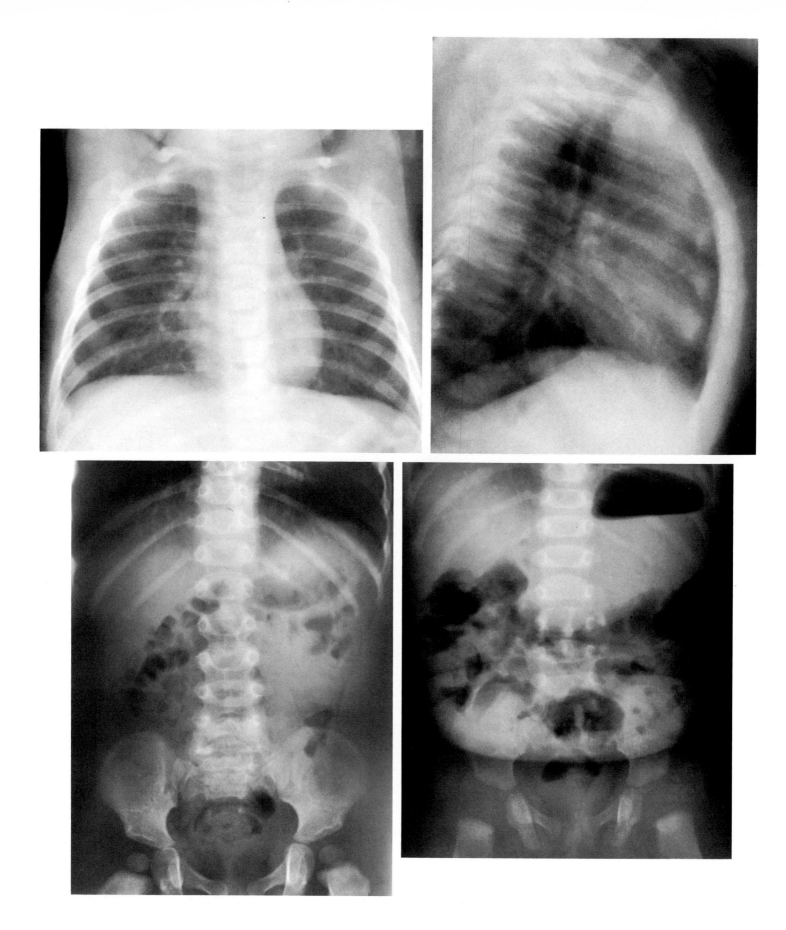

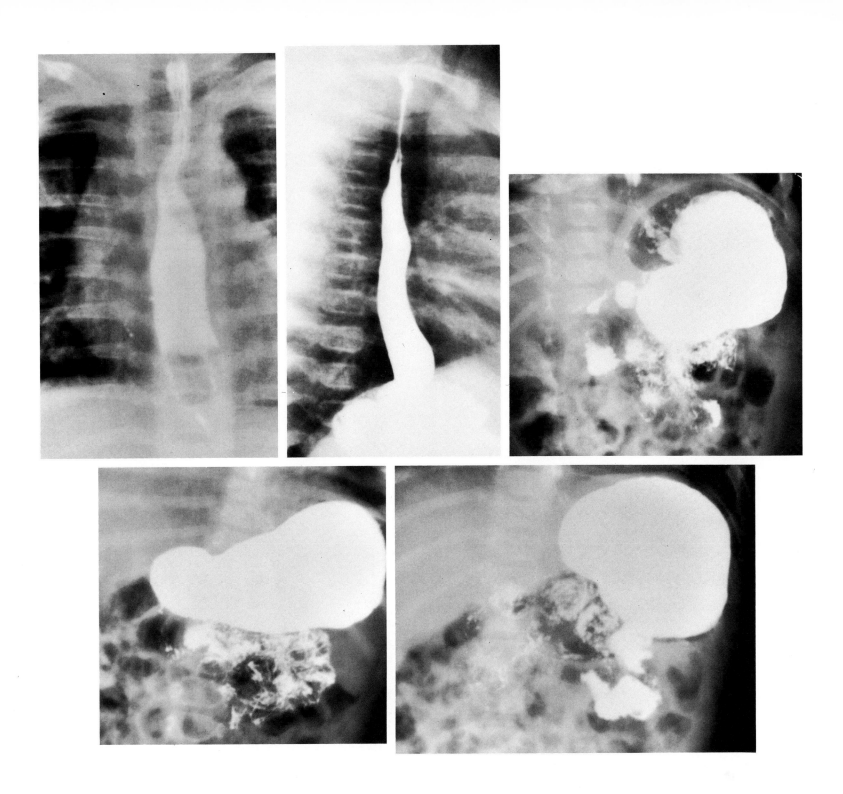

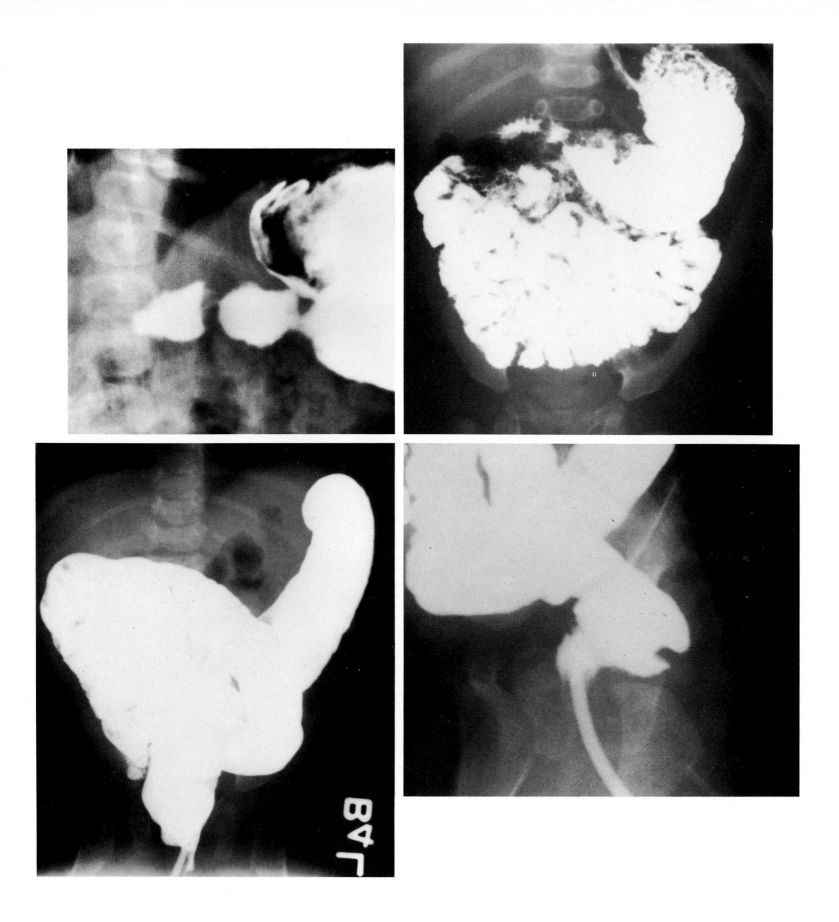

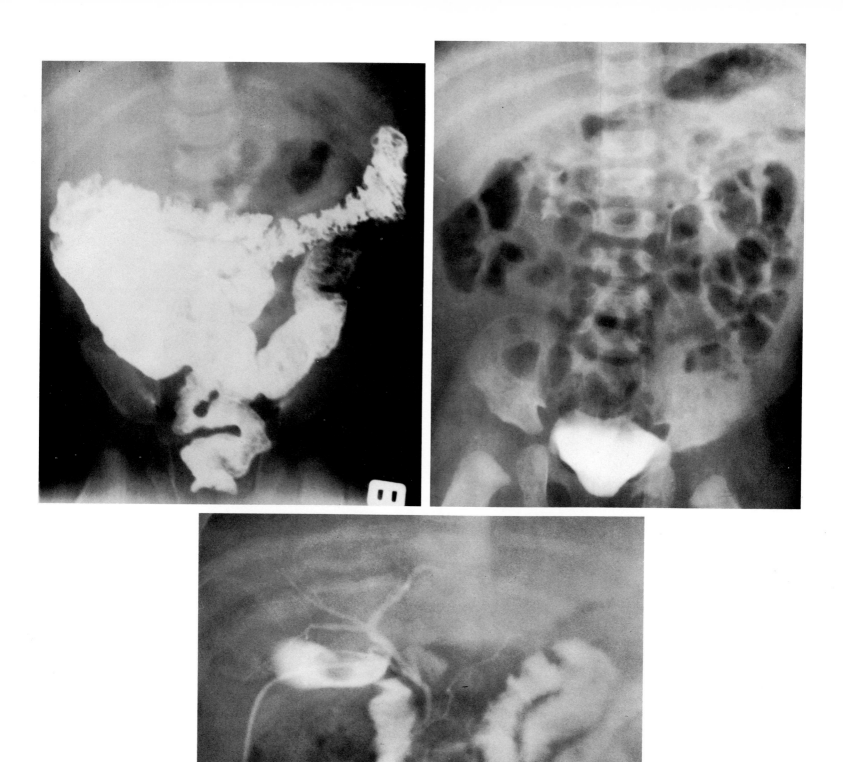

4

6 MONTHS

The calvarial sutures and fontanels are now clearly defined. Pneumatization of the maxillary and ethmoid sinuses is becoming evident. The cervical spinal canal is still relatively large, particularly as seen in the frontal projection. The vertebrae have assumed a more rectangular appearance. Cervical and lumbar lordosis is present. The vertebral ring now appears complete.

The cortices of the long bones are relatively thicker and more sharply defined. The talus and calcaneus are enlarging. Two carpal centers are present. The proximal humeral epiphysis may be duplicated. In the frontal plane, the shafts of the radius and ulna may have a bowed configuration.

The pattern of the small bowel is becoming more regular and shows better delineation of the valvulae conniventes. The bladder appears disproportionately large compared with the size of the child.

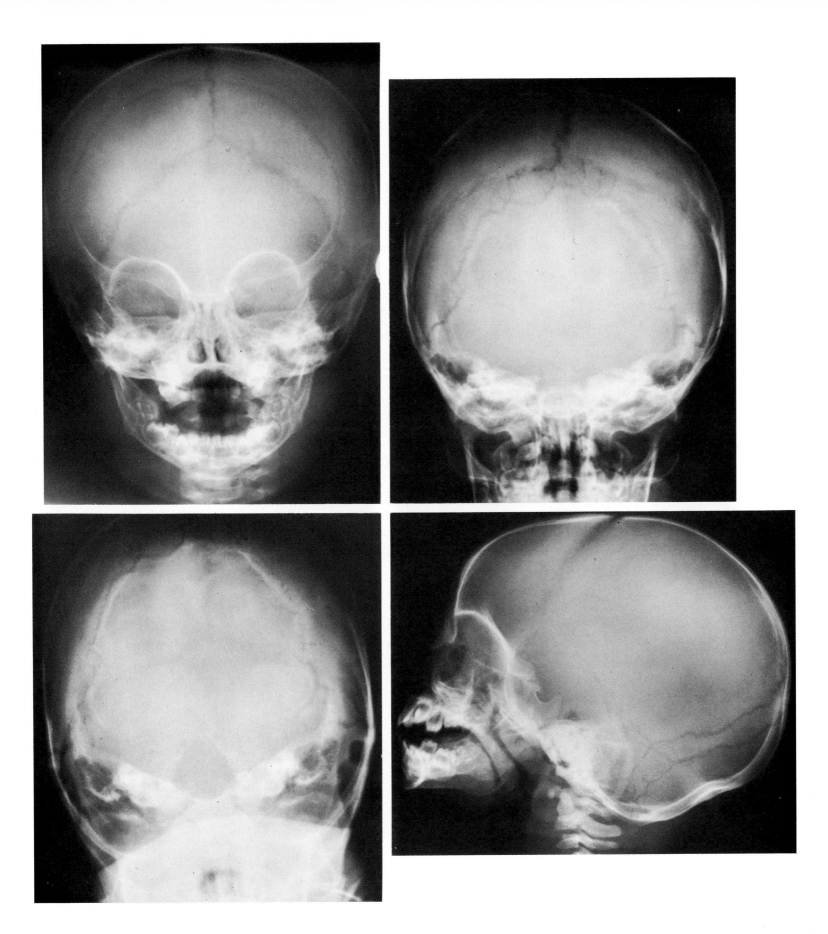

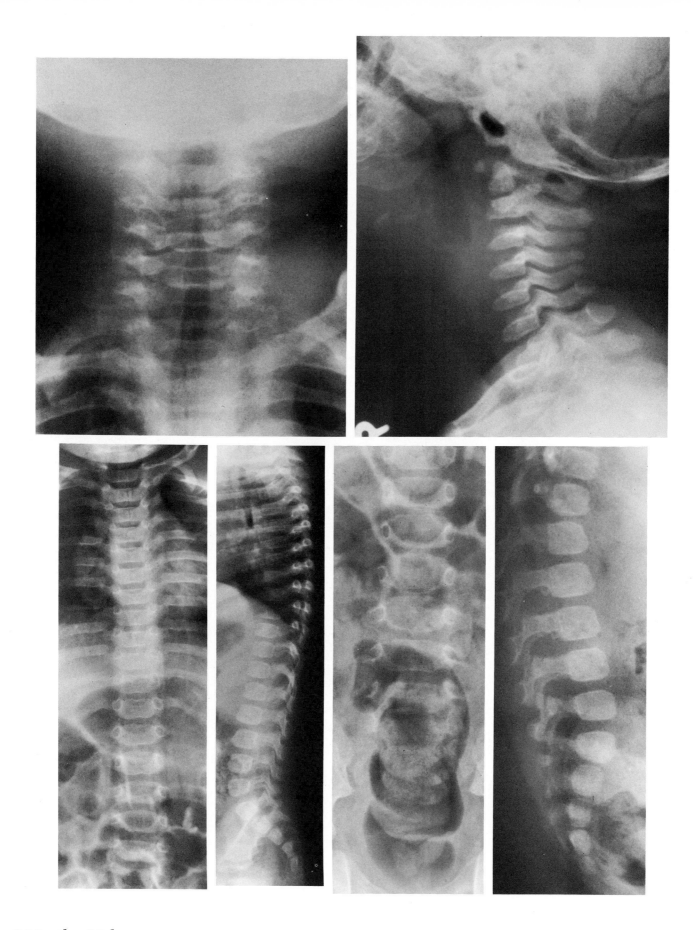

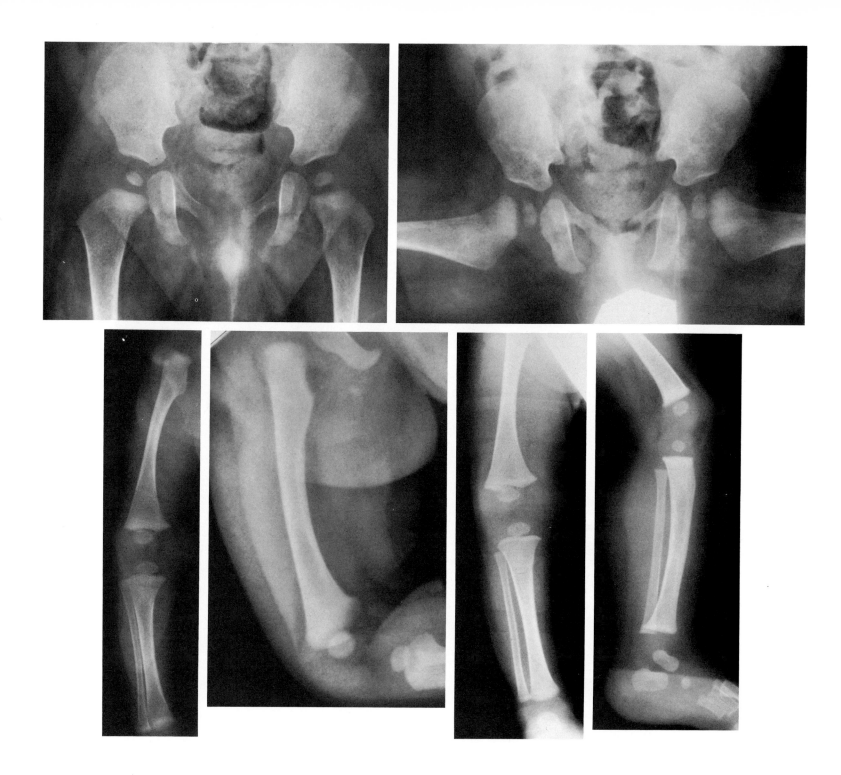

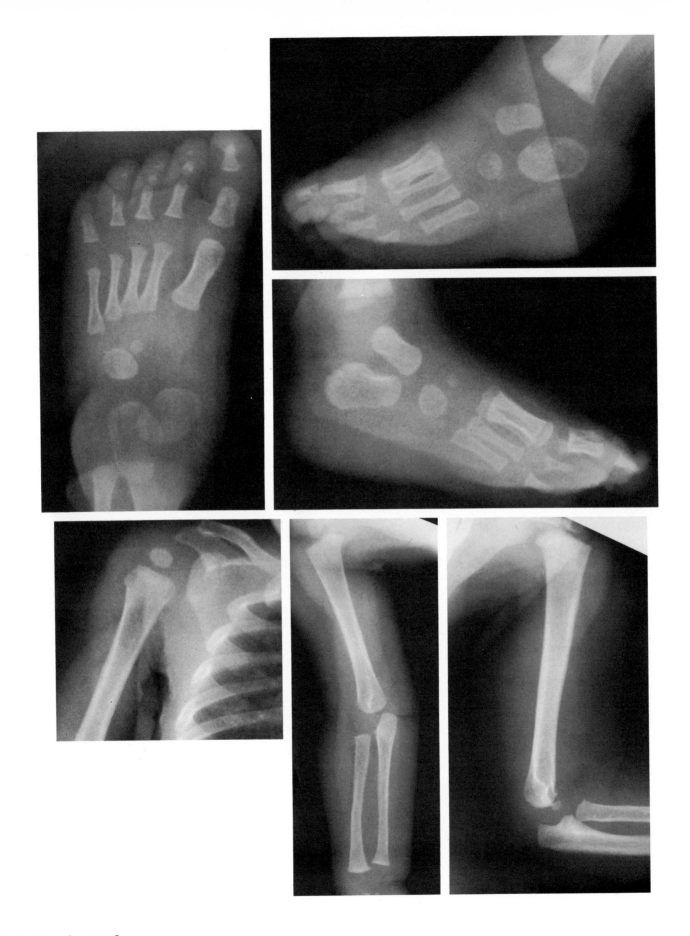

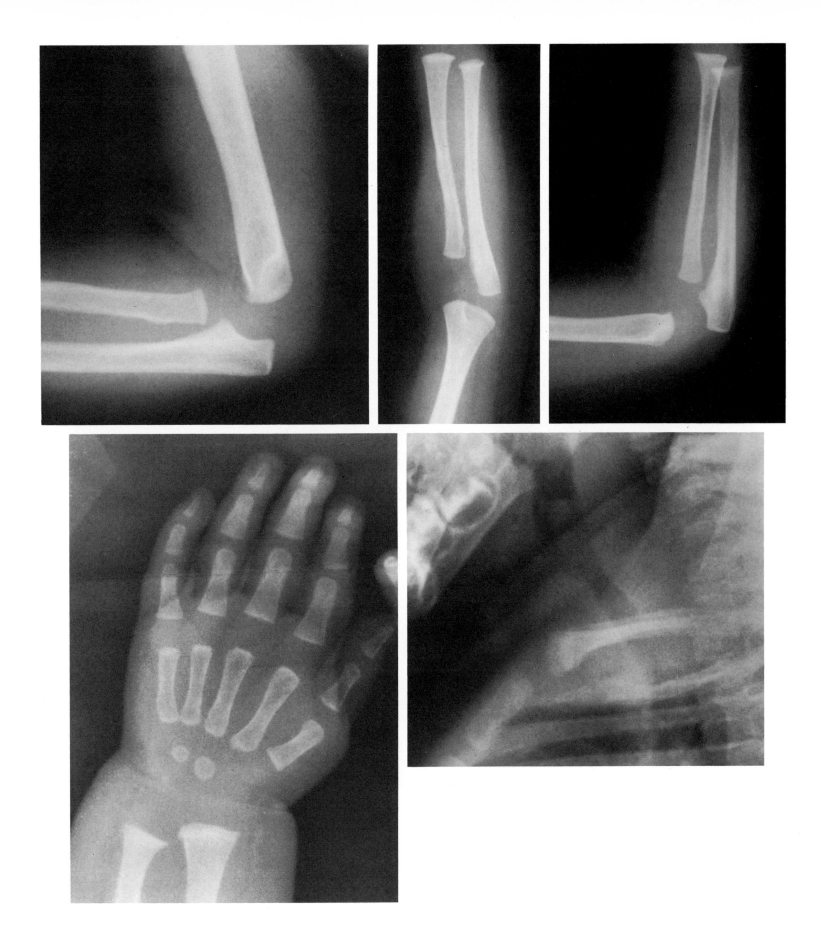

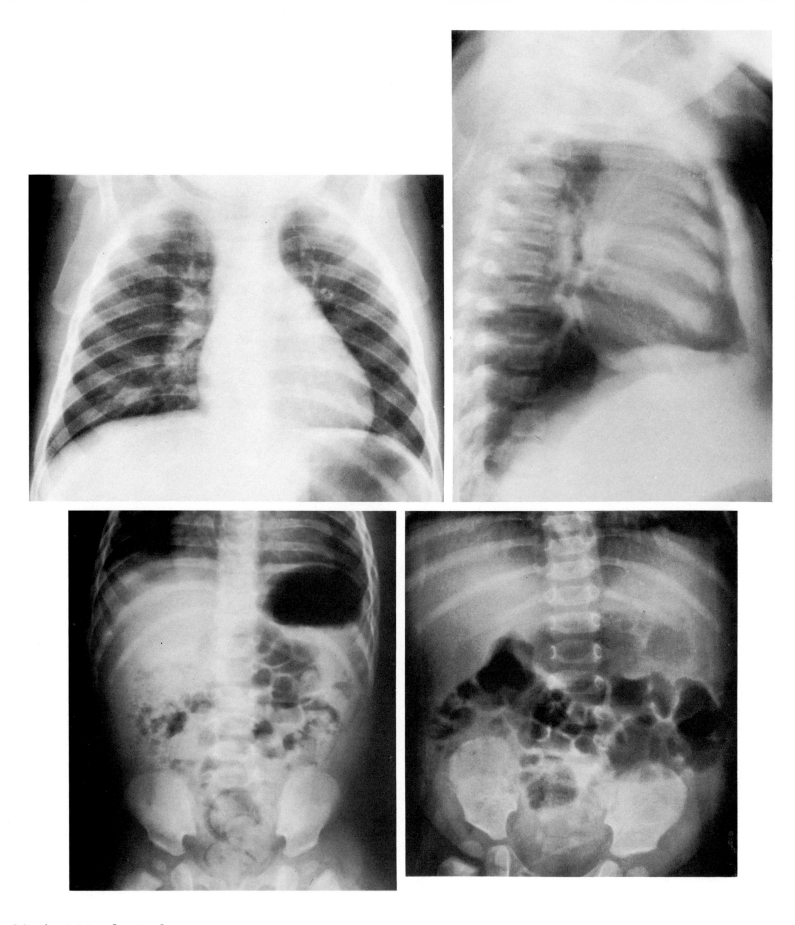

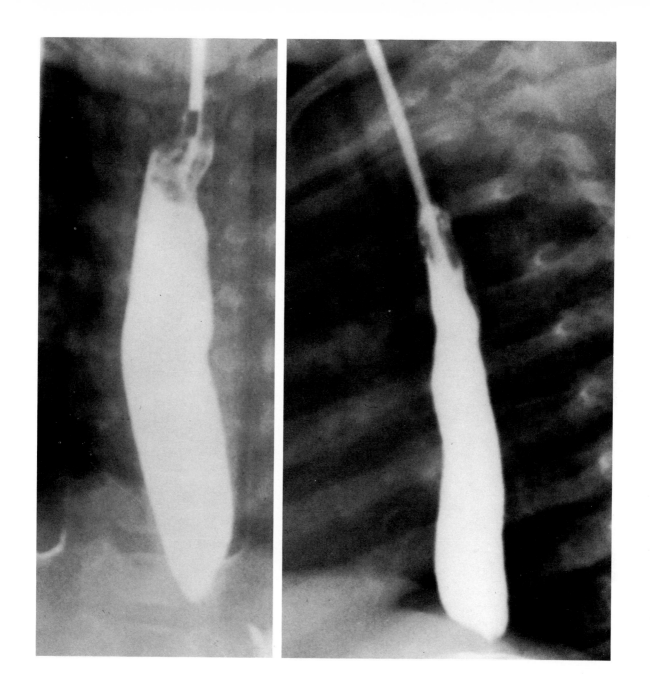

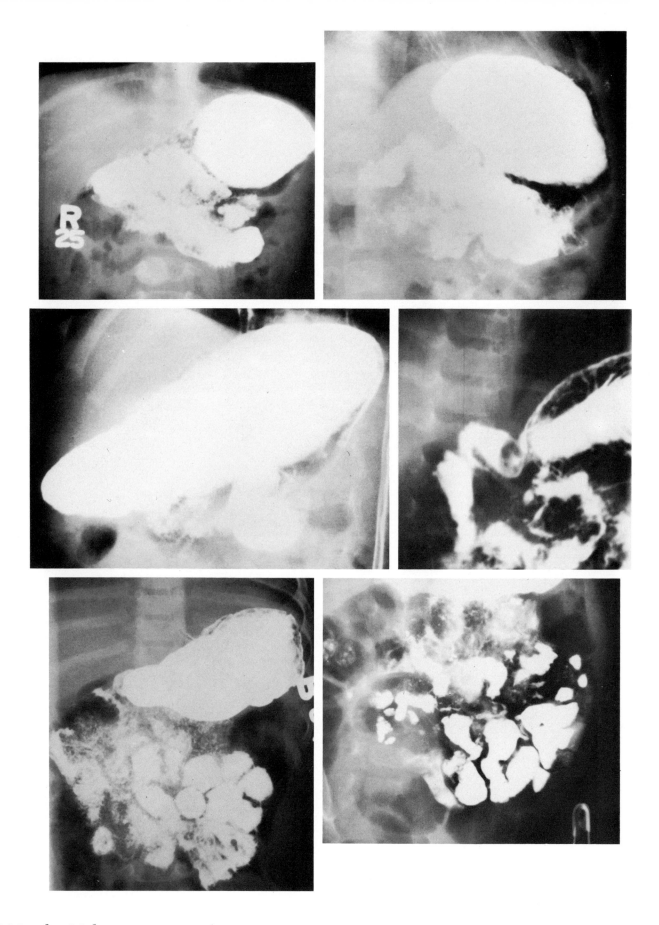

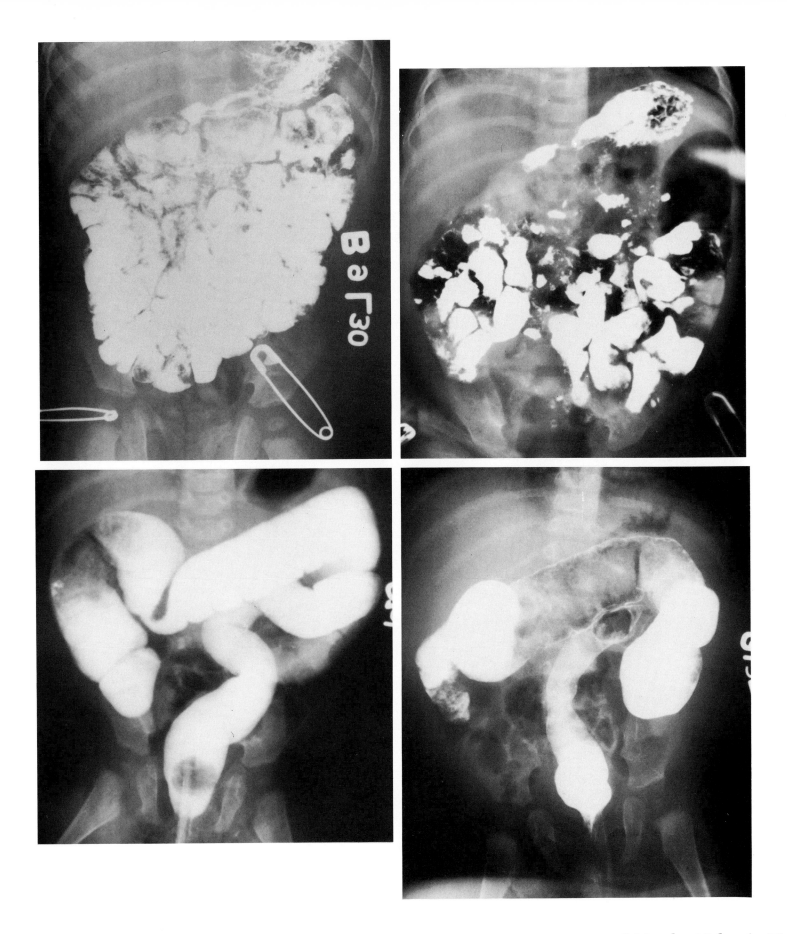

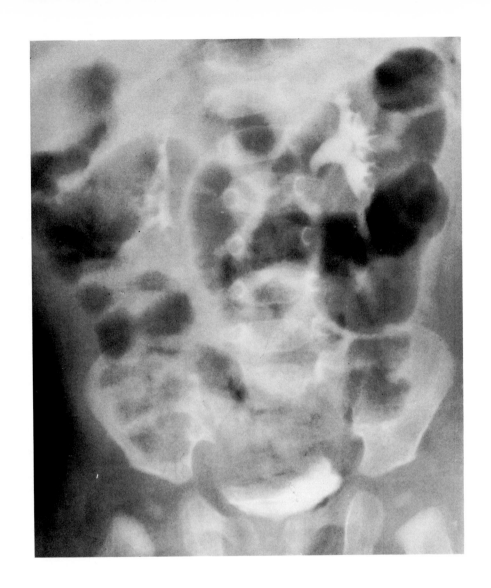

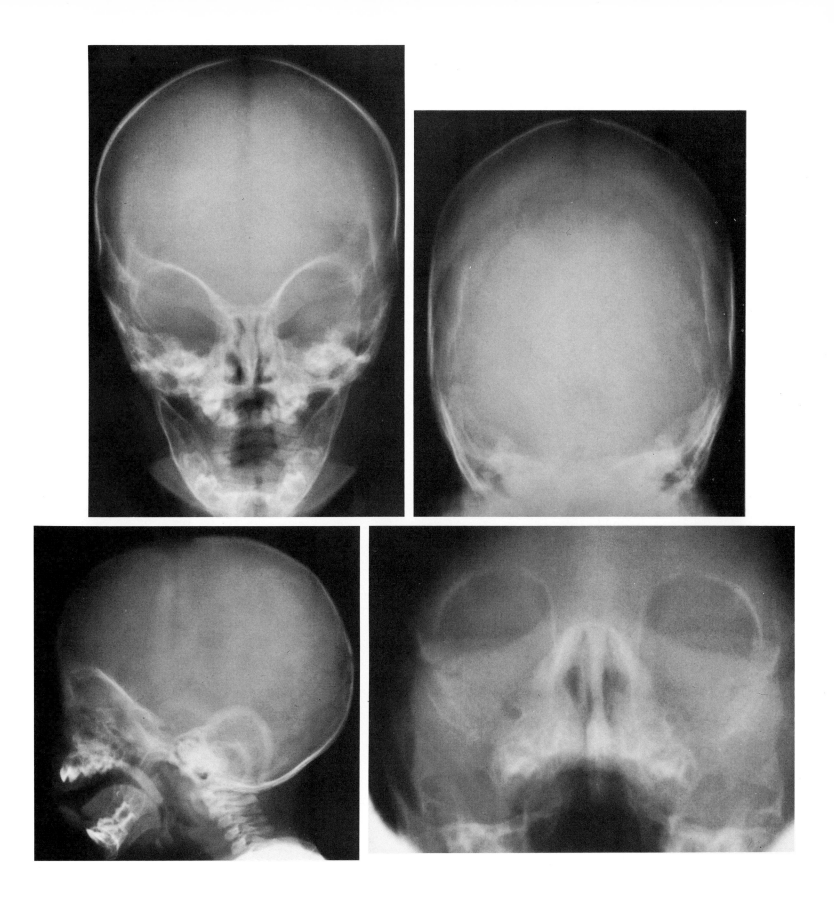

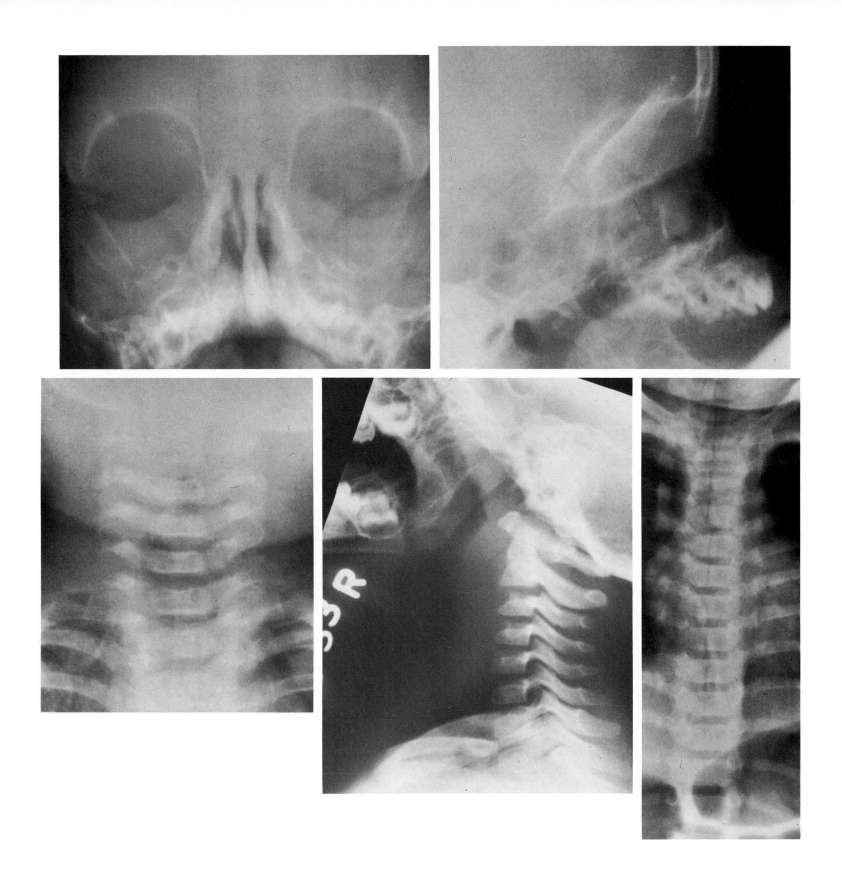

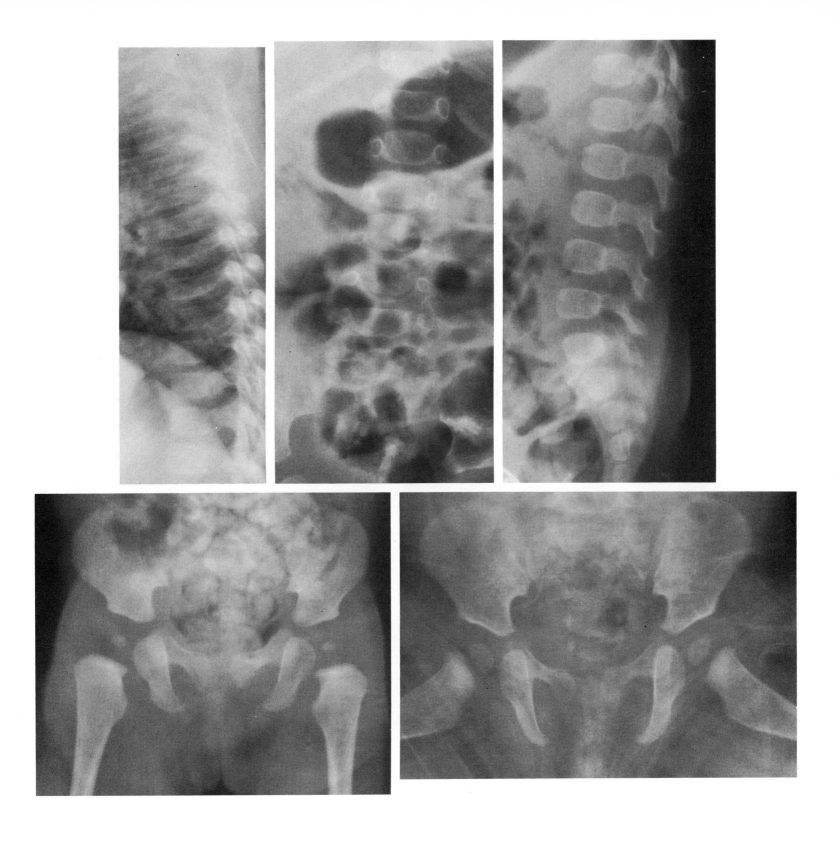

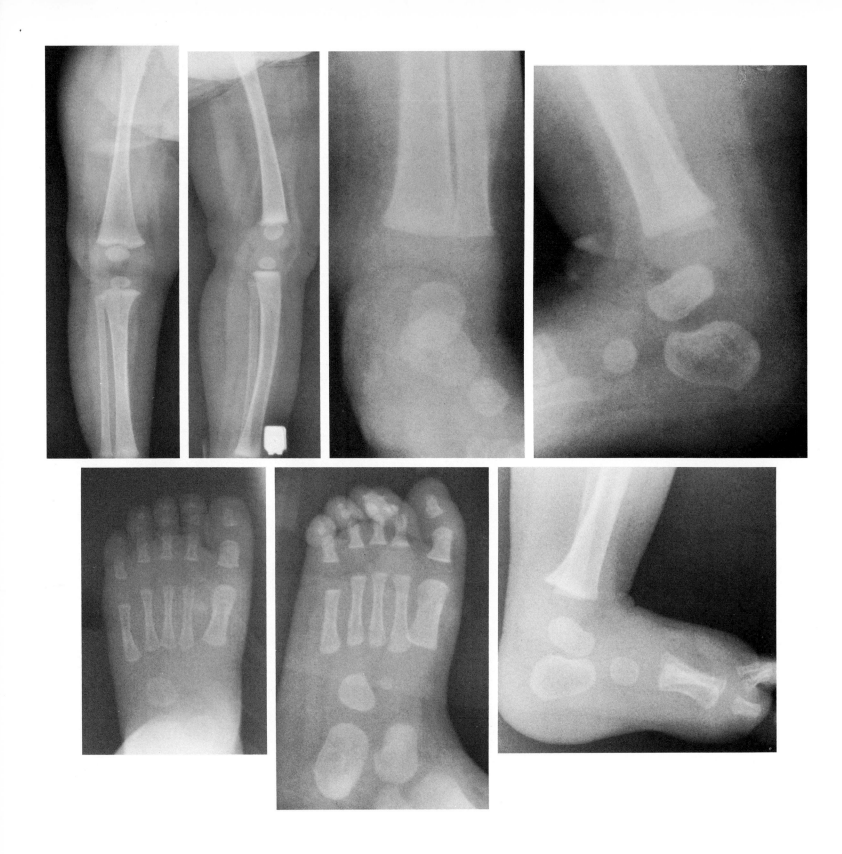

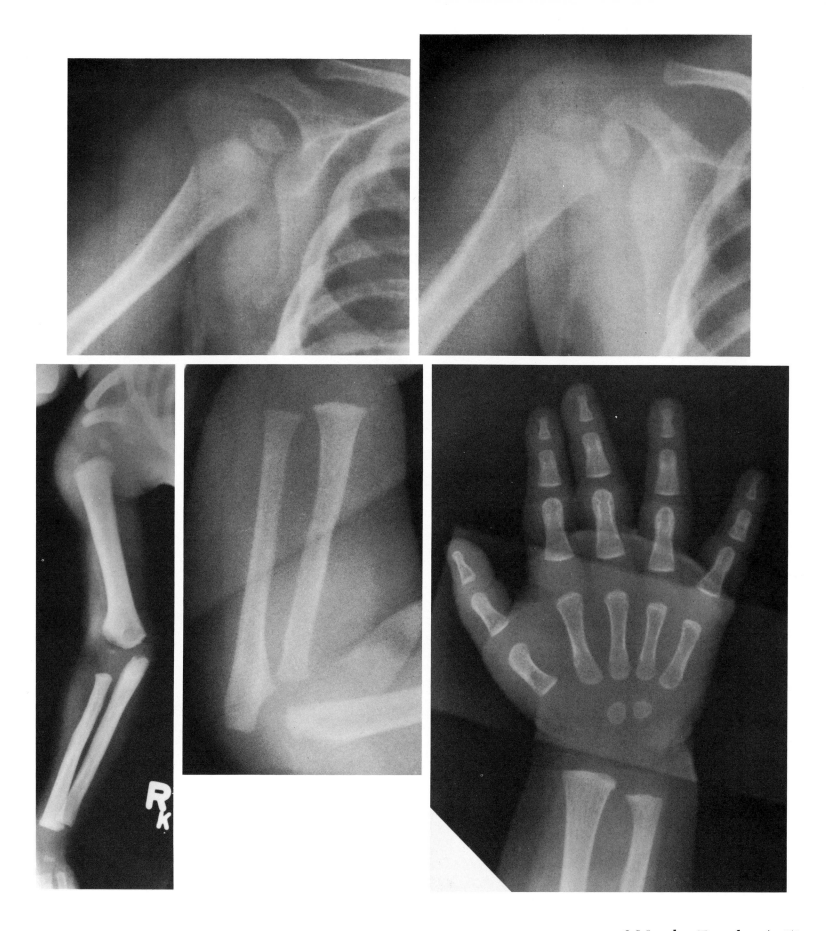

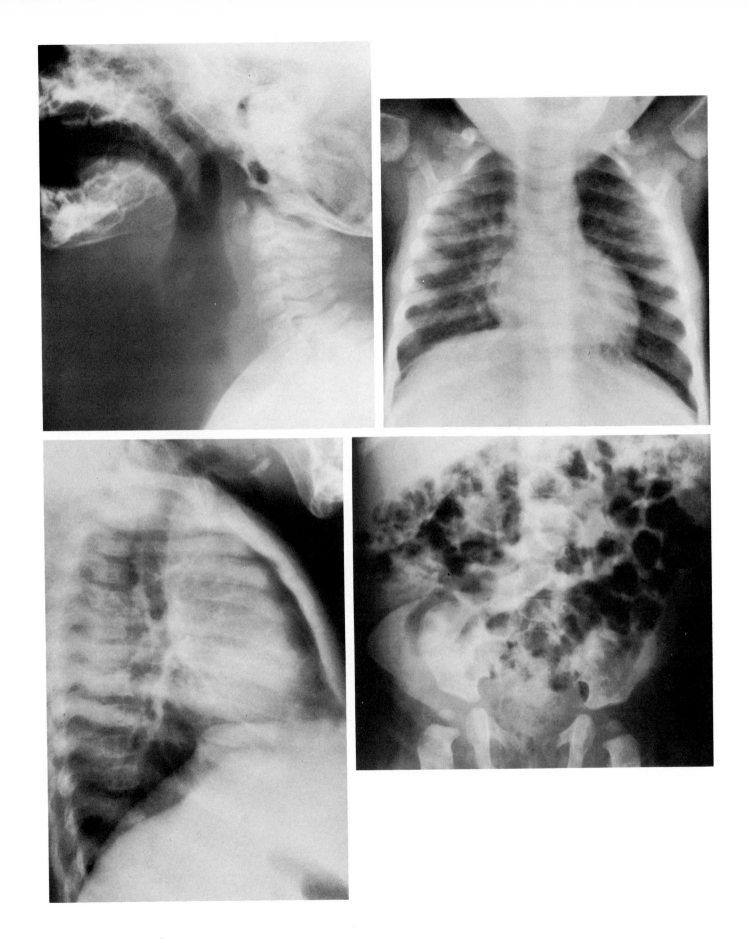

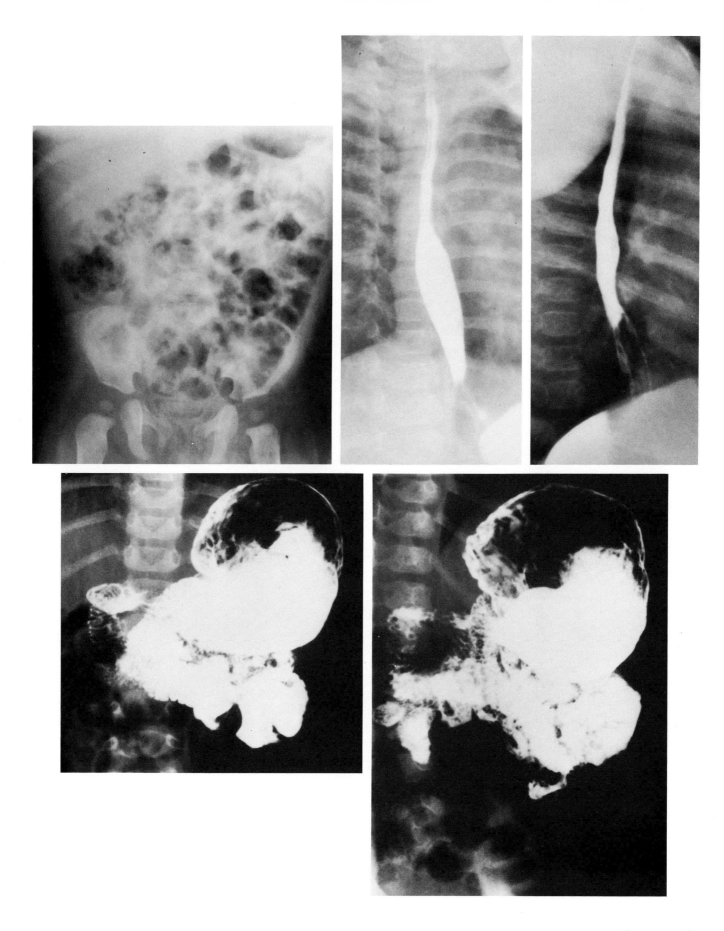

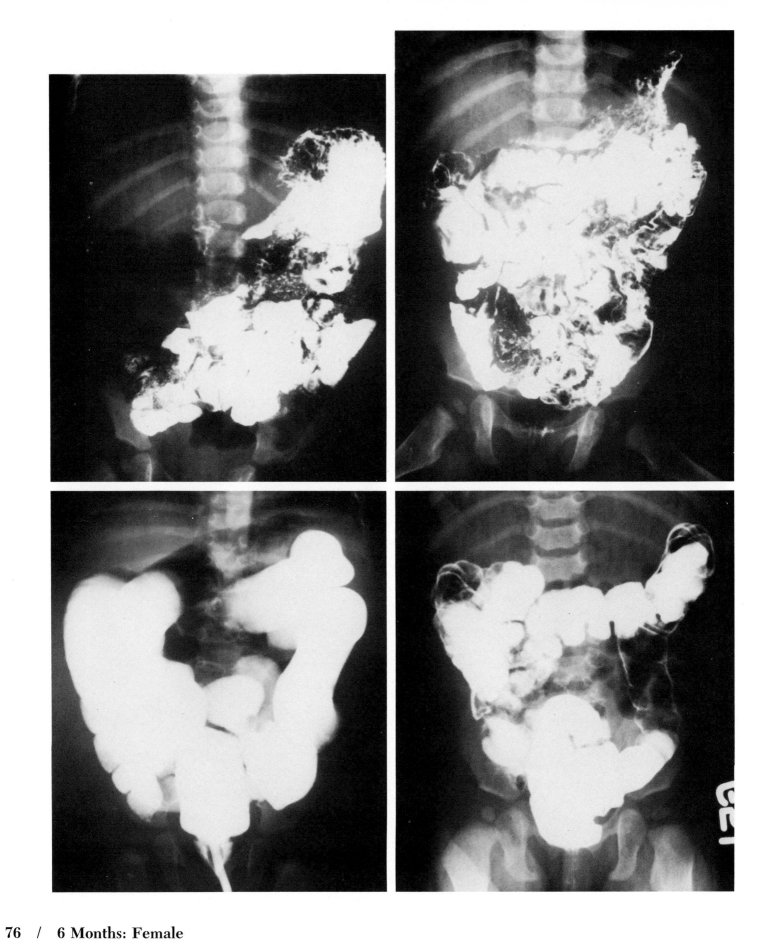

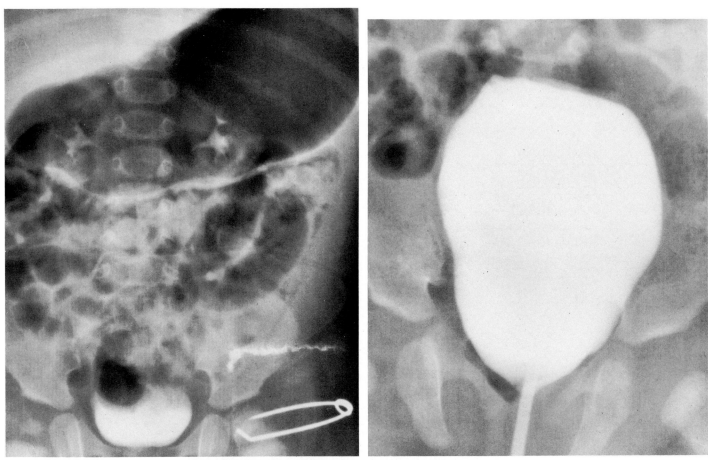

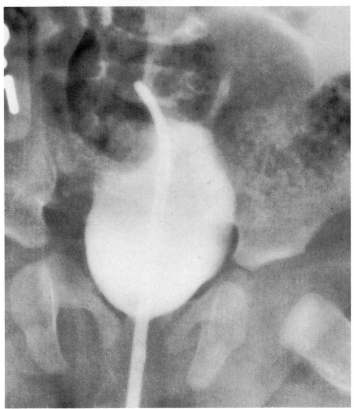

5

9 MONTHS

The skull to face ratio is changing towards the adult. Wormian bones may still be evident. The anterior fontanel is clearly defined. The cervical spinal canal still appears large. The ring of the ischium and pubis is beginning to close. The ossification center of the distal femoral epiphysis is indenting the distal metaphysis, which begins to widen. The second ossification center for the humeral head has become evident.

The retropharyngeal soft tissues are becoming thinner. The small bowel and colon now closely resemble their adult appearance.

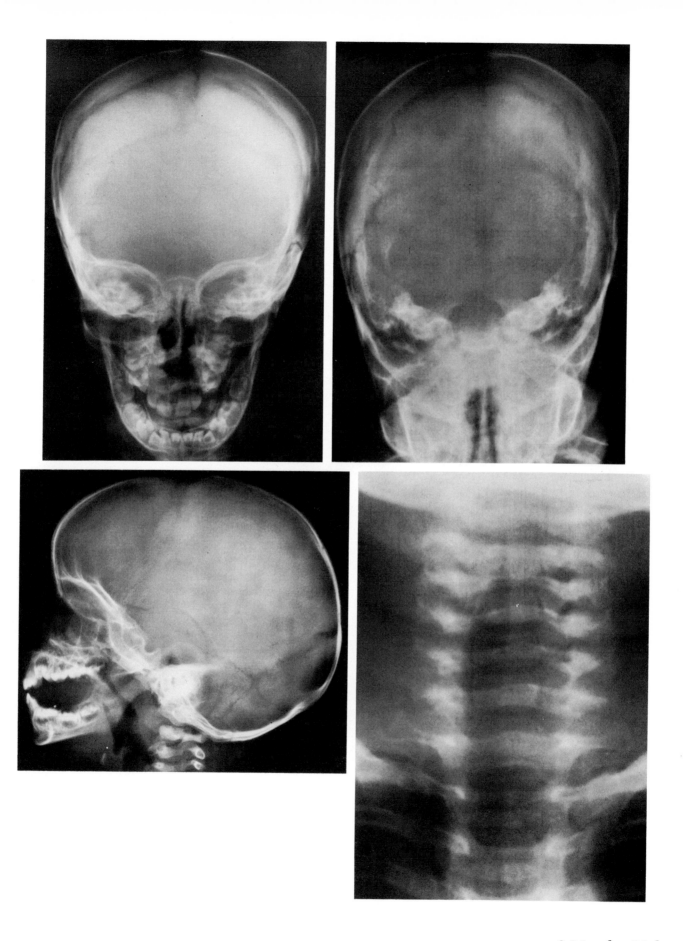

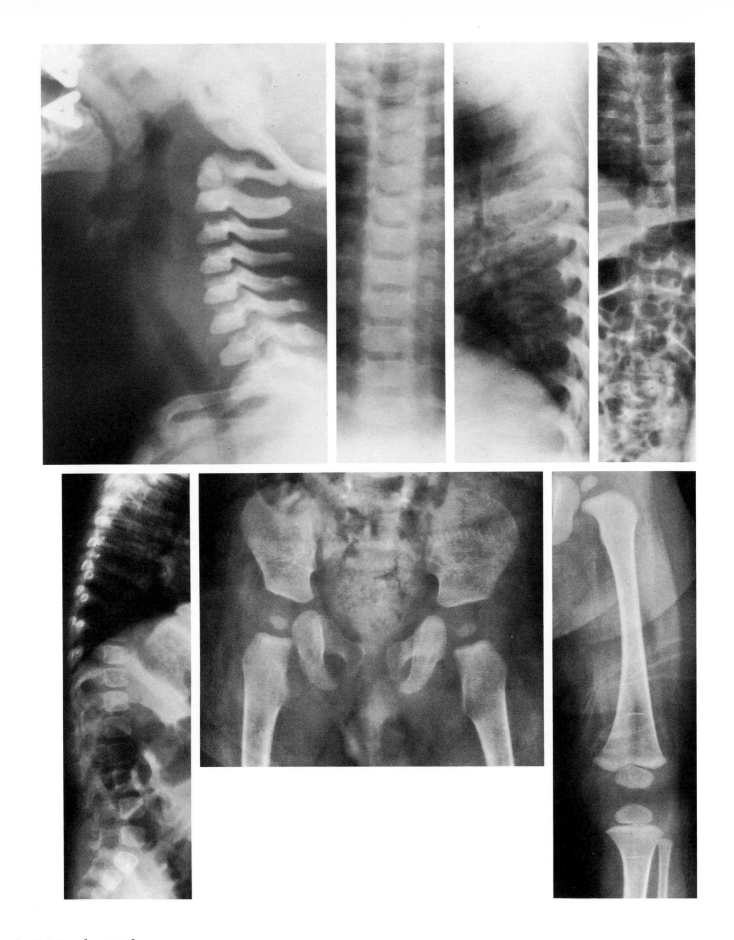

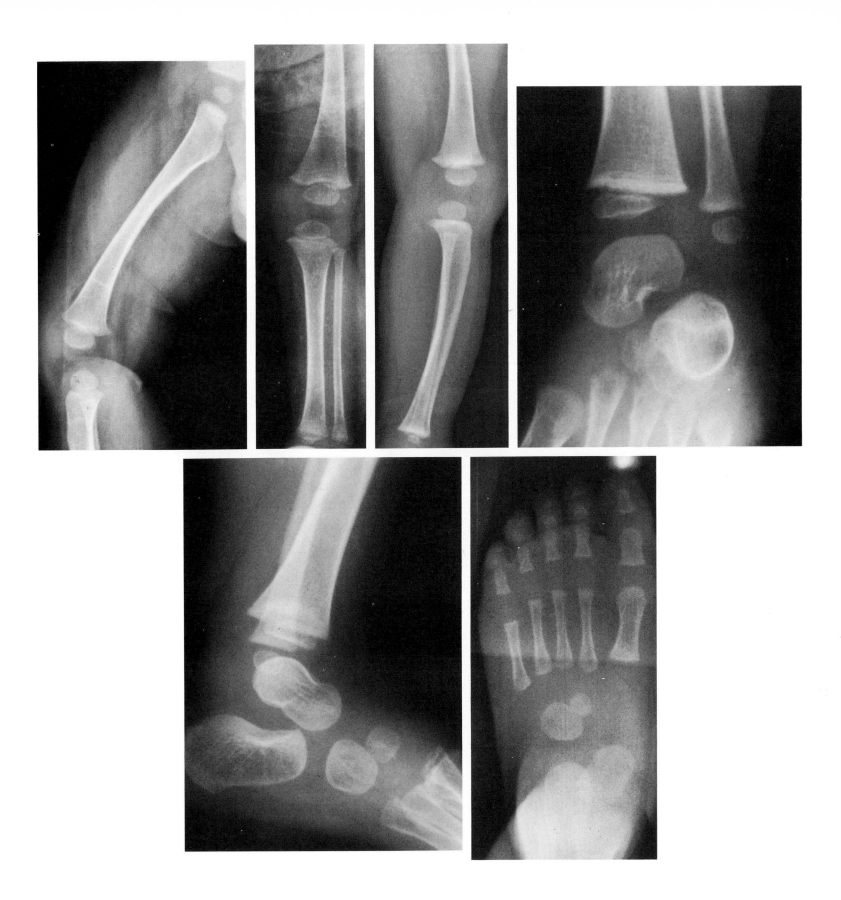

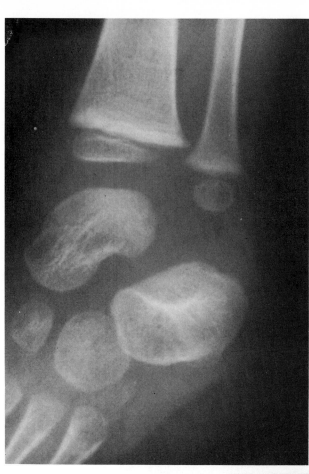
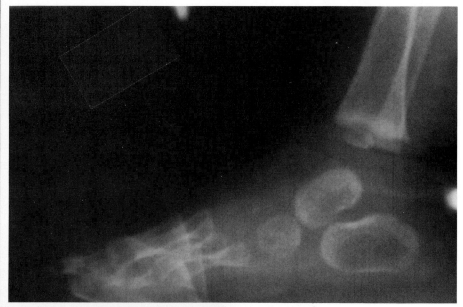
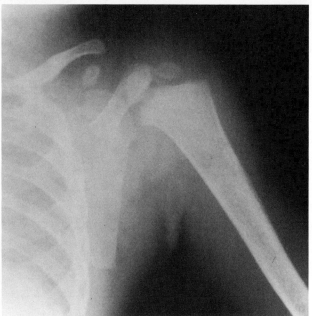

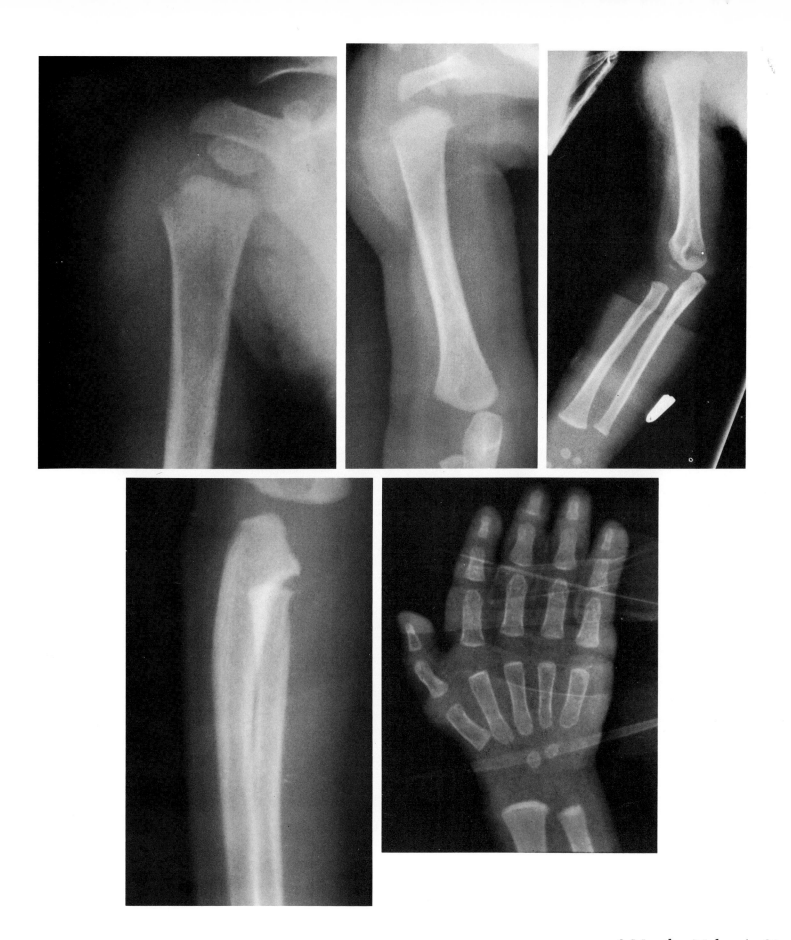

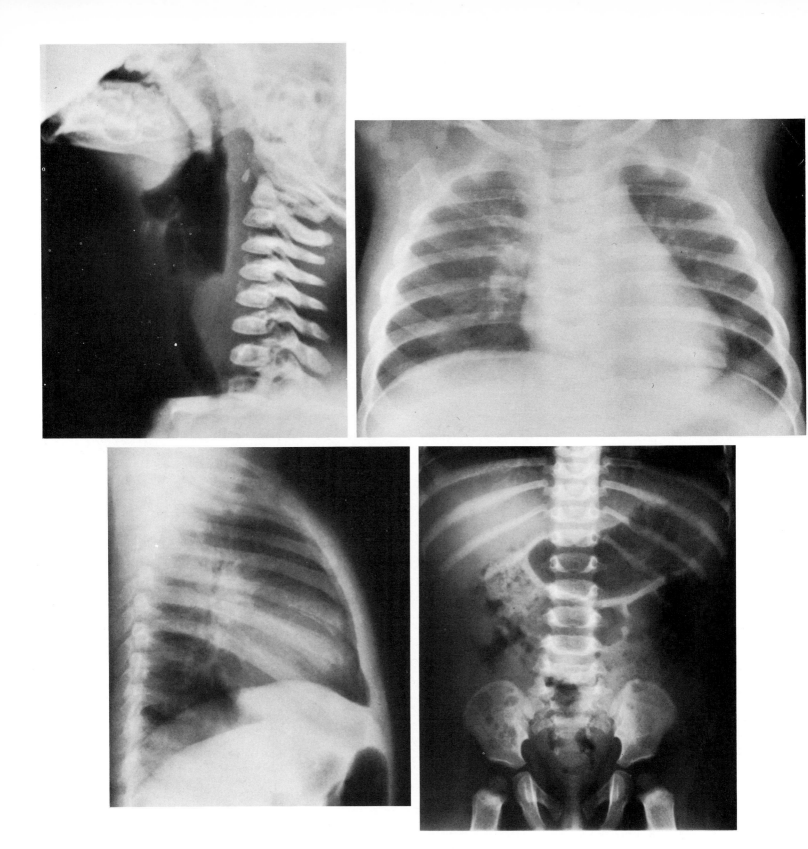

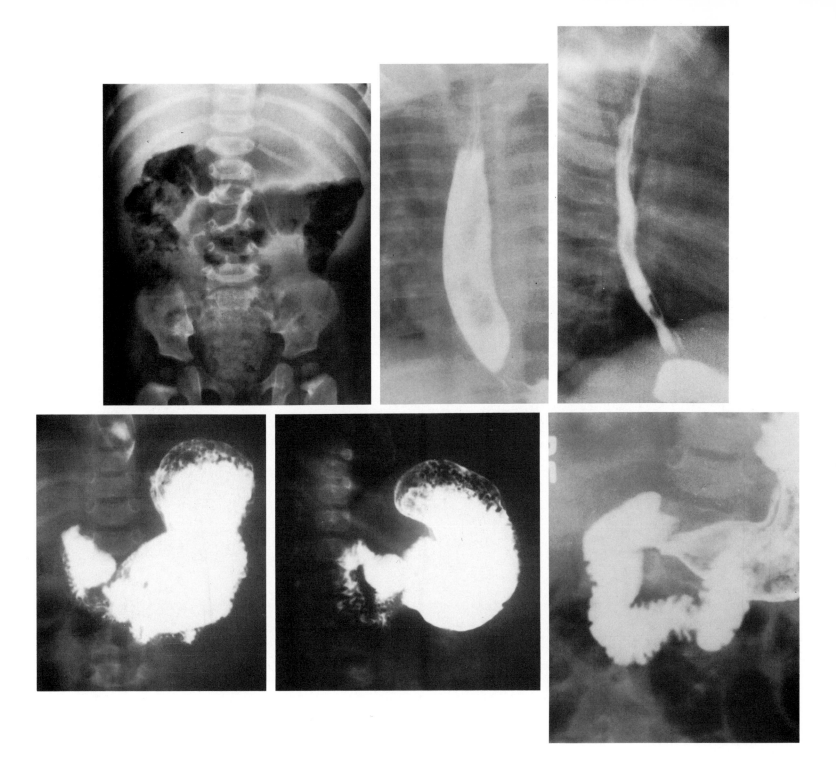

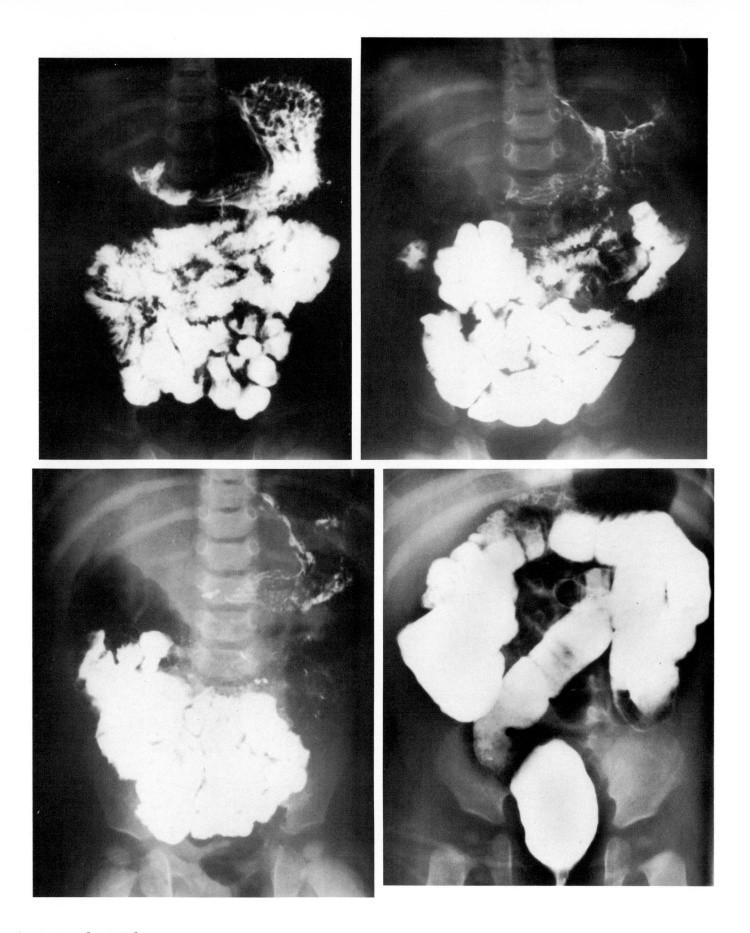

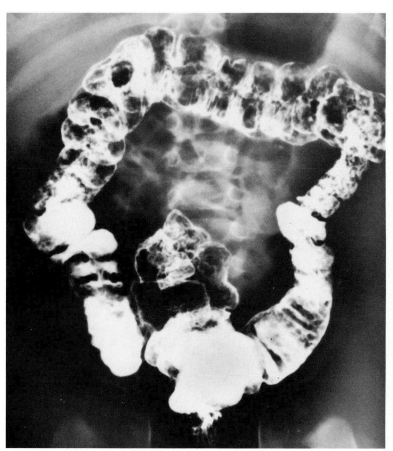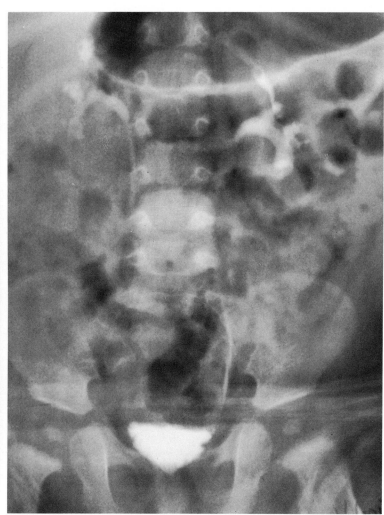

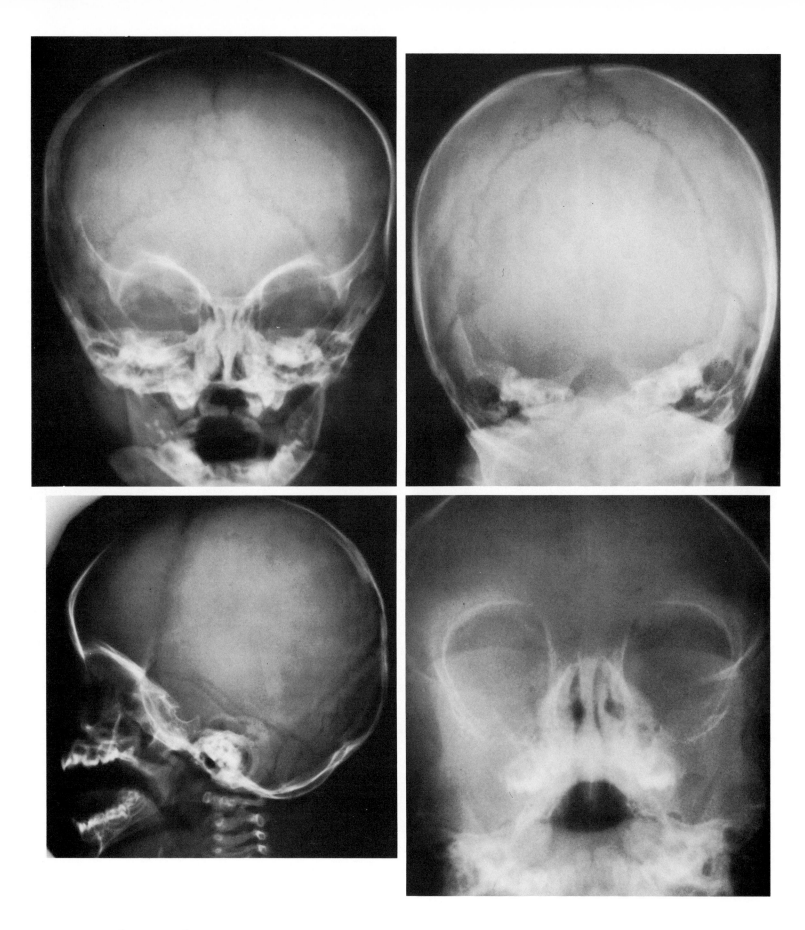

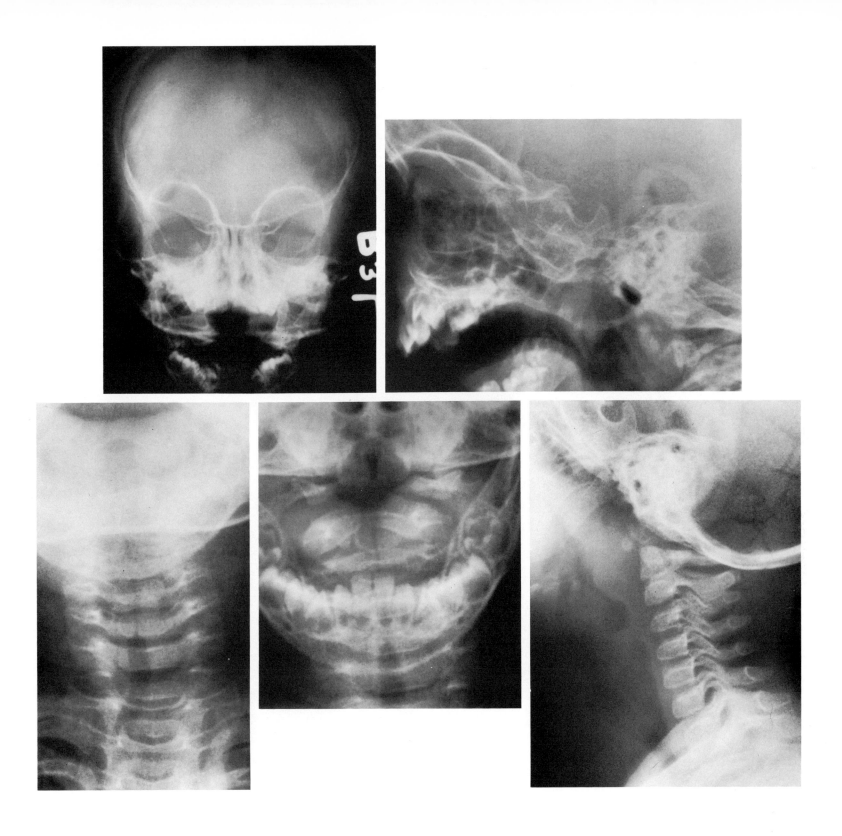

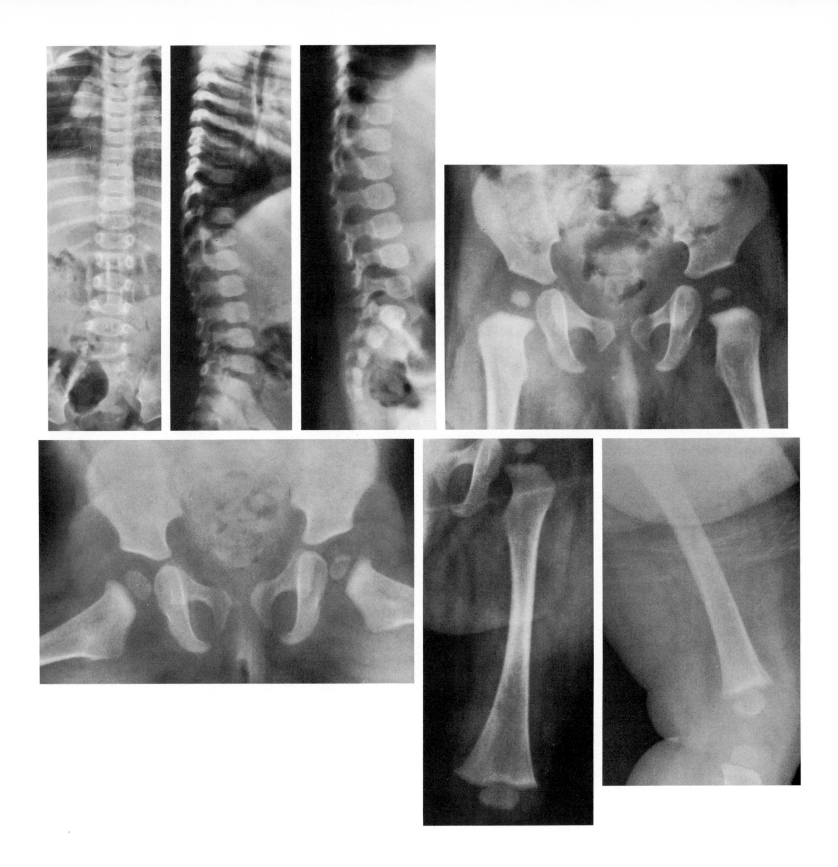

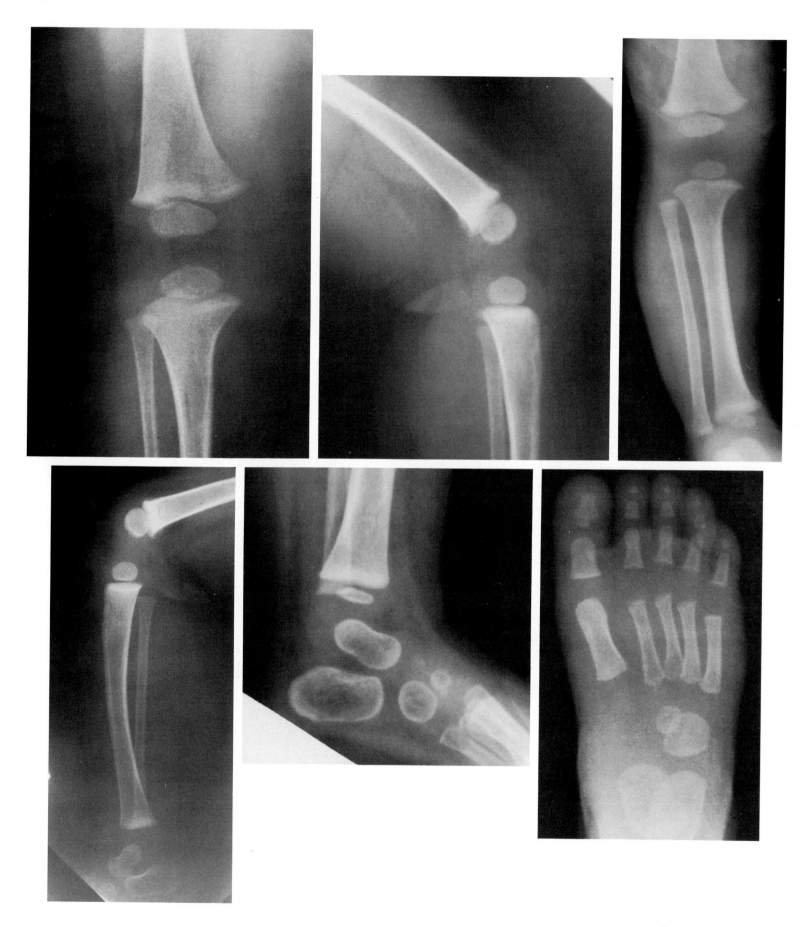

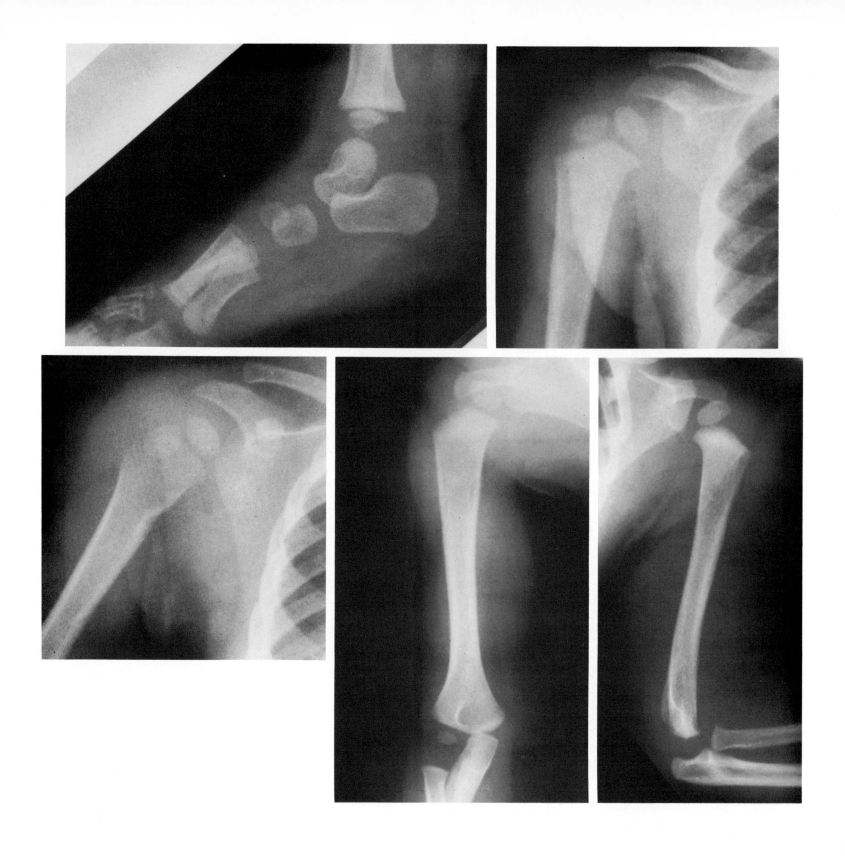

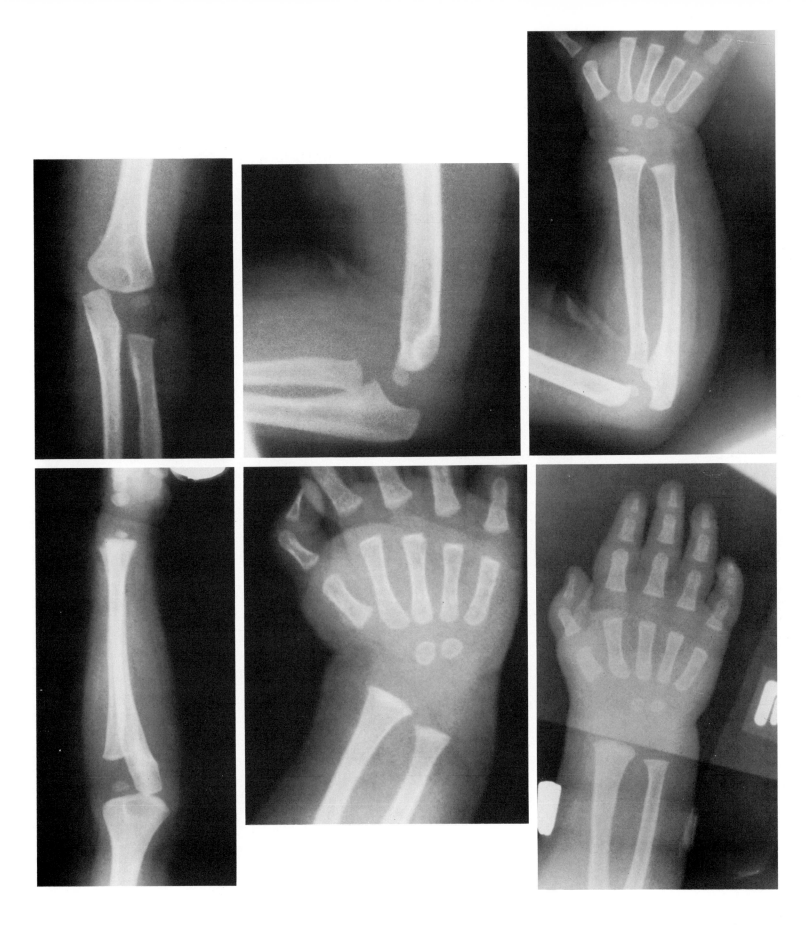

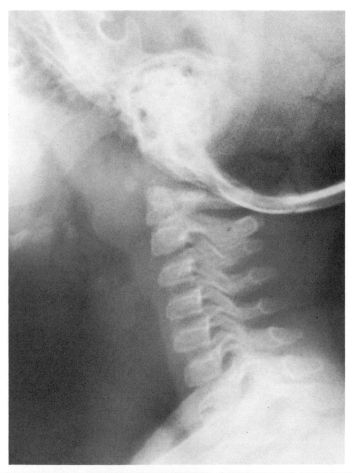

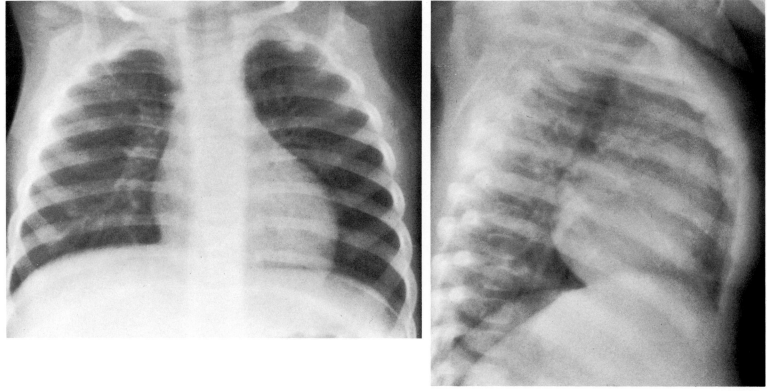

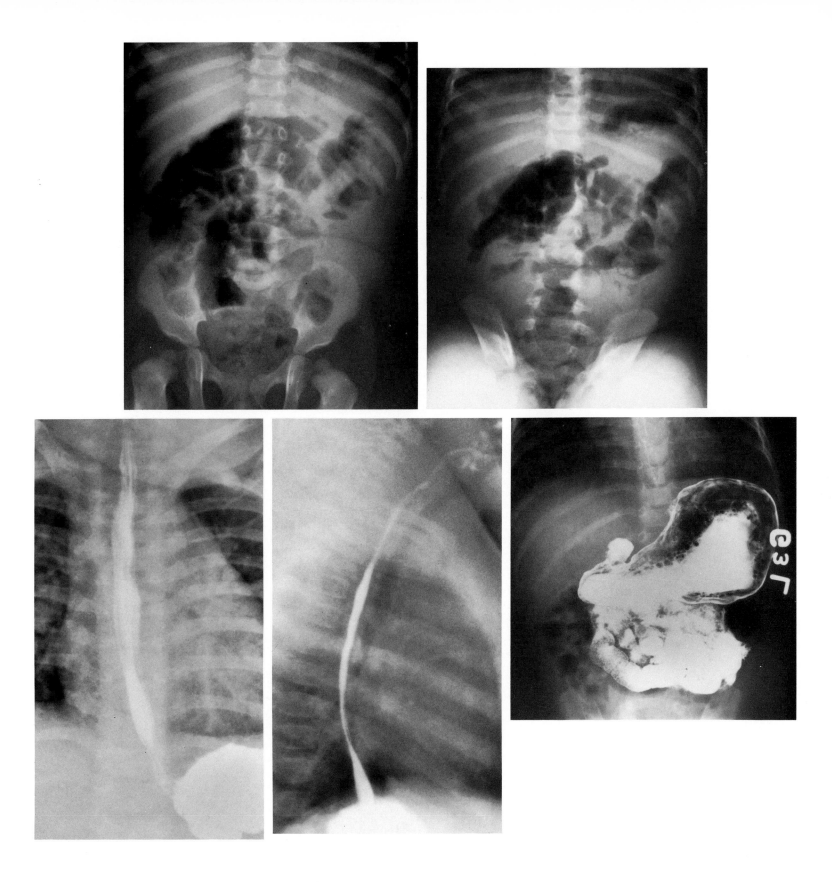

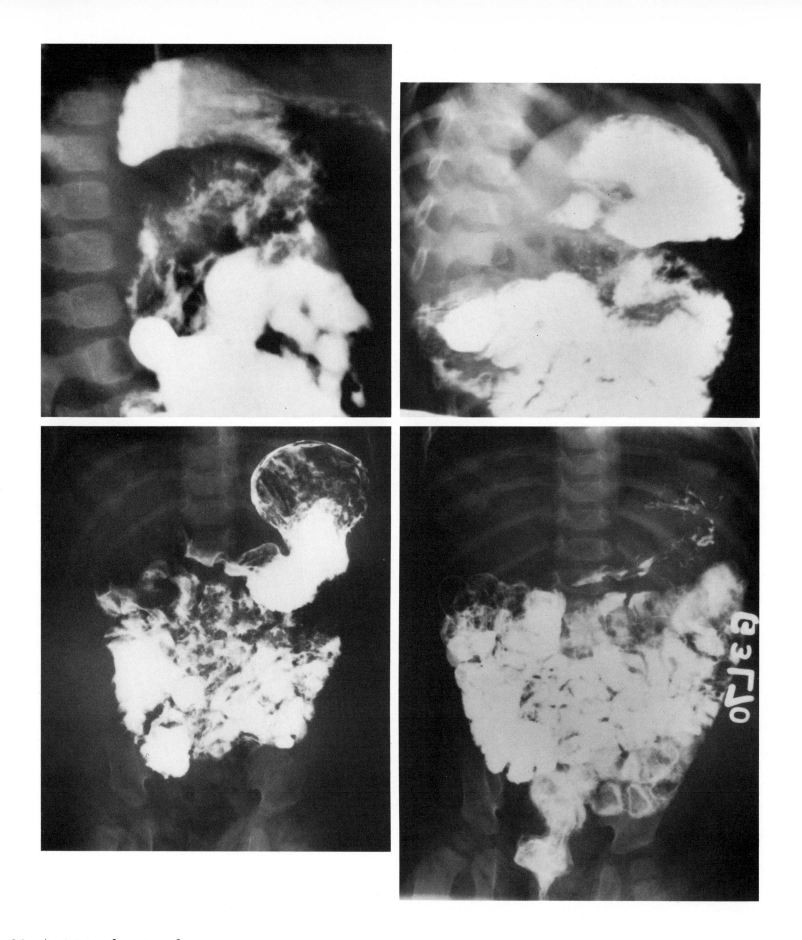

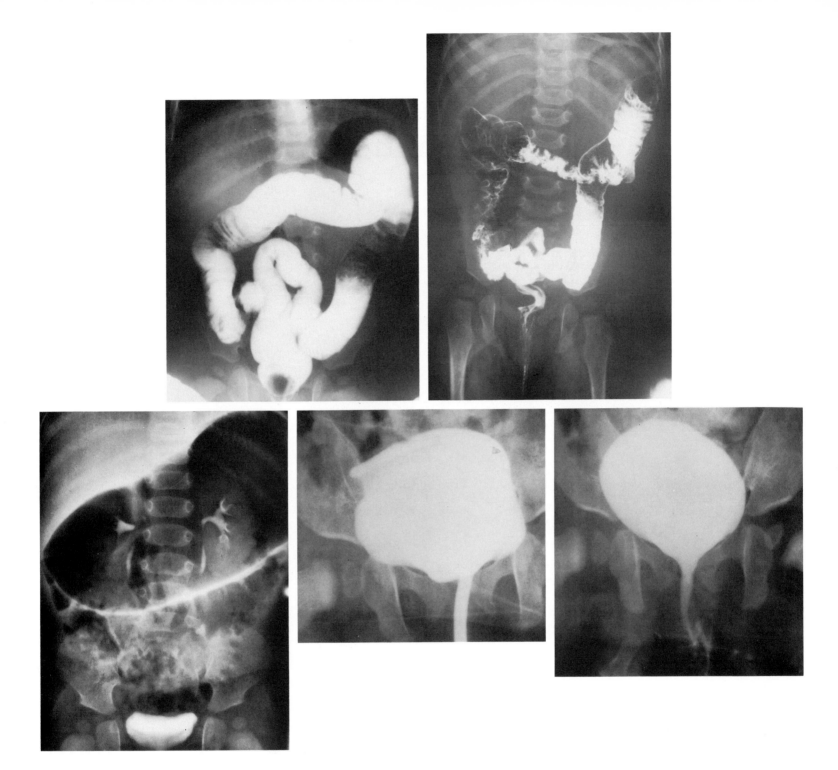

6

12 MONTHS

The anterior fontanel is starting to close. The cranial sutures are narrower. Paranasal sinus pneumatization may be well established. The size of the cervical spinal canal is not as disproportionate as before. The vertebrae now show anterior beaking, particularly in the lumbar region.

Rather dense zones of provisional calcification appear in the long bones. The capital femoral epiphysis covers most of the adjacent metaphysis. The medial margin of the metaphysis of the tibia may show a spur-like configuration. The ossification center for the capitellum is evident. Epiphyseal centers for the phalanges may be seen in the female.

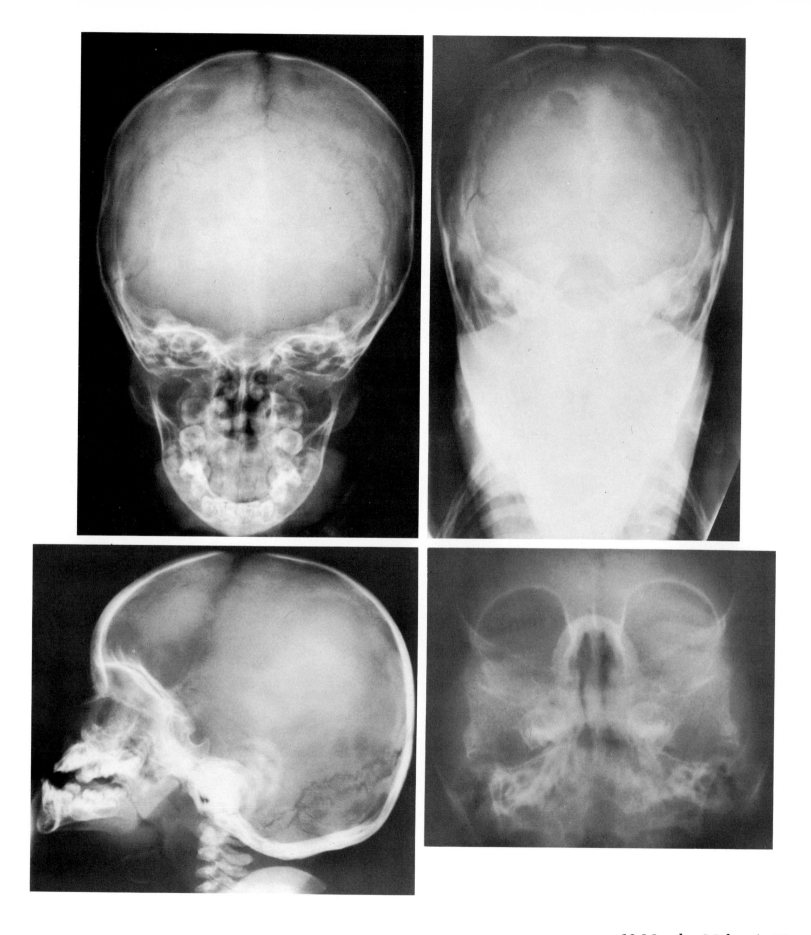

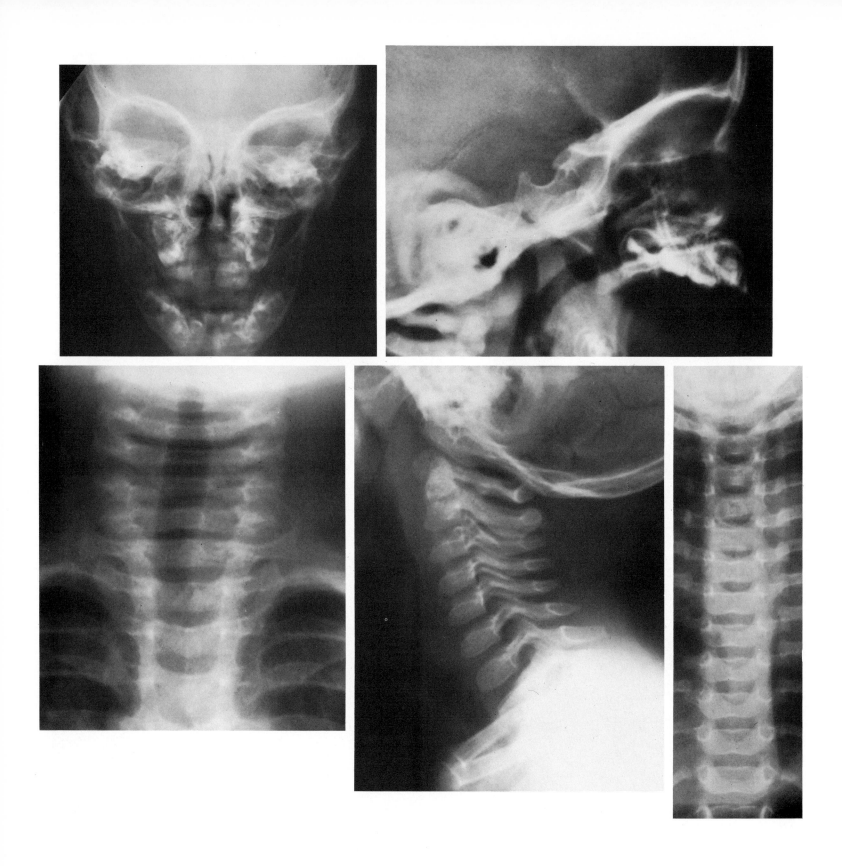

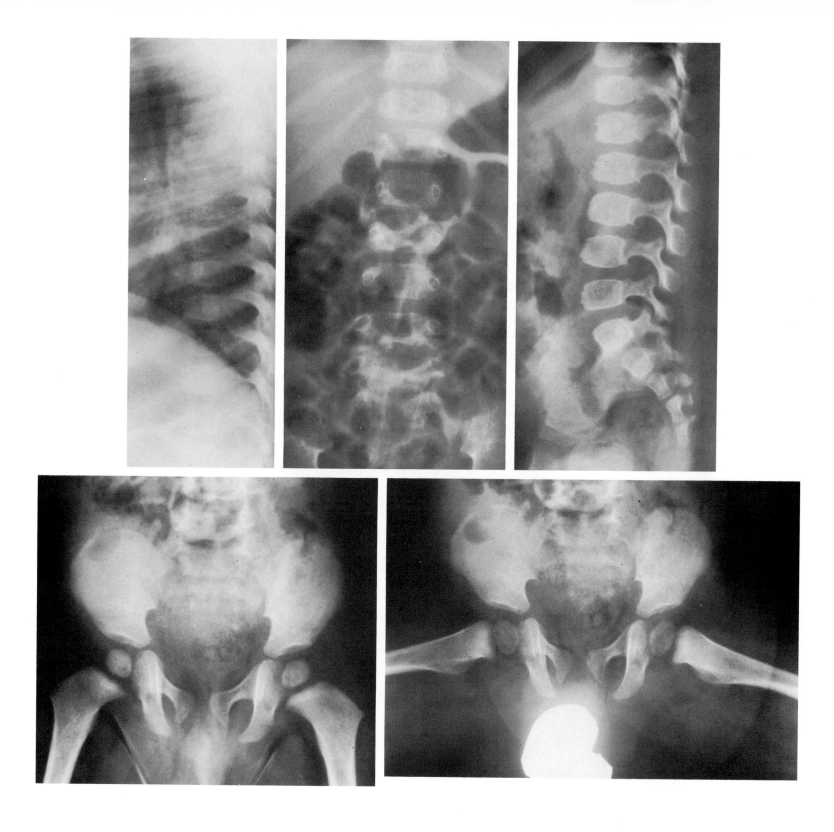

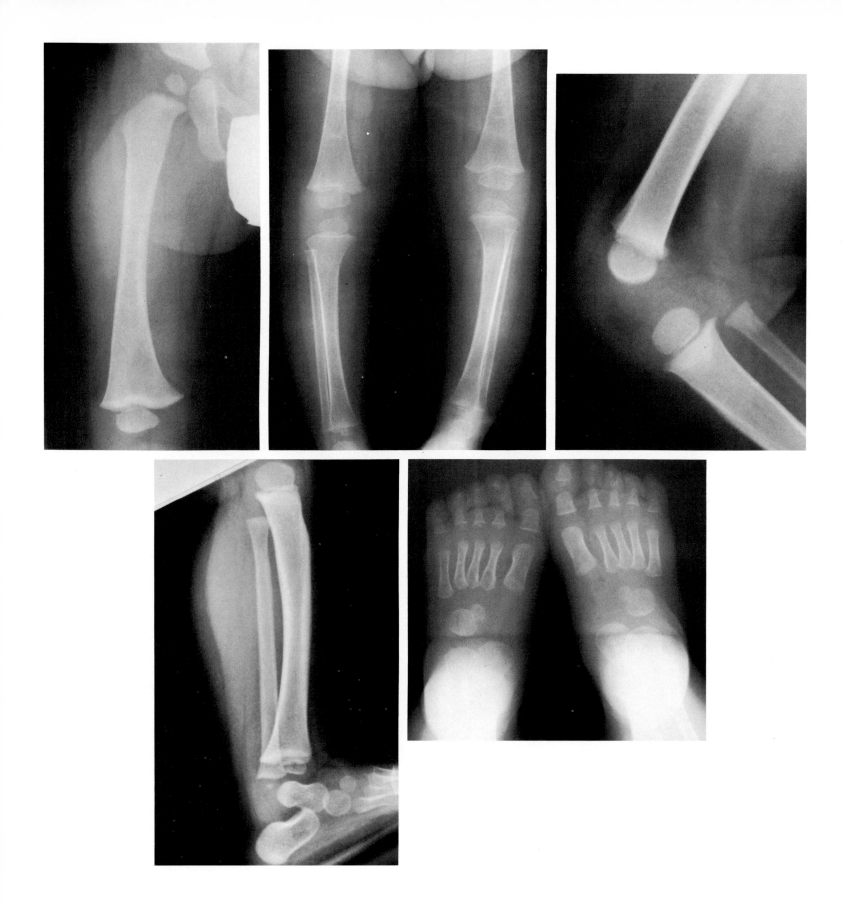

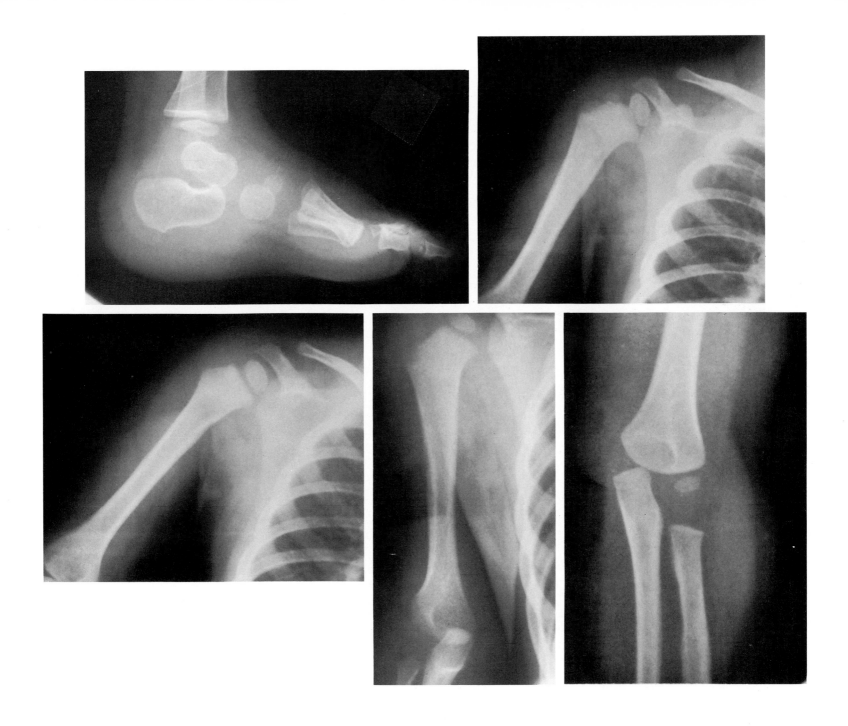

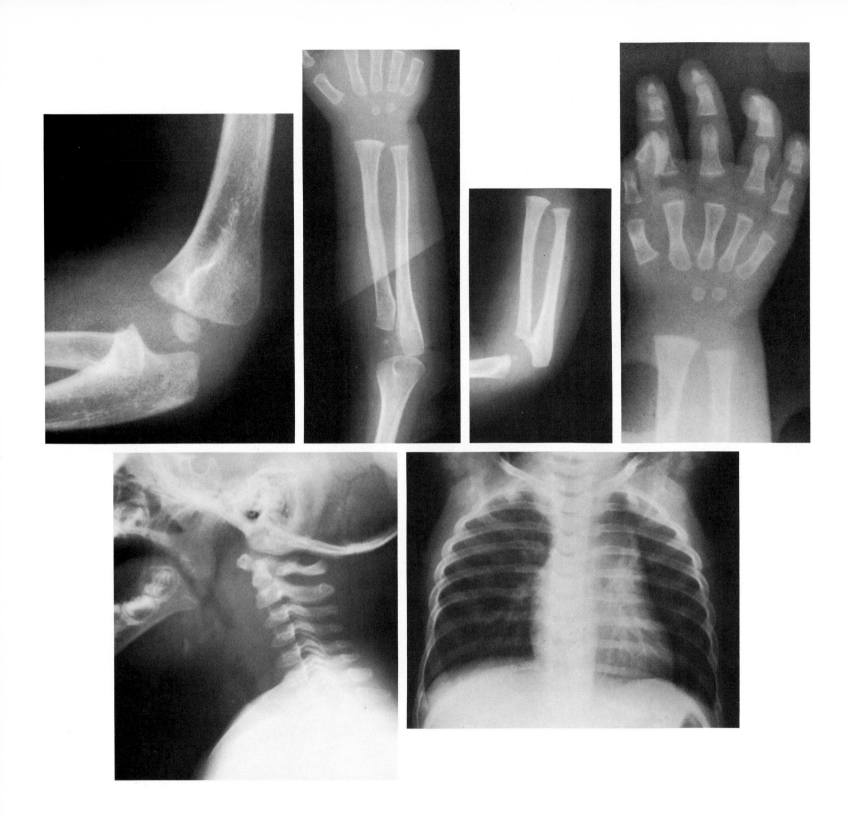

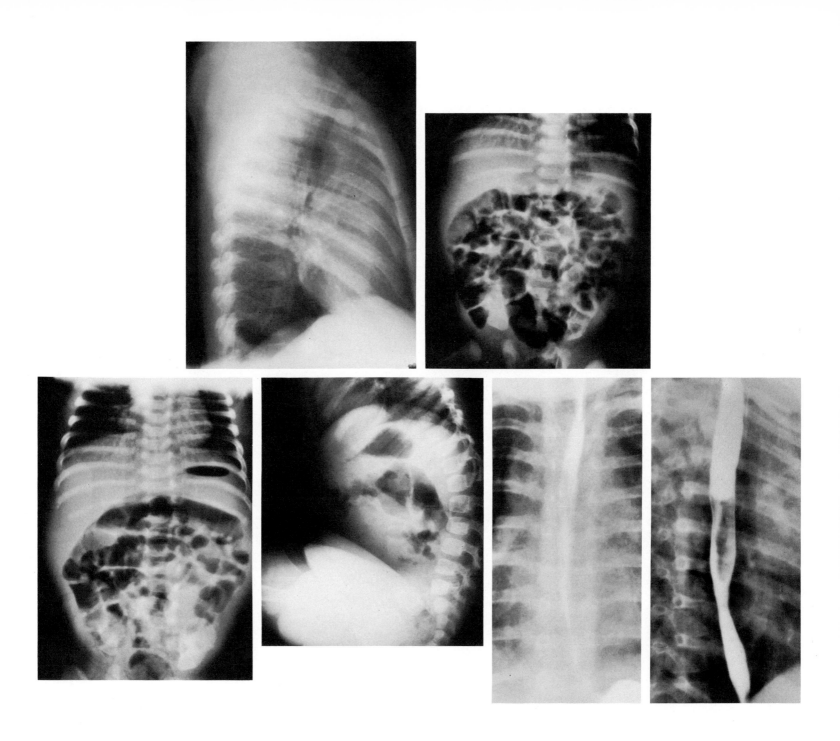

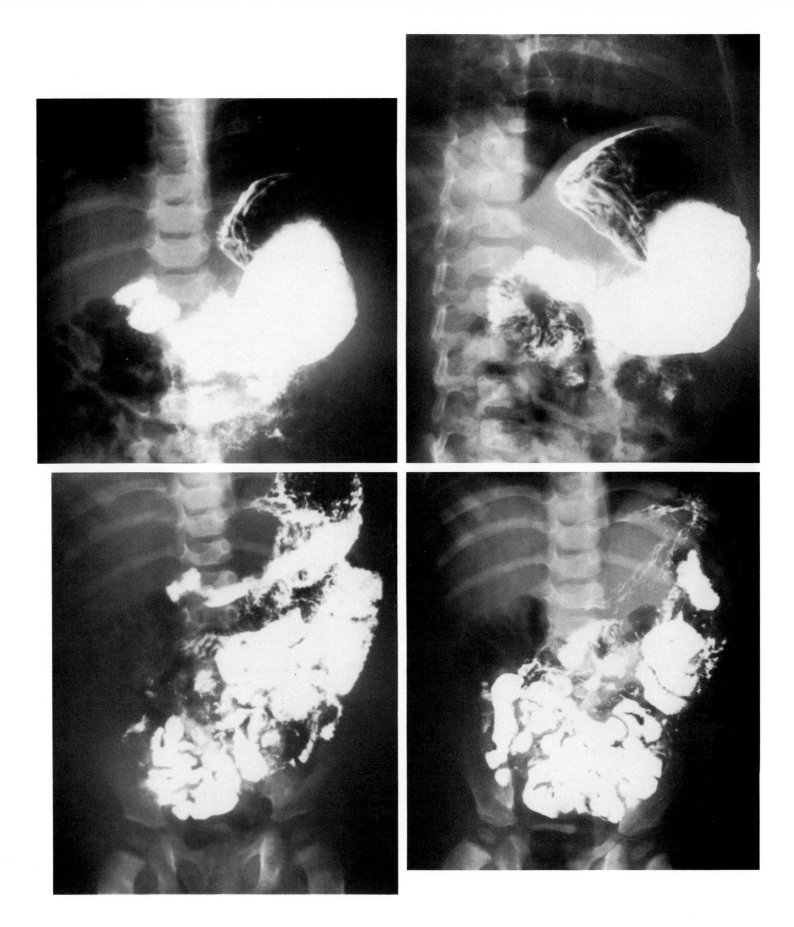

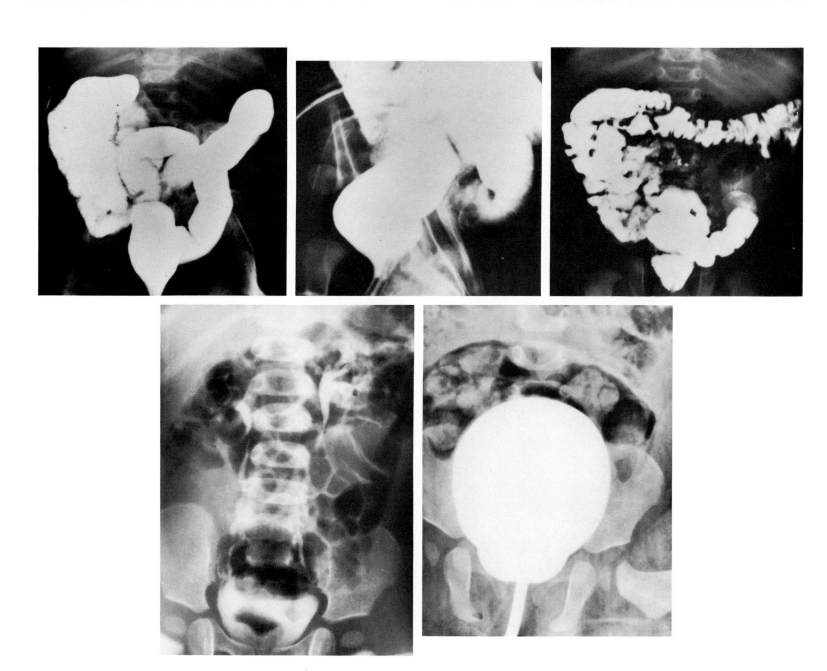

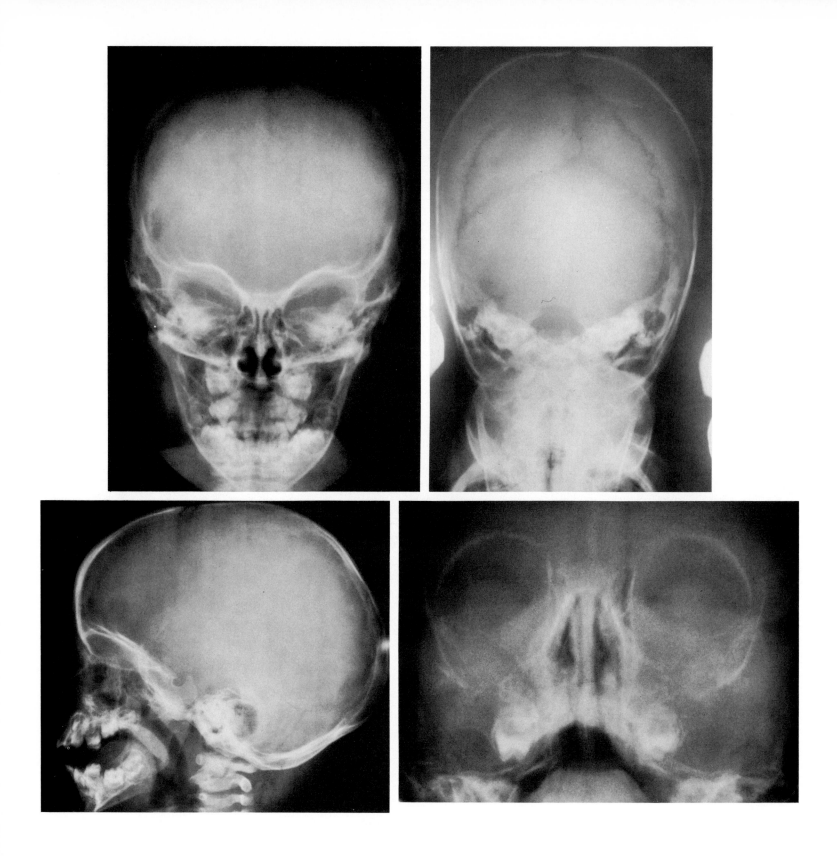

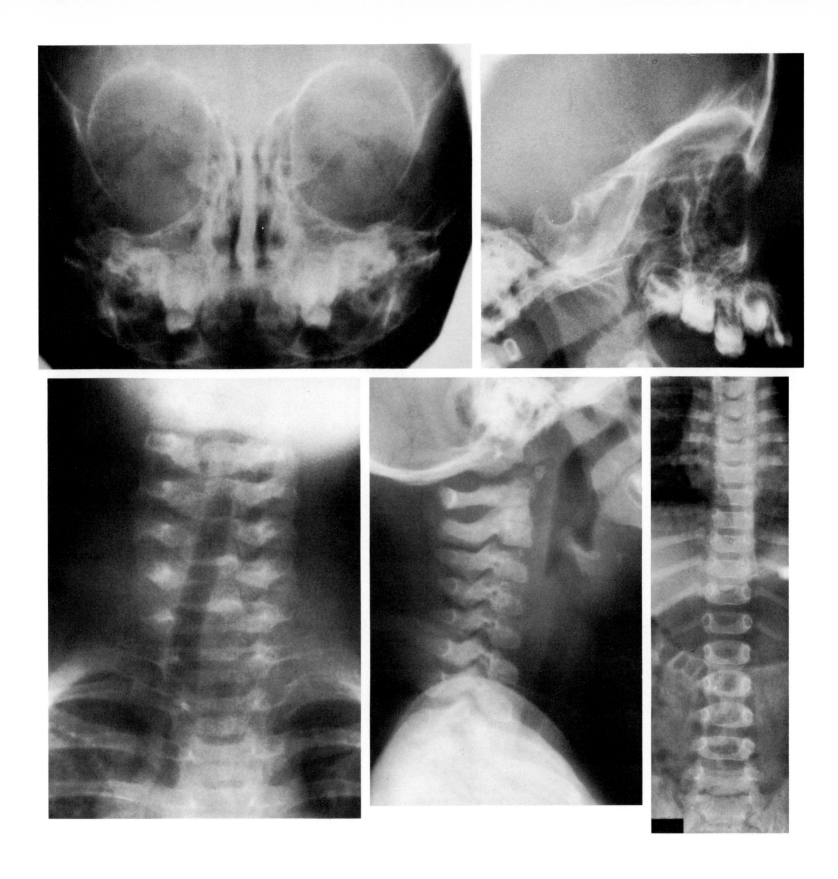

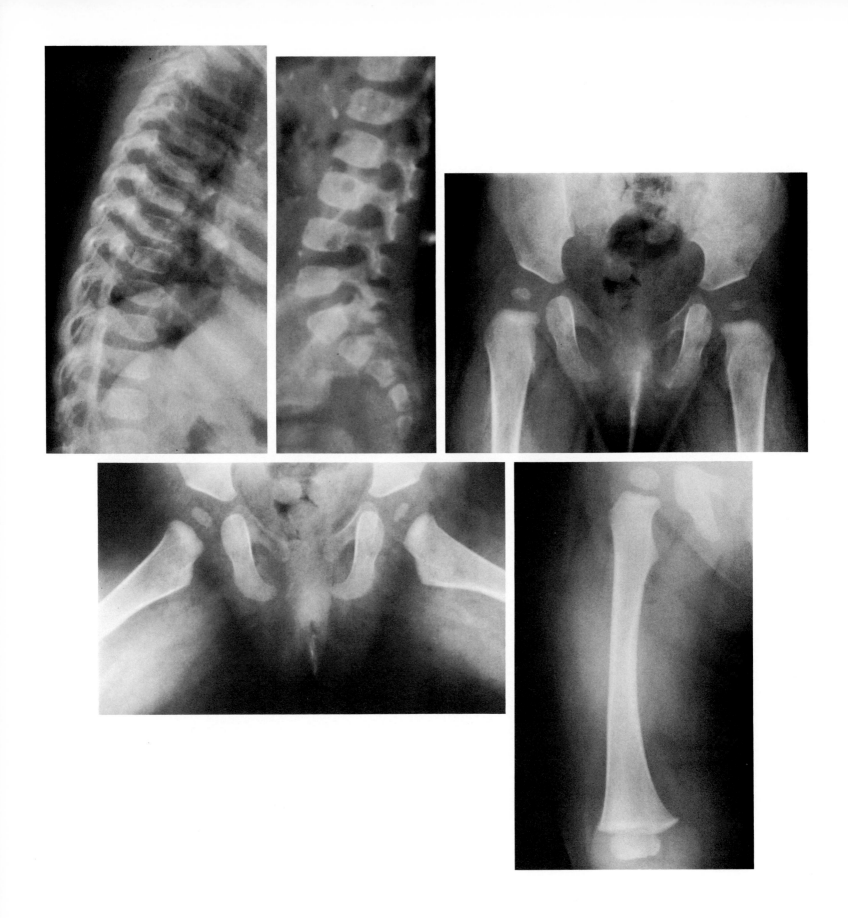

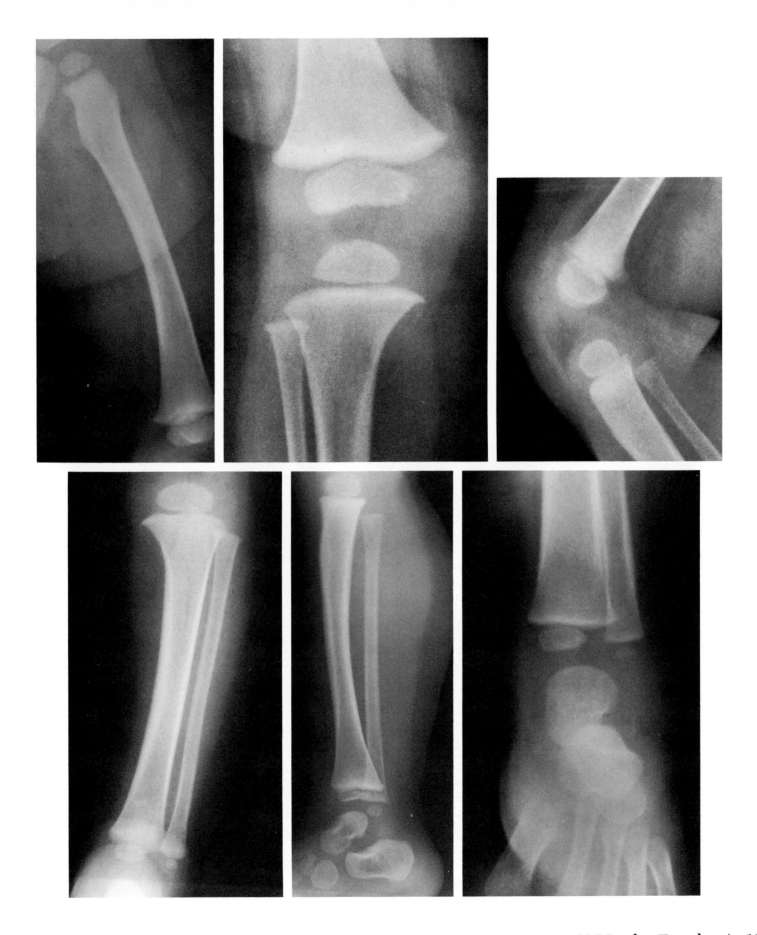

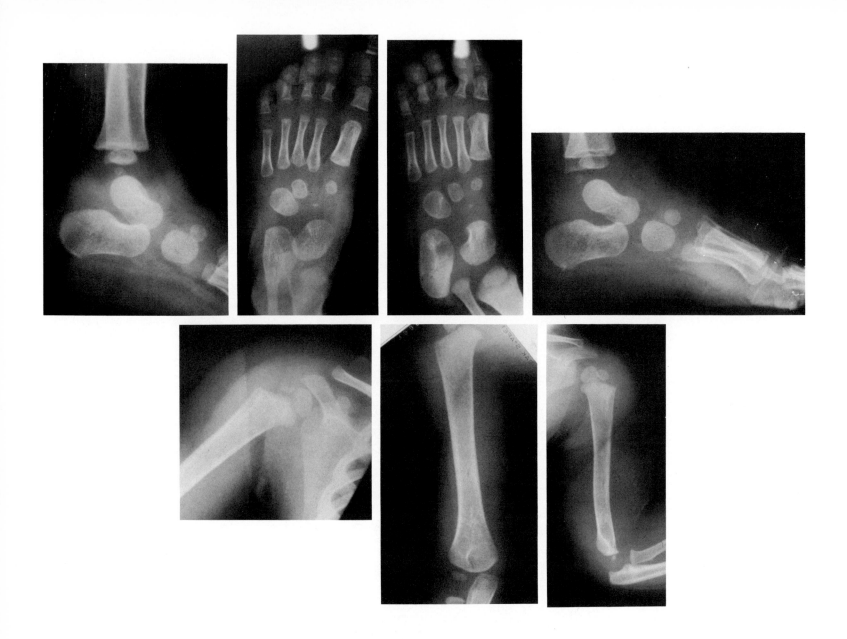

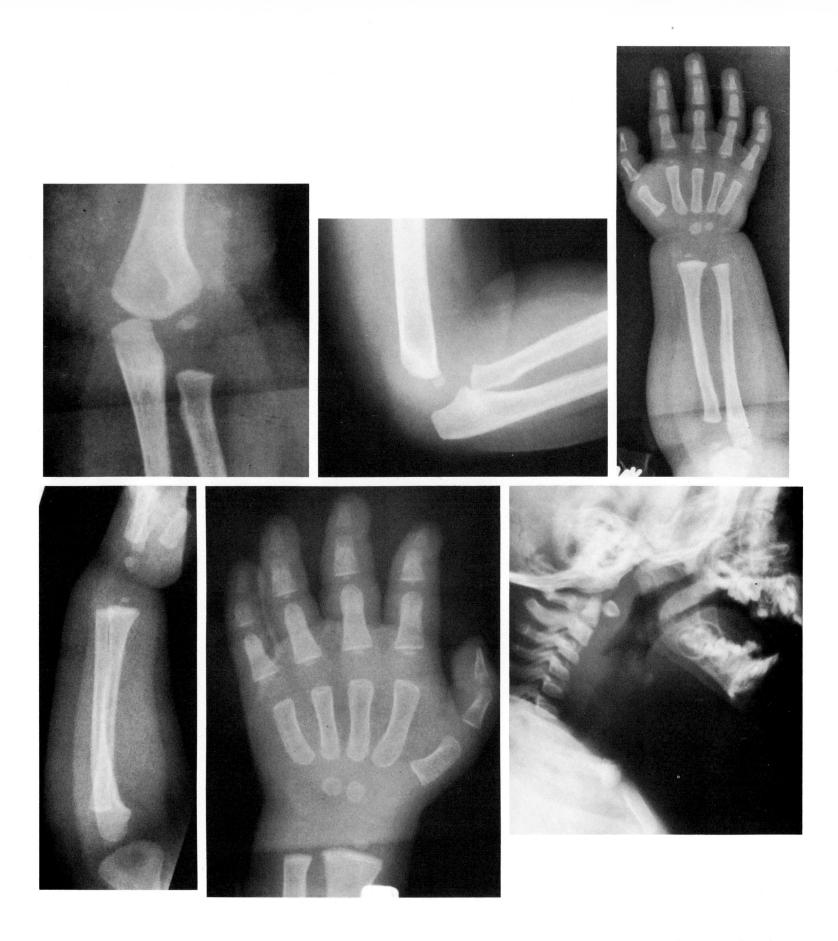

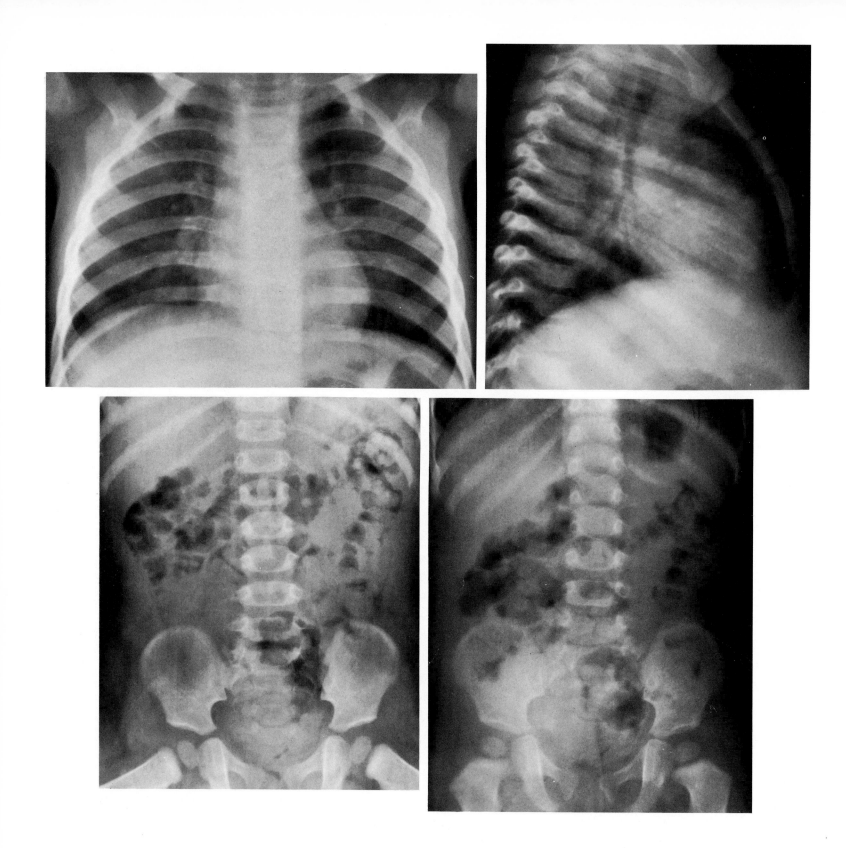

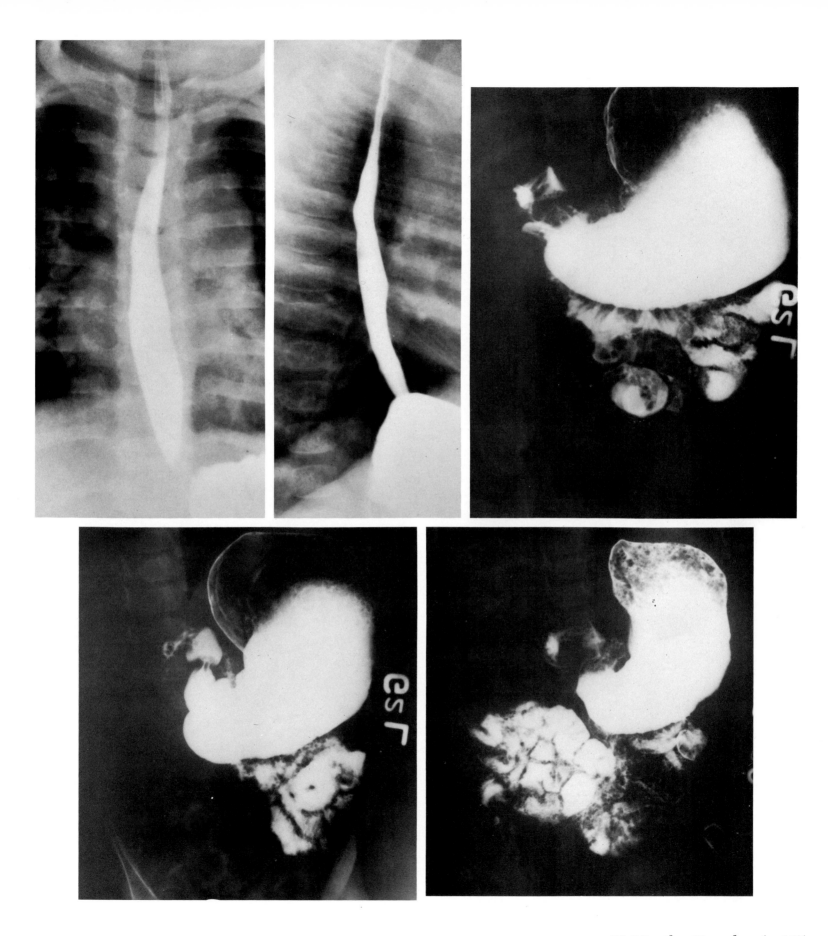

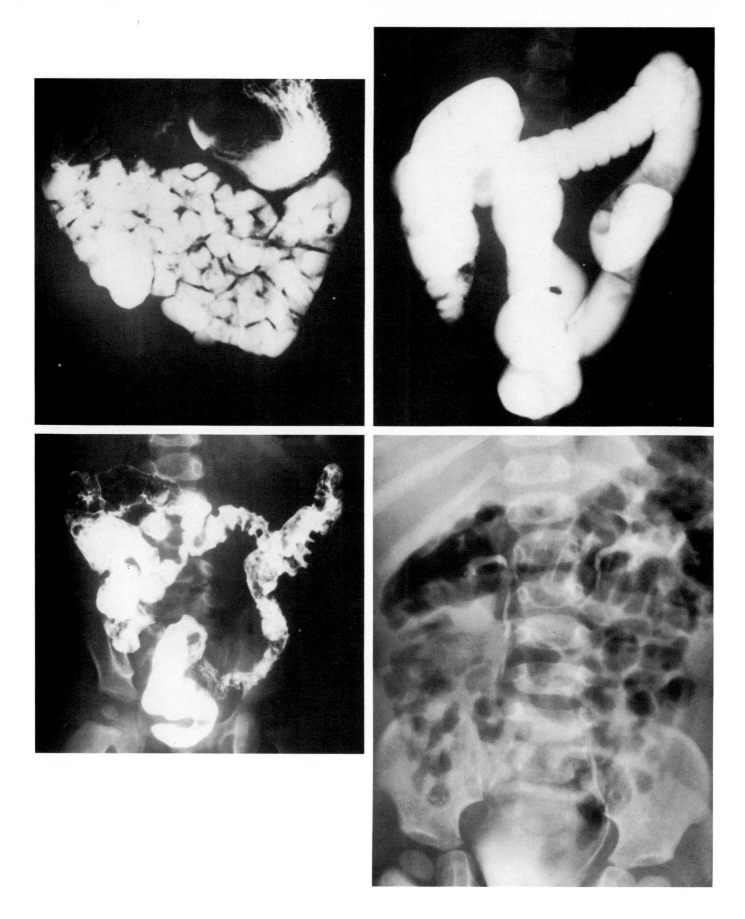

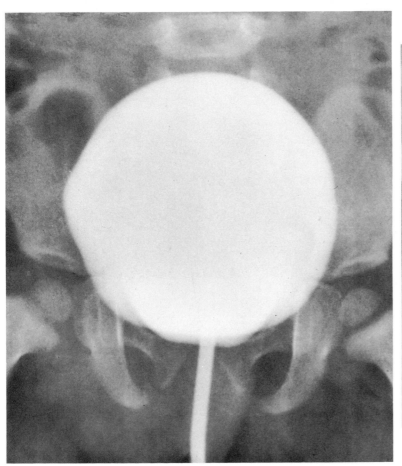
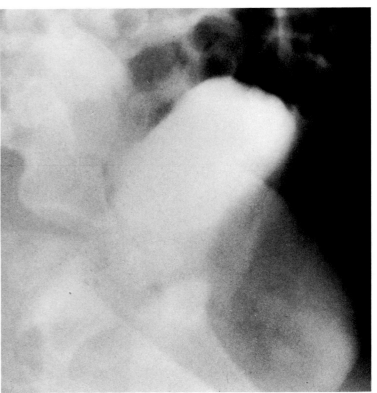

7

15 MONTHS

The skull has assumed a more adult configuration, and the paranasal sinuses may be well pneumatized. The anterior fontanel is still open. The sutures are less clearly defined. The cervical spinal canal is still relatively large. Physiologic posterior scalloping of the lumbar vertebrae becomes visible for the first time.

The ilia are enlarging. In the long bones, the zones of provisional calcification are still dense but less than they were previously. The femurs are relatively long and more adult-like. Irregularity of the medial aspect of the distal femoral epiphysis is evident. Distal metacarpal epiphyses and phalangeal epiphyses may be present in the hands and feet of the female.

The chest is more adult-like. Gas is still present in the small bowel. The colon is less redundant. The elongating kidneys may now be defined. The filled bladder does not occupy as much of the abdomen as it did at the earlier ages.

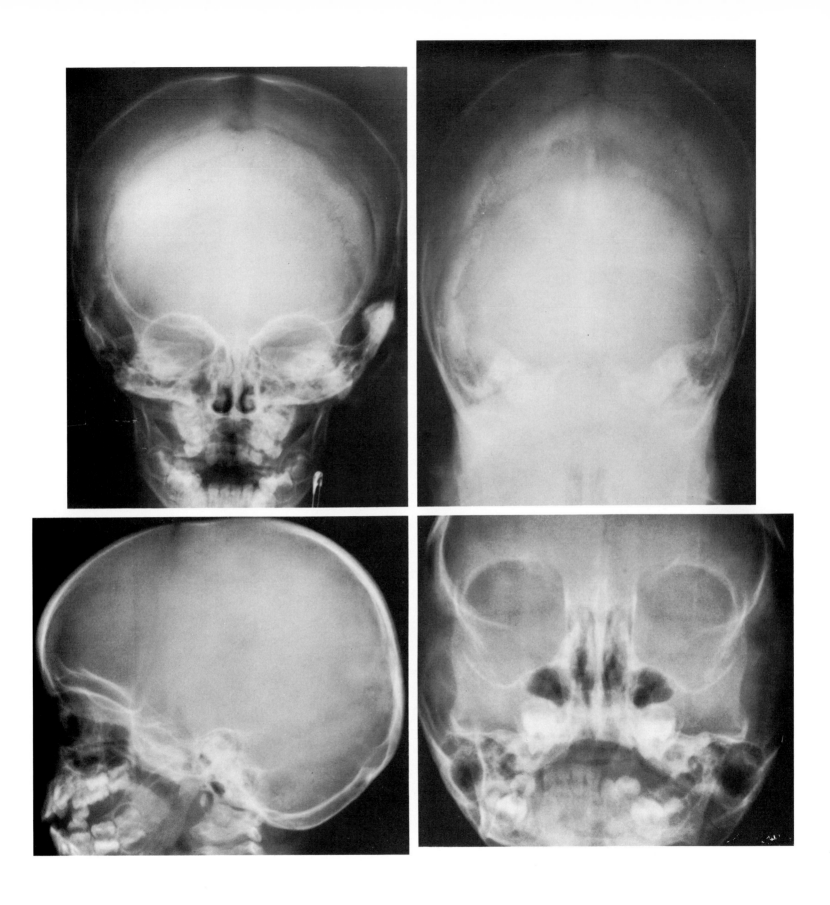

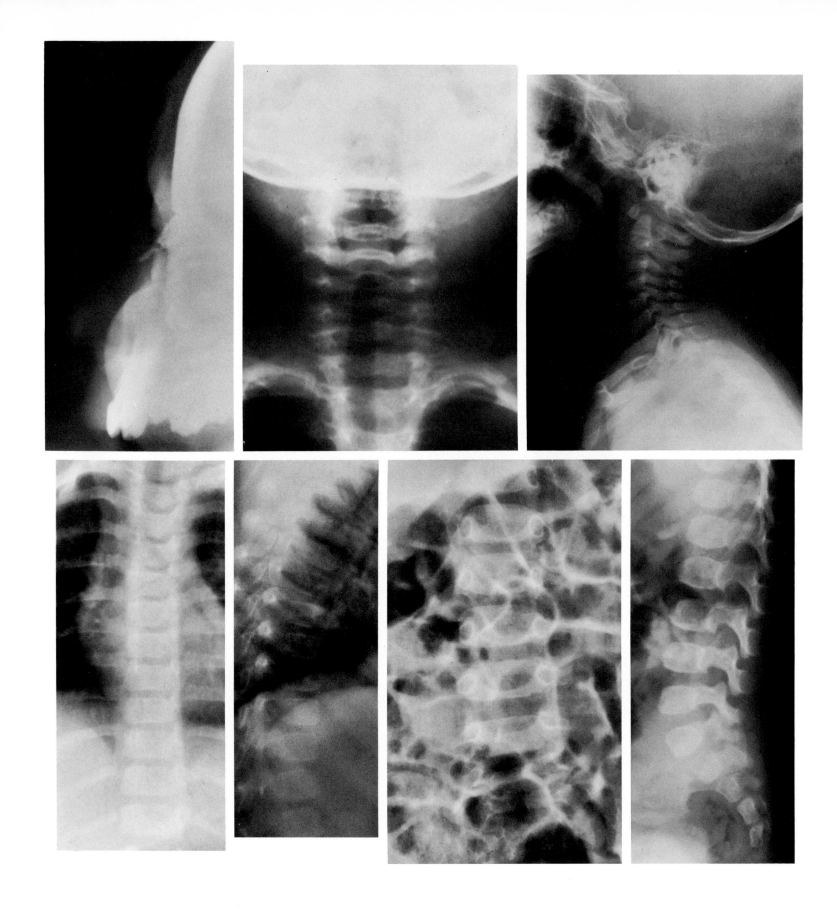

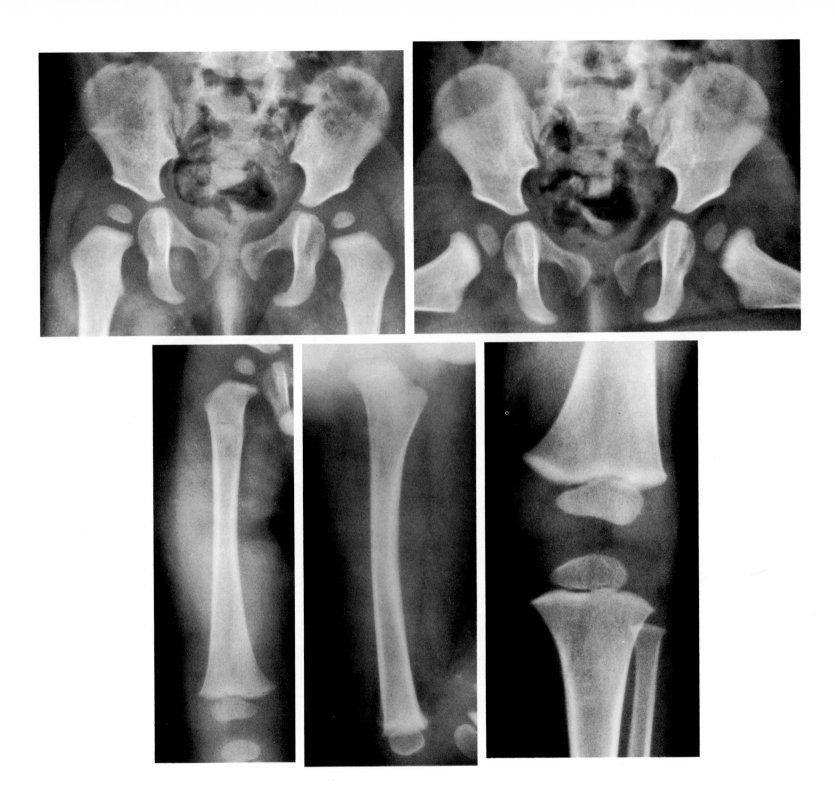

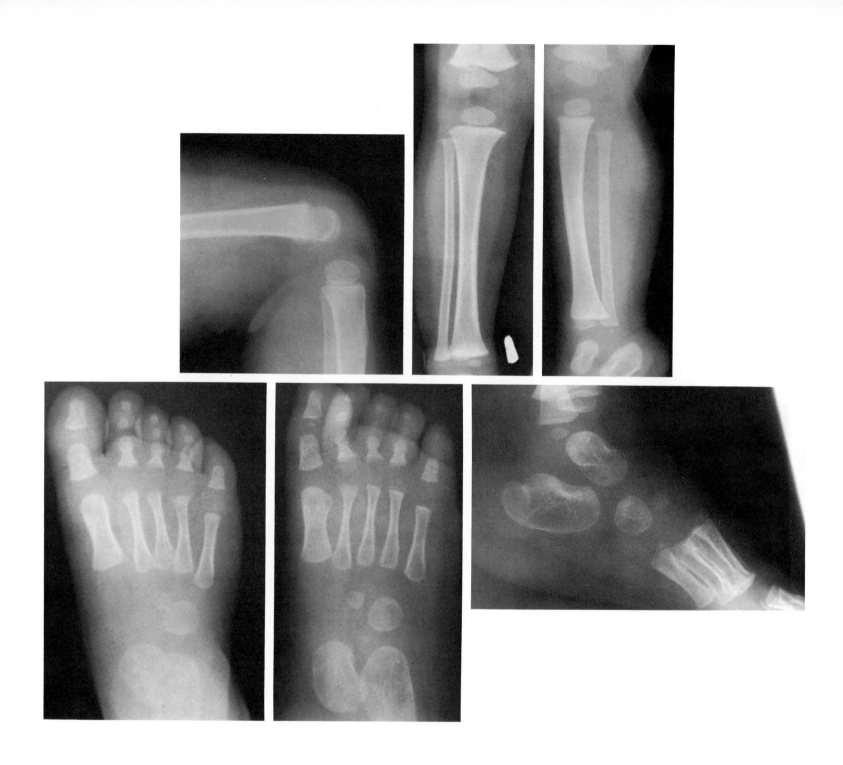

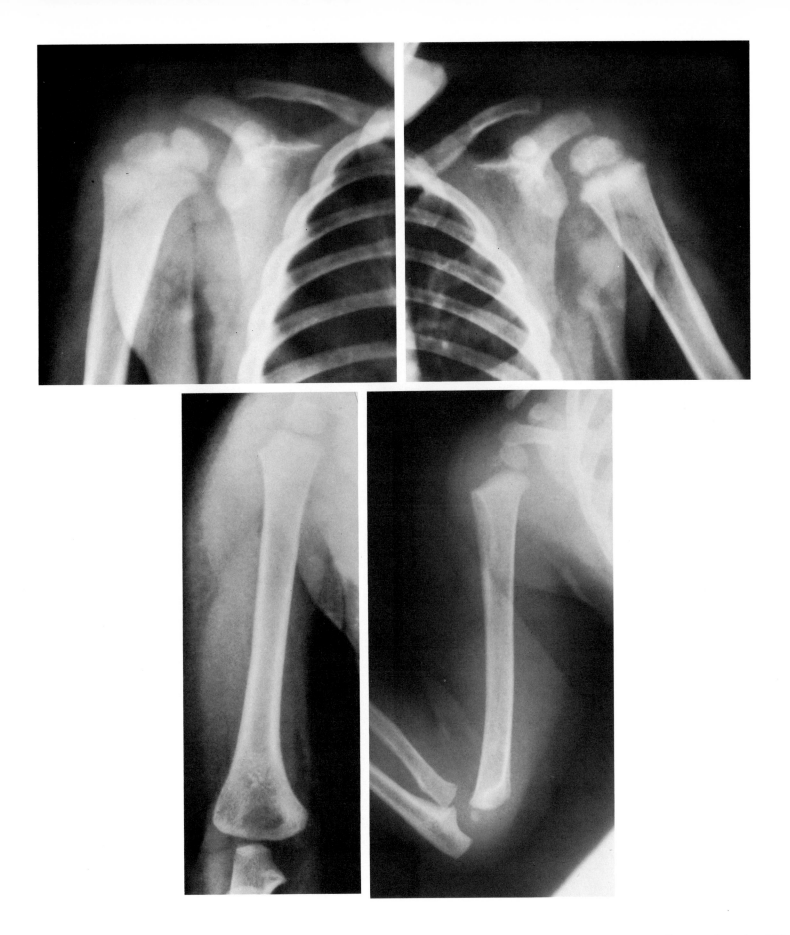

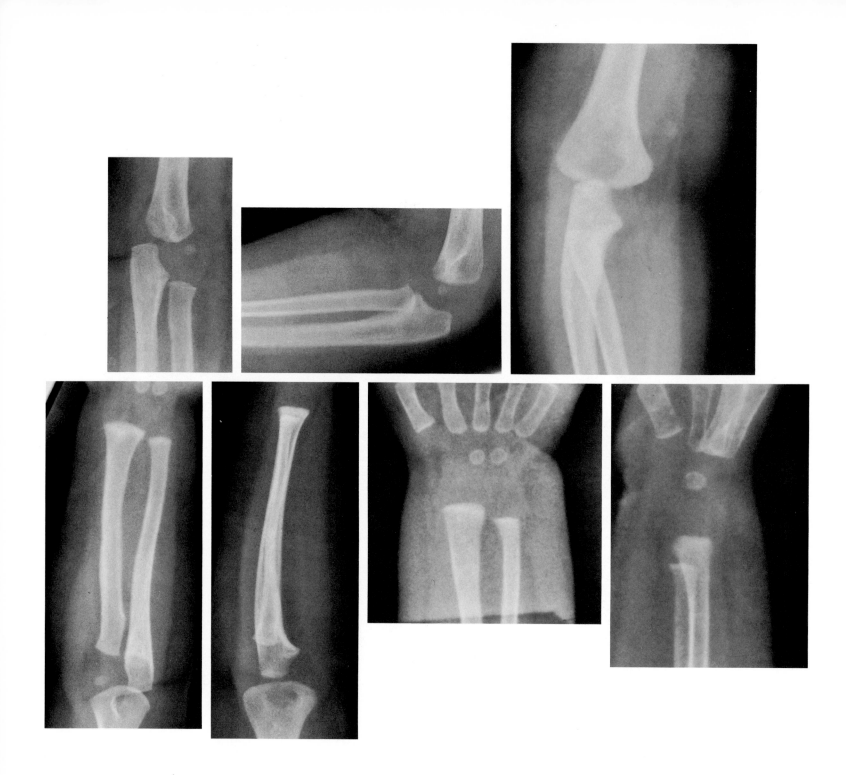

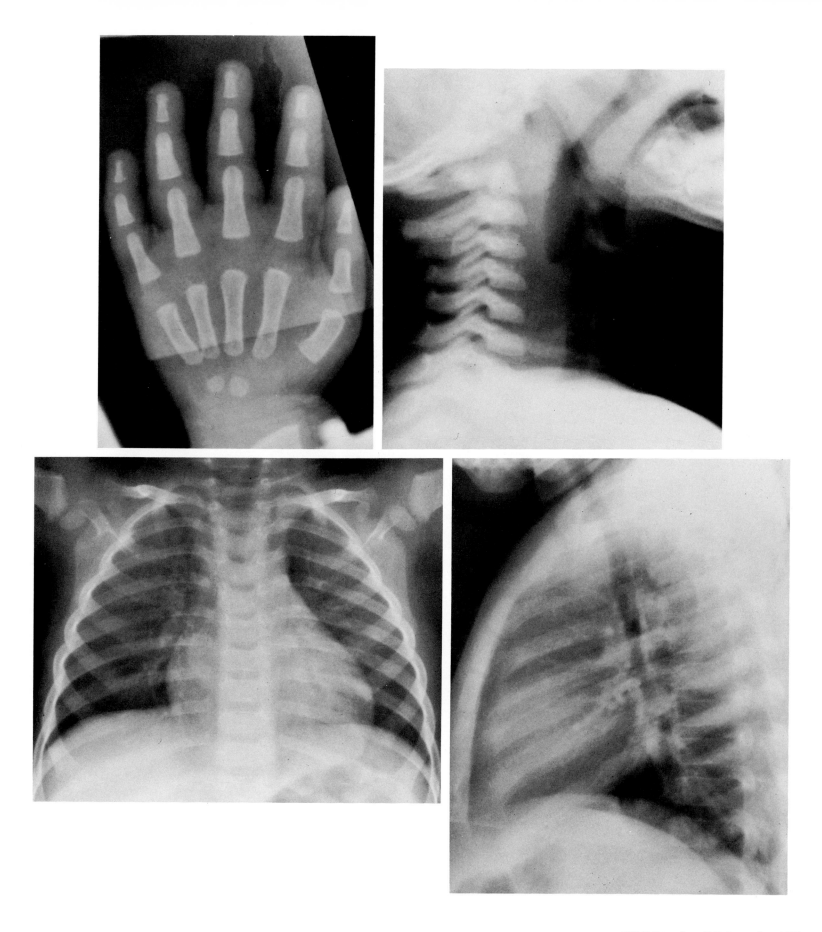

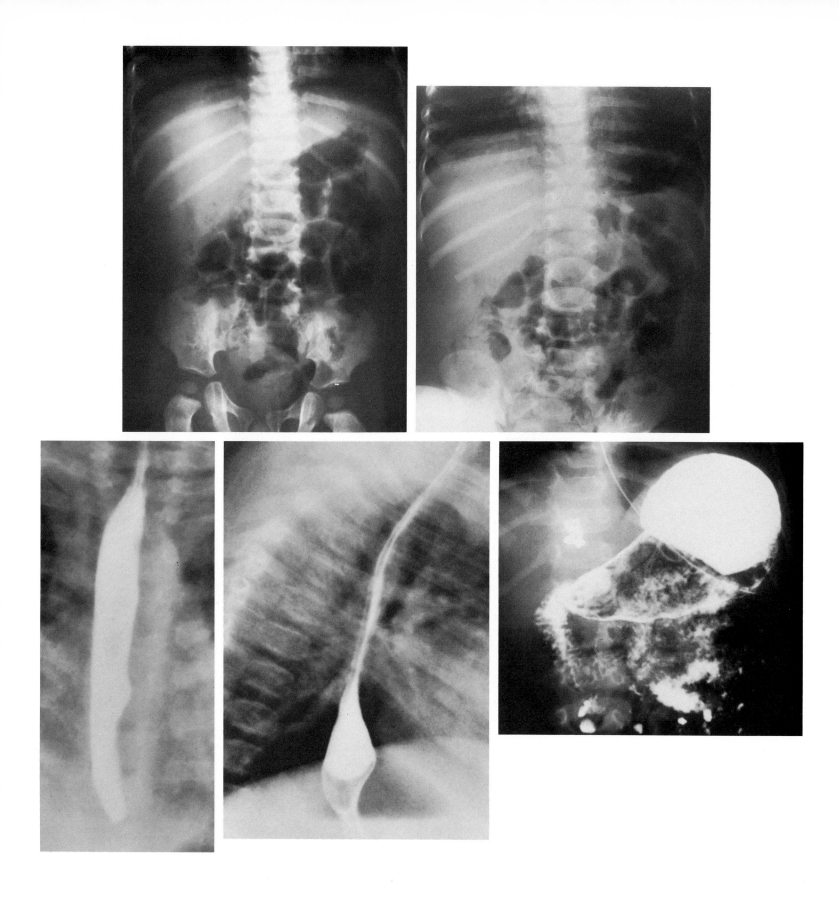

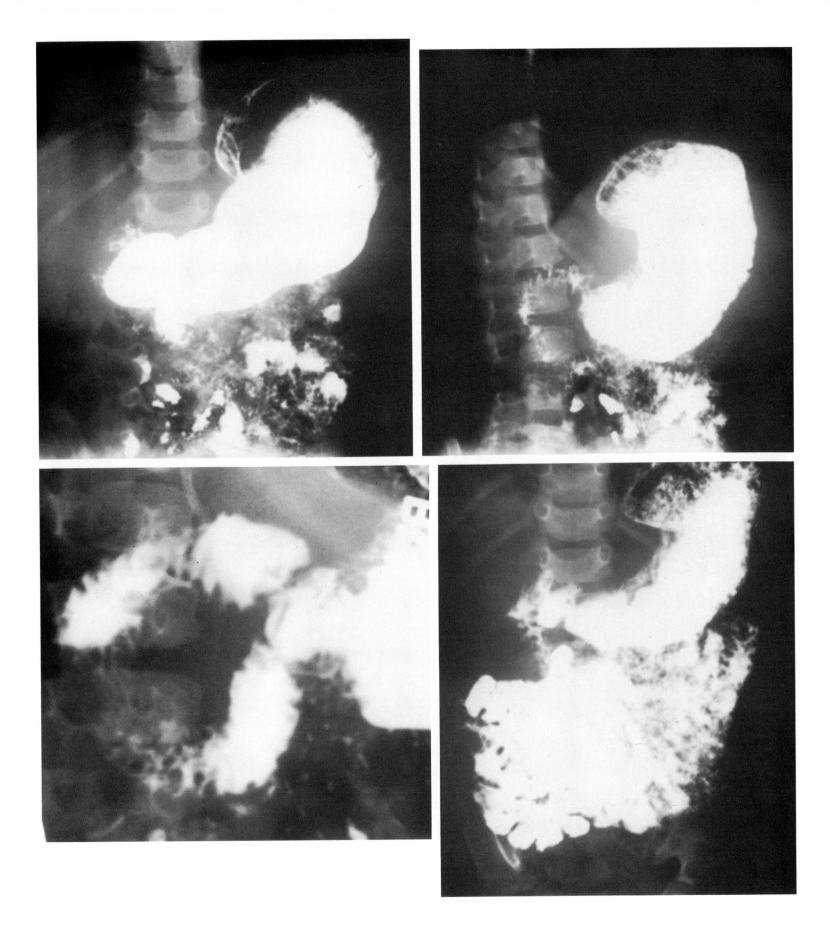

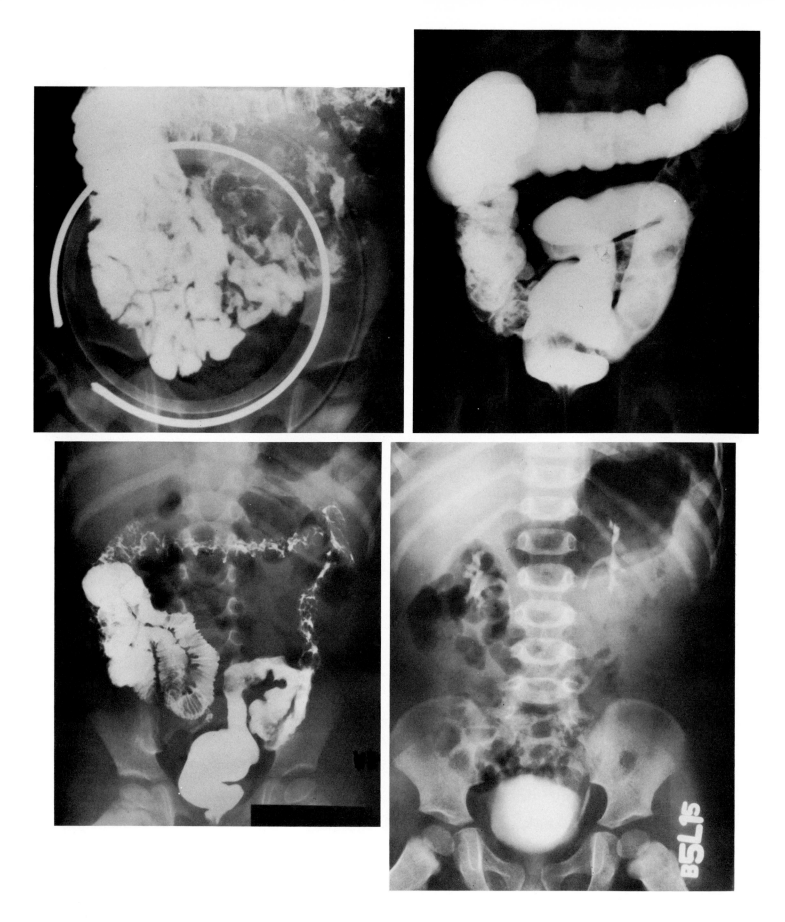

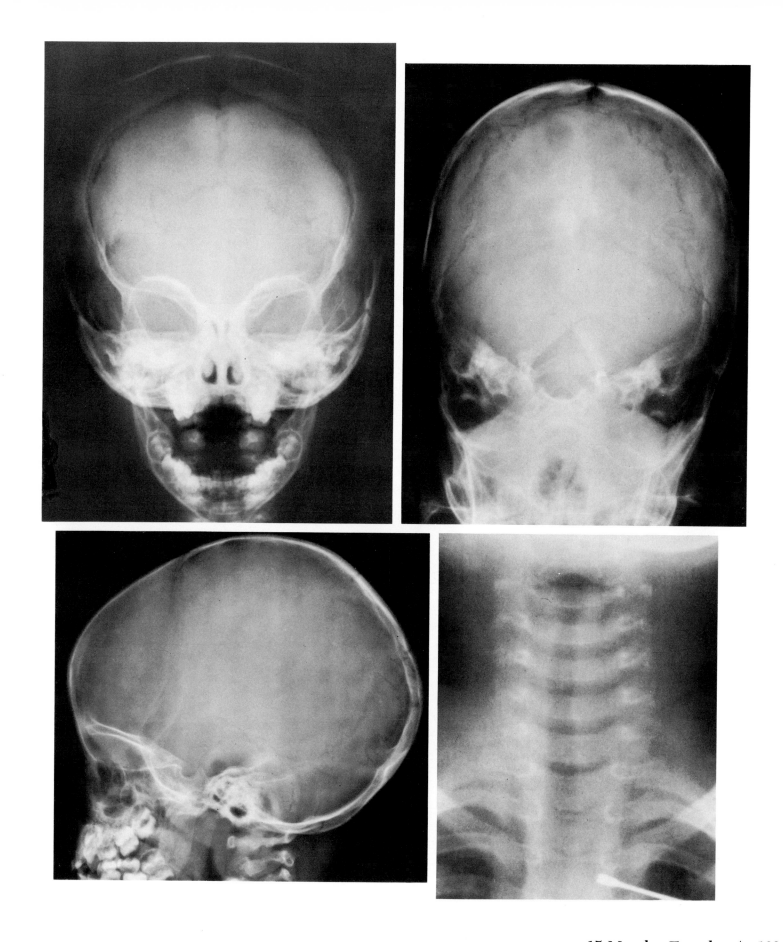

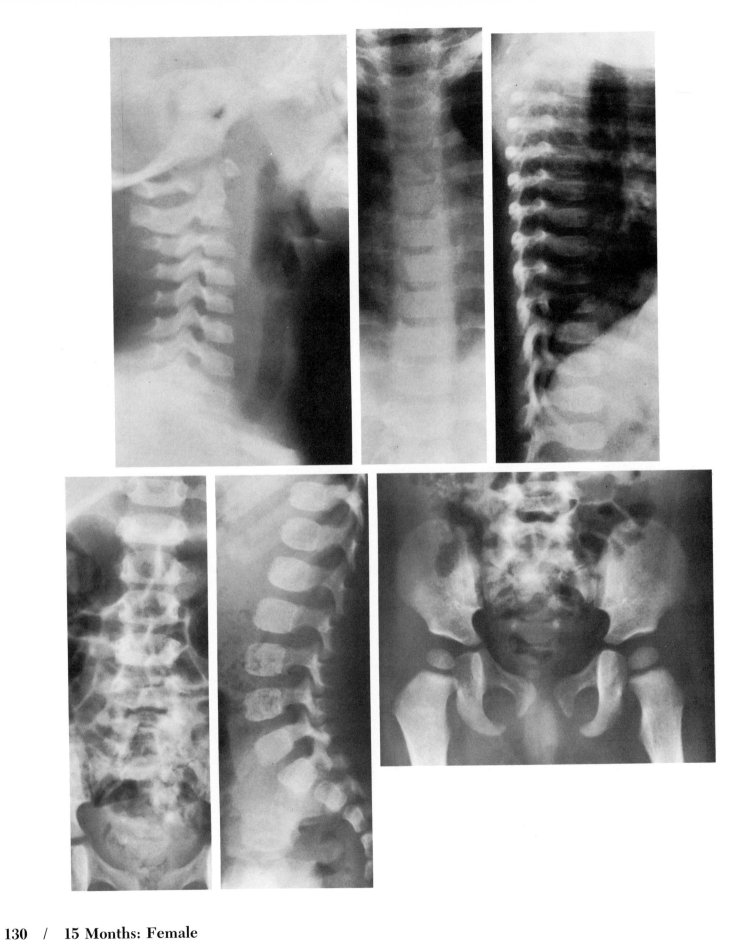

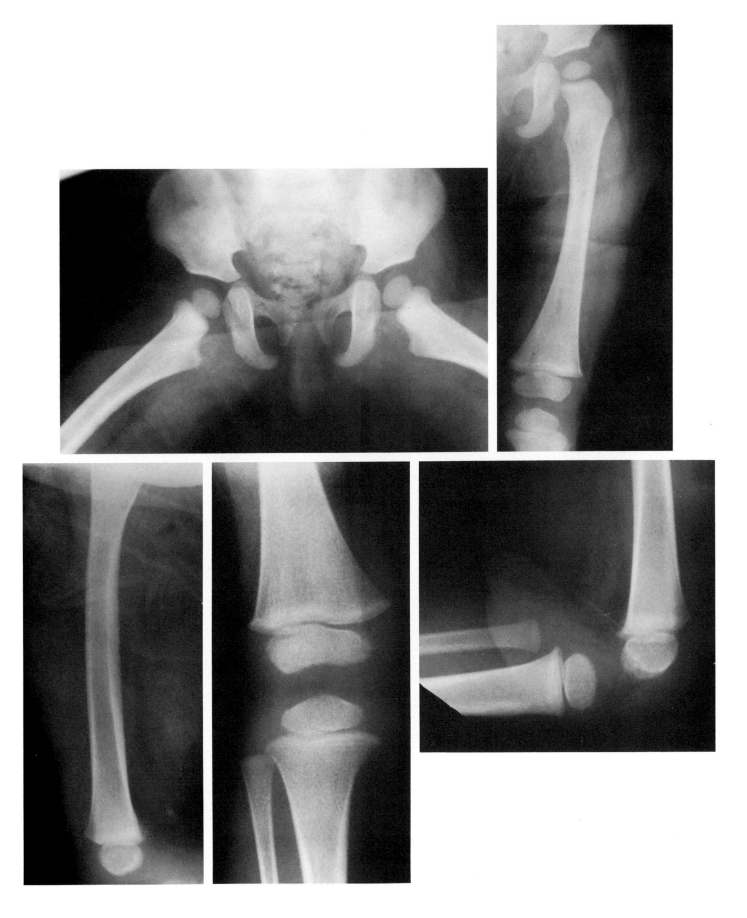

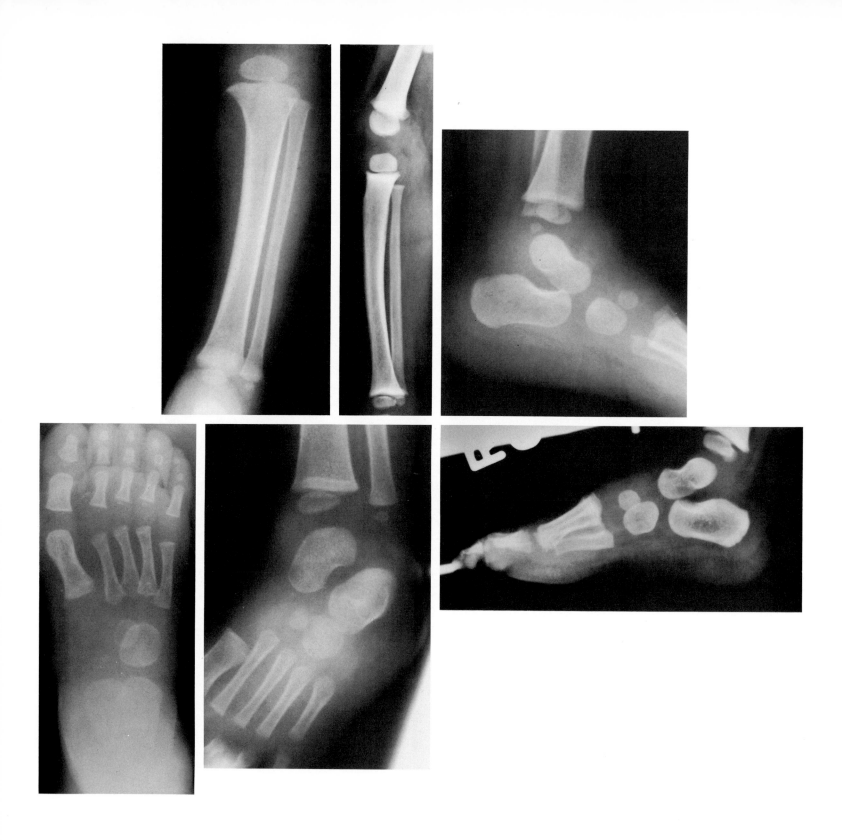

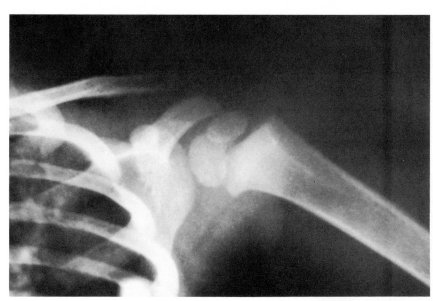

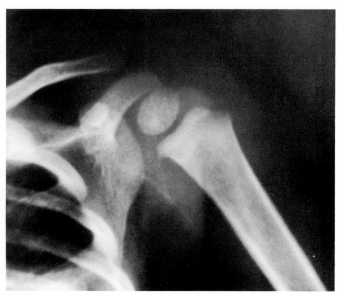

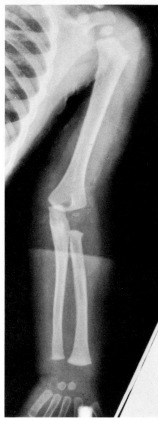

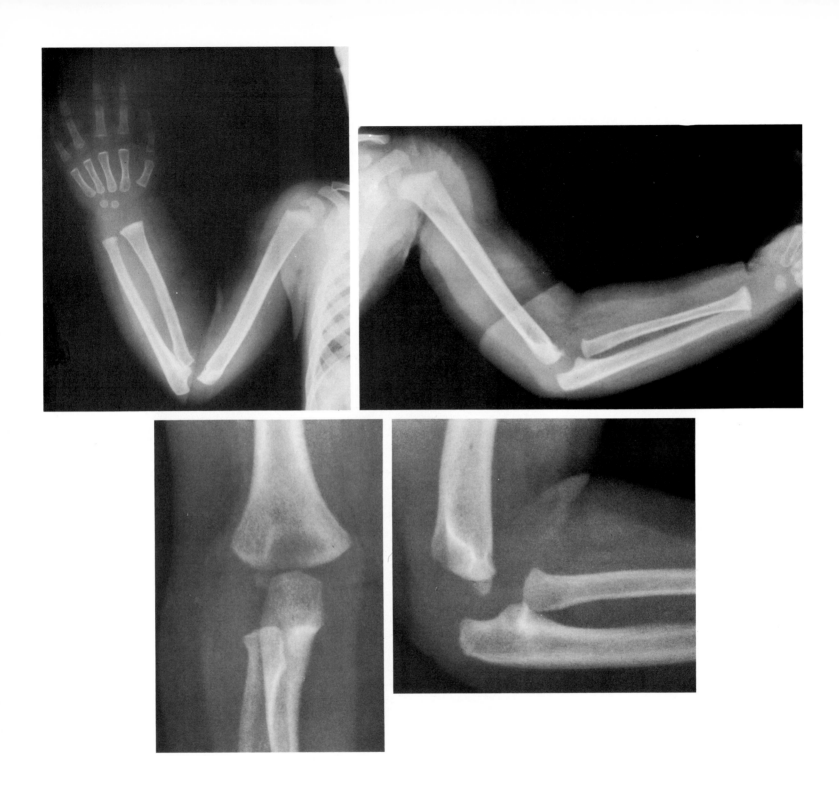

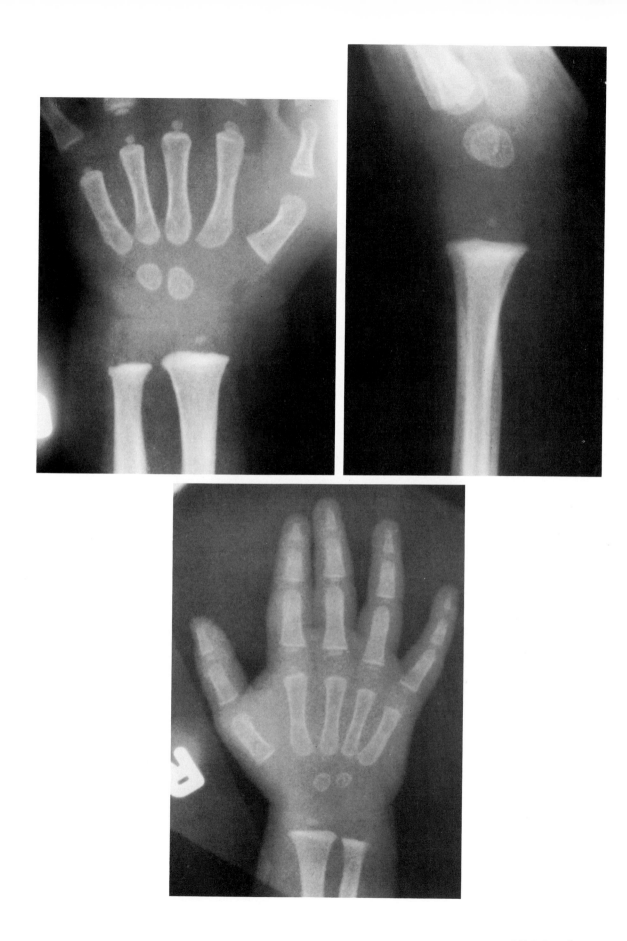

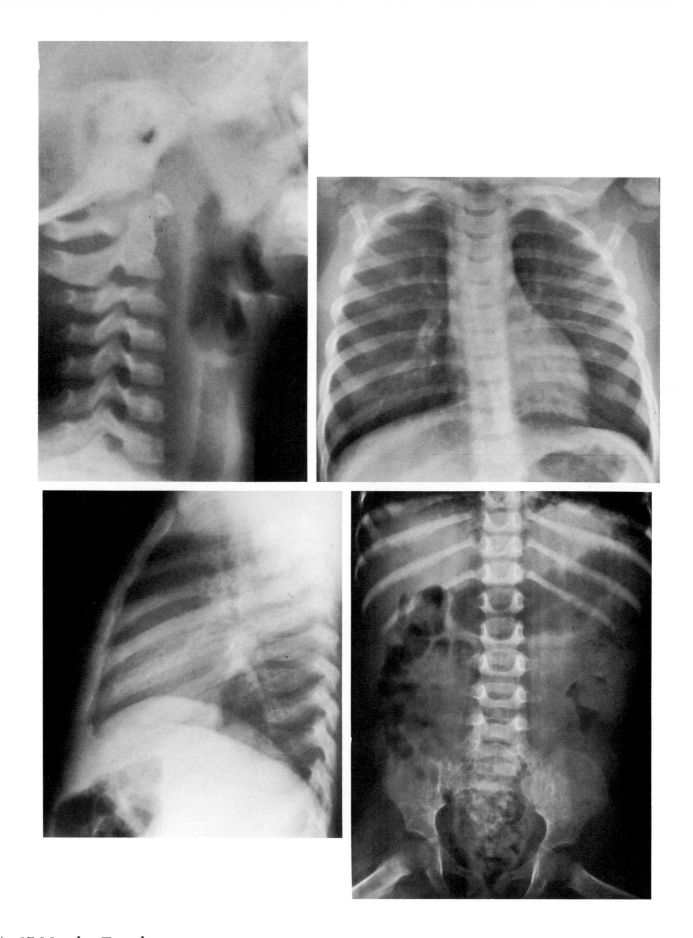

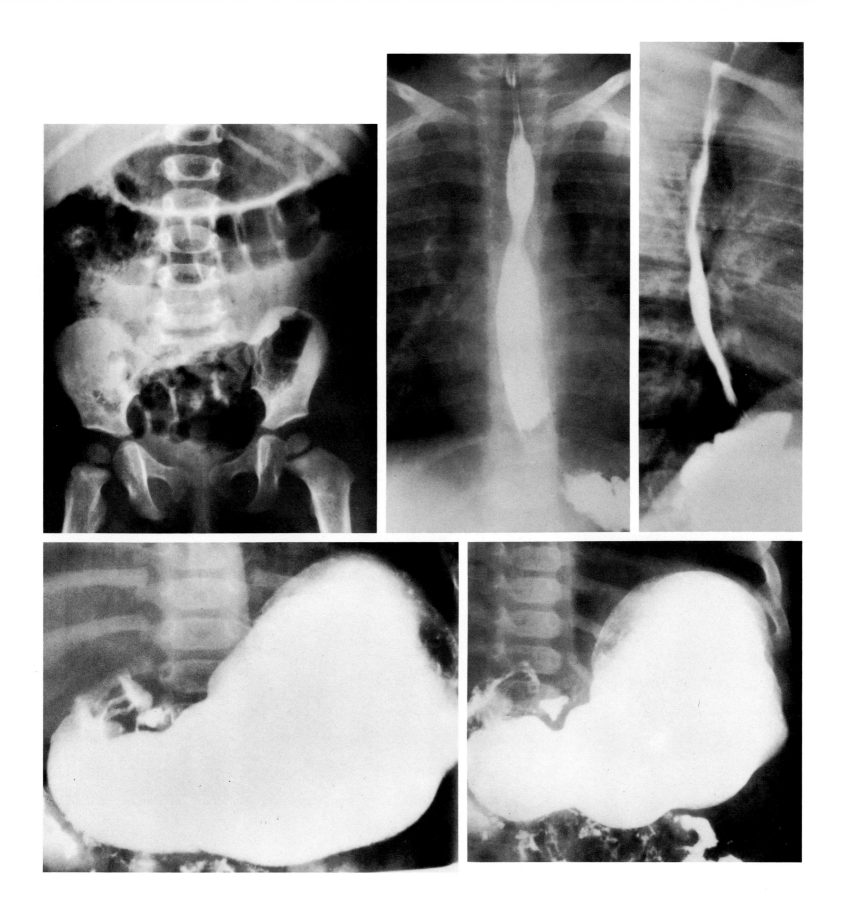

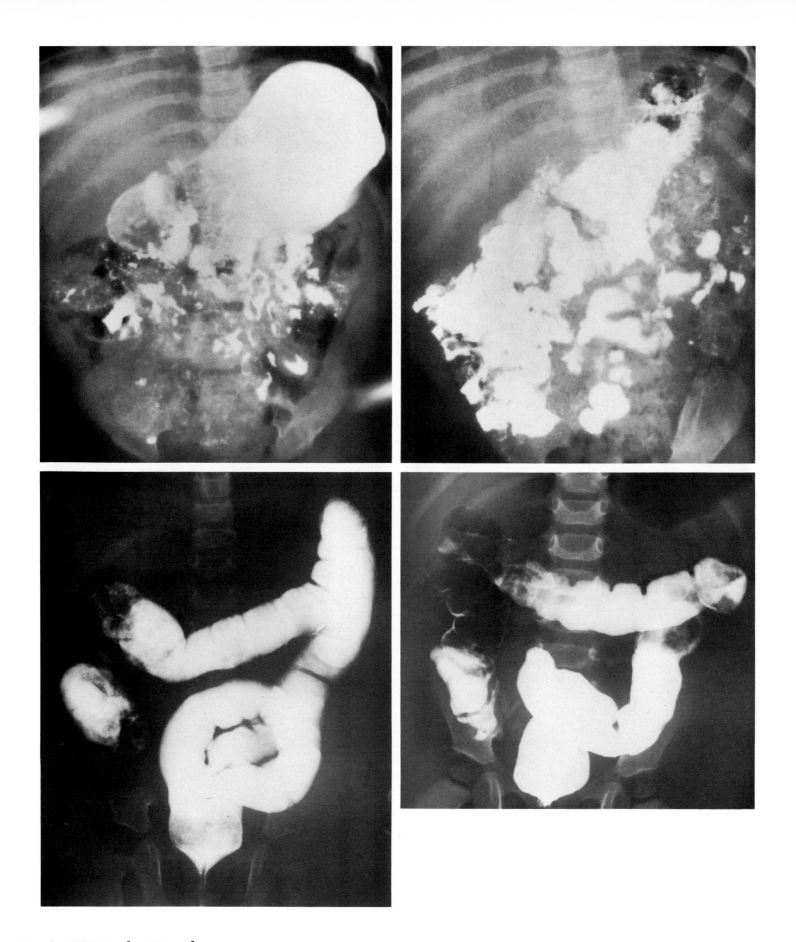

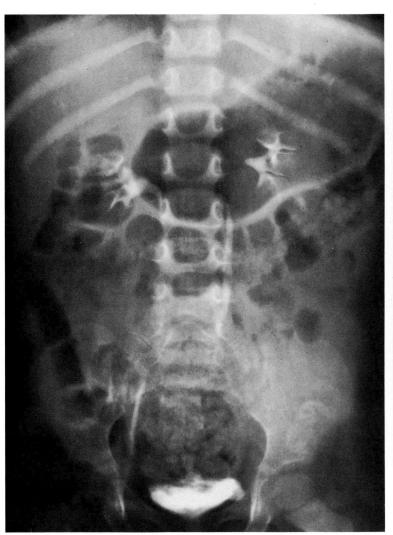

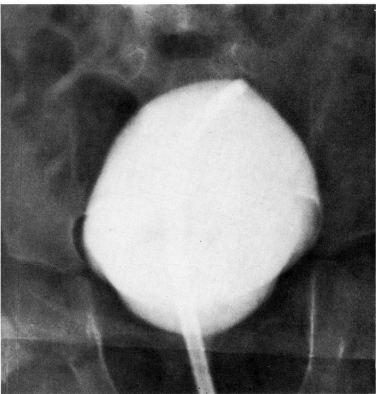

8

18 MONTHS

The anterior fontanel is still visible in varying degrees. The cervical spinal canal has a more adult configuration. The zones of provisional calcification are less dense, except at the knee, where they may still be quite prominent.

The relatively accelerated maturation of the female compared with the male is particularly noticeable in the hands and feet. The distal fibular epiphysis may now be seen.

The adenoids are evident.

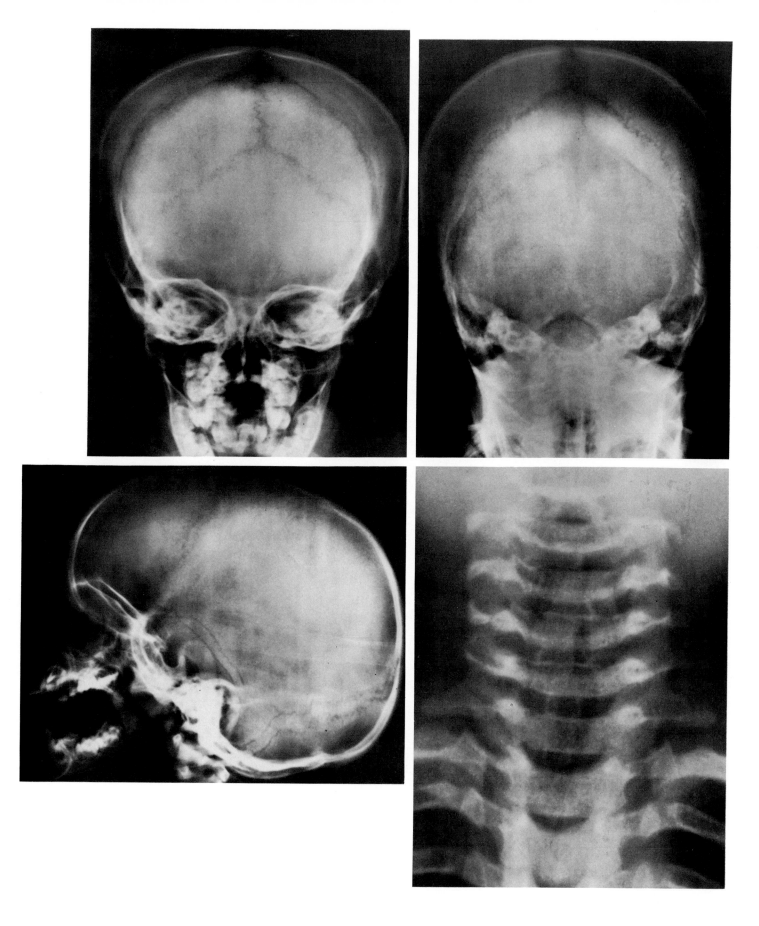

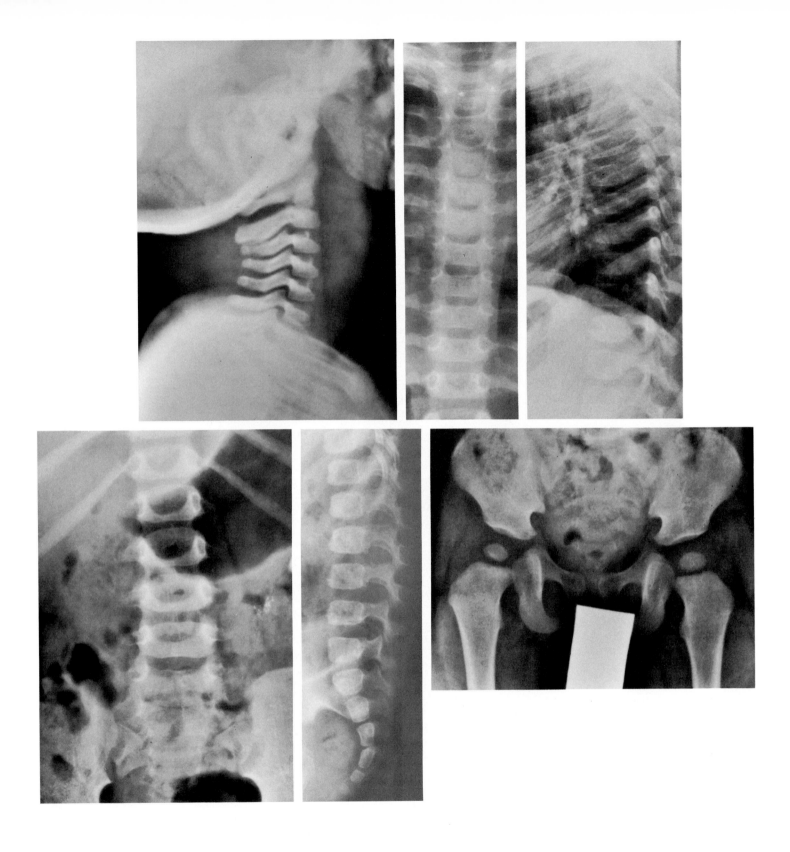

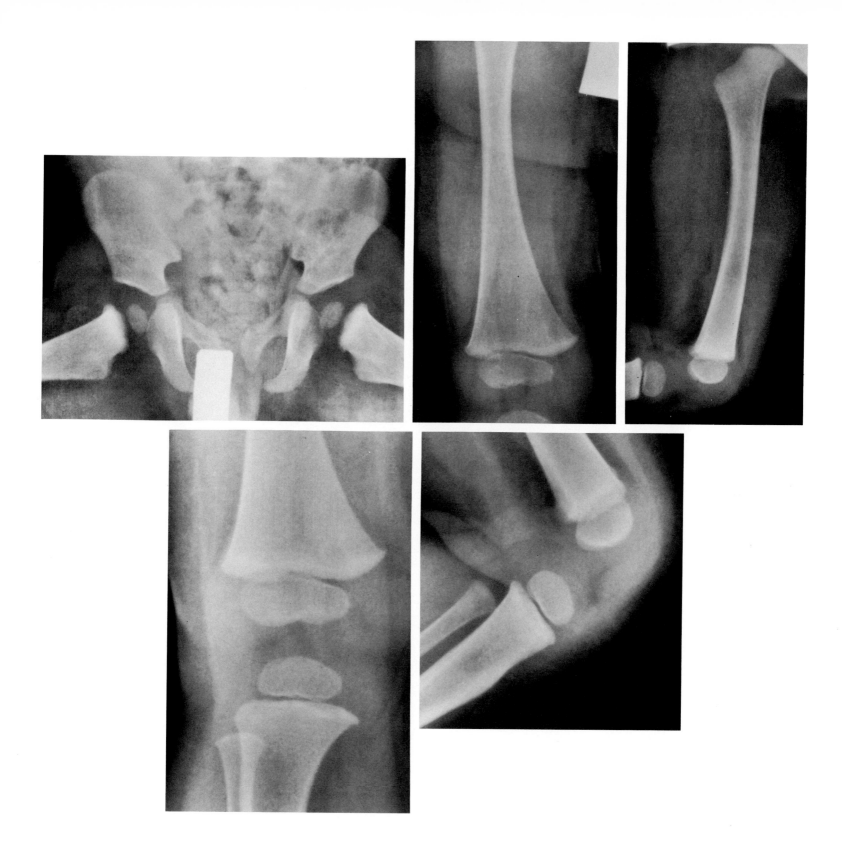

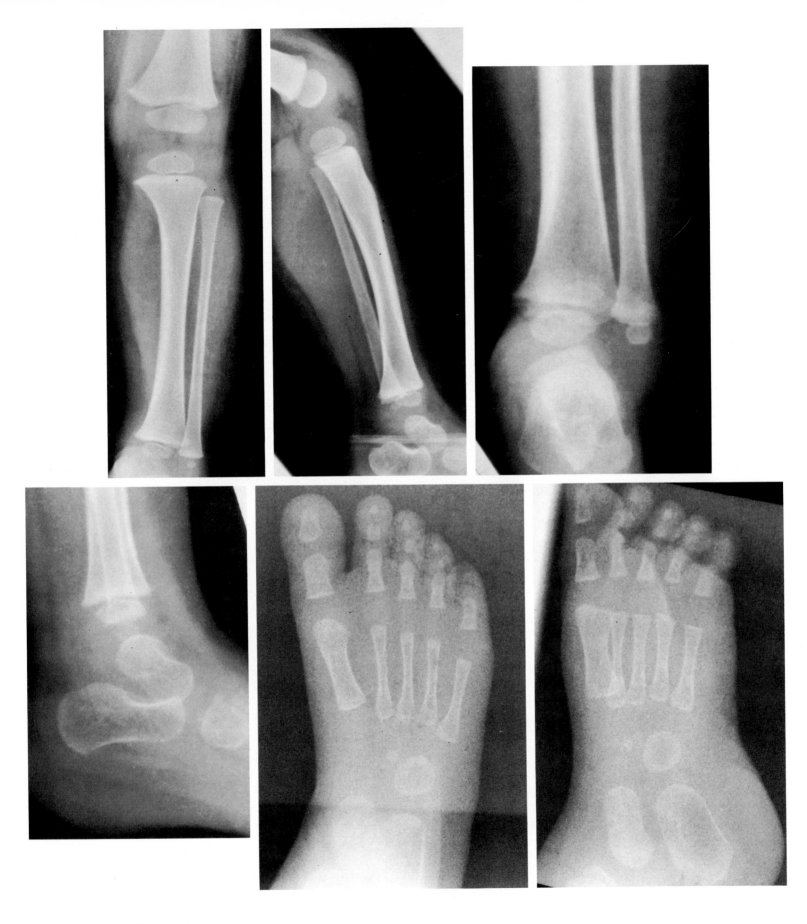

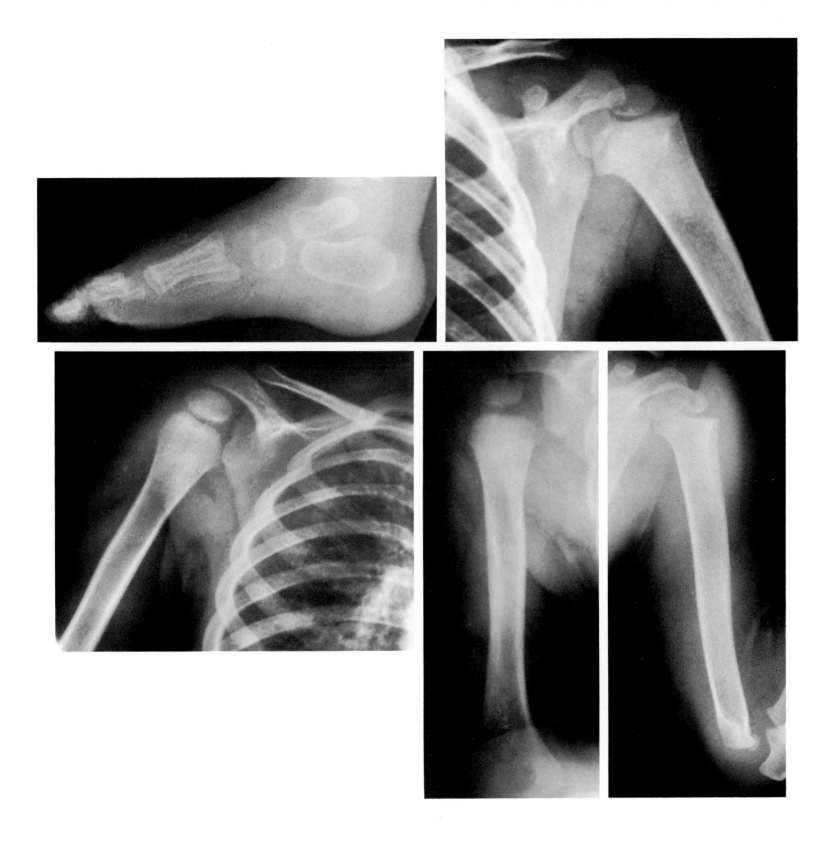

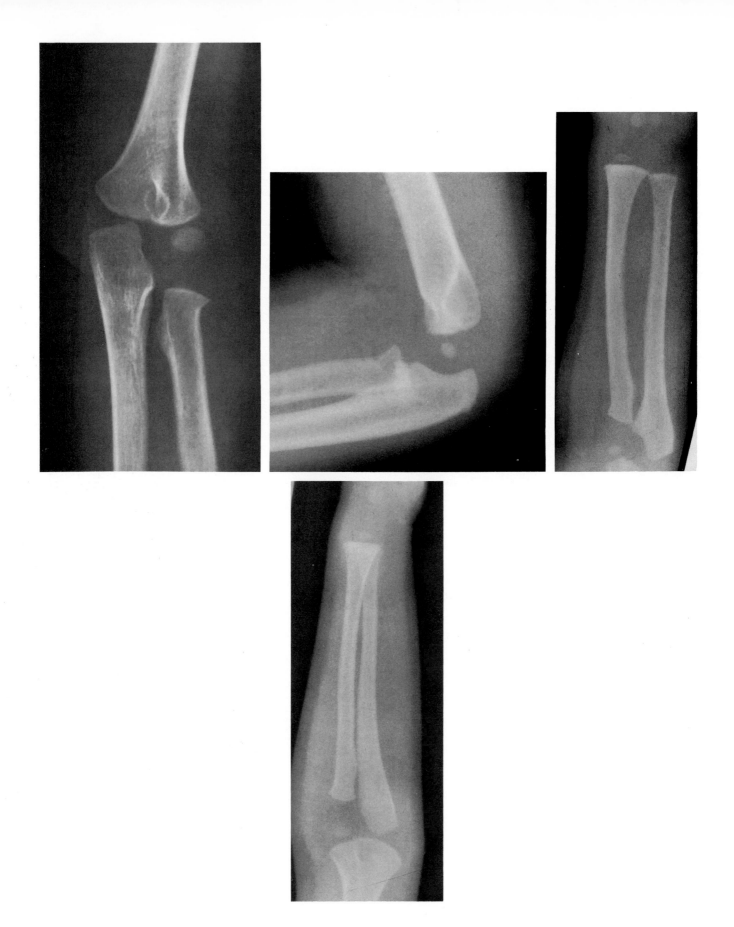

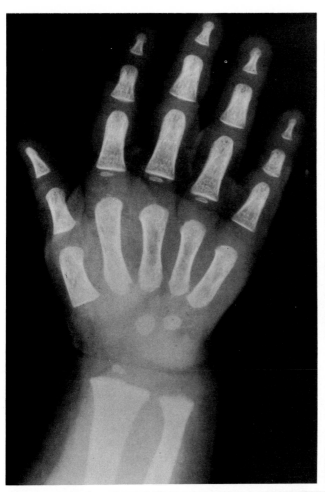

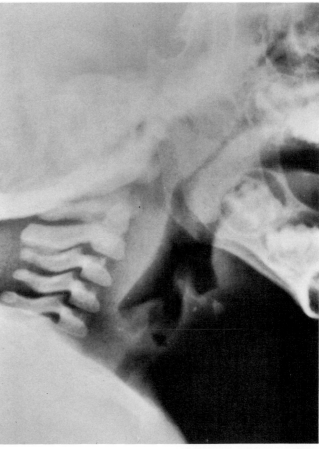

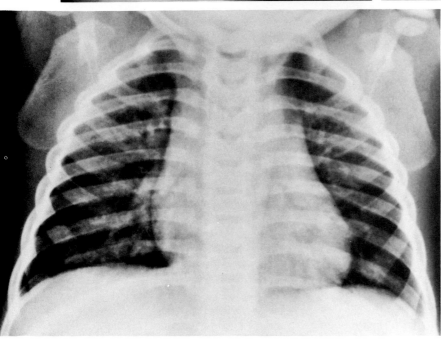

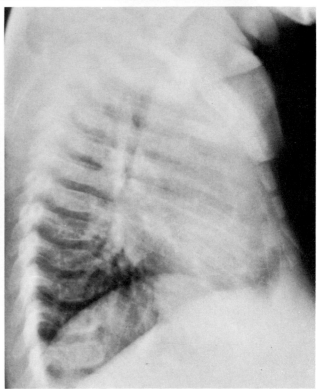

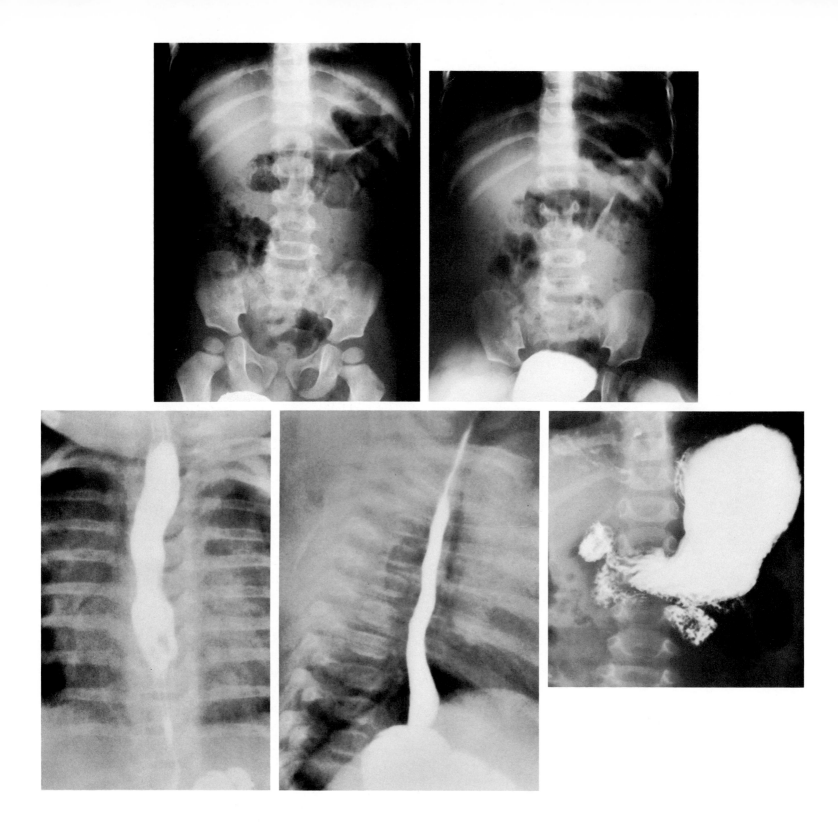

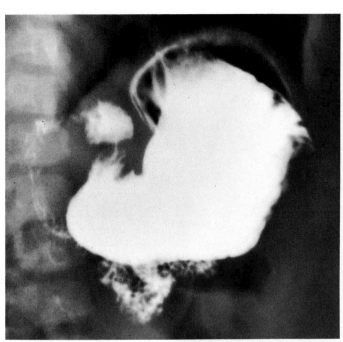

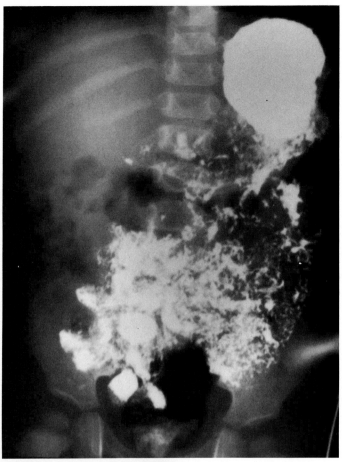

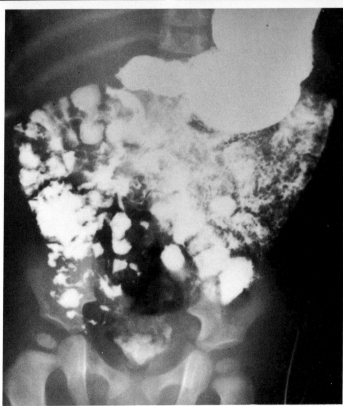

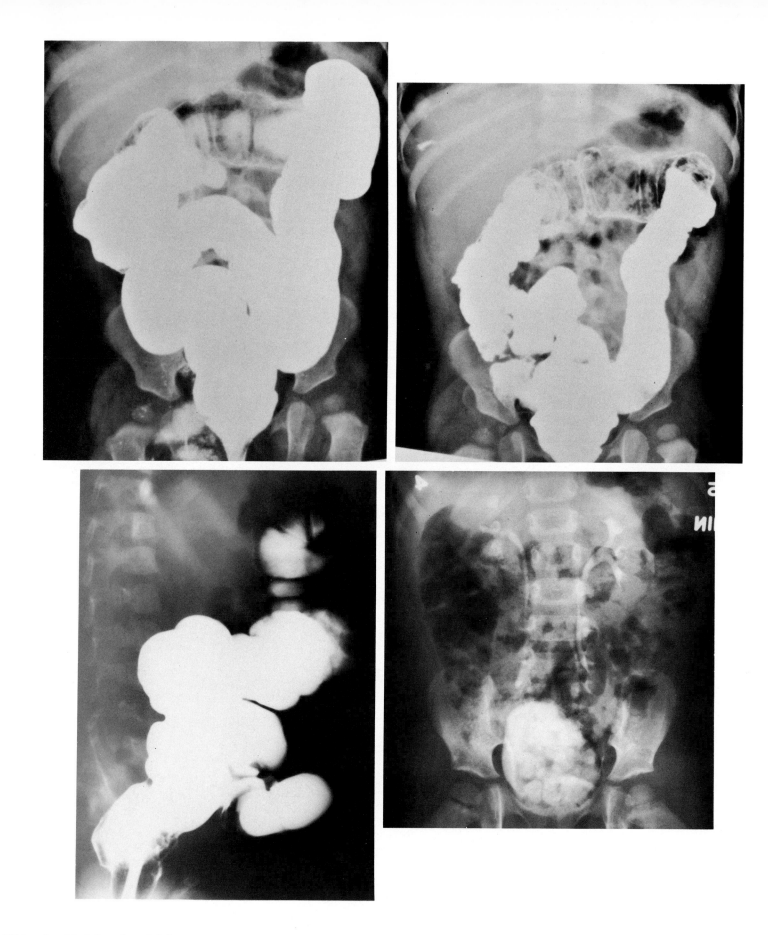

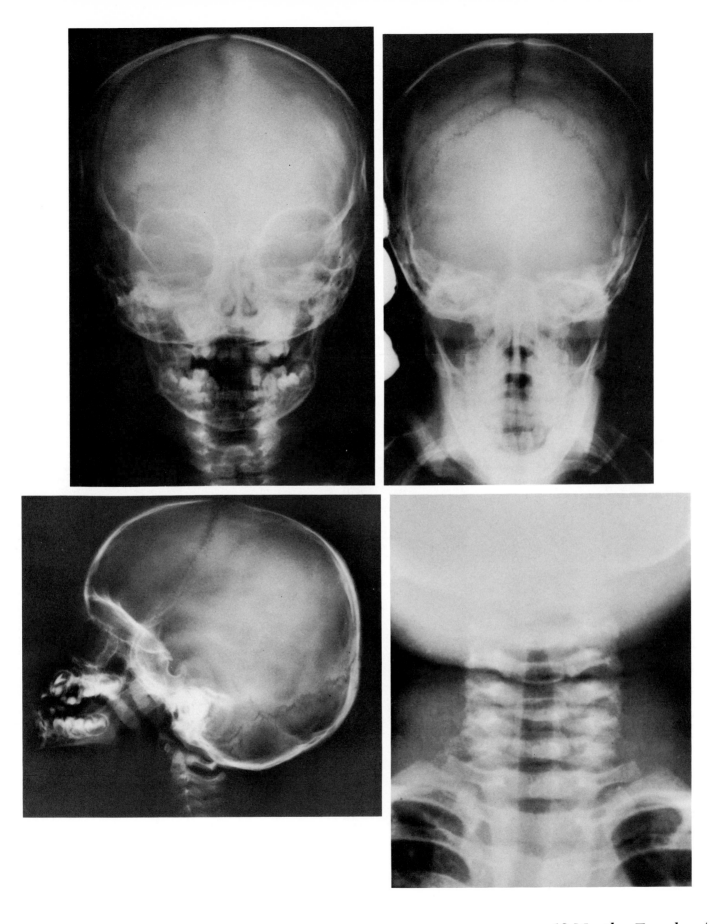

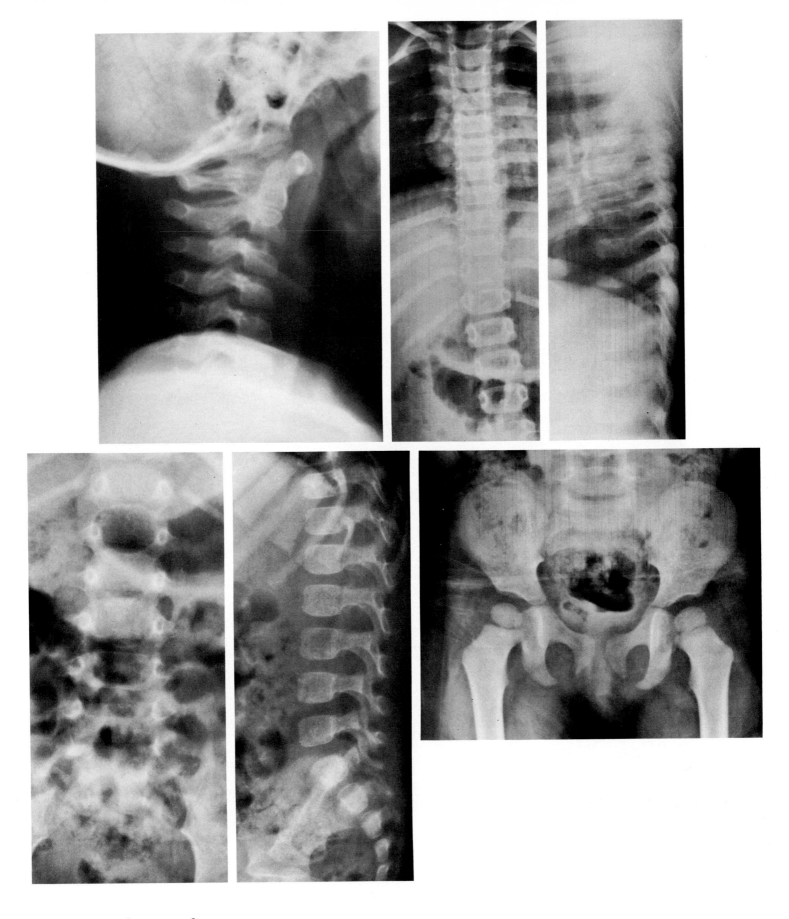

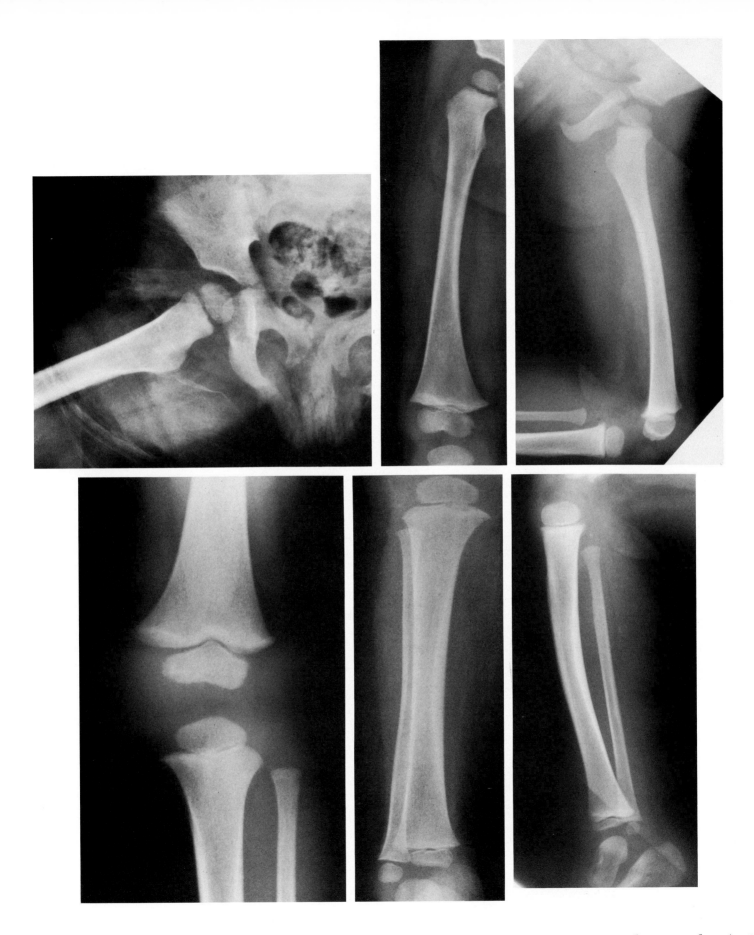

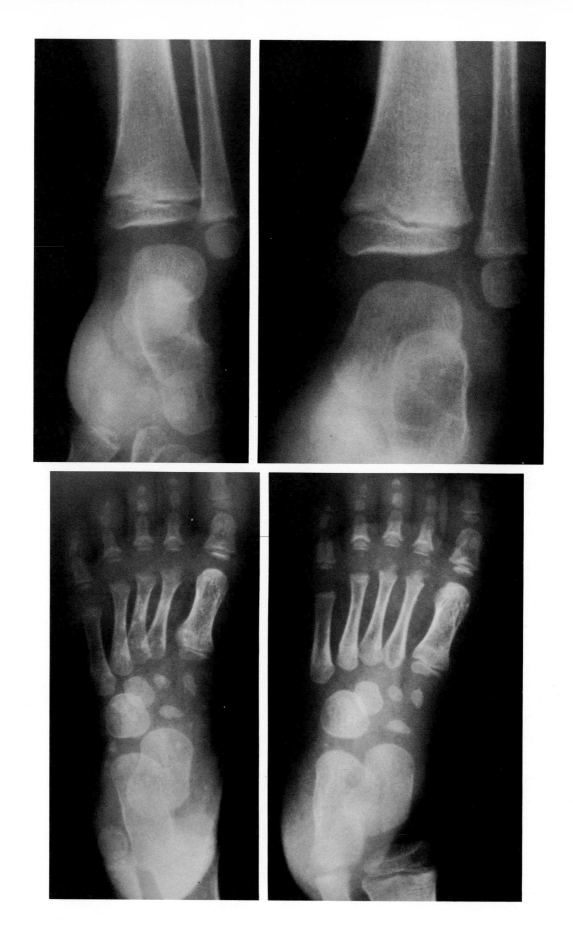

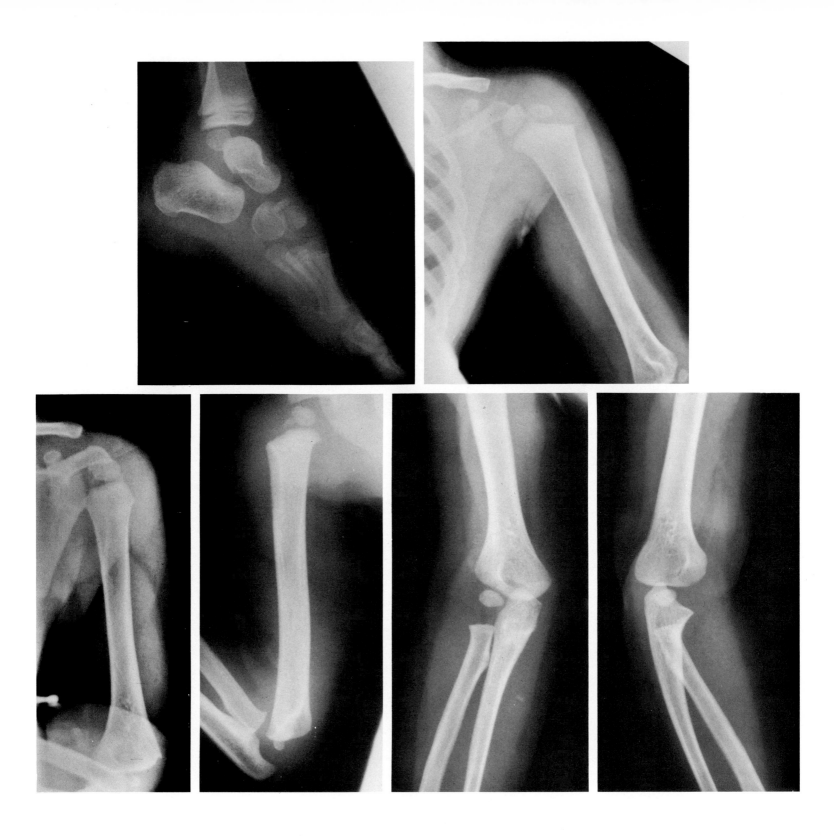

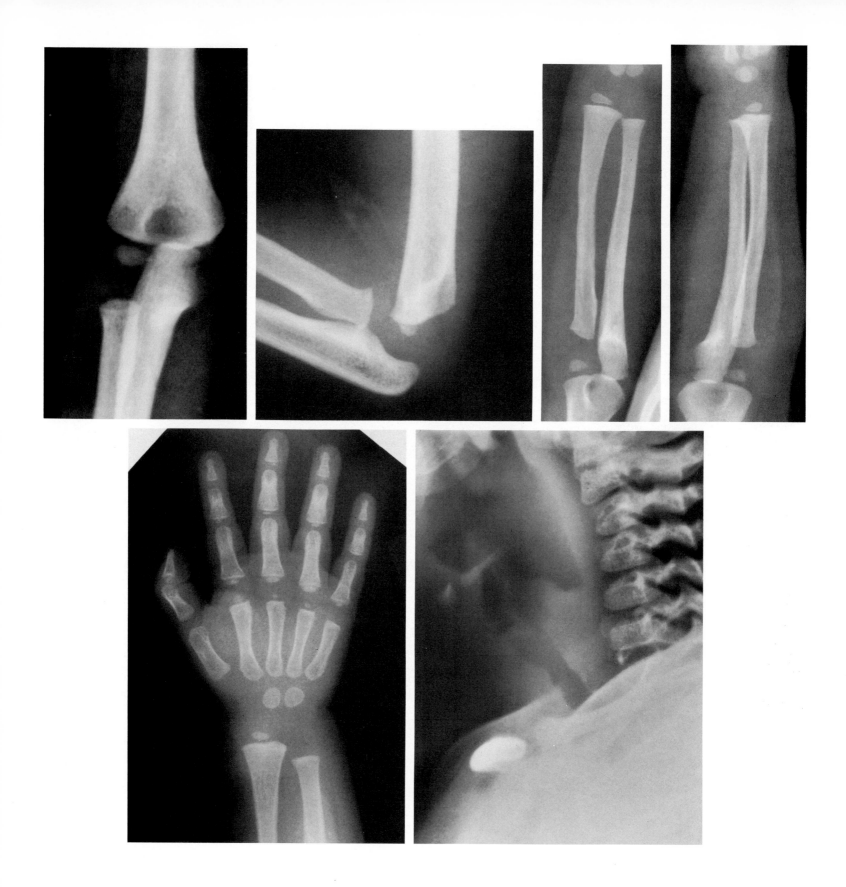

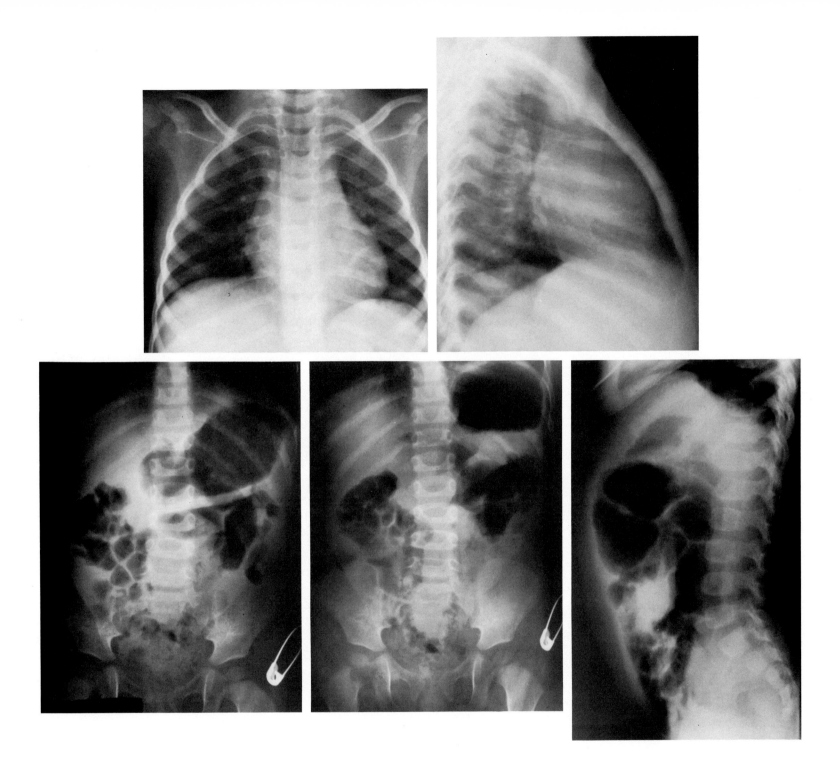

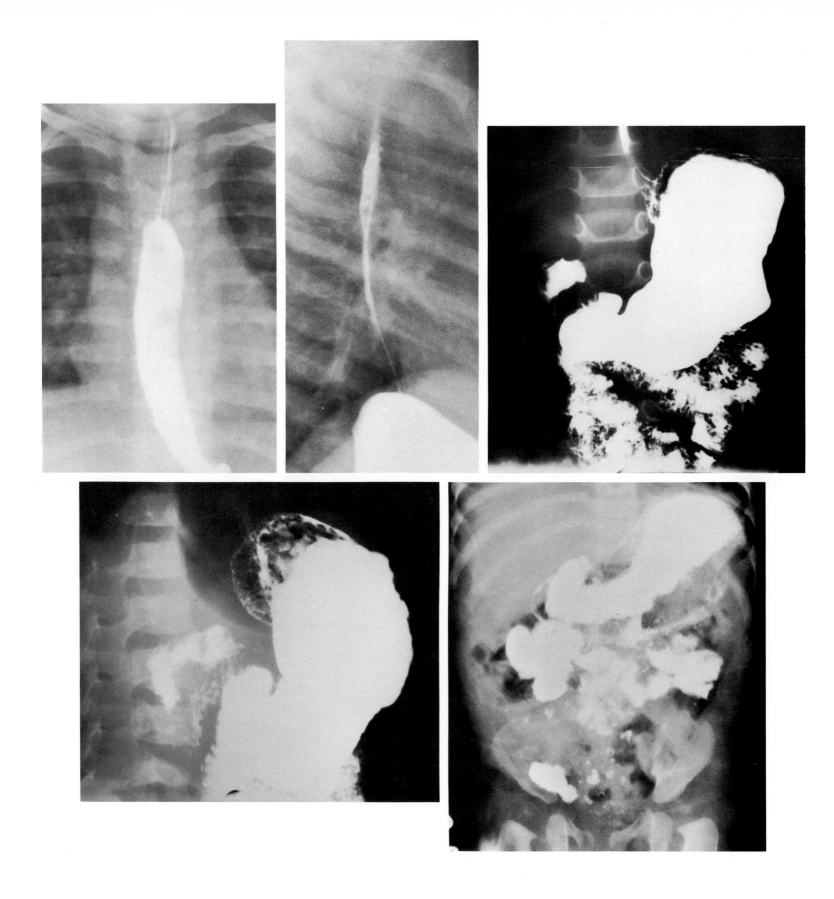

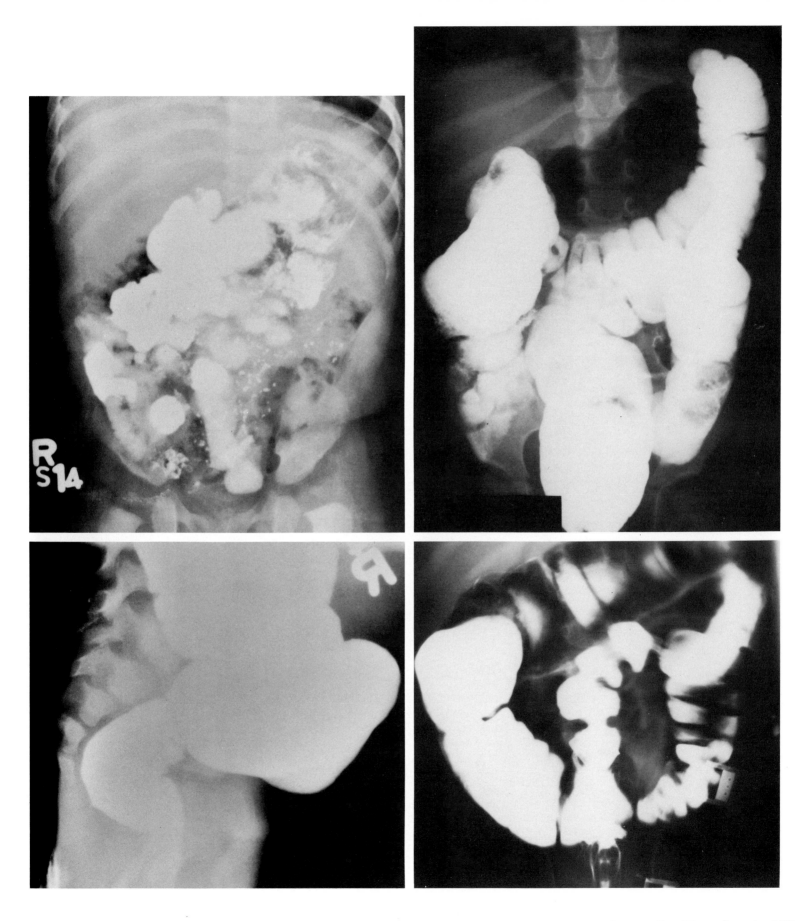

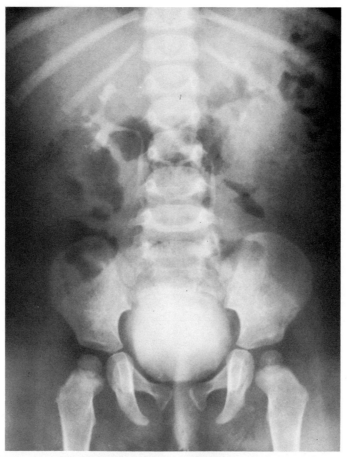

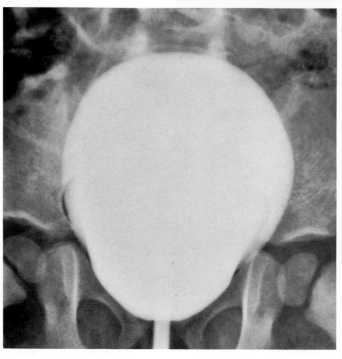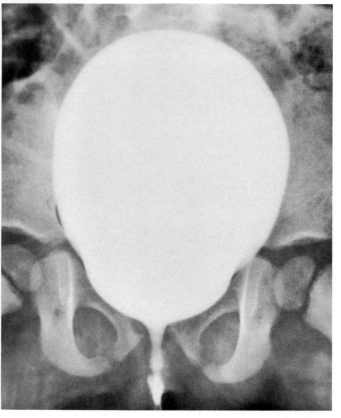

160 / 18 Months: Female

9

21 MONTHS

The fontanels are closed. The nasal bone is well formed and, radiographically, easily recognizable. The ethmoid and maxillary sinuses are well pneumatized.

The ilia continue to enlarge. The proximal femoral epiphysis now conforms to the metaphysis. Rapid growth lines may be seen. Physiologic bowing of the tibias and femurs are apparent at this age. The distal femoral epiphysis is irregular and asymmetric. Early appearance of the metatarsal epiphysis occurs in the female. The distal tibial epiphysis is more rectangular in shape. The metacarpal epiphyses are appearing.

The adenoids may be quite large. The psoas shadows are barely visible.

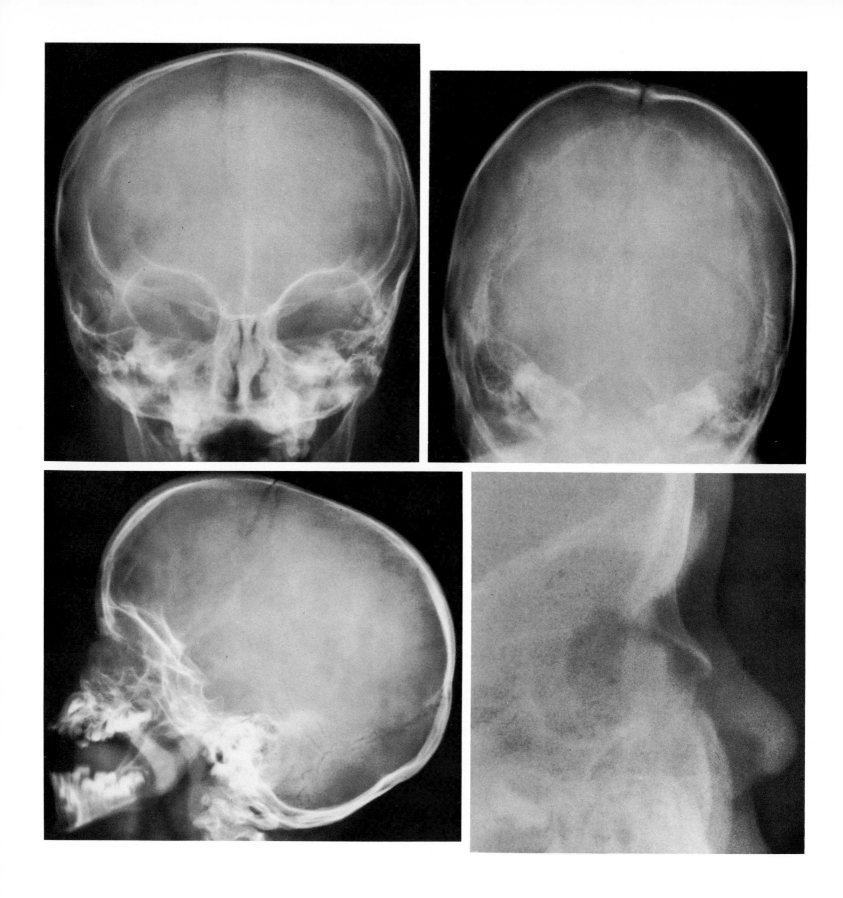

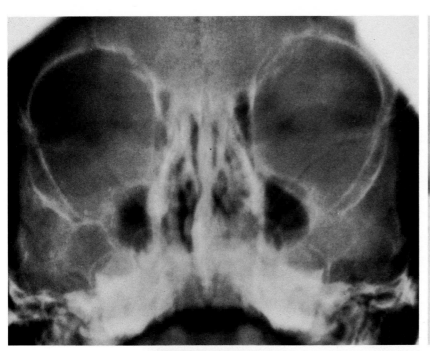
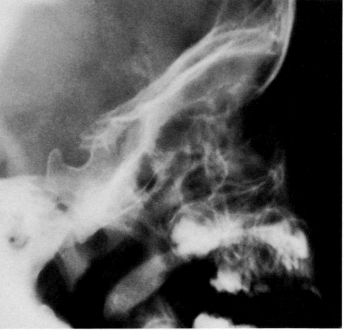
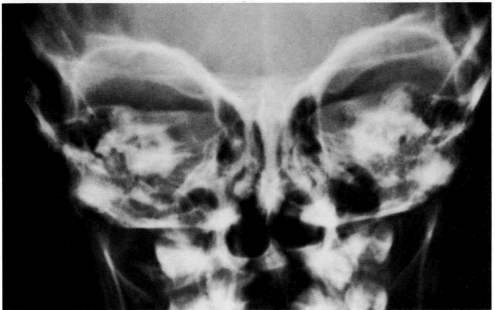

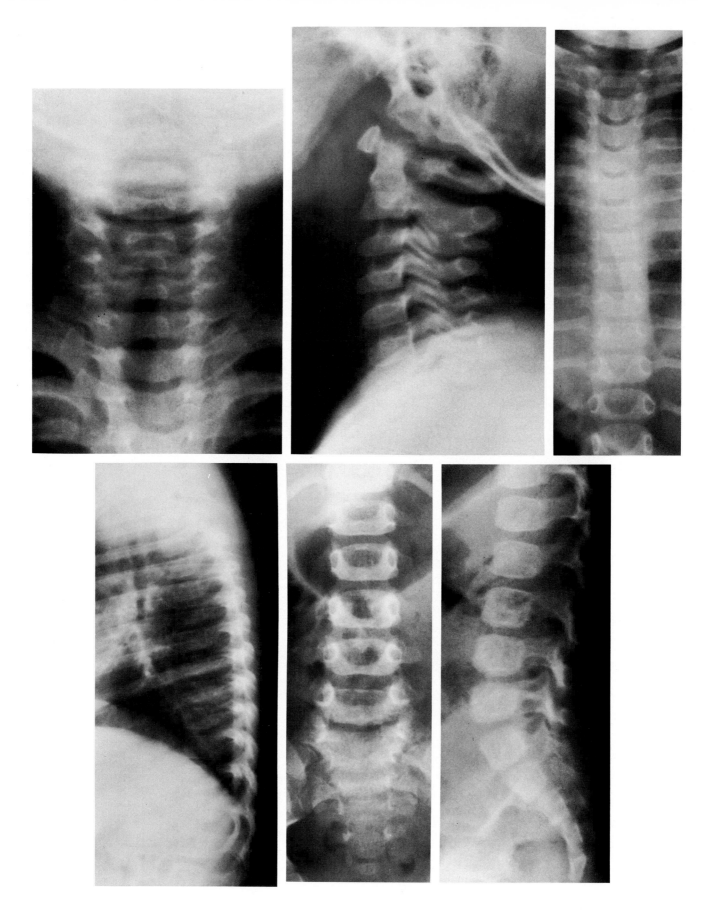

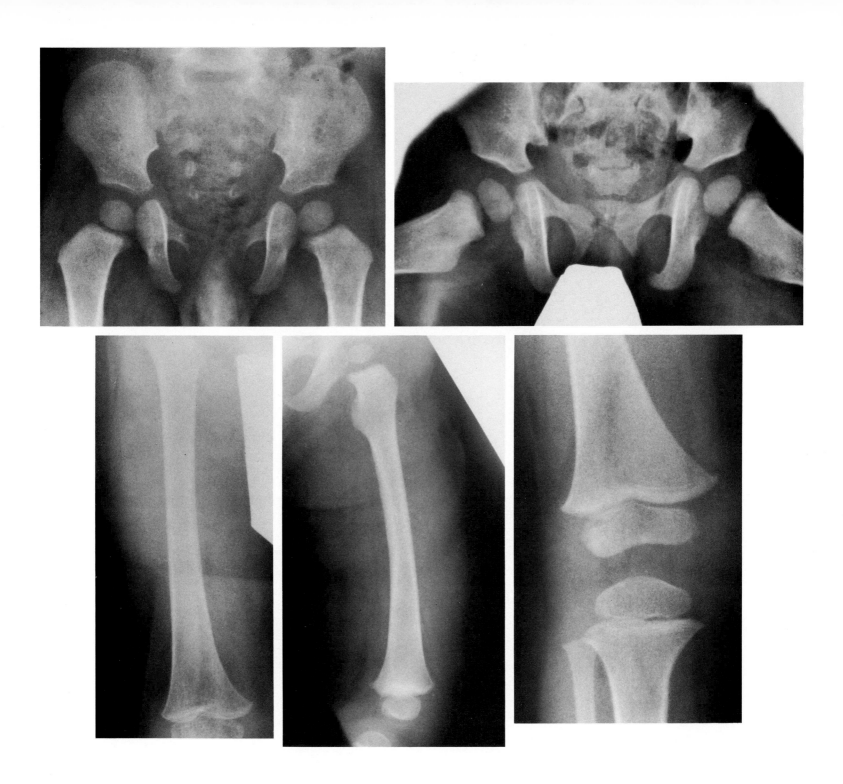

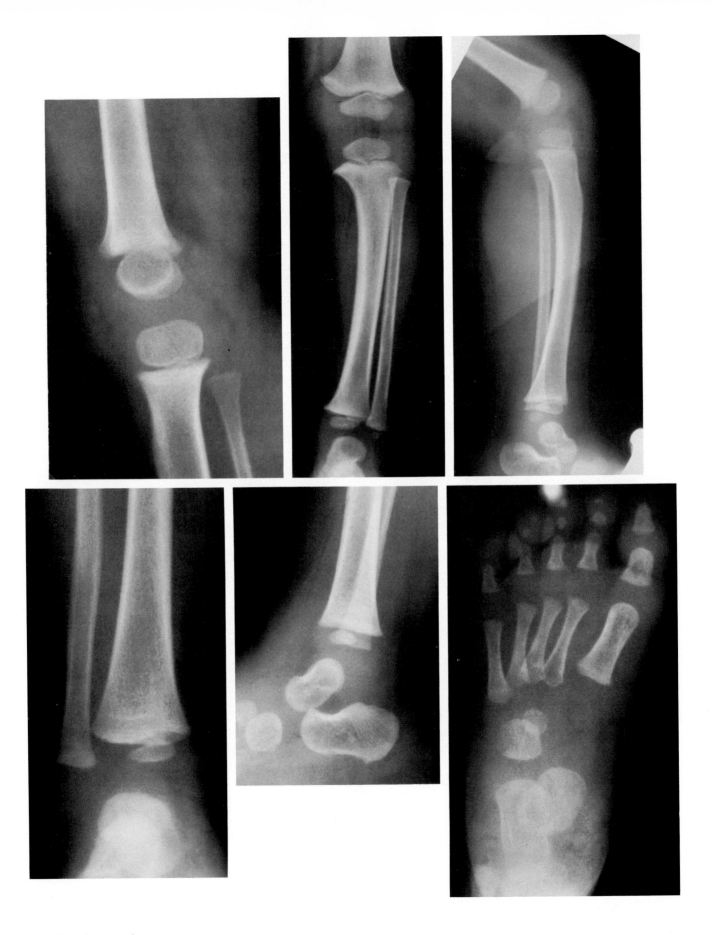

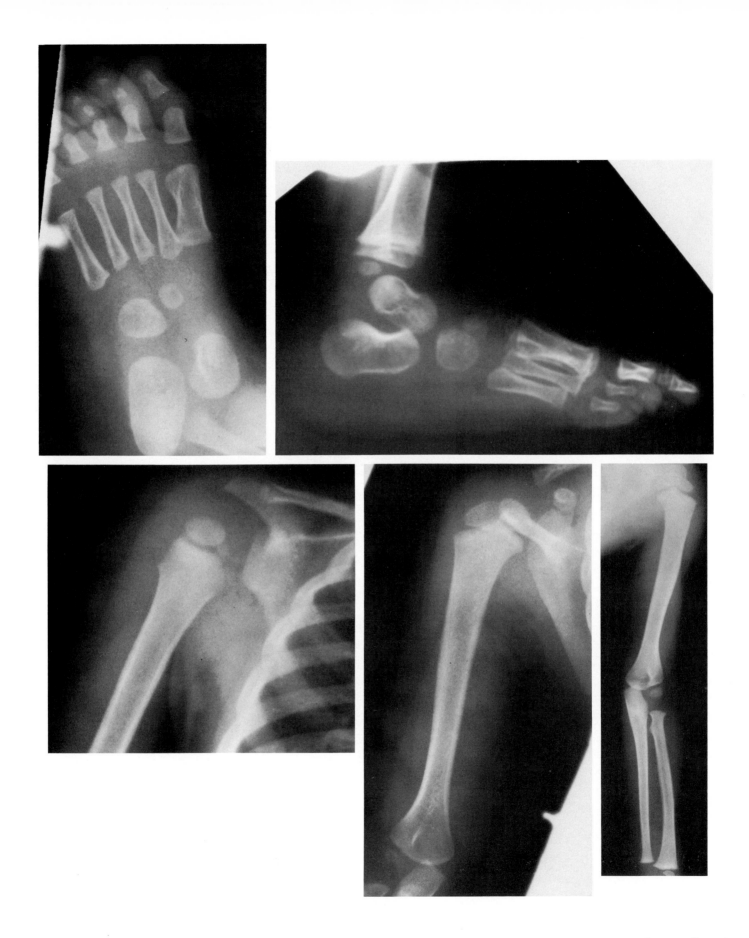

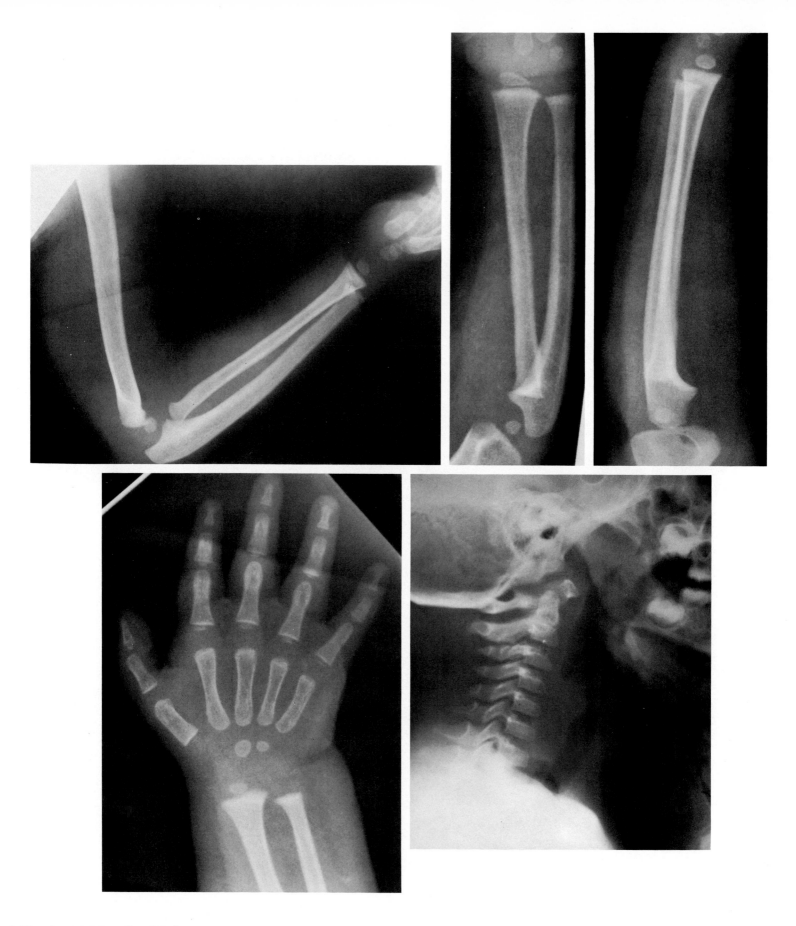

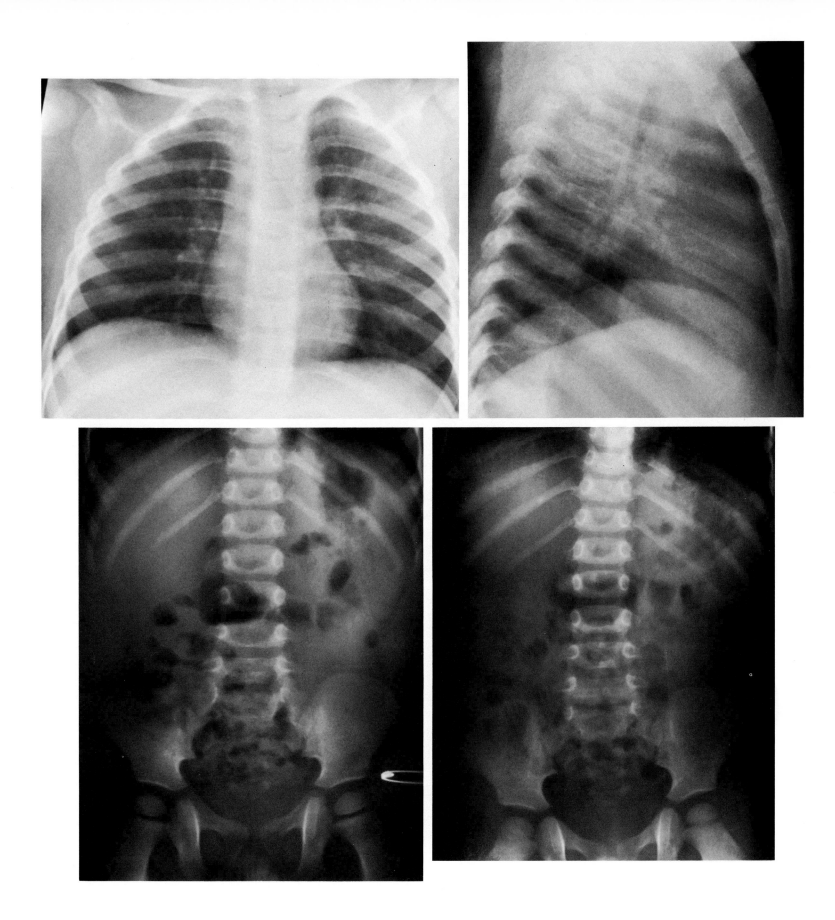

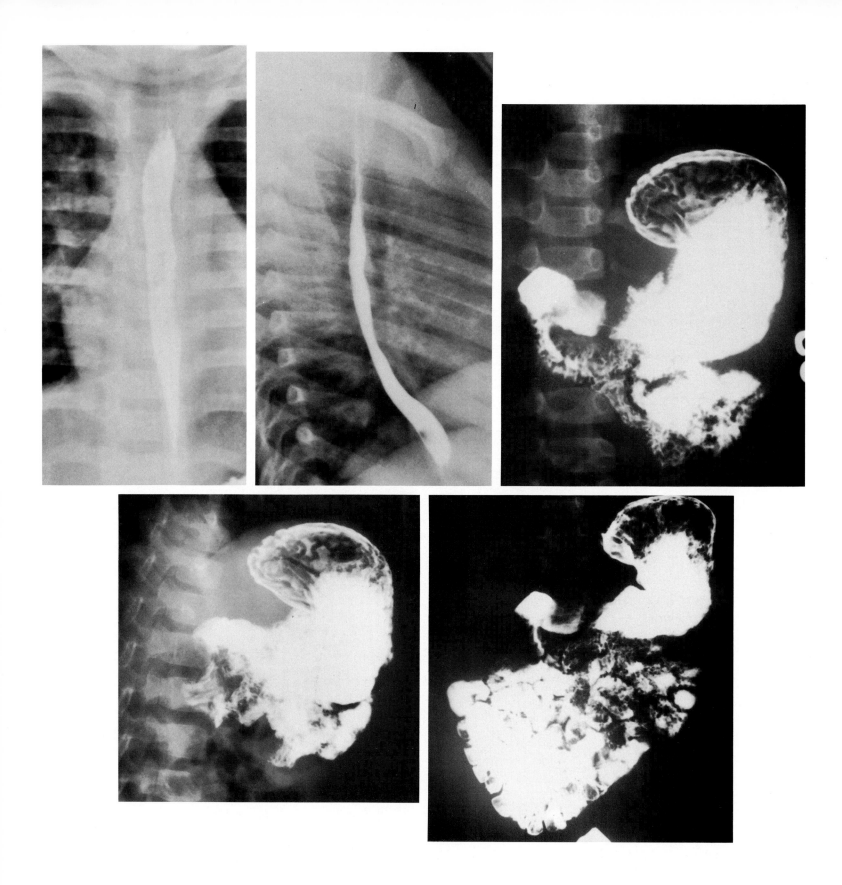

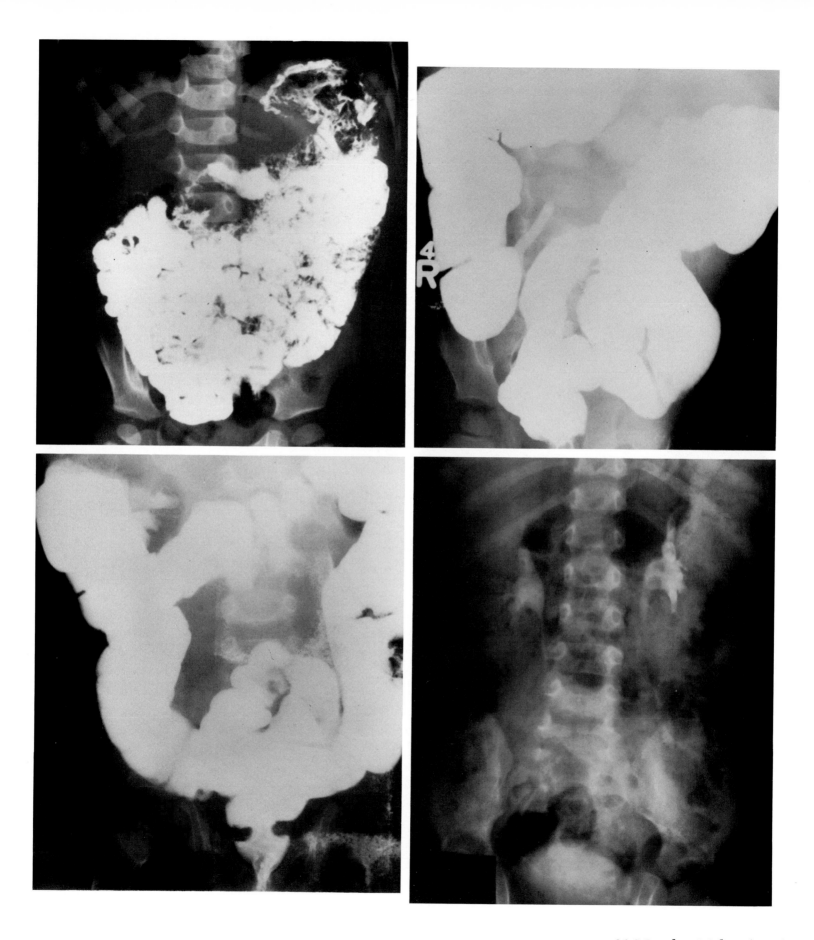

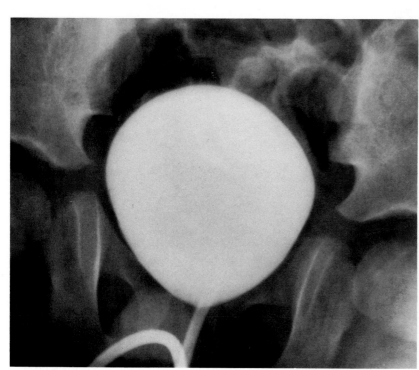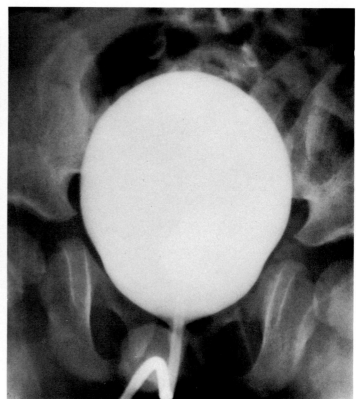

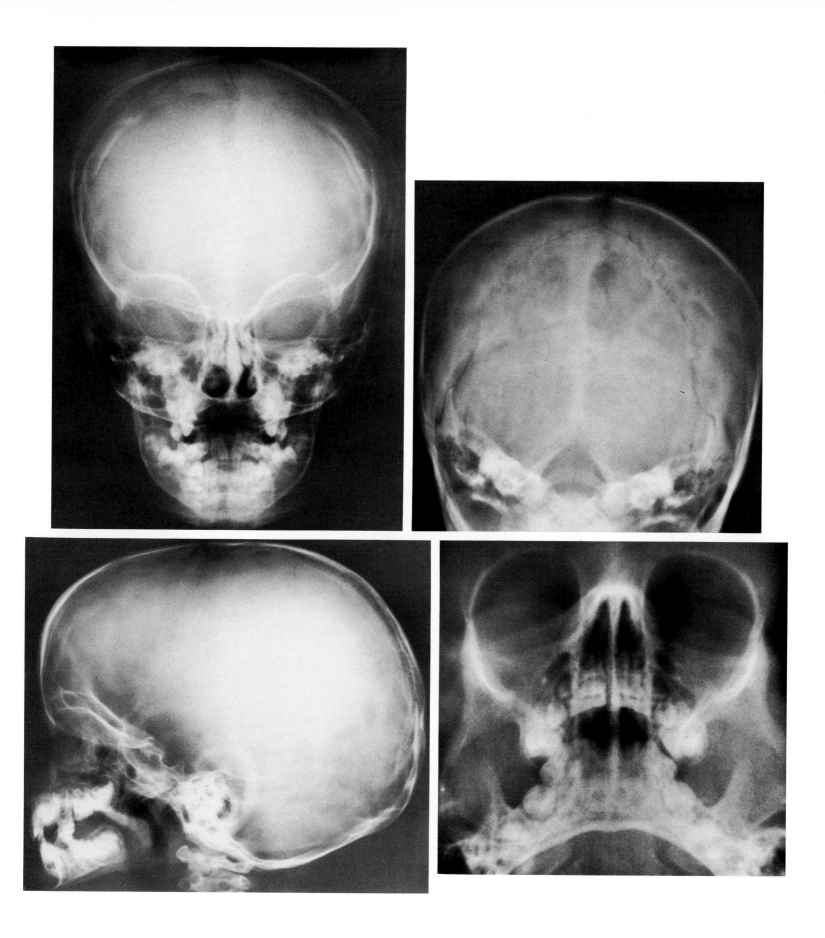

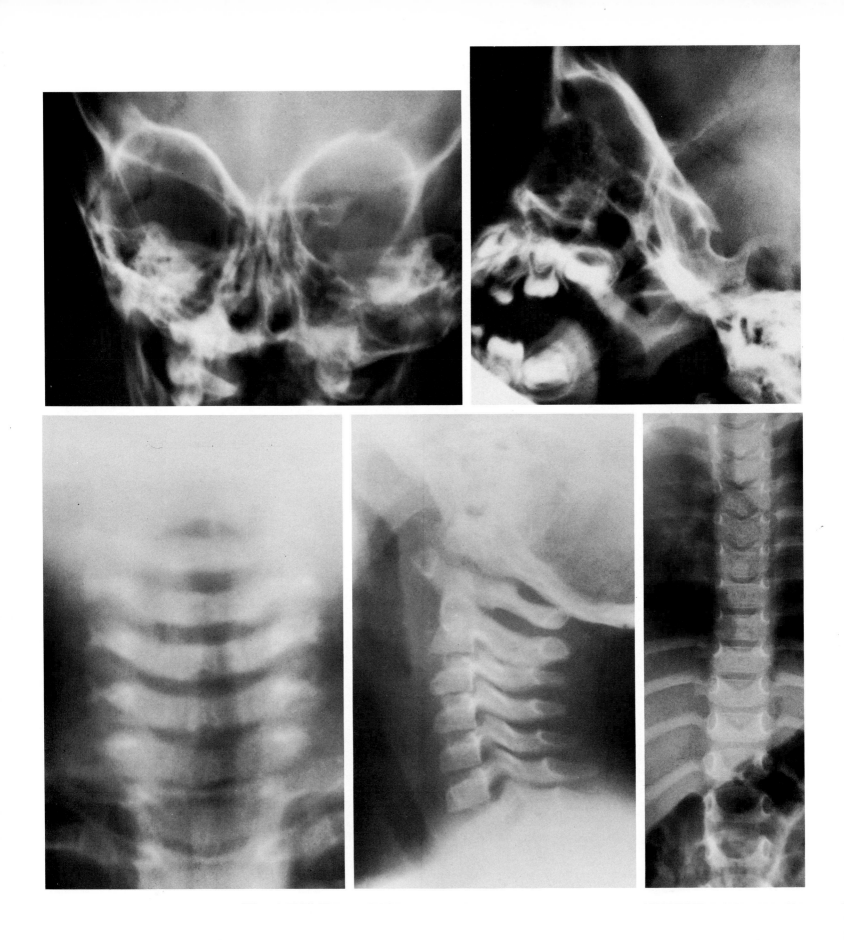

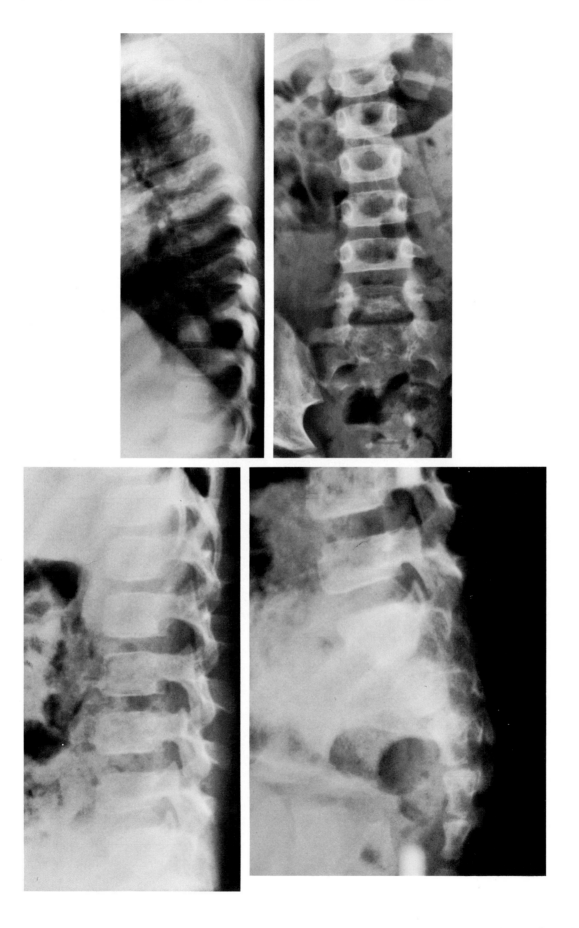

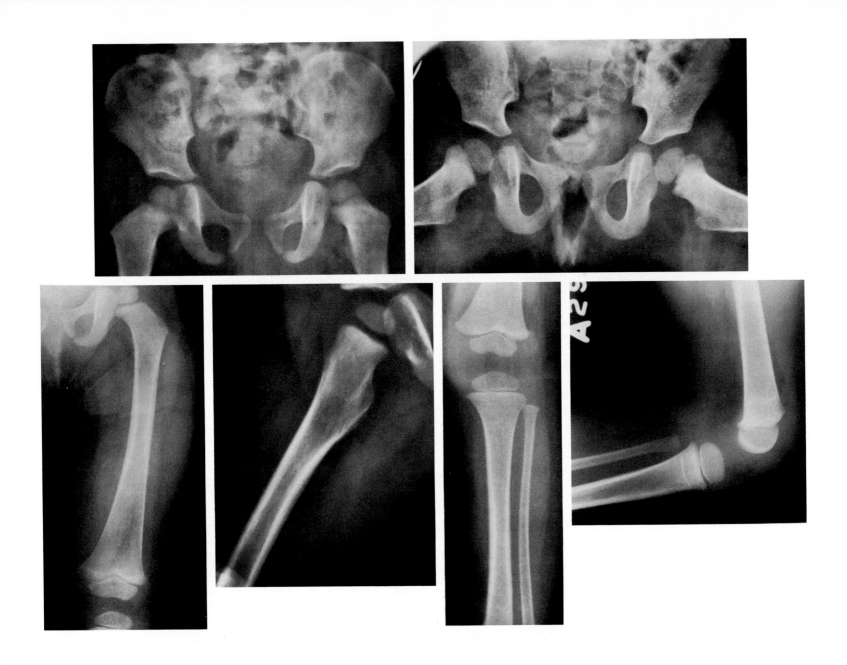

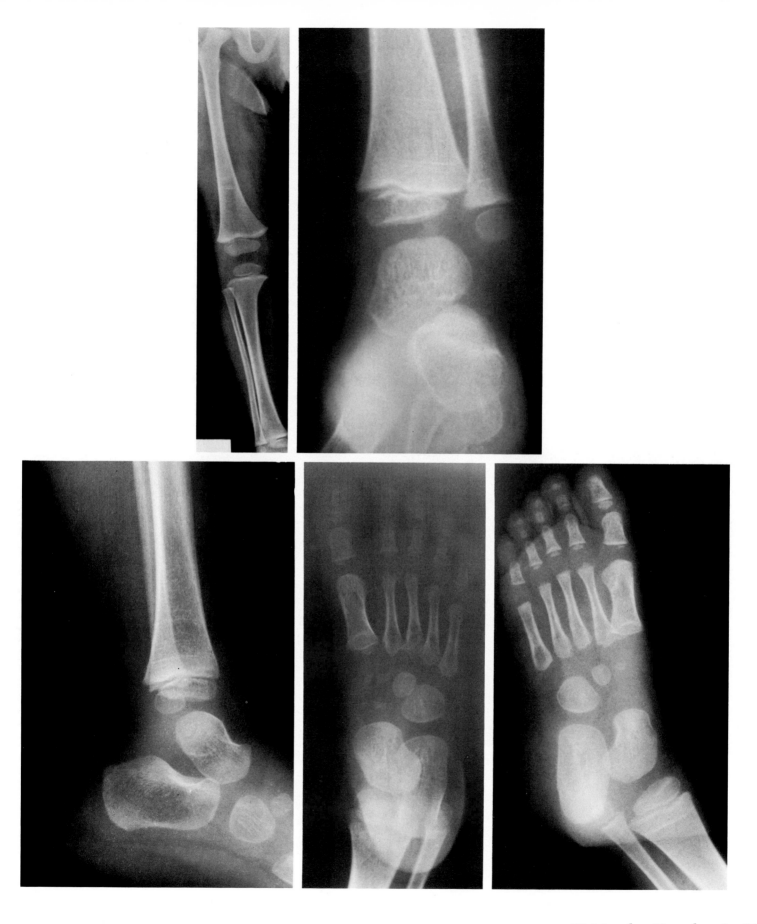

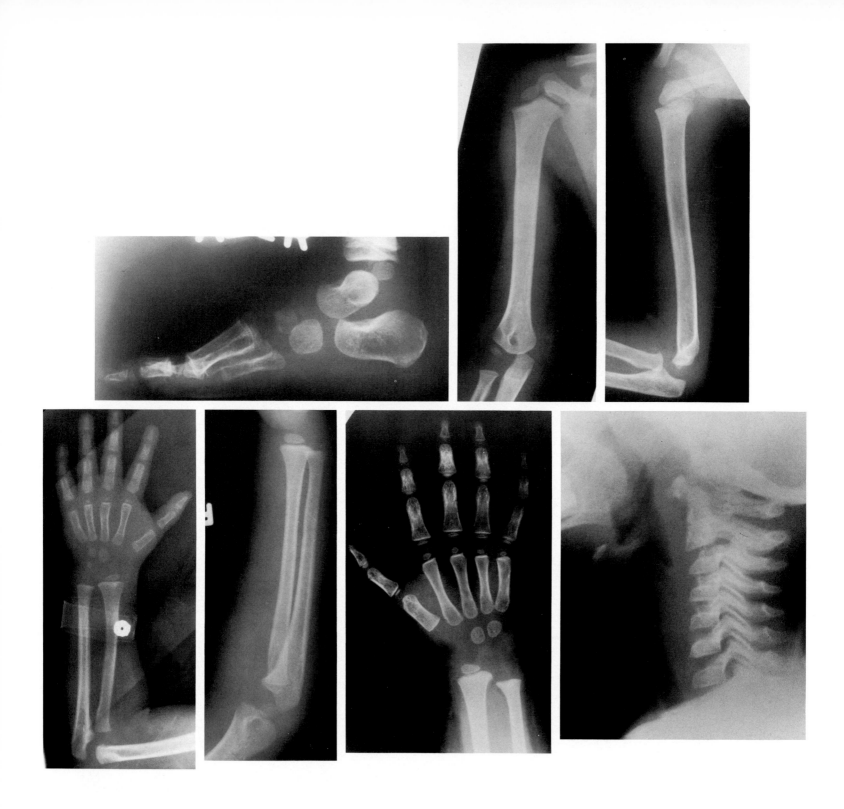

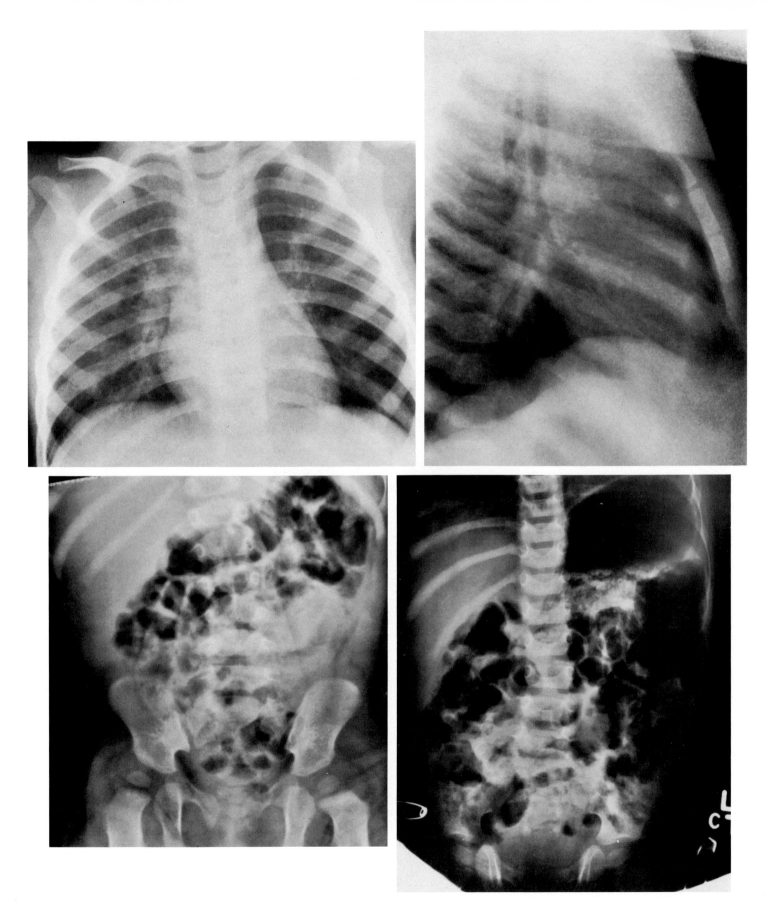

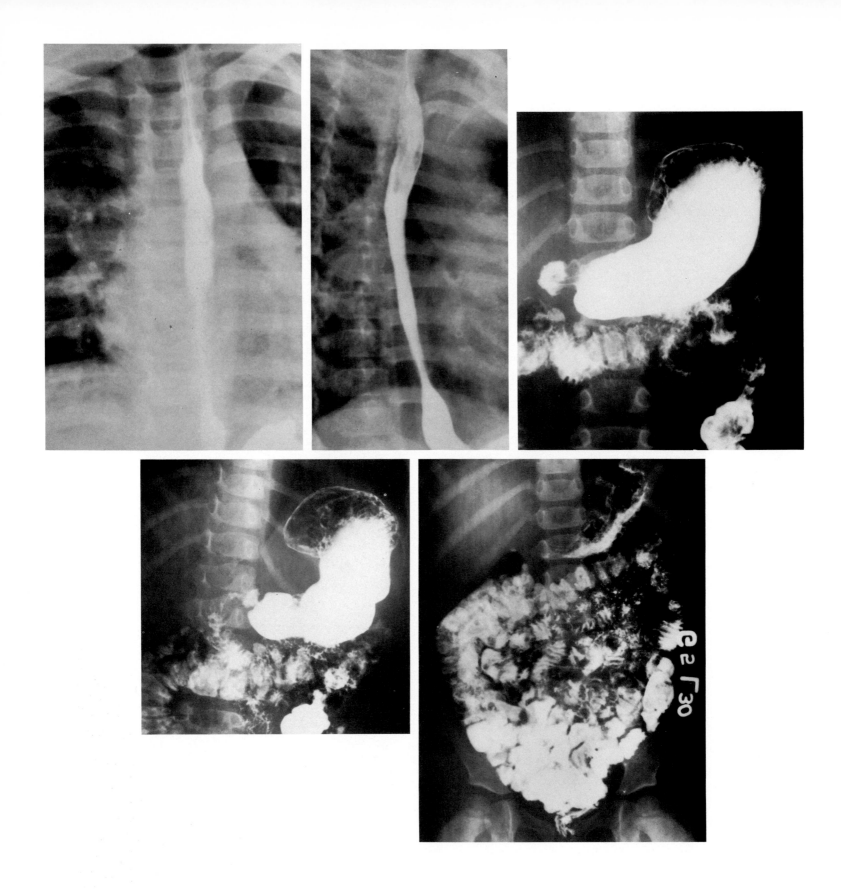

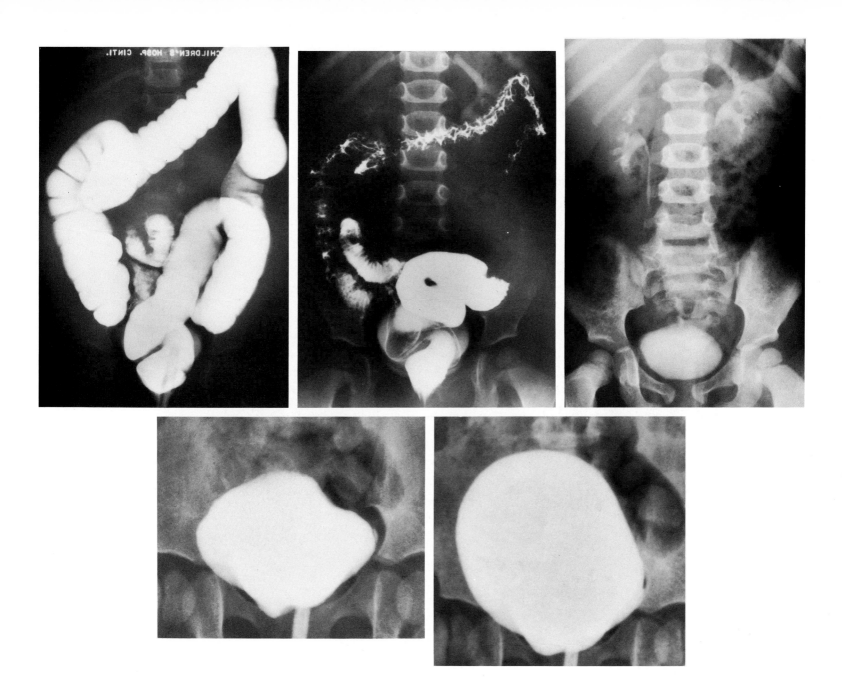

10

2 YEARS

The anterior fontanel is closed. Pneumatization of the sinuses and mastoids is well established, except for the sphenoid, which is partially pneumatized.

The proximal femoral epiphyses and metaphyses have molded to each other. The distal femoral metaphyses may appear somewhat irregular at this age, particularly posteriorly. Metatarsal epiphyses now appear in the male. The tarsal centers are increasing in size and number.

The stomach has become more like the adult, both in its appearance and in its relationship to the duodenum. The bladder is still relatively large.

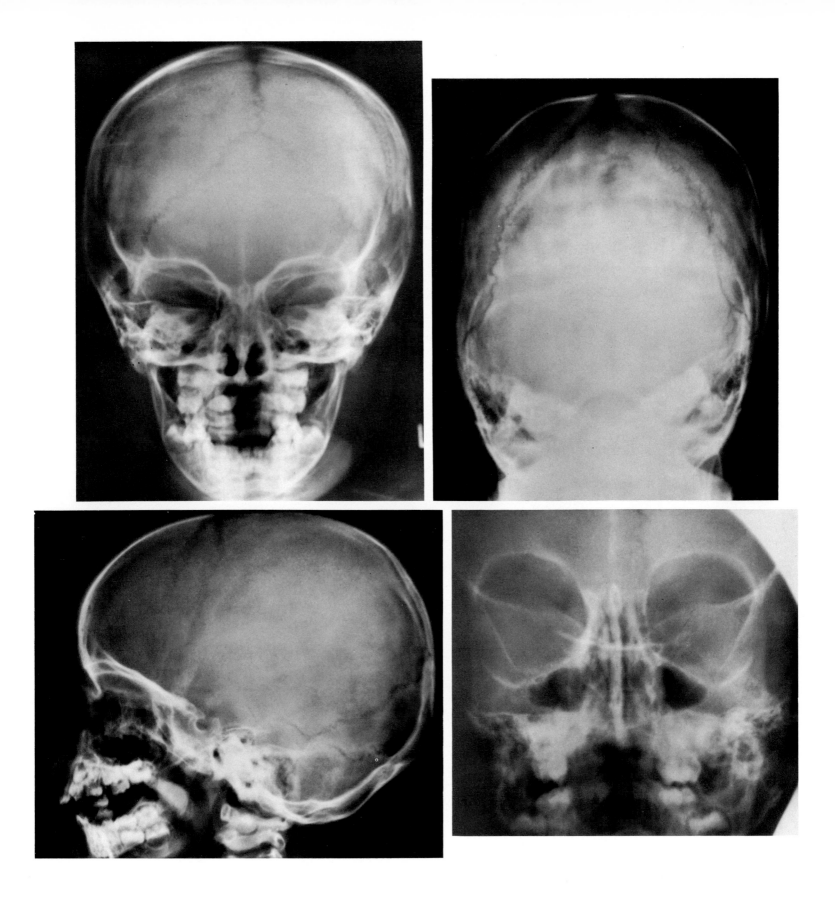

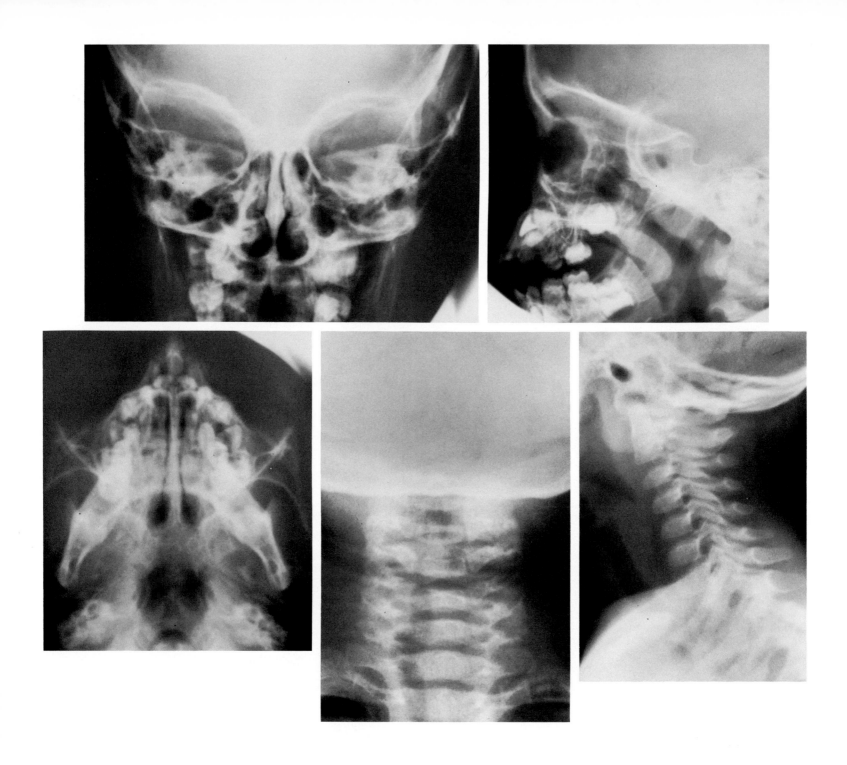

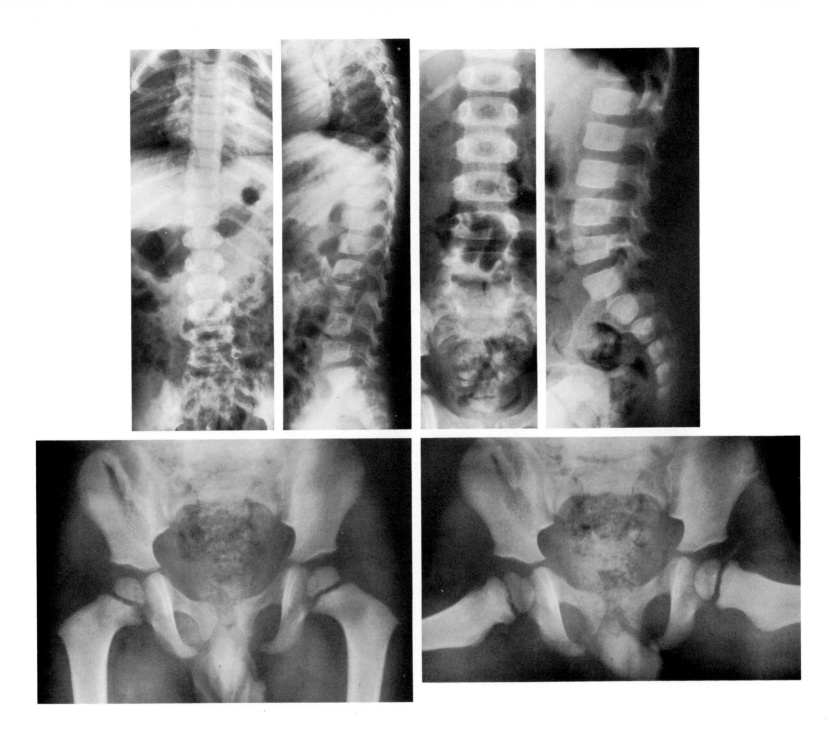

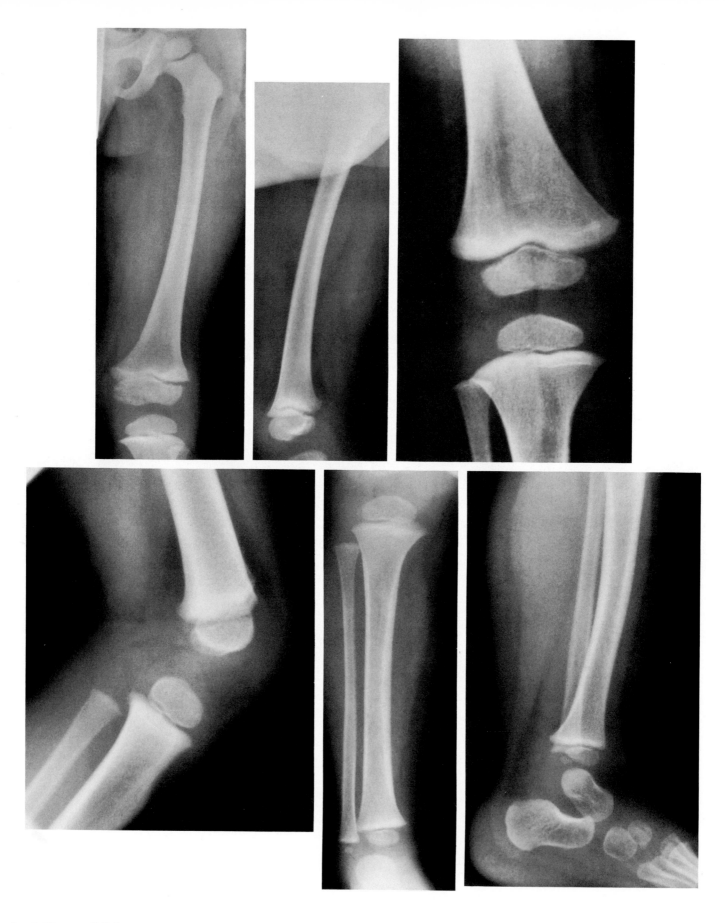

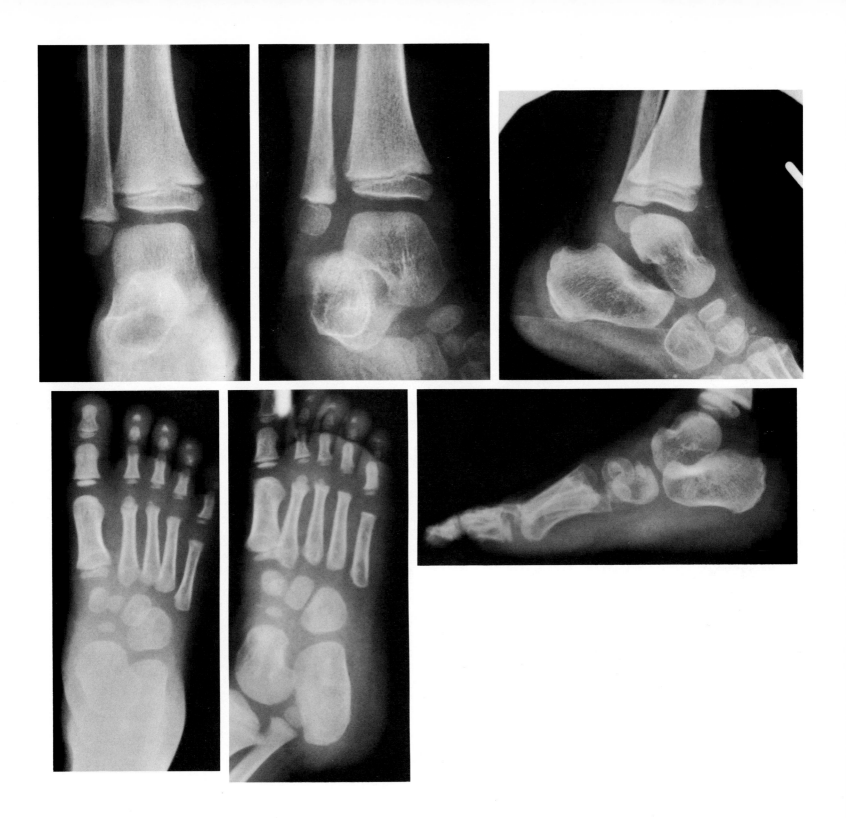

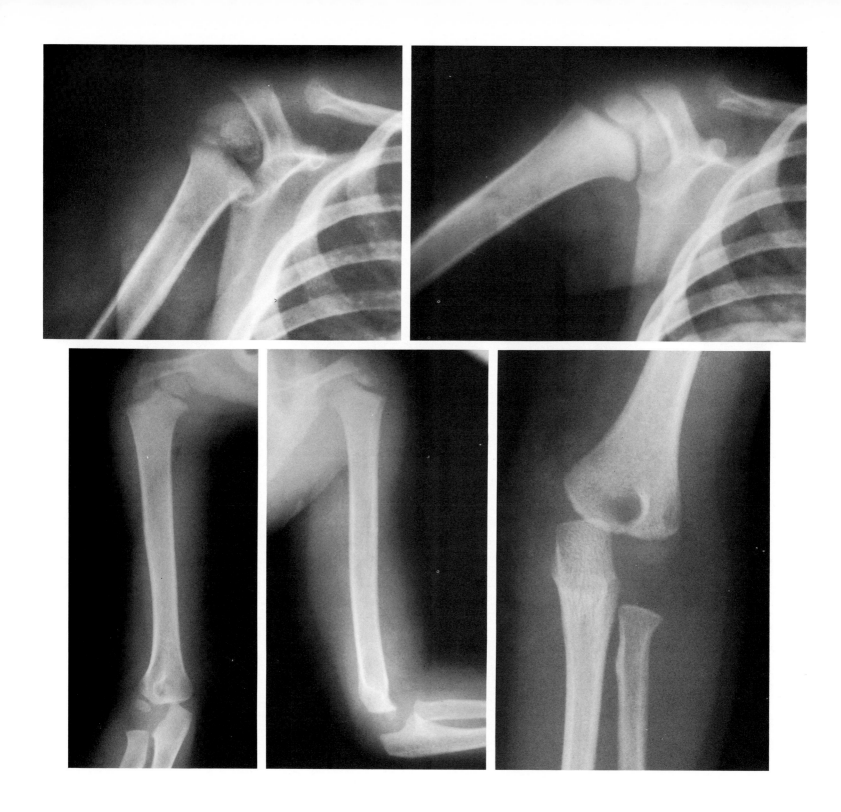

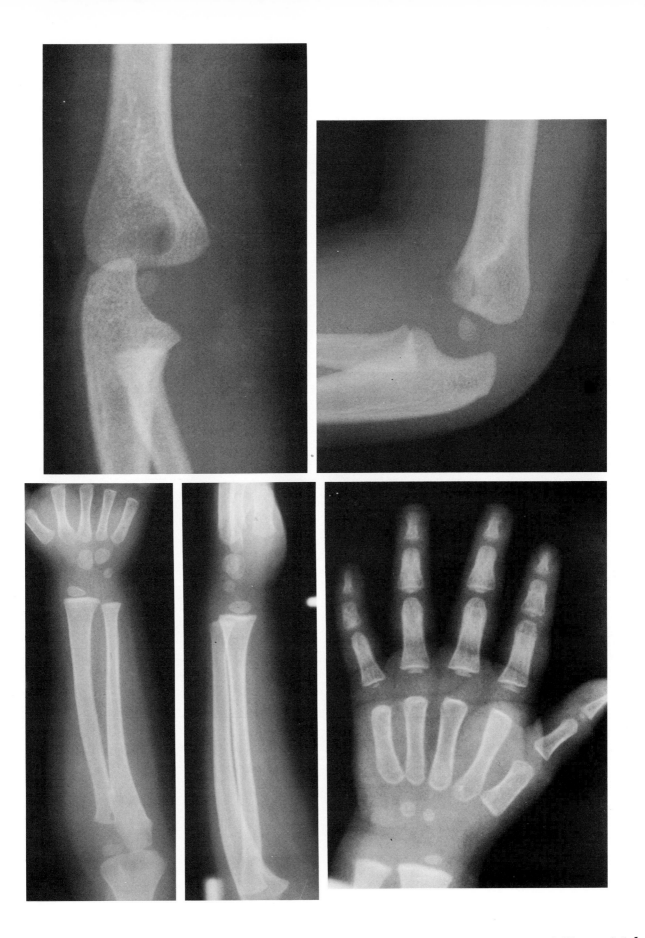

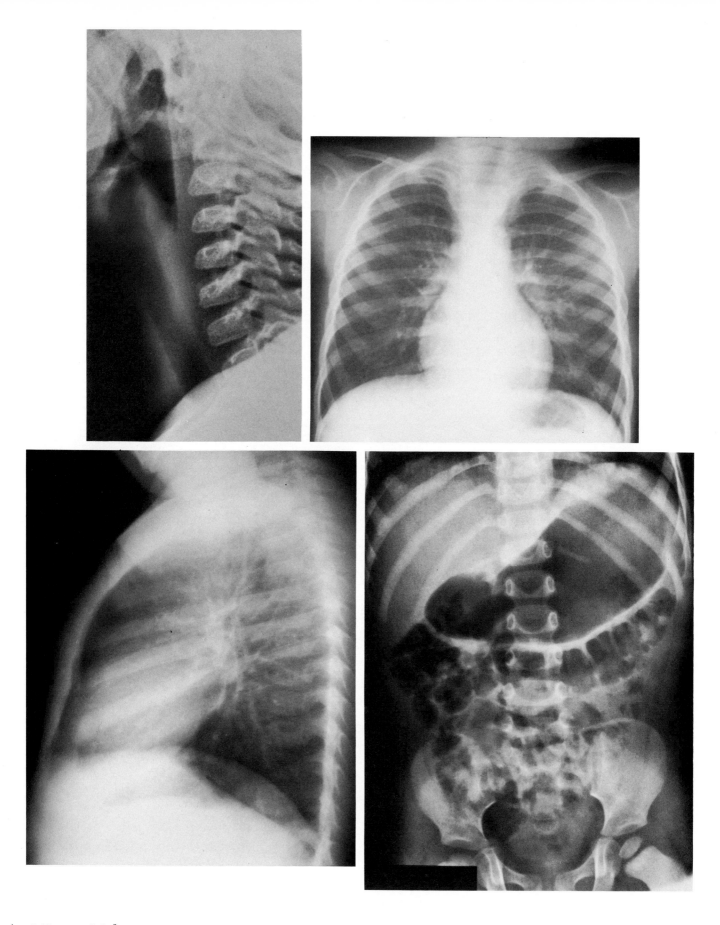

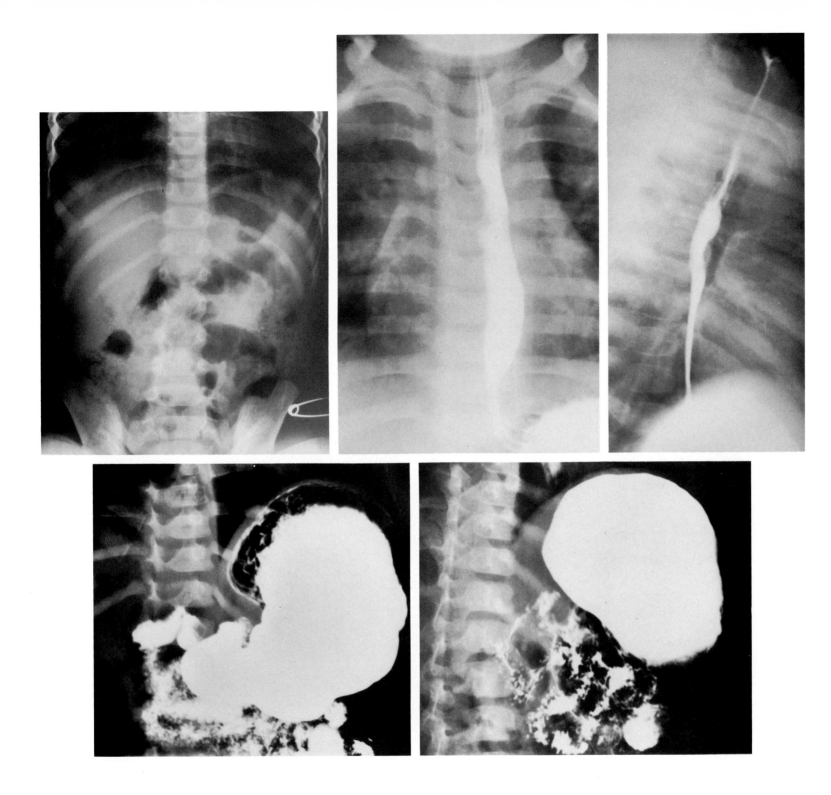

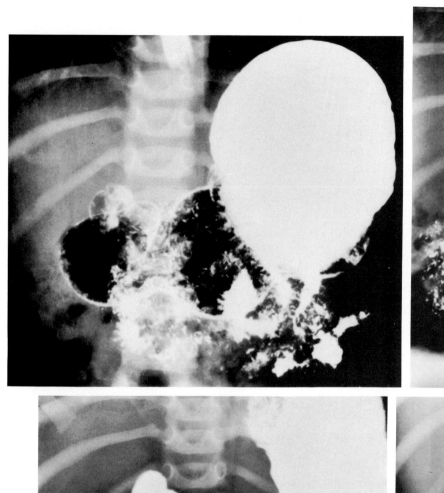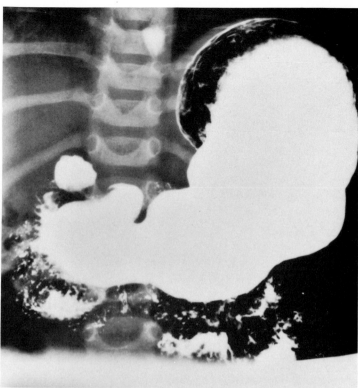
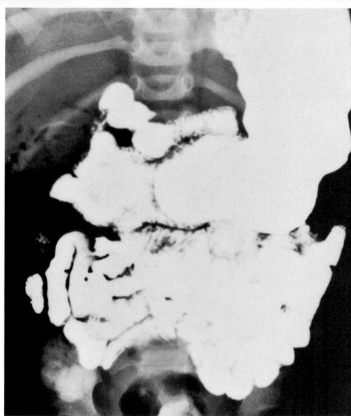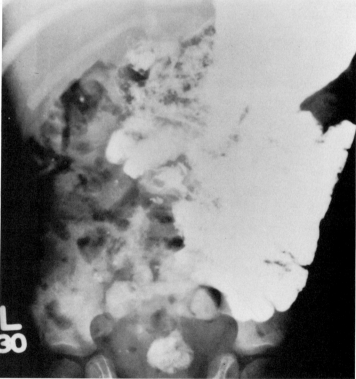

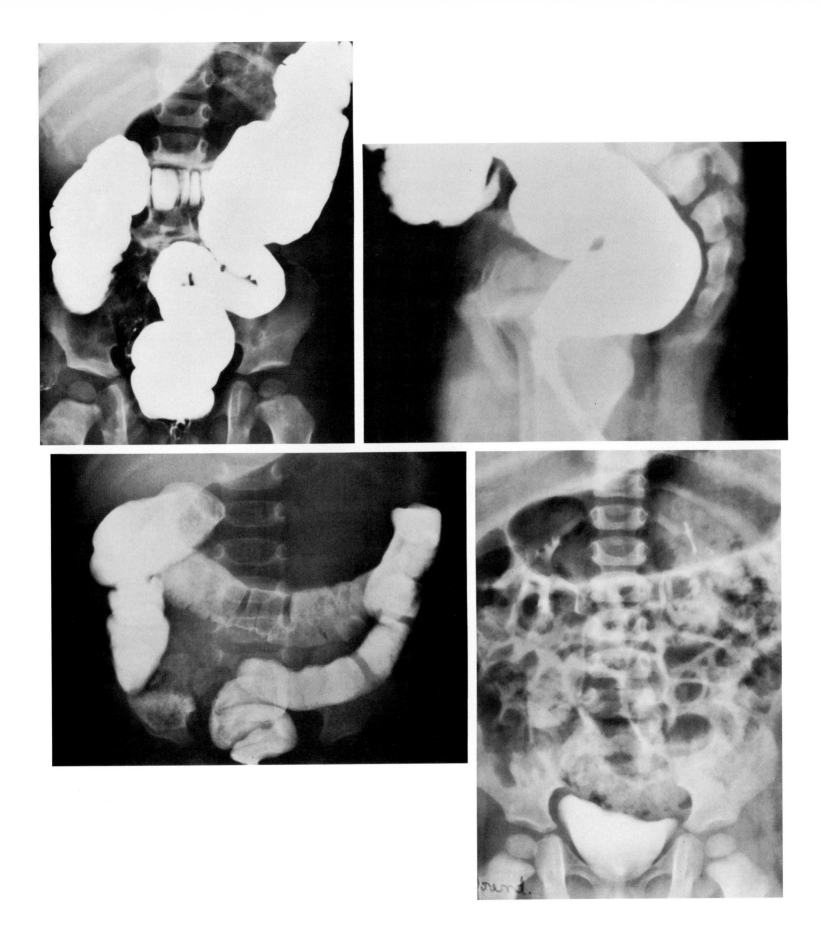

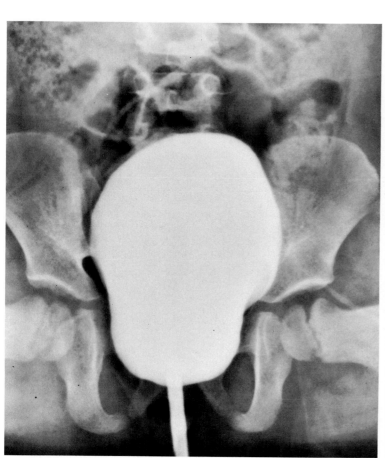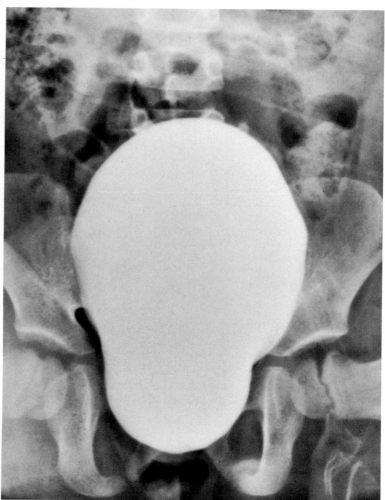

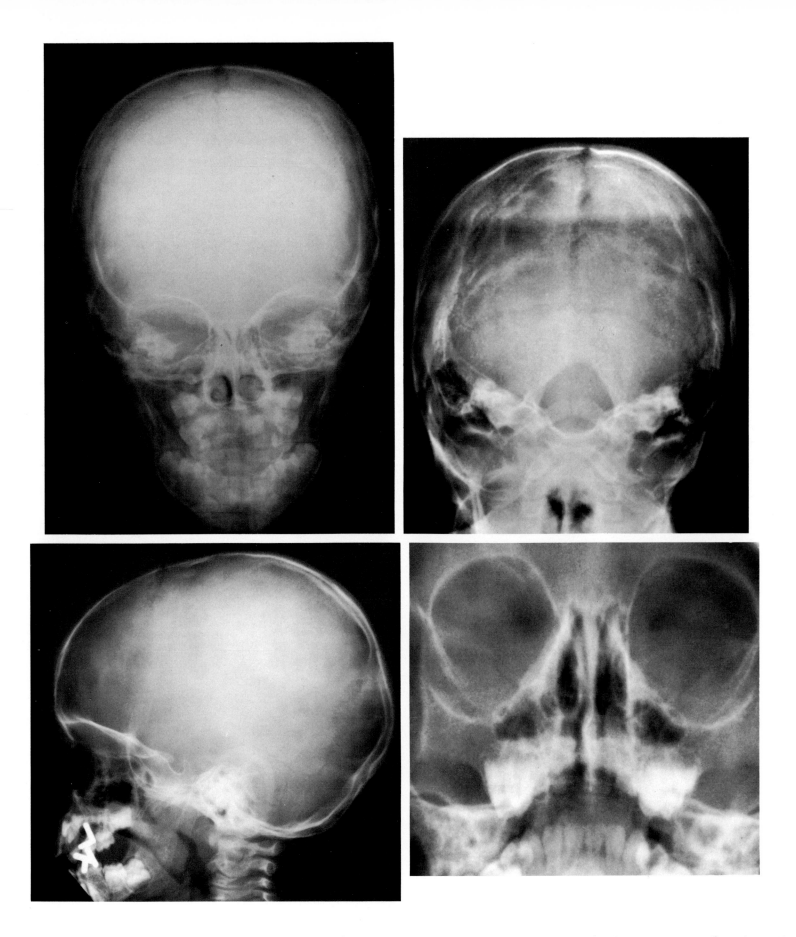

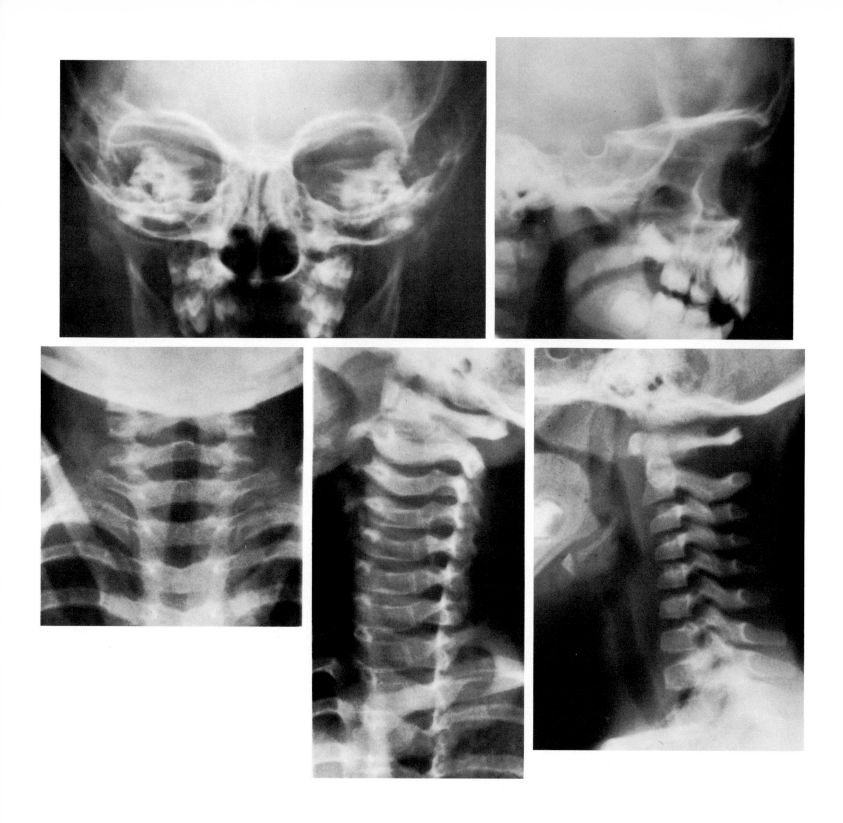

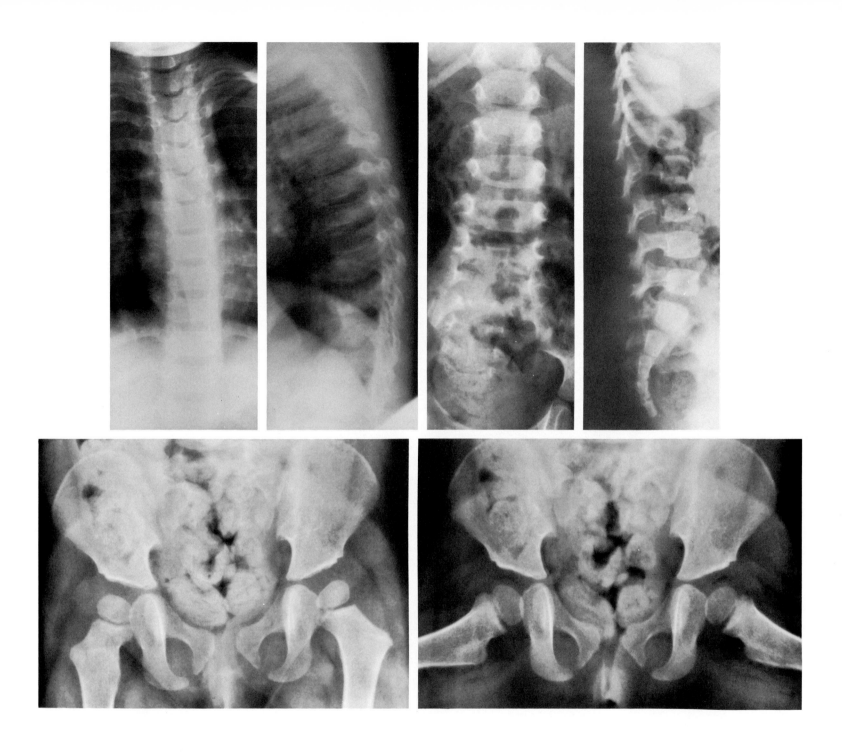

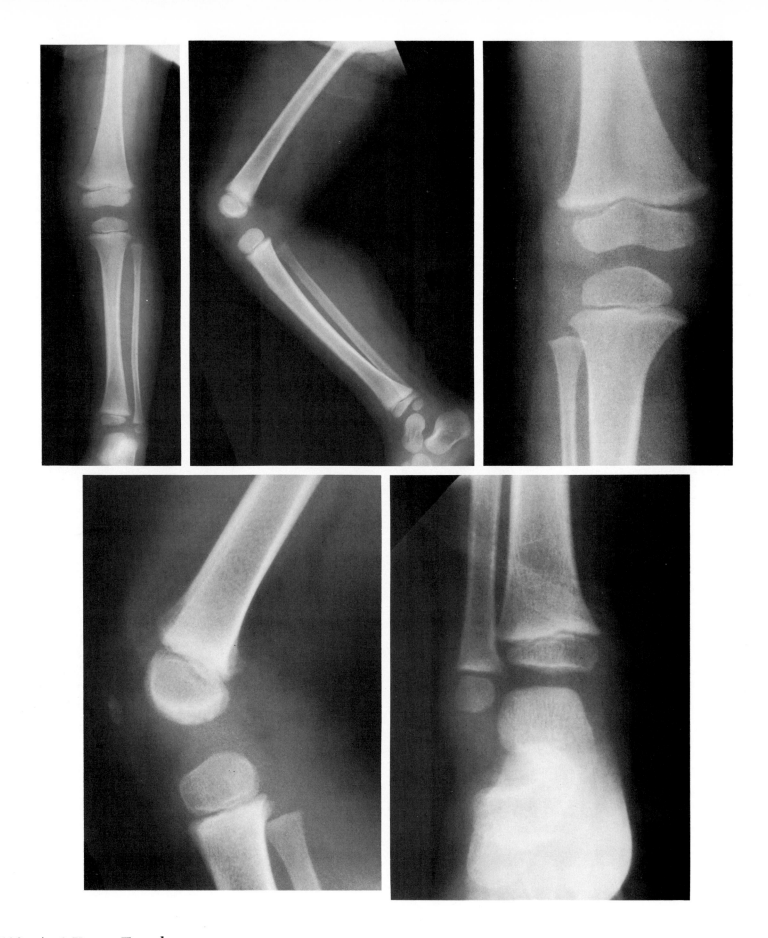

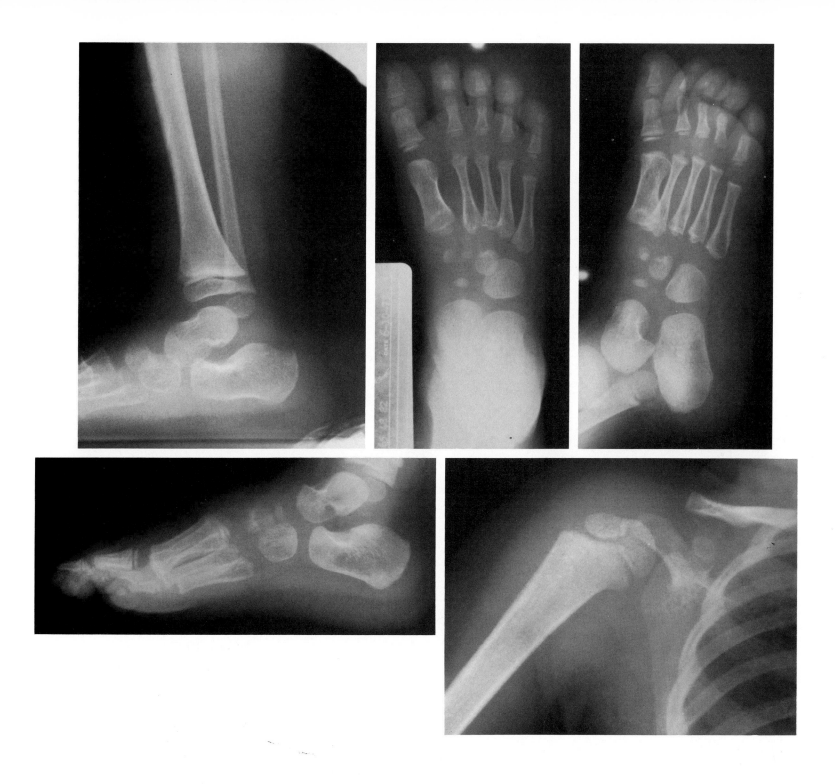

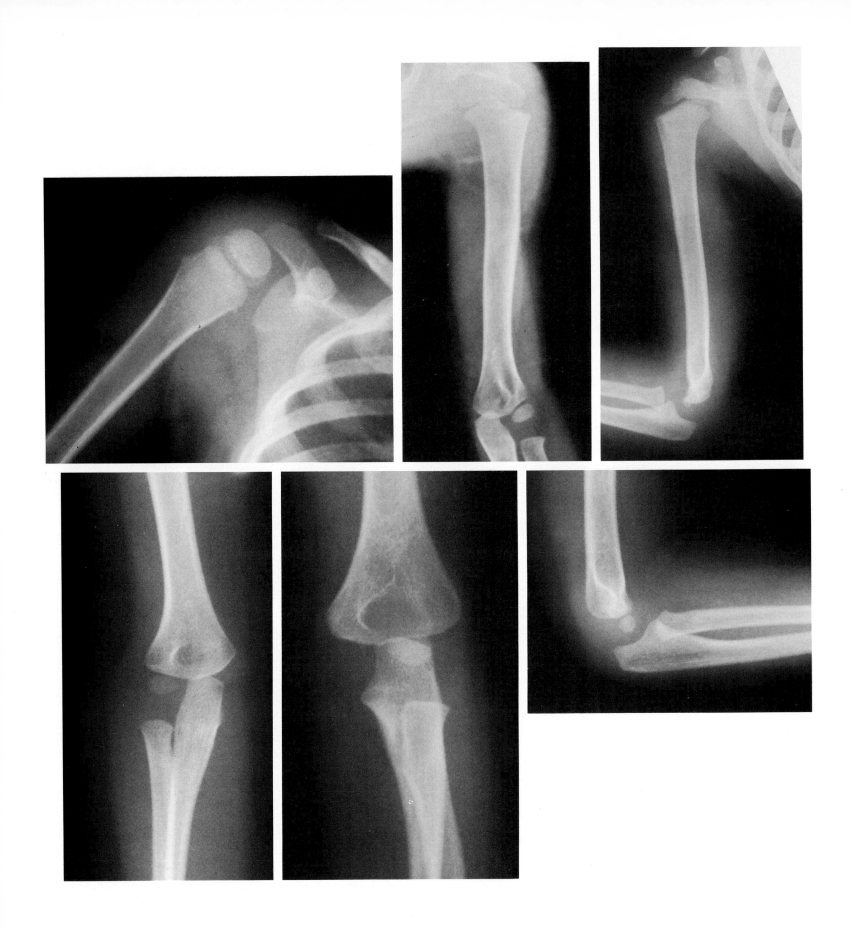

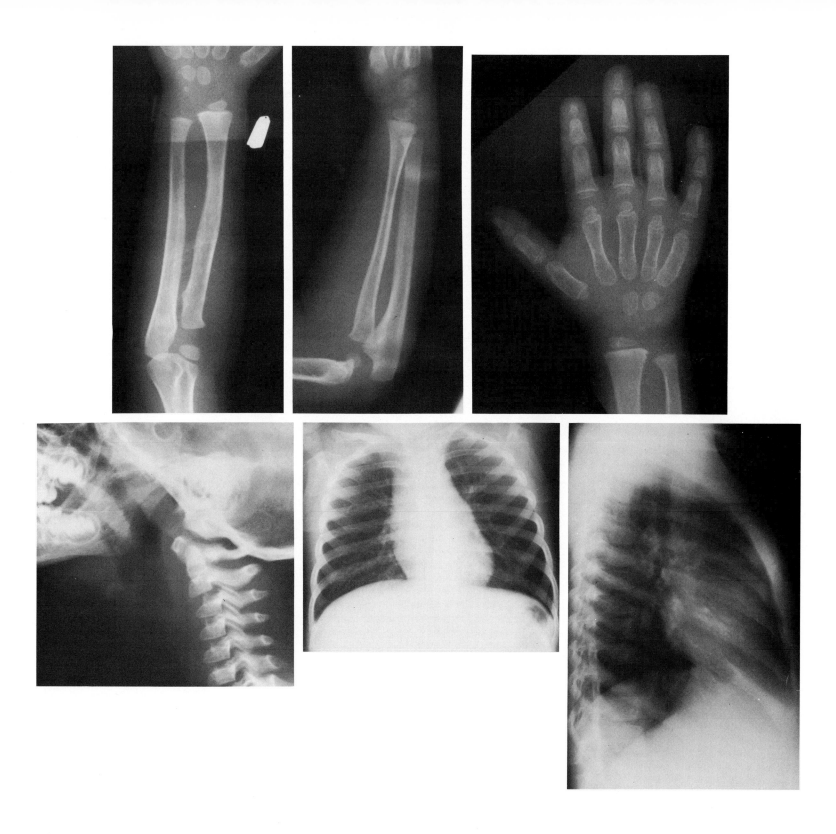

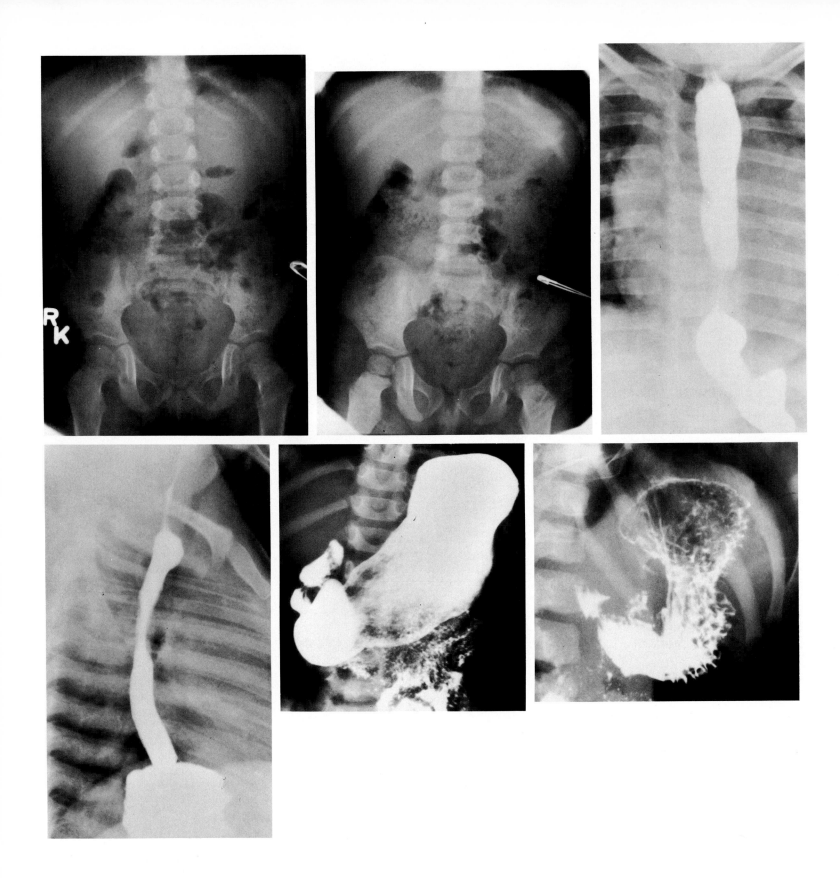

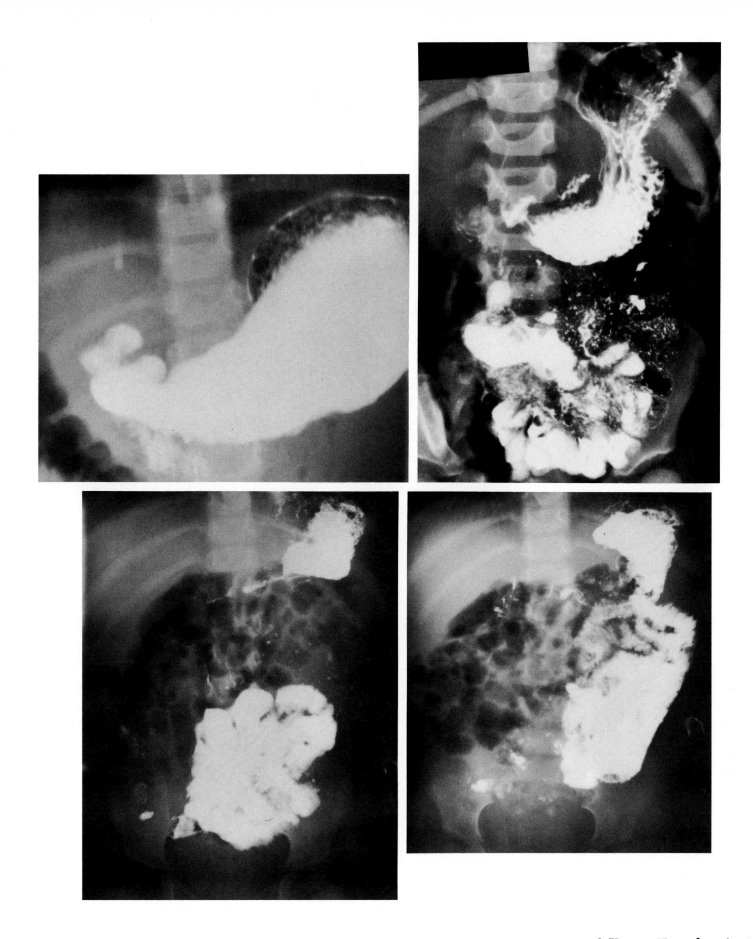

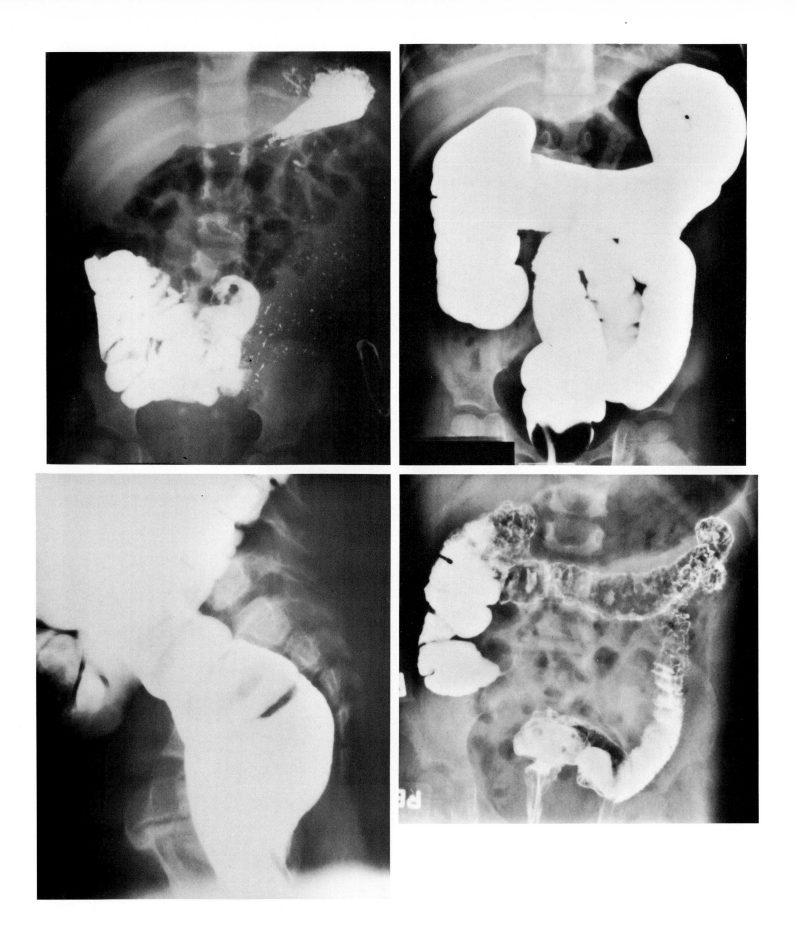

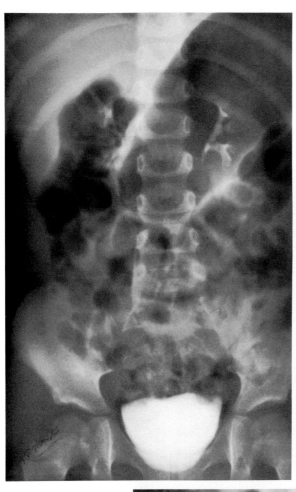

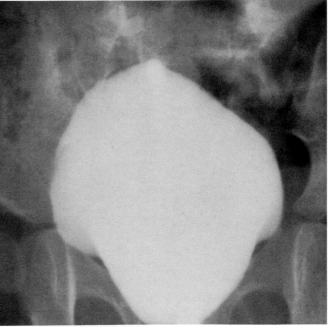

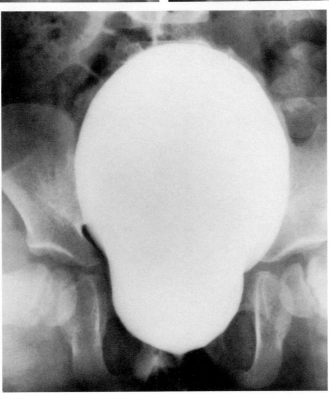

11

3 YEARS

The cranial sutures are less pronounced. Pneumatization of the sphenoid sinus is evident in varying degrees. The nasofrontal suture may no longer be evident.

The ischiopubic synchondrosis is in the process of closing. Irregularities in the outline of the distal femoral epiphysis are seen. The ossification center for the patella is first apparent. The fat planes now permit excellent definition of the muscles. The ossification centers of the proximal humerus are fusing and conform to the metaphyses.

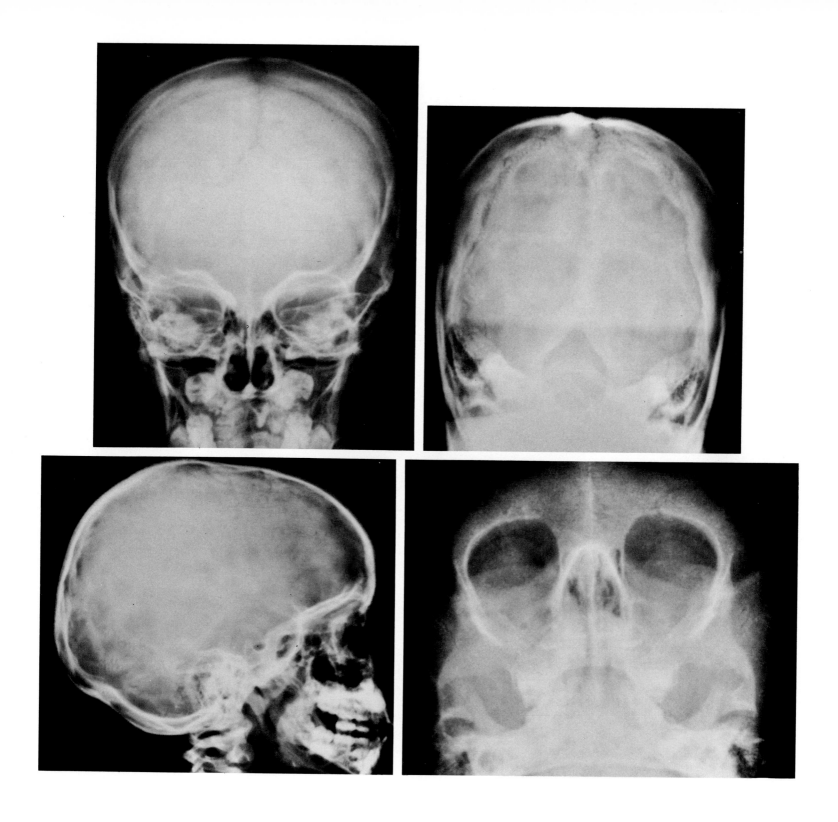

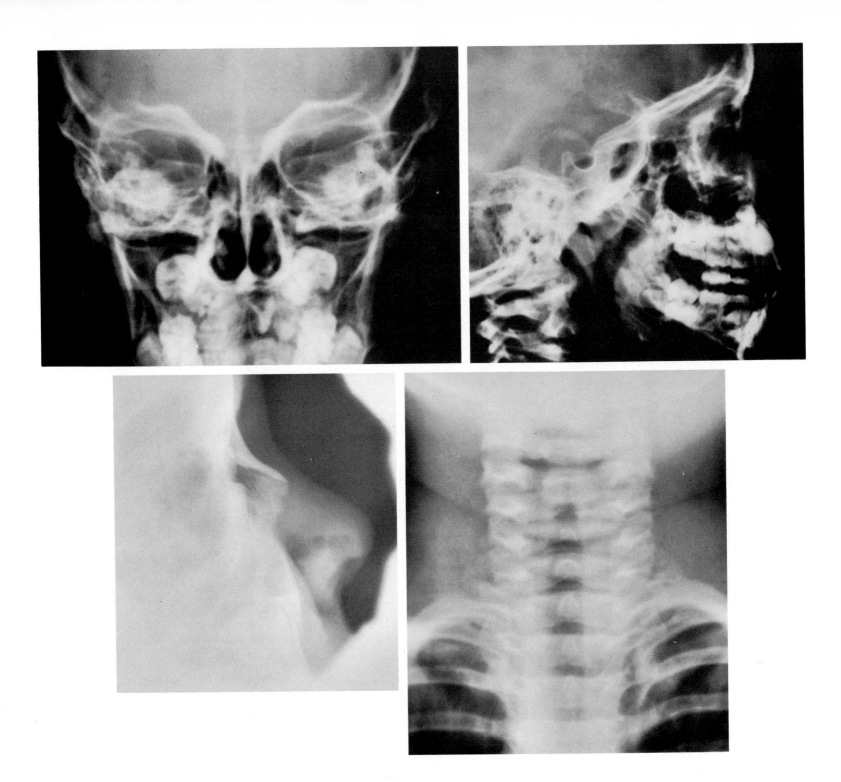

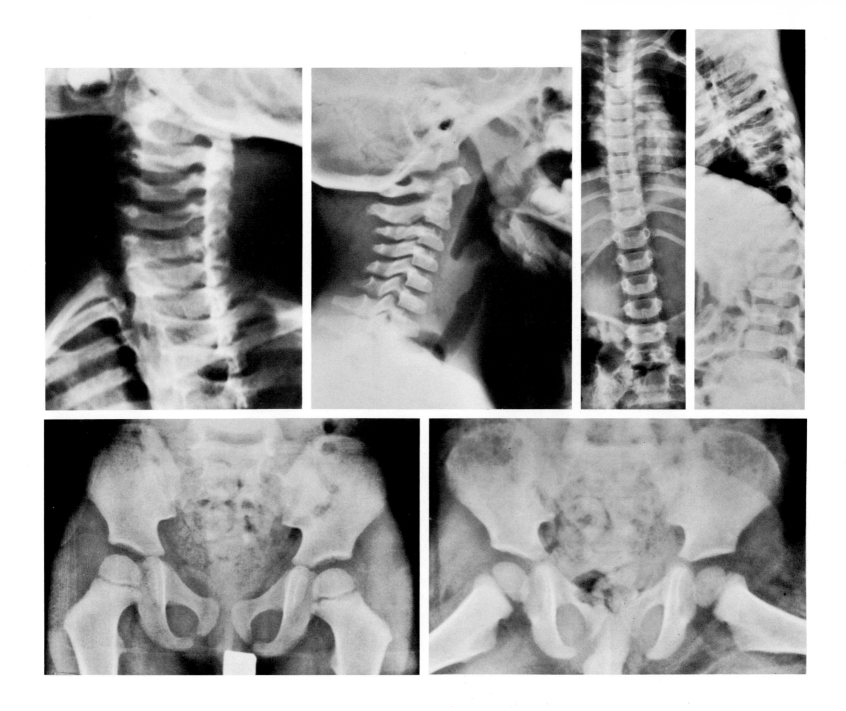

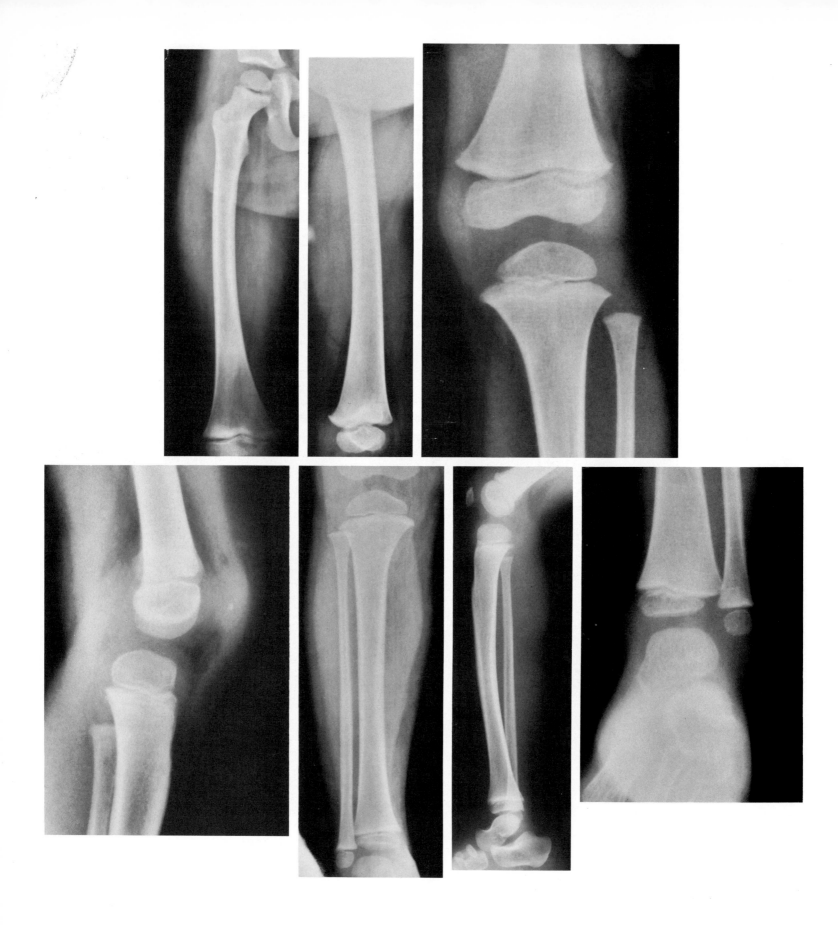

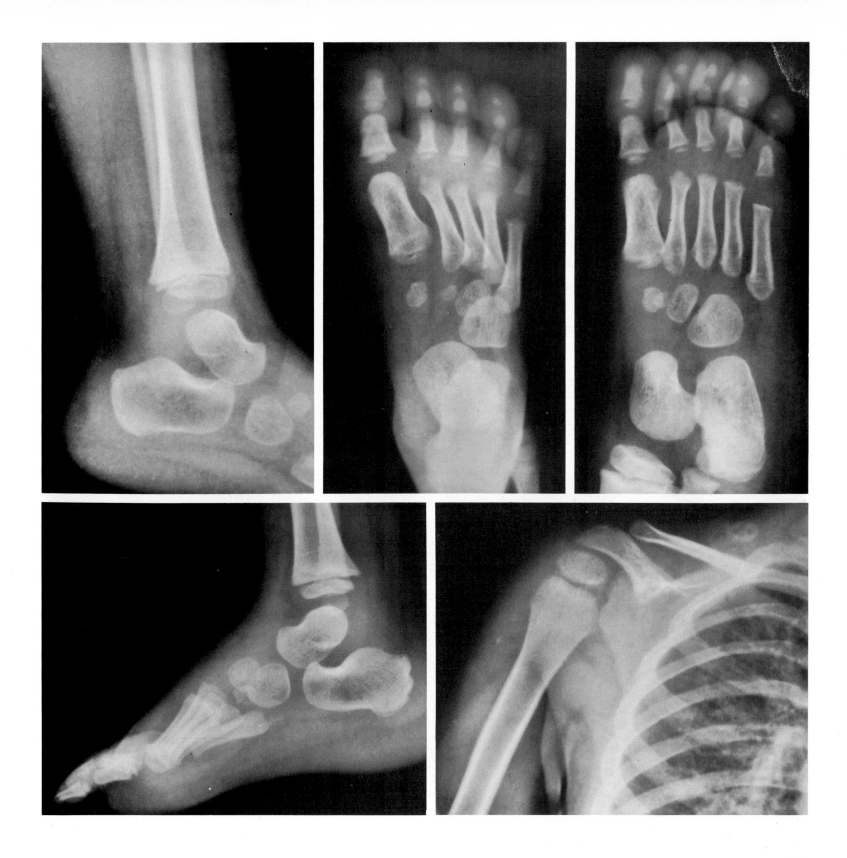

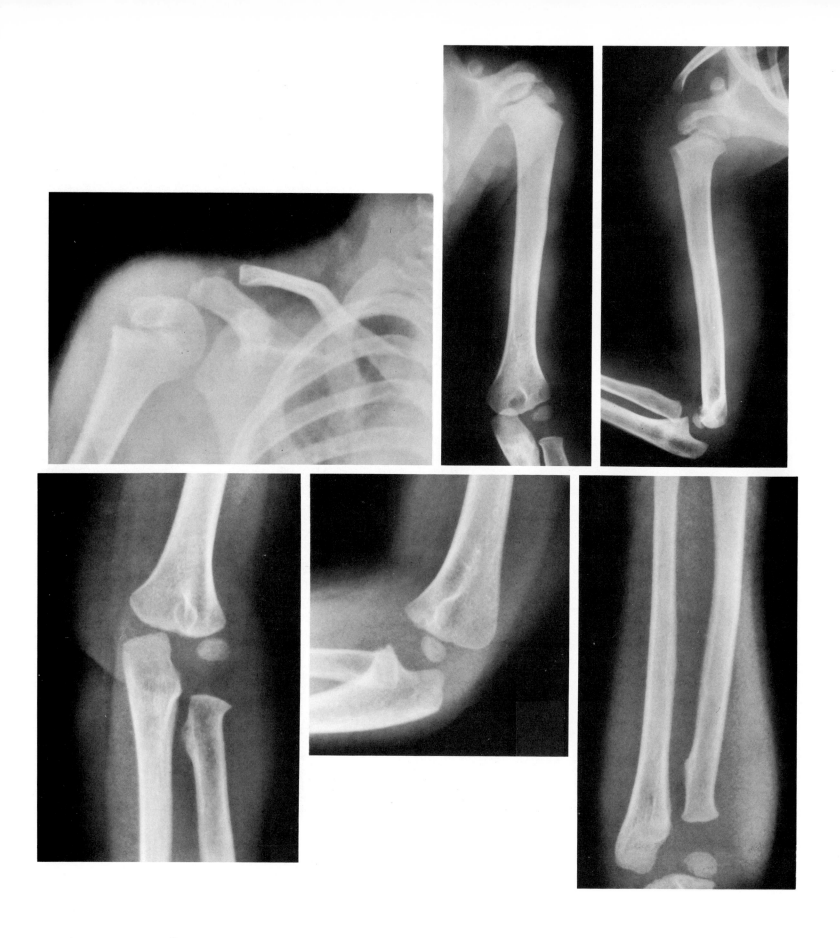

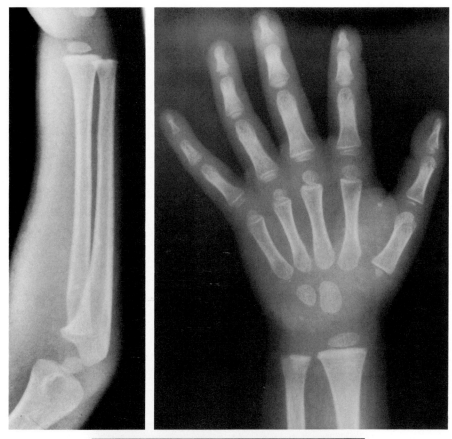

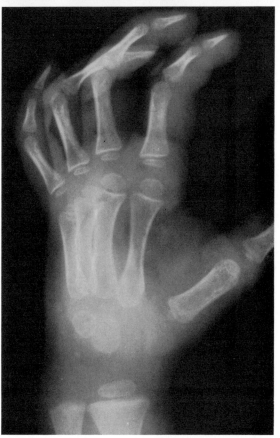

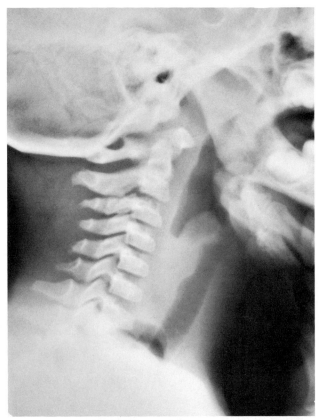

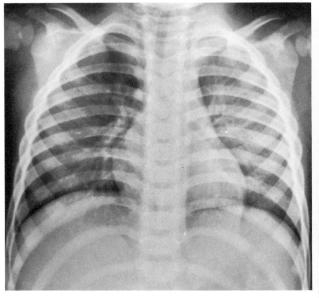

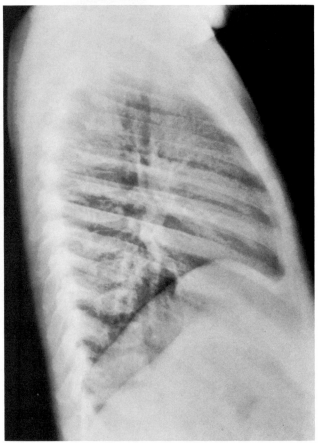

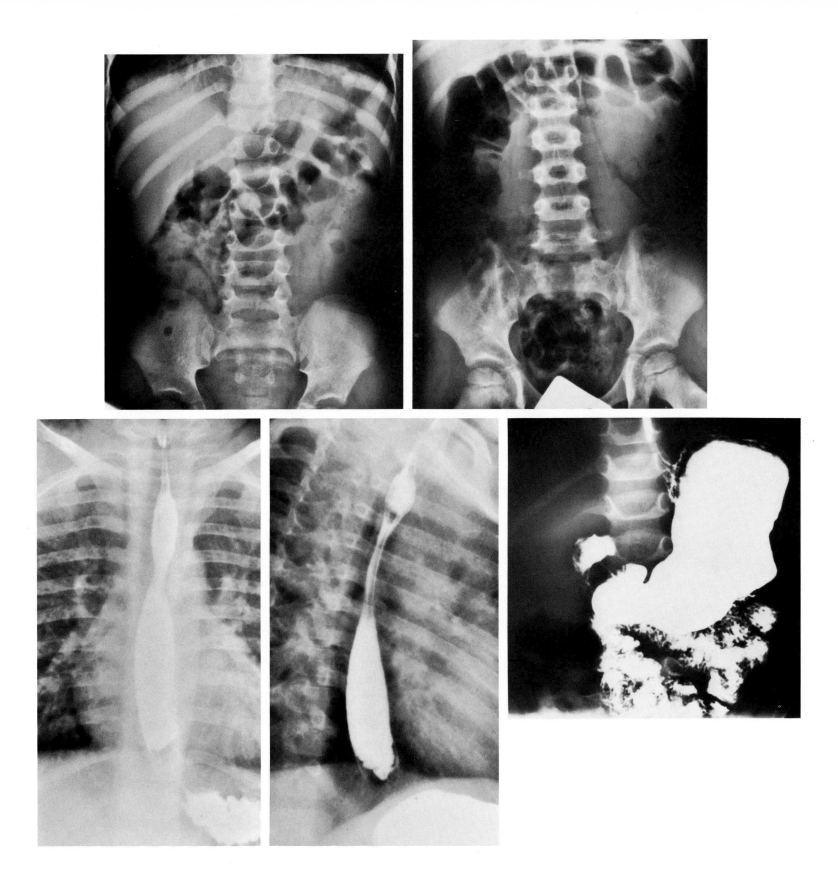

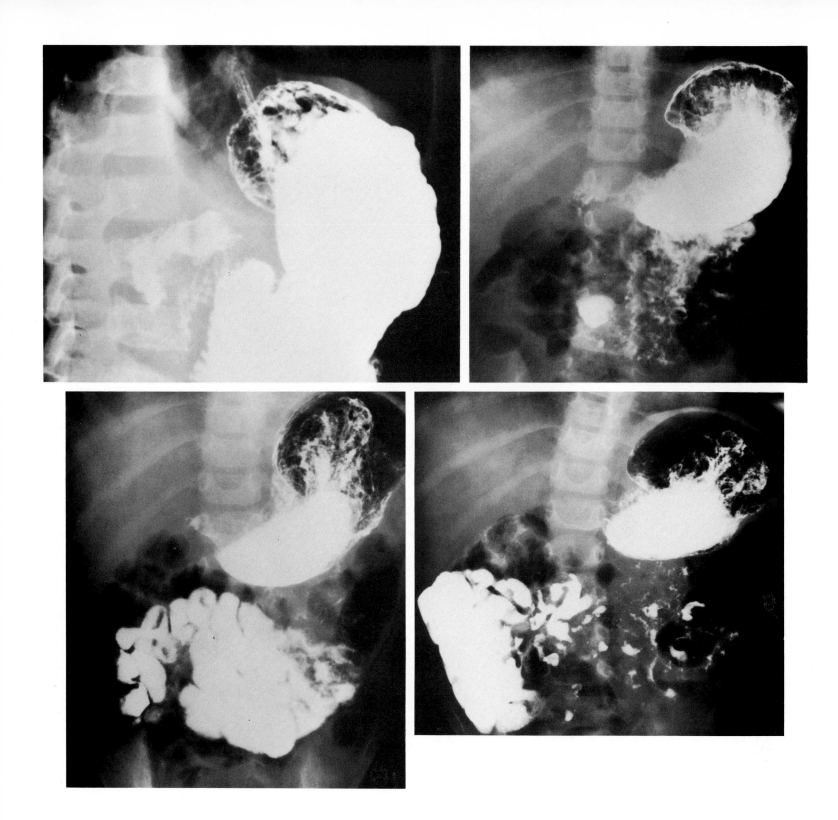

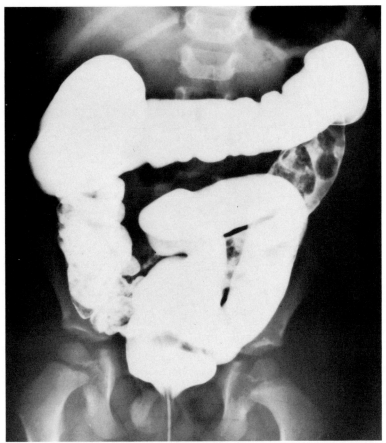

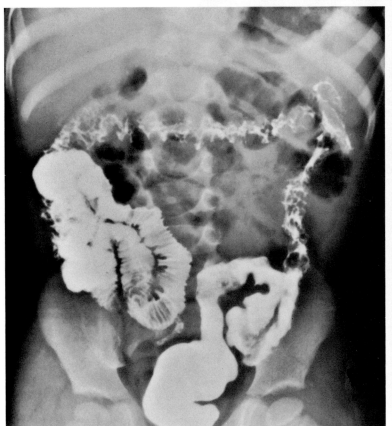

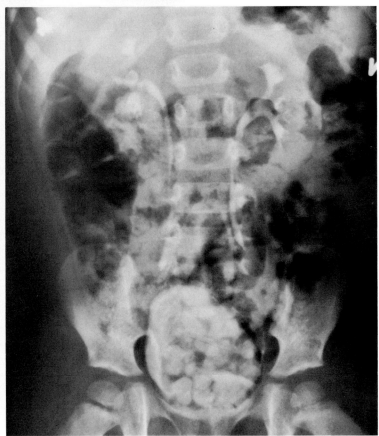

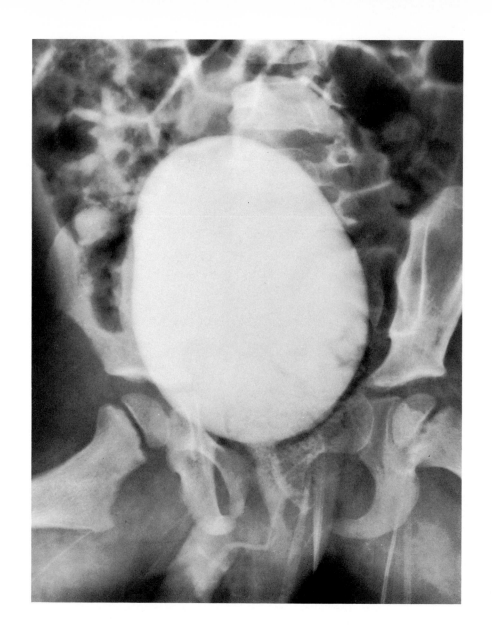

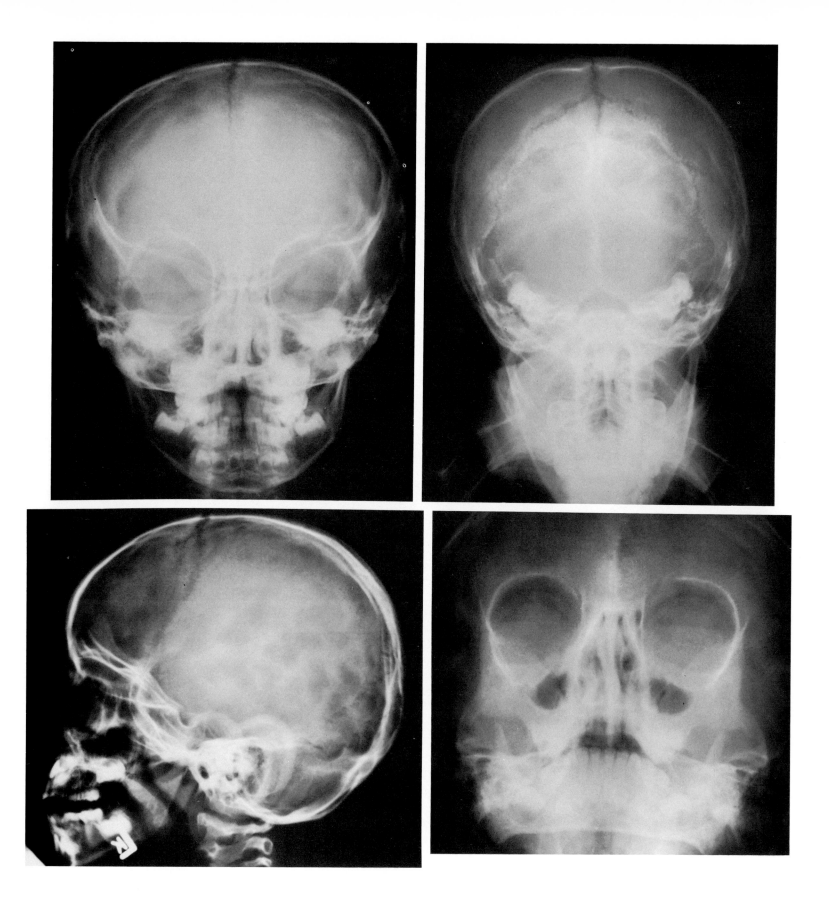

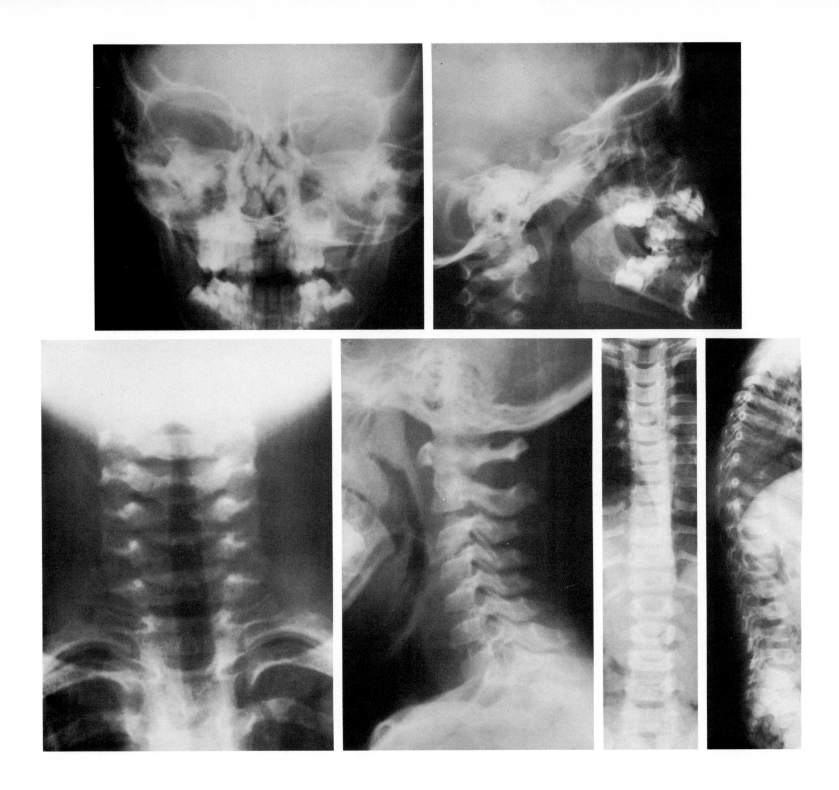

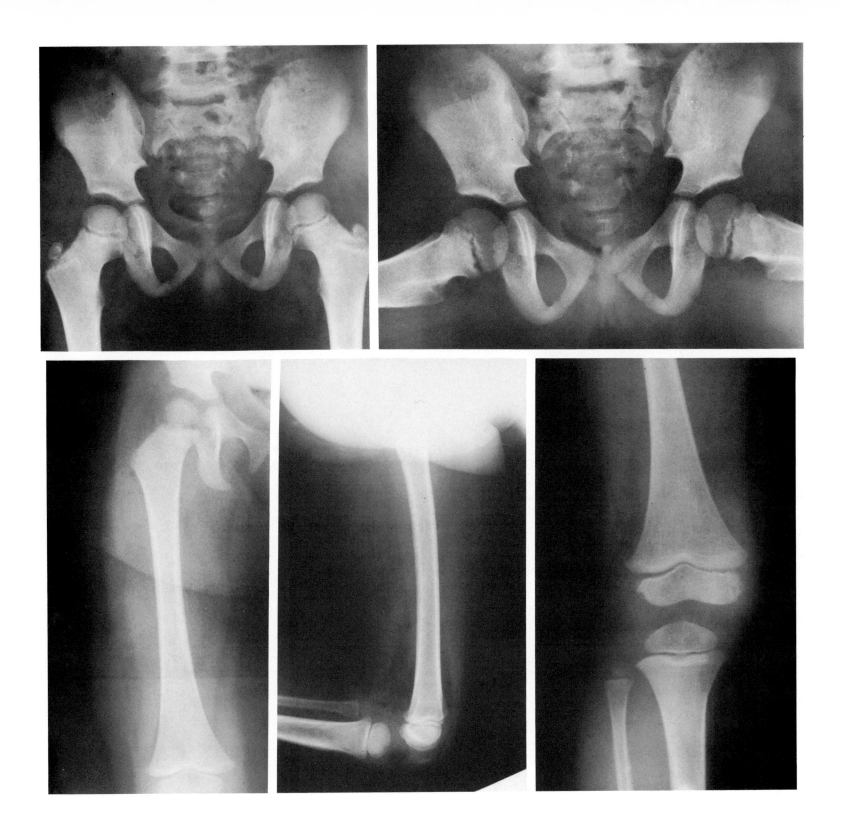

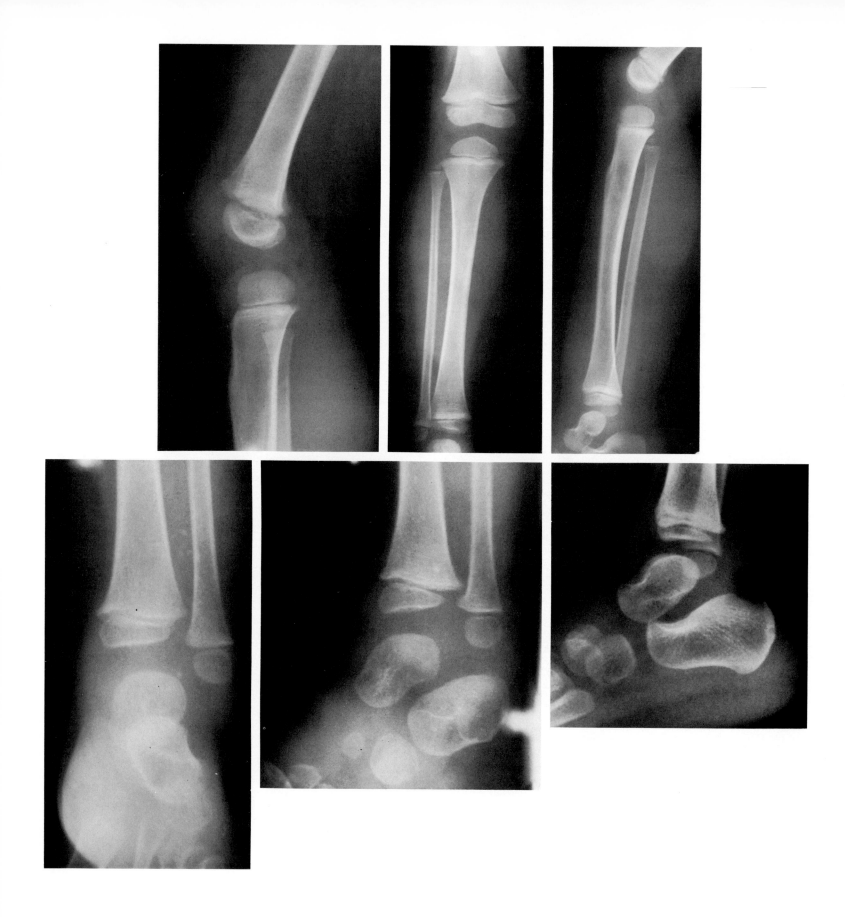

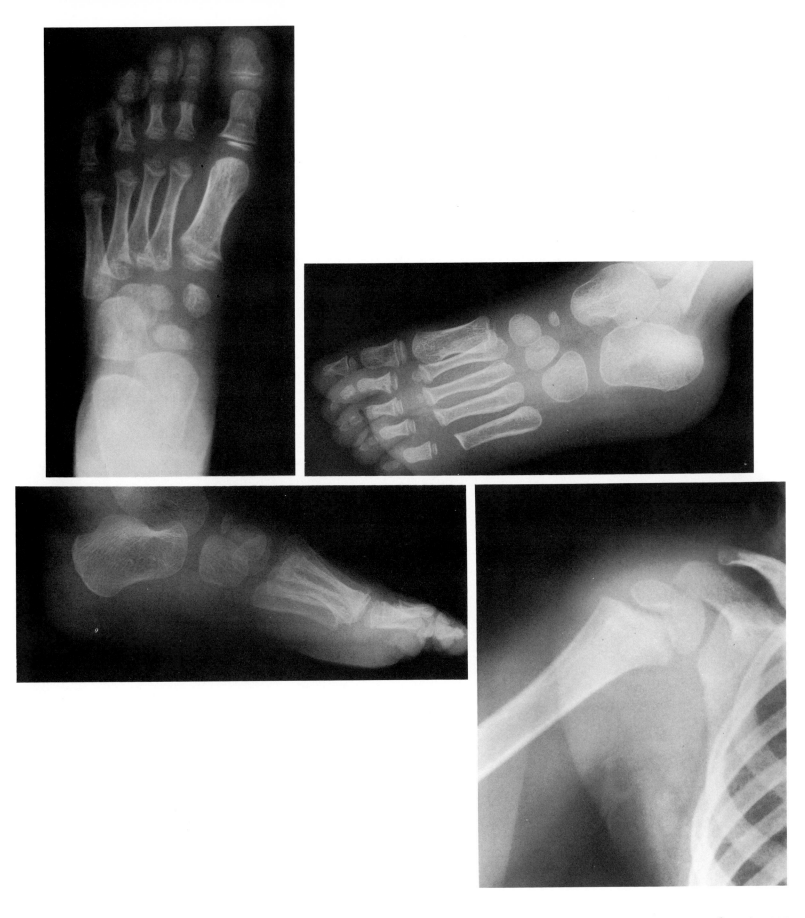

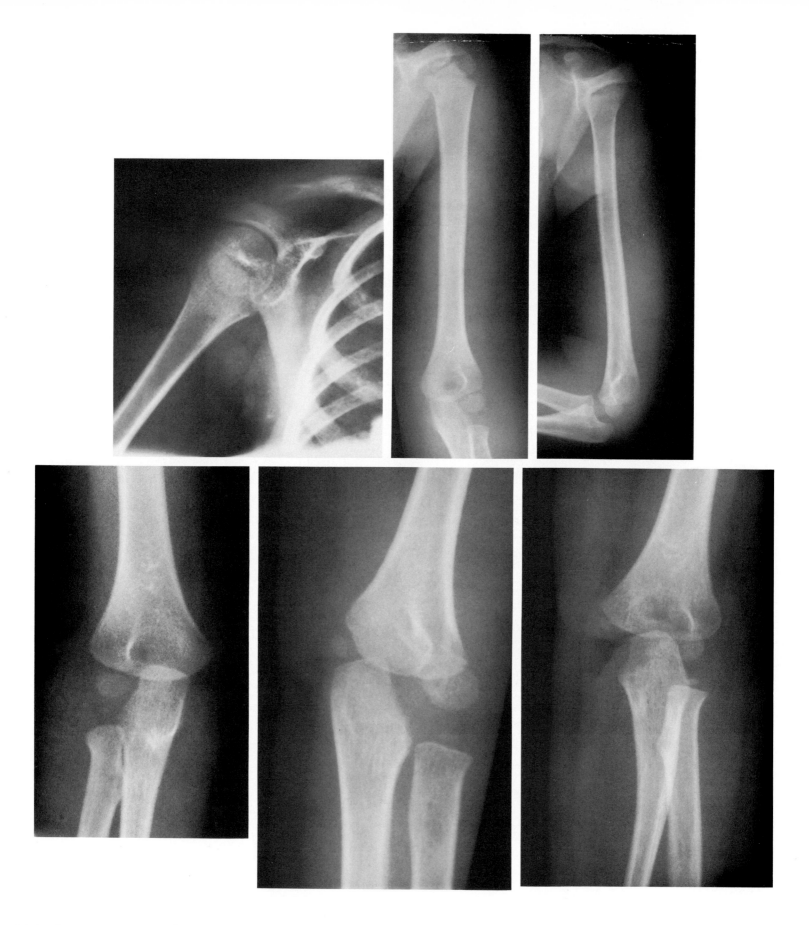

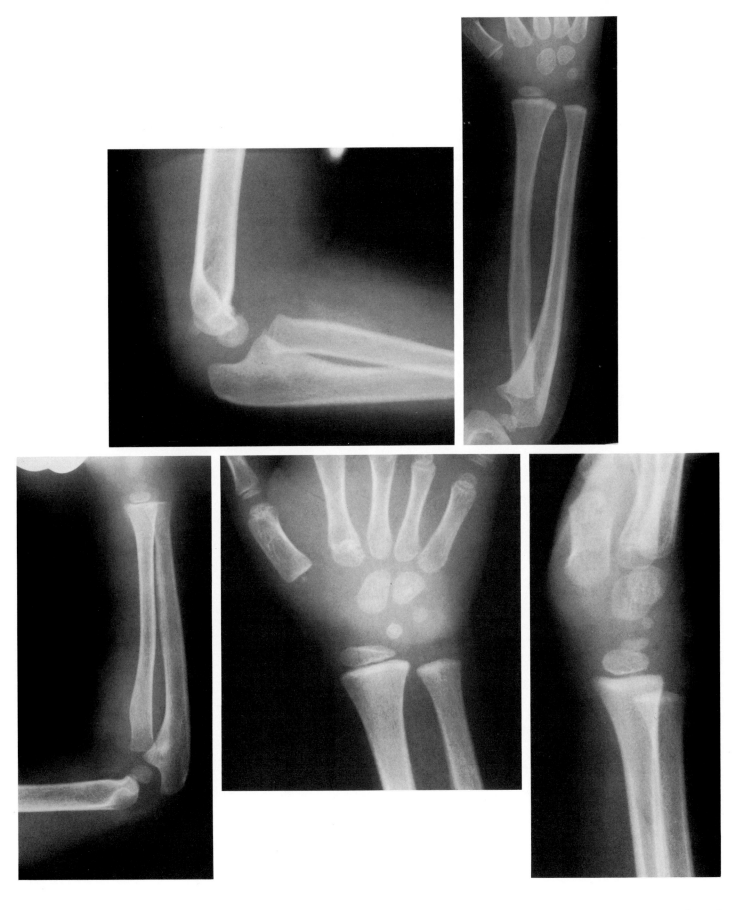

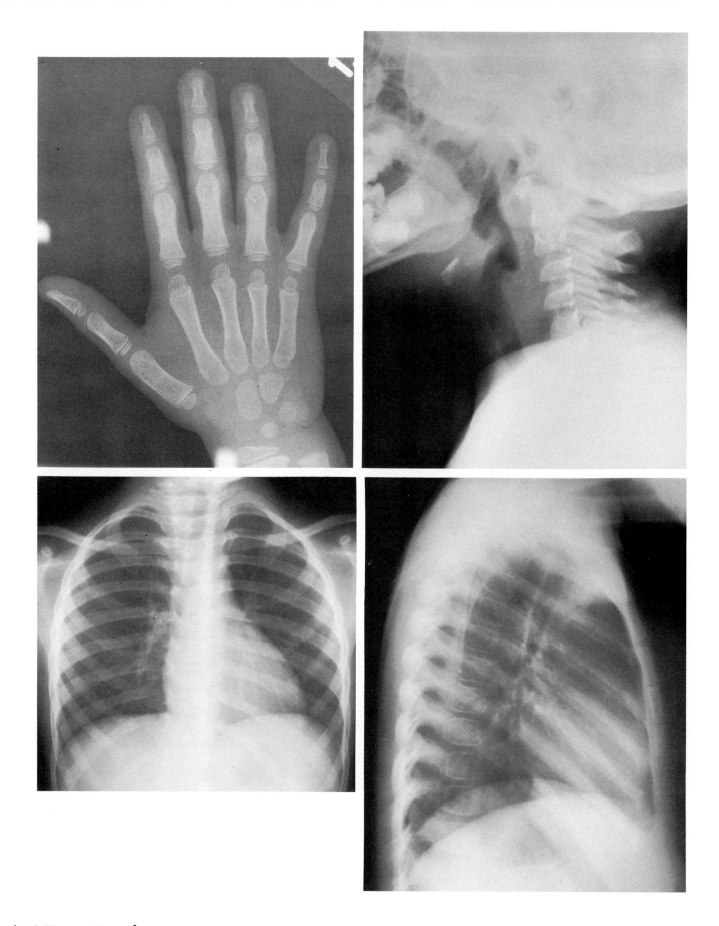

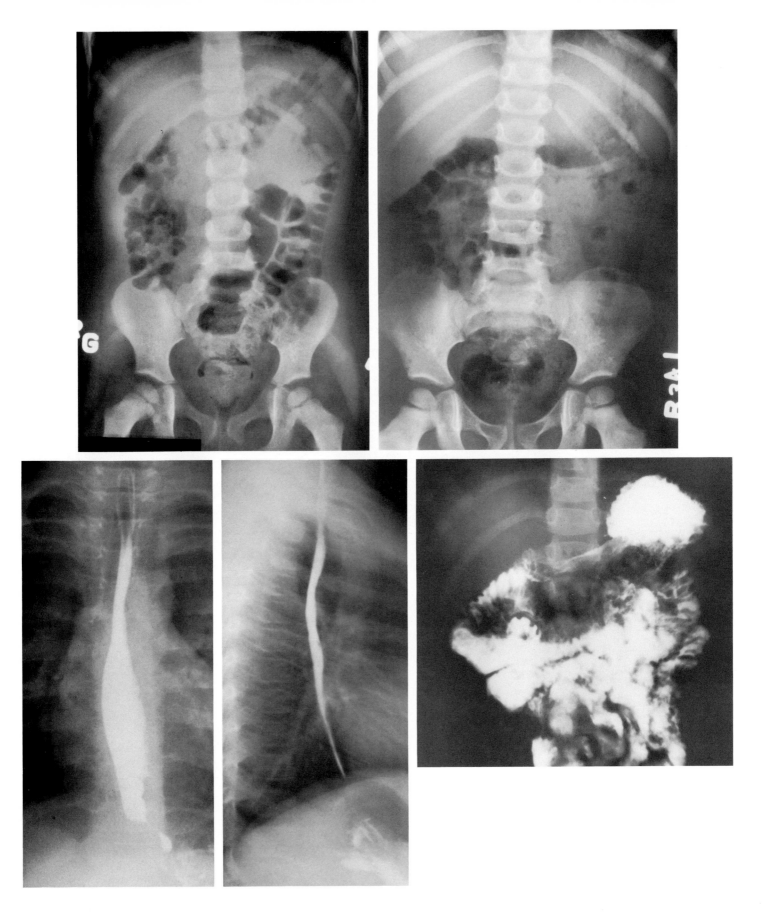

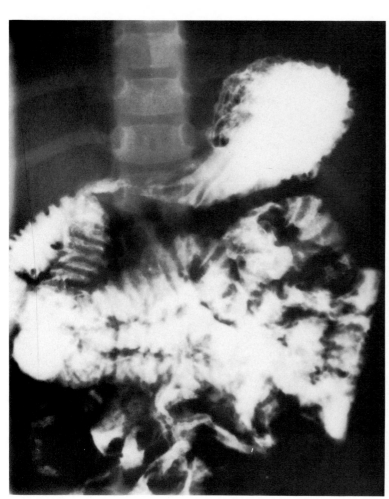
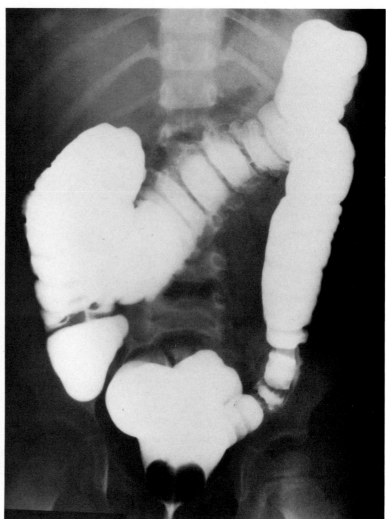

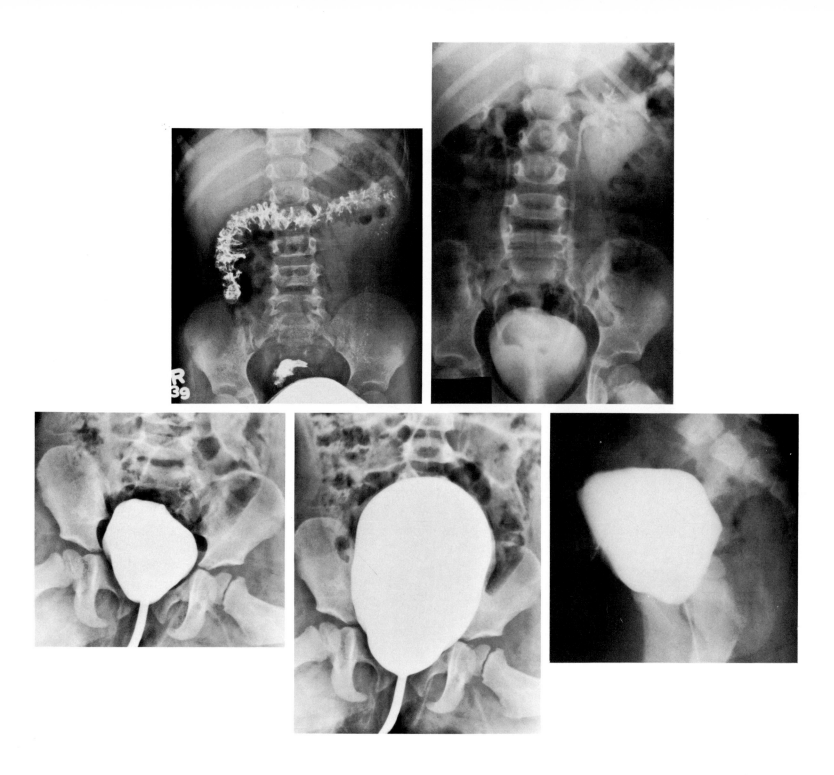

12

4 YEARS

Cranial sutures are barely visible. The skull to face ratio is adult-like. Digital markings in the calvarium are evident. The lumbar vertebrae show shallow fossae anteriorly. The lumbar lordosis is less marked.

Condensing bone changes about the acetabulum are seen. The posterior aspect of the calcaneus is irregular. All of the tarsal bones are evident in the male and are beginning to assume adult propor-tions. Irregularity of the distal femoral metaphysis is still present, as is the irregularity of the medial aspects of the distal femoral epiphyses.

Air may still be seen in the small bowel. Colon and small bowel are easily differentiated. The "spinning top" configuration of the female vesical outlet is evident.

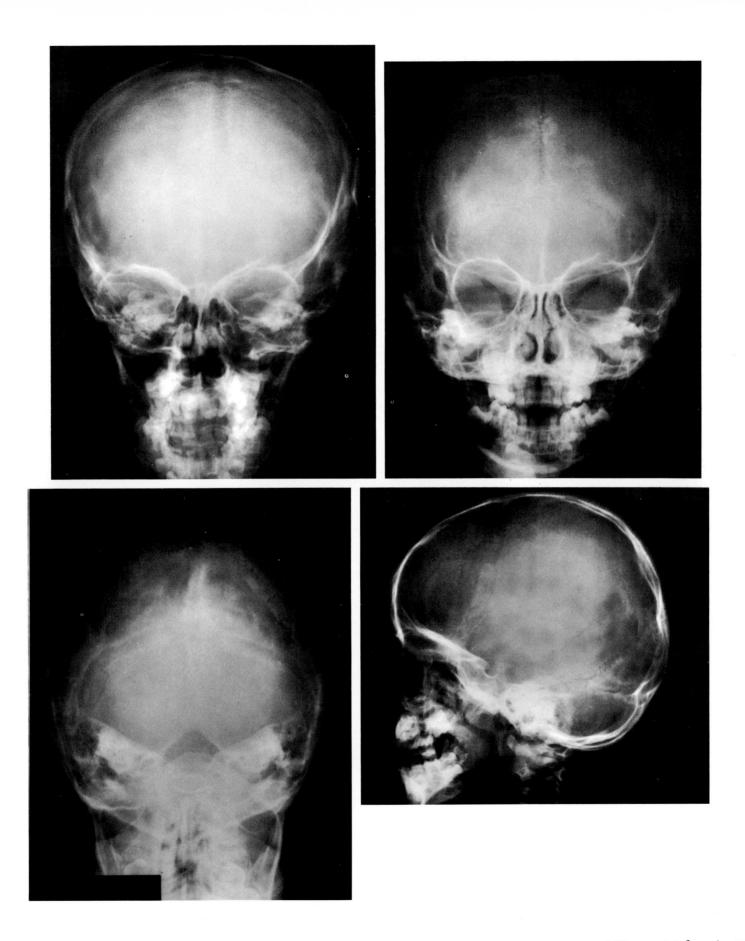

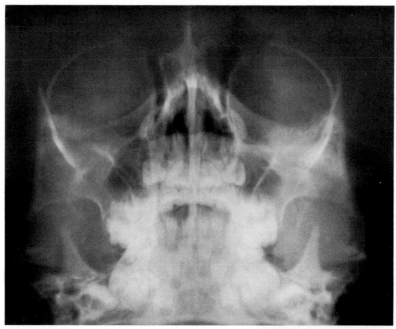

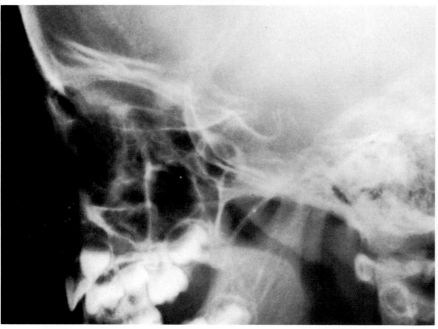

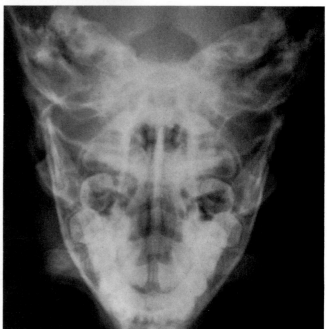

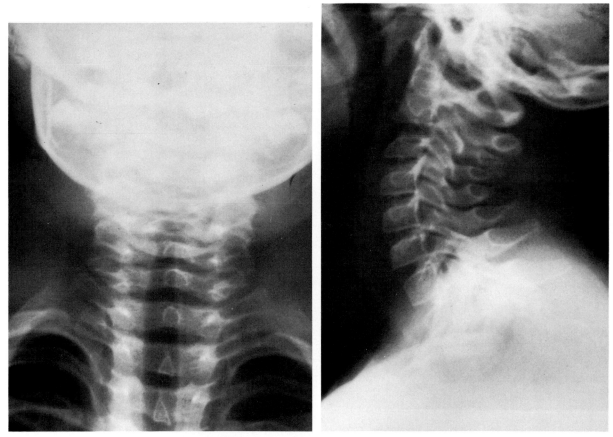

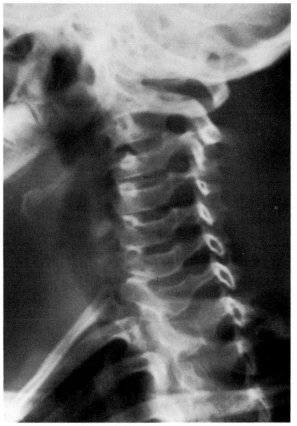

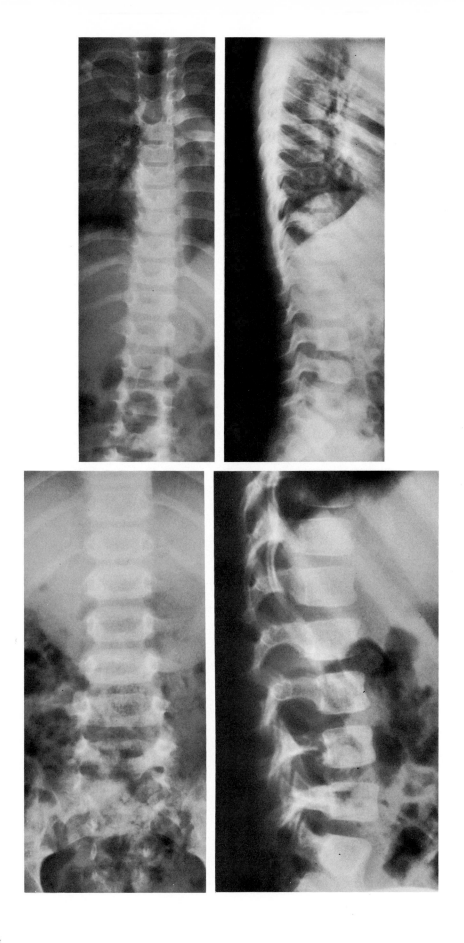

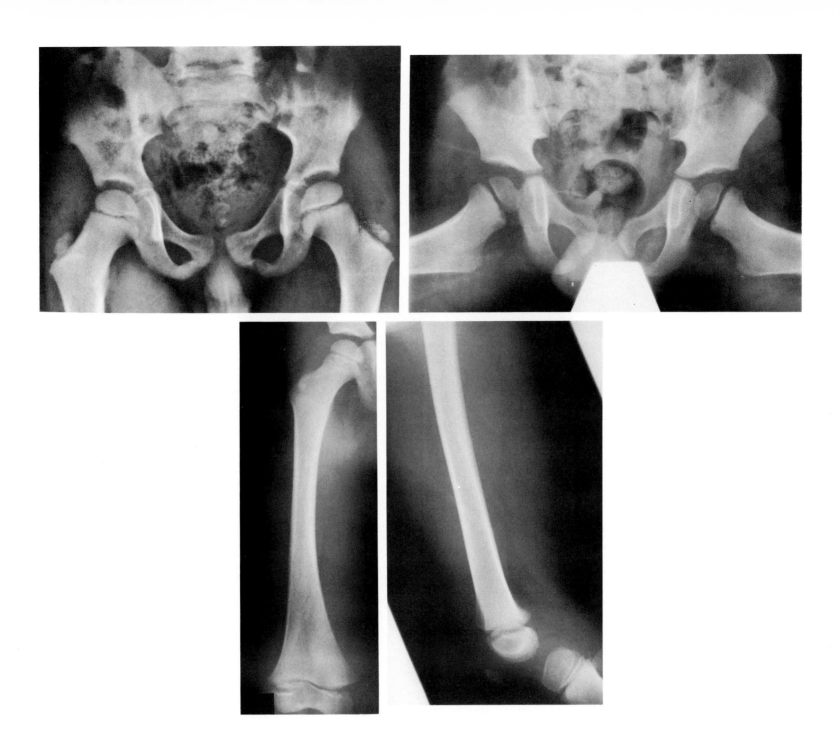

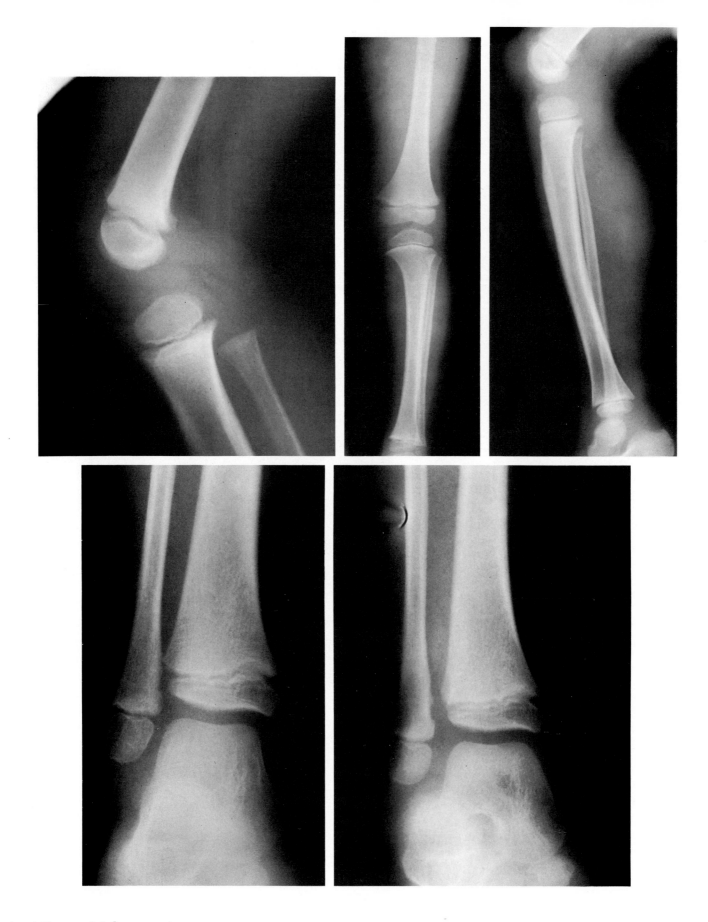

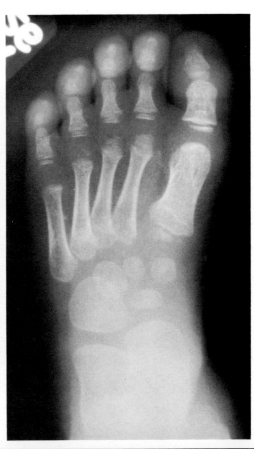

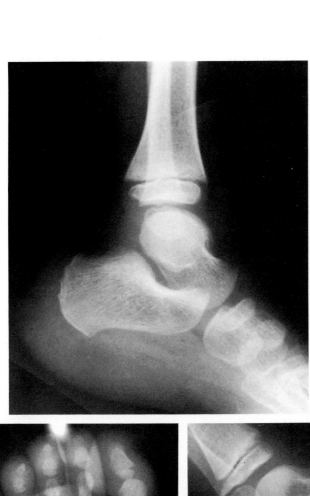

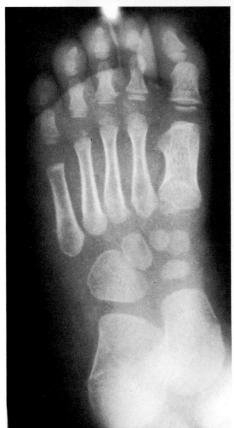

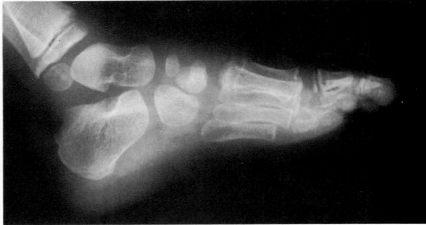

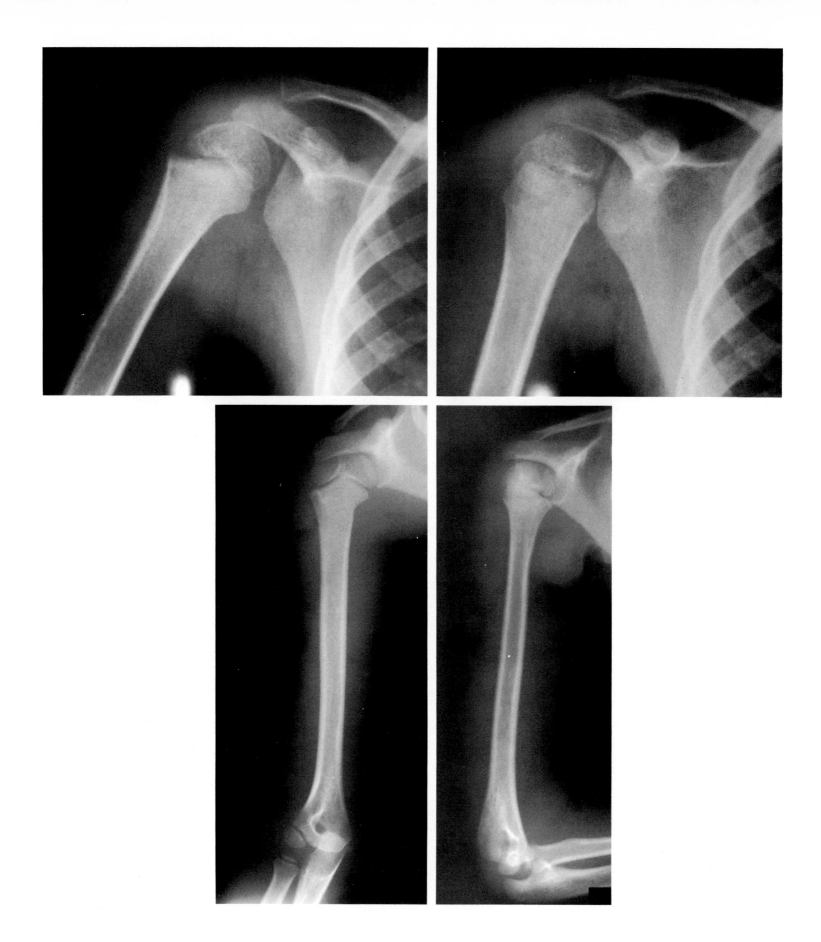

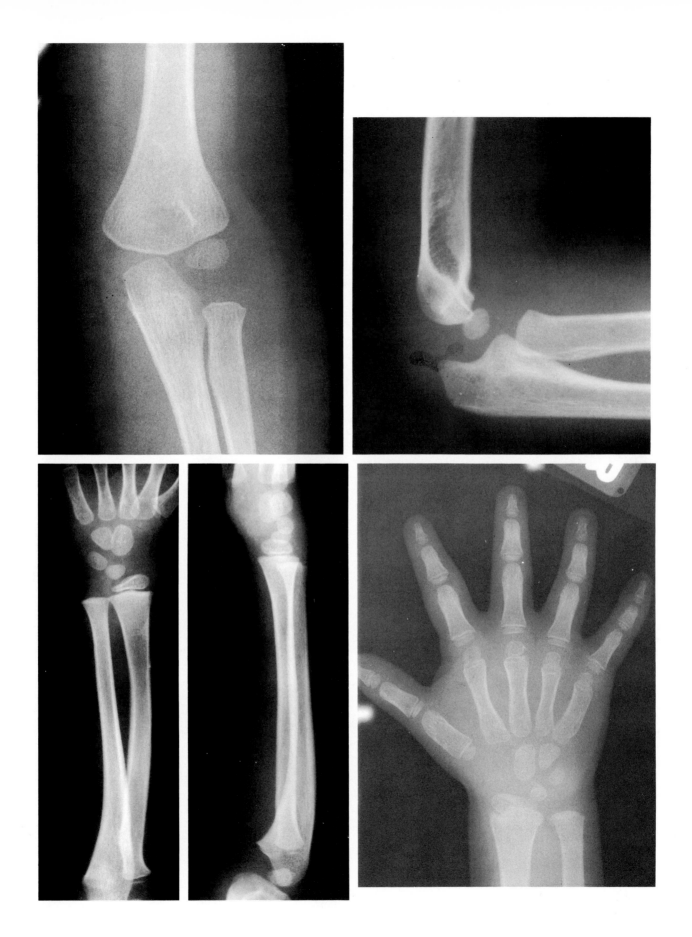

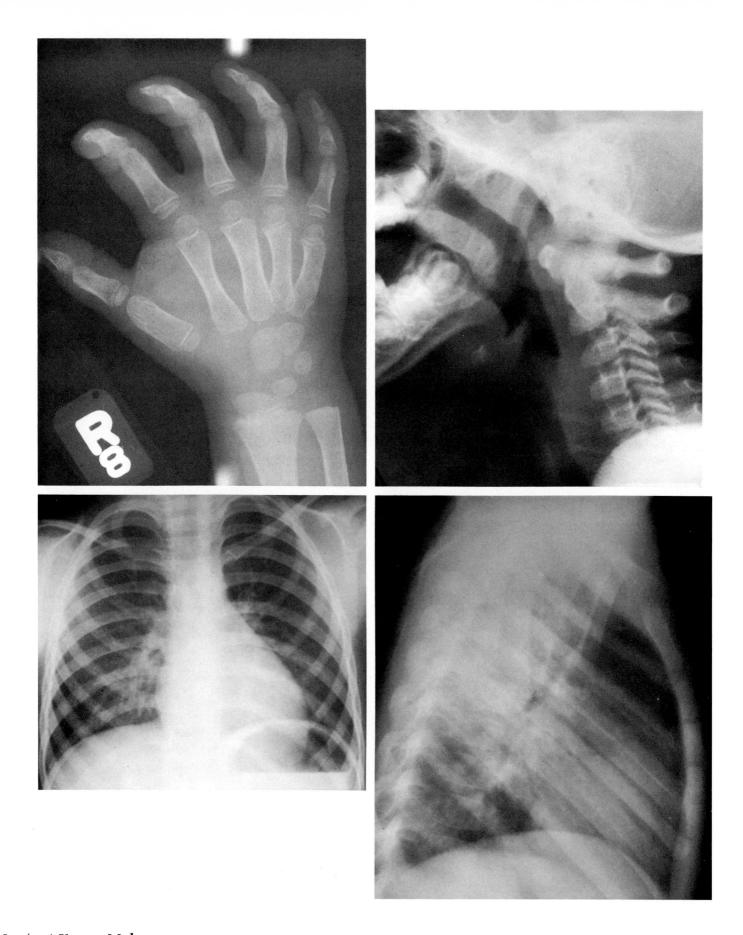

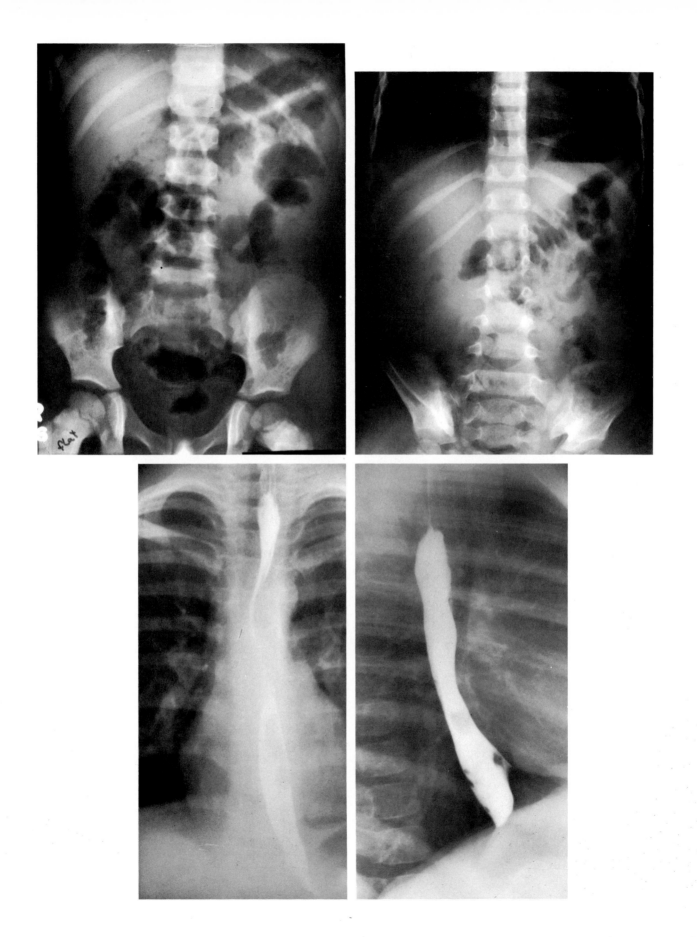

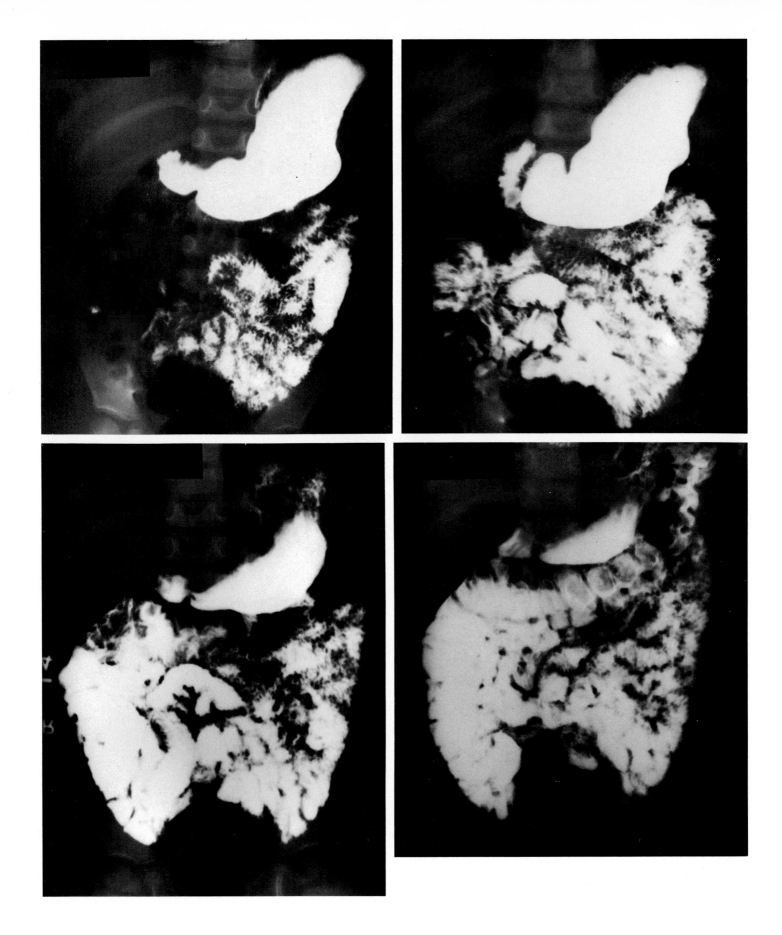

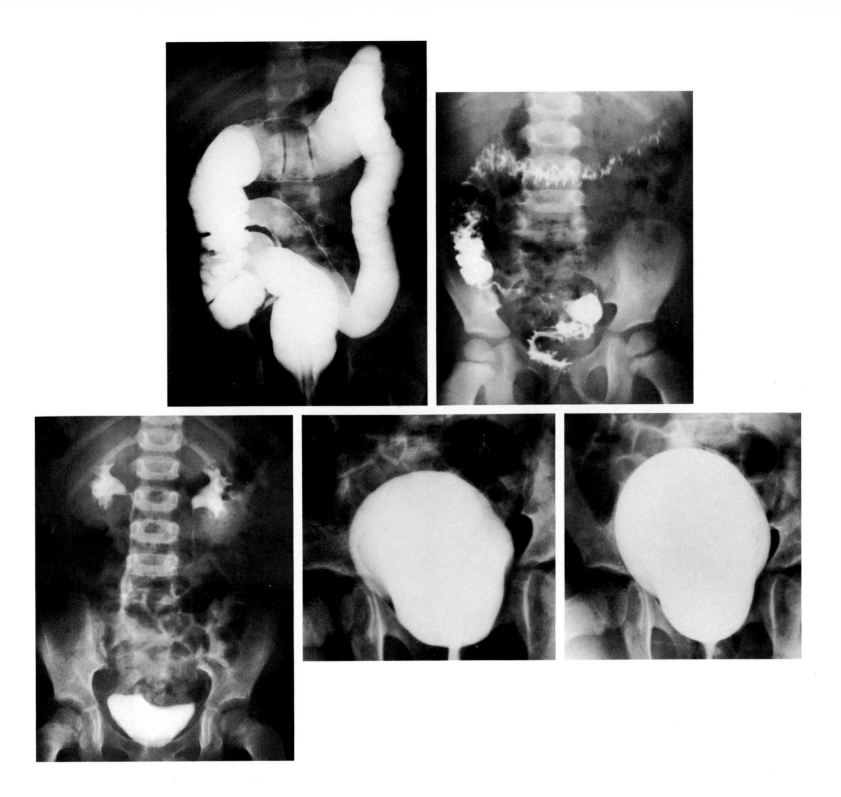

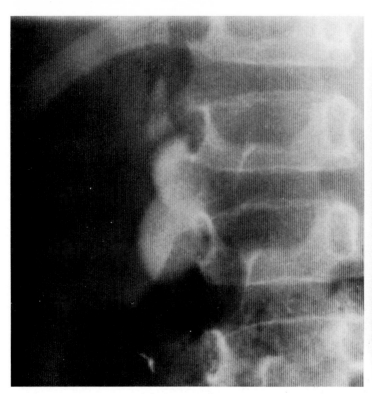 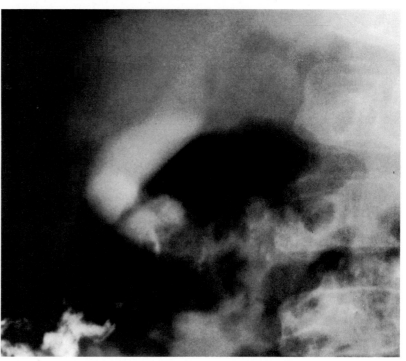

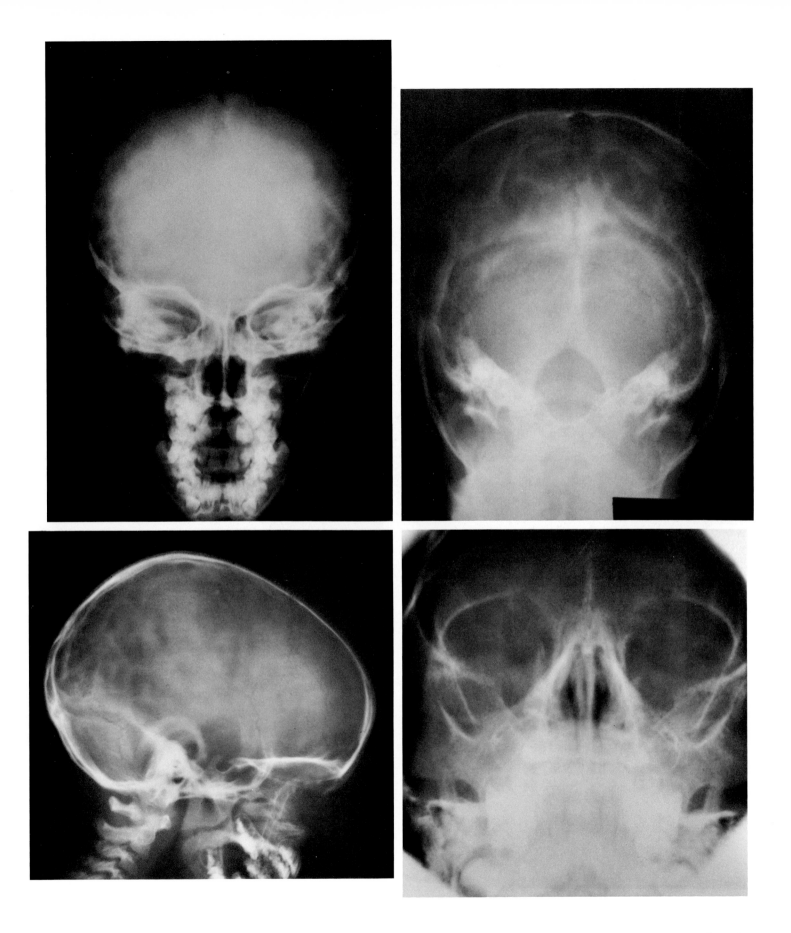

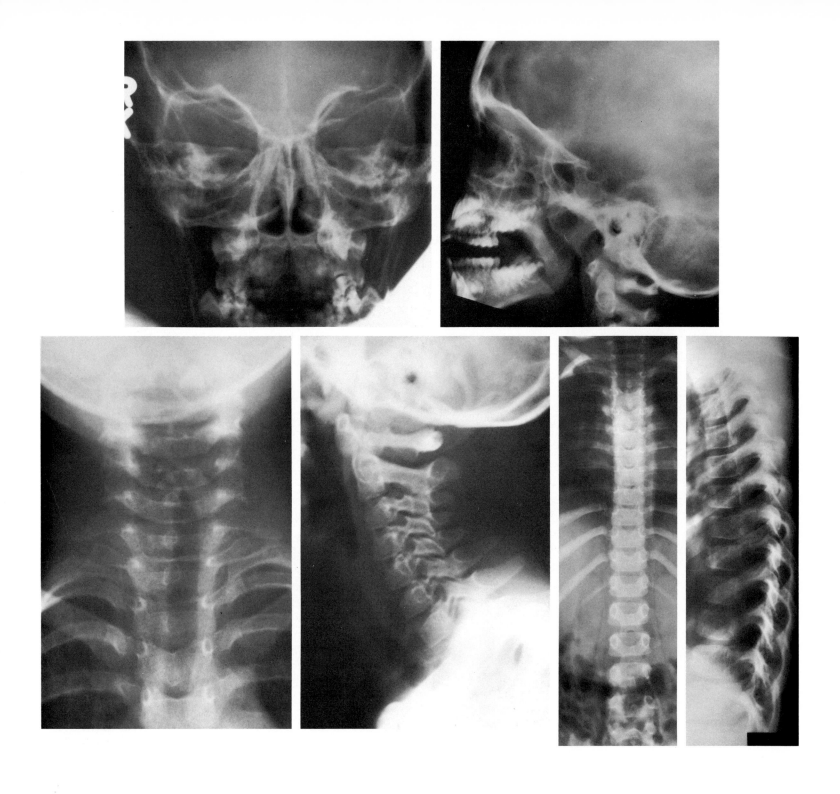

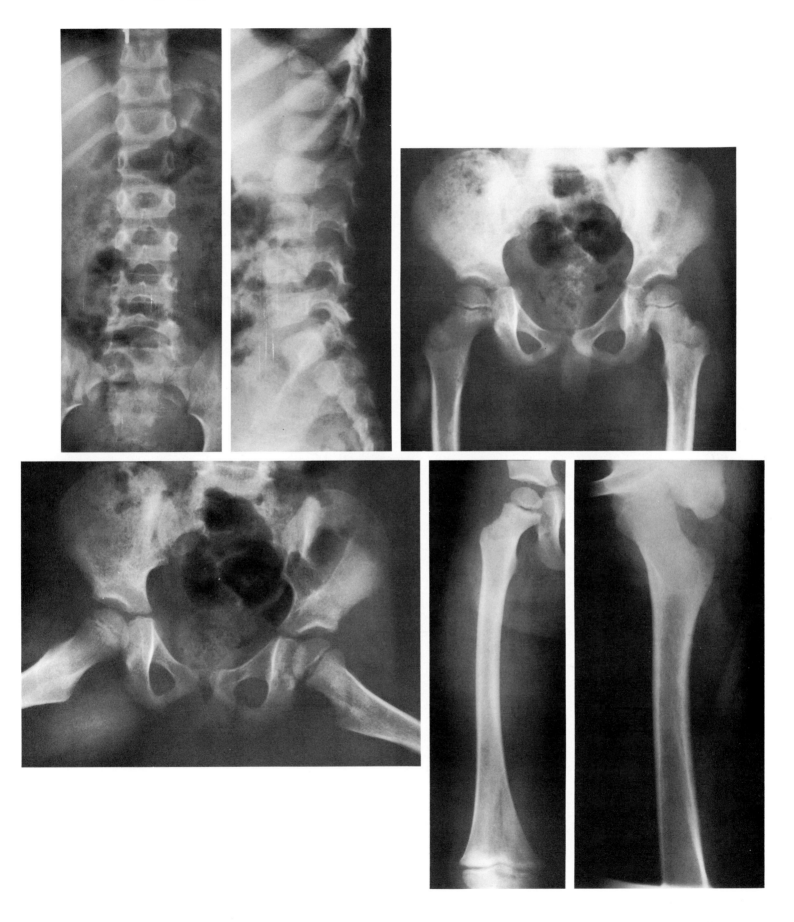

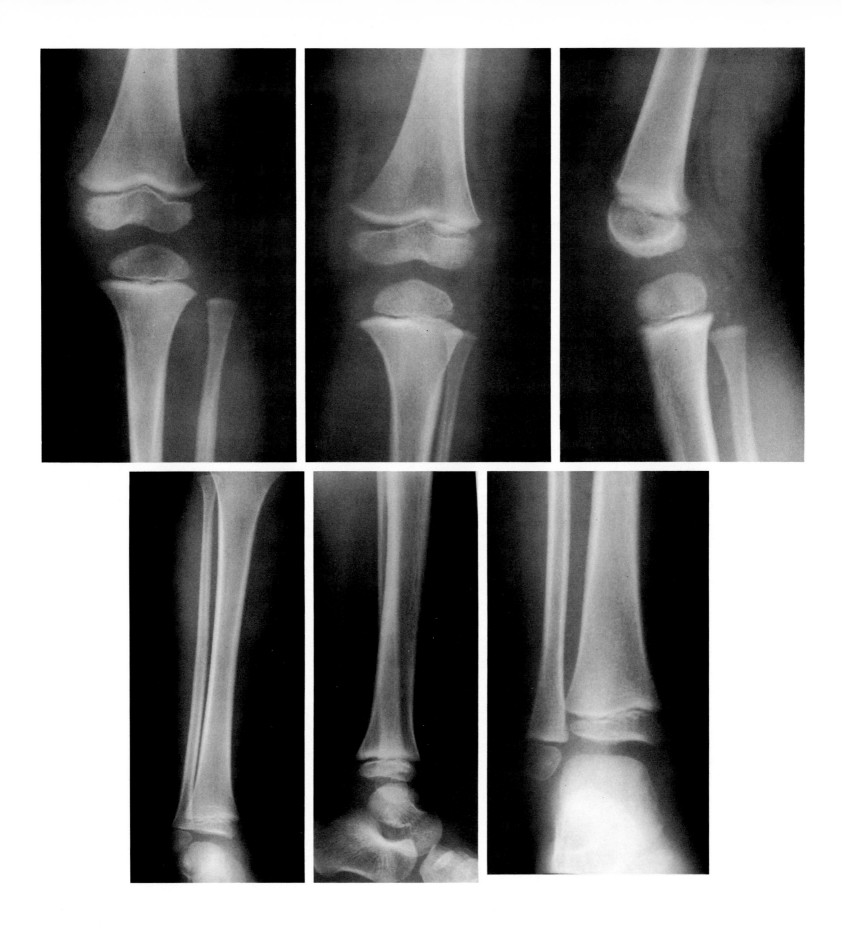

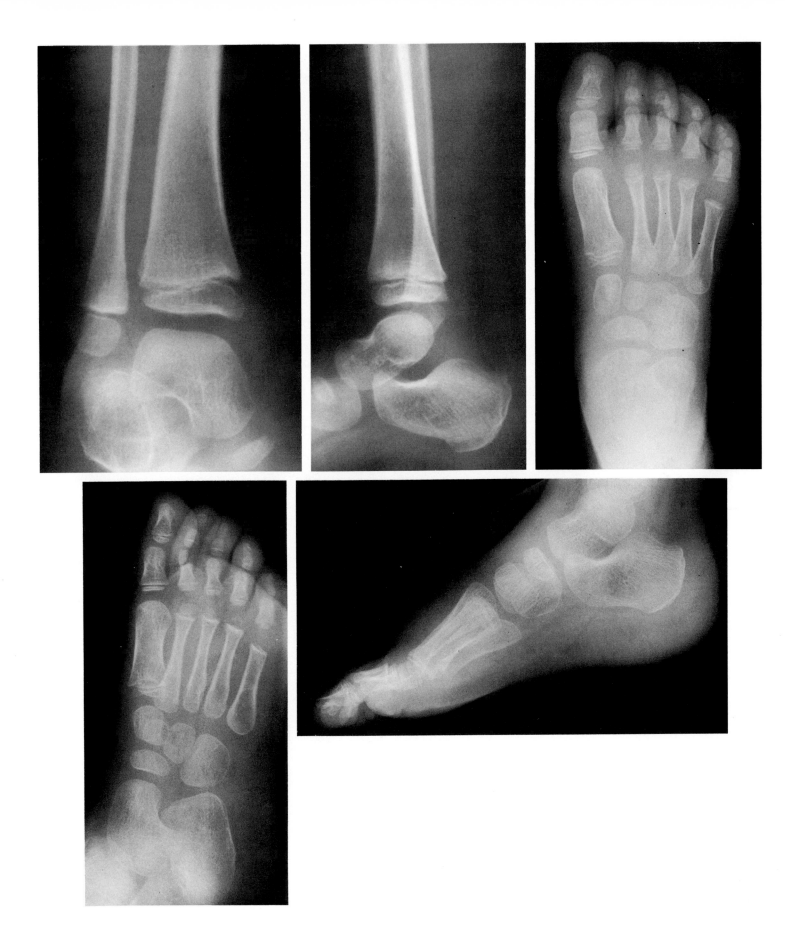

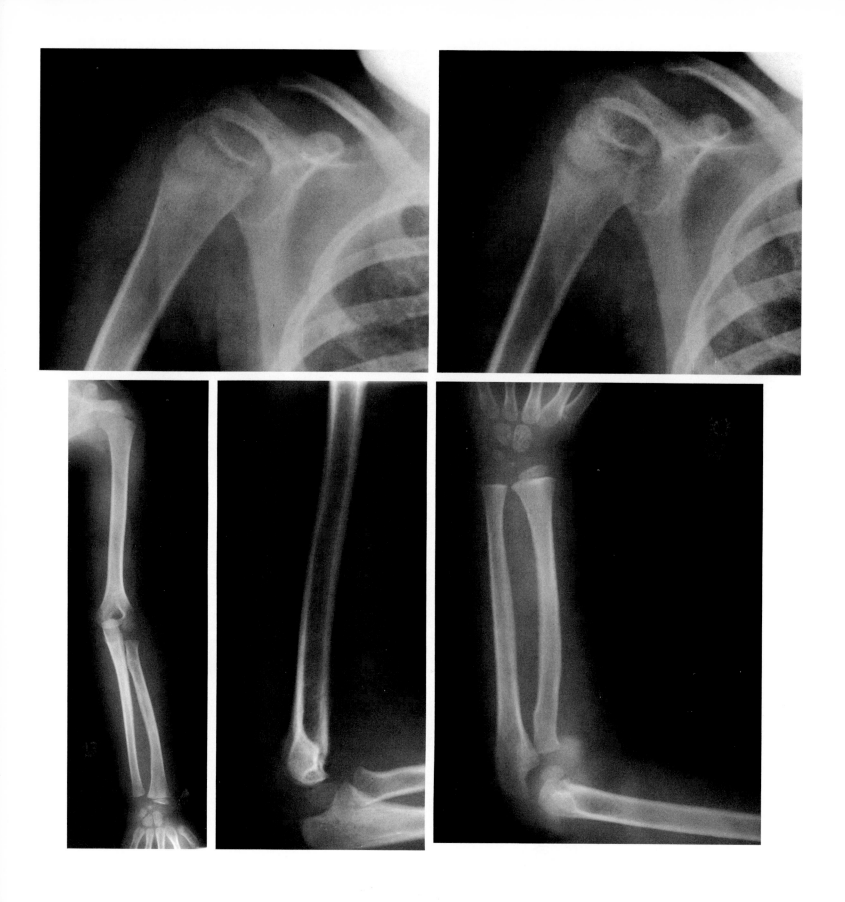

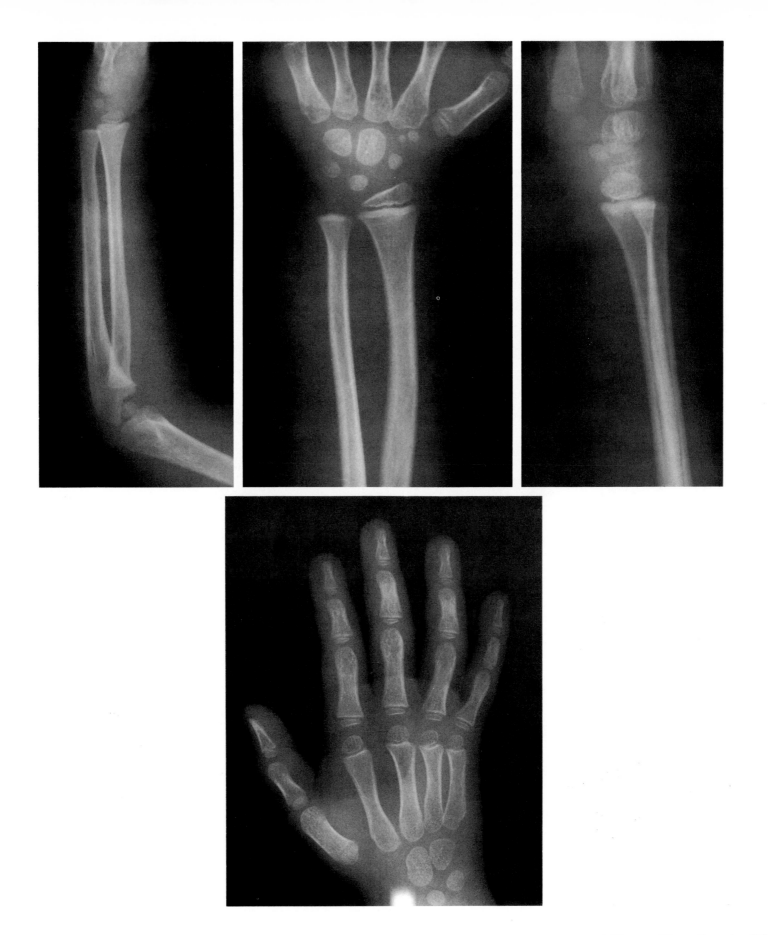

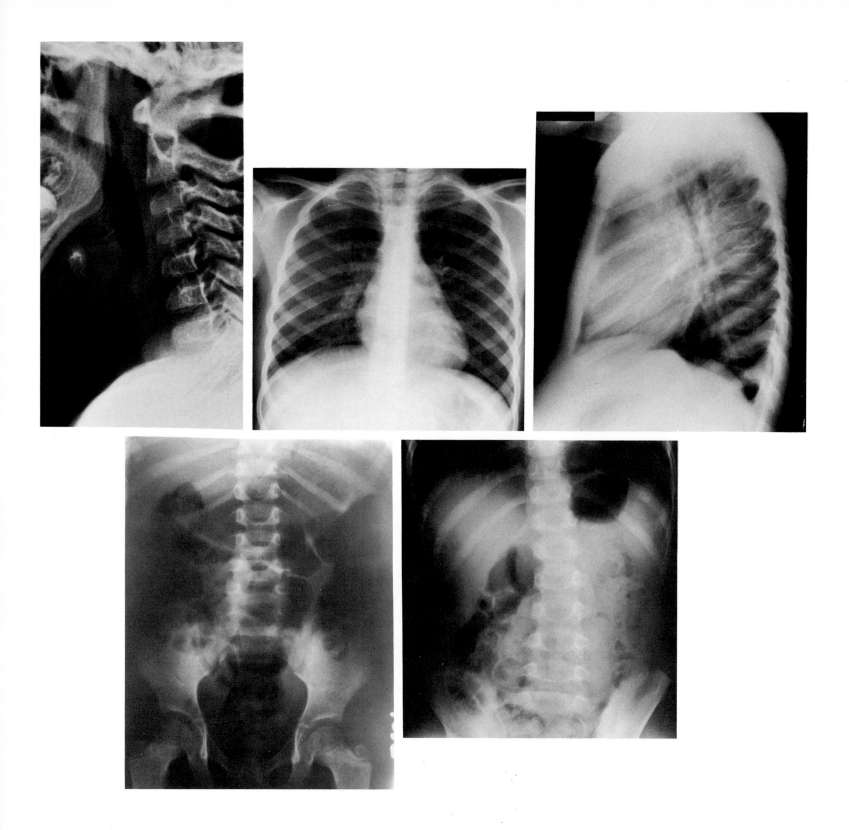

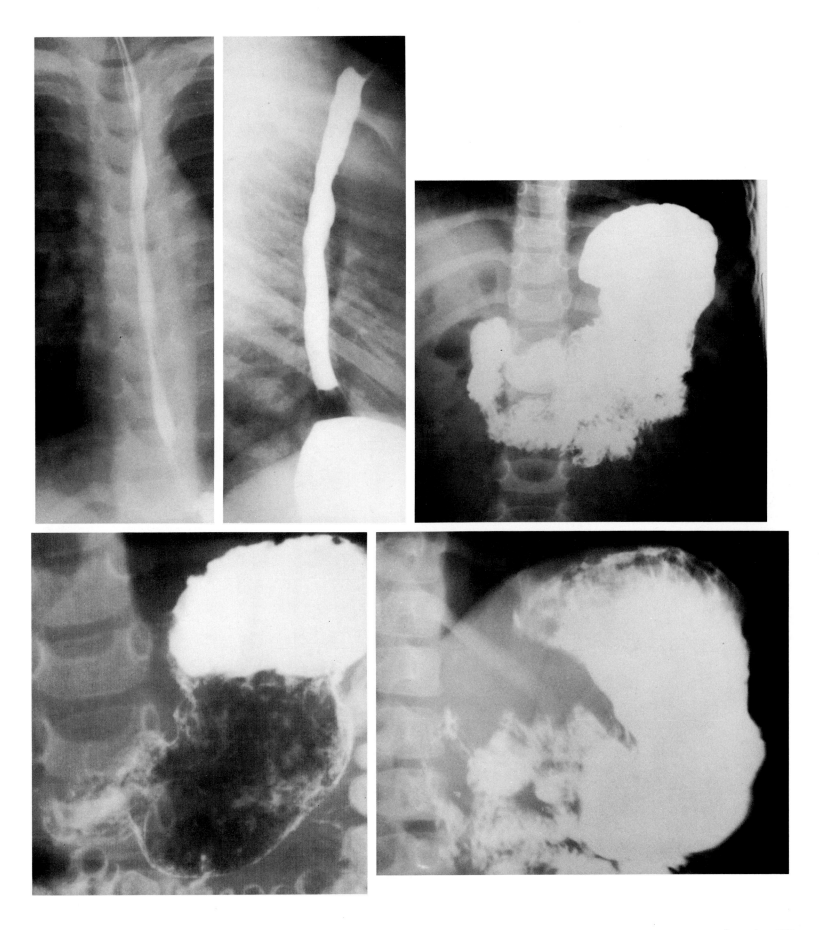

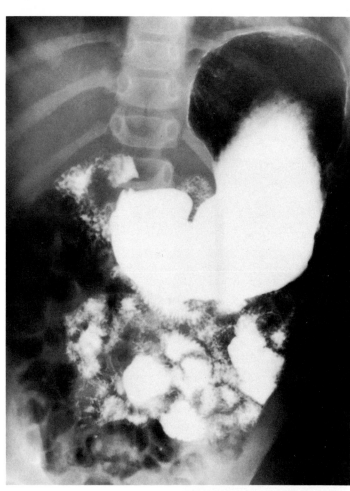
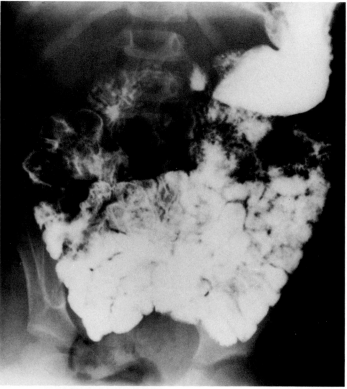
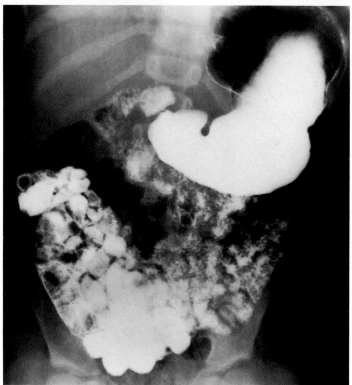

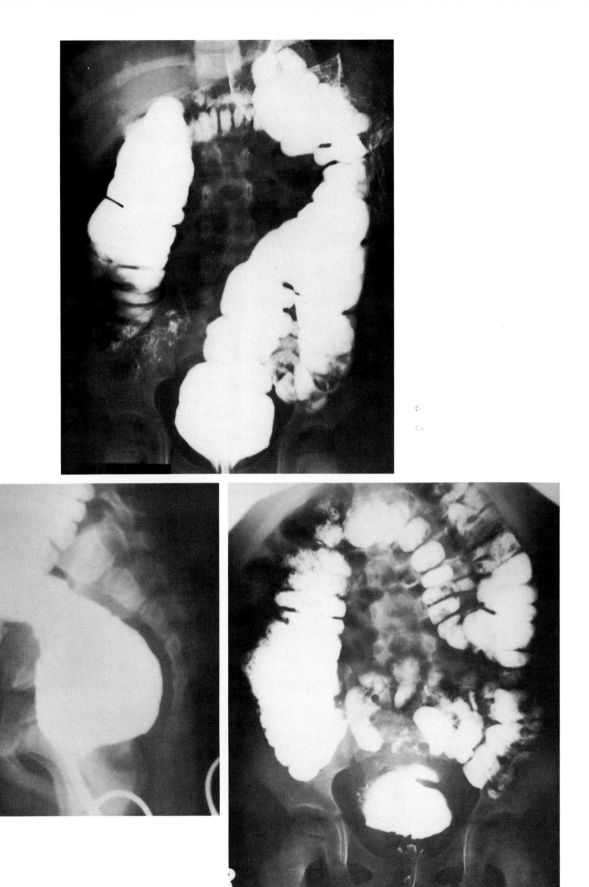

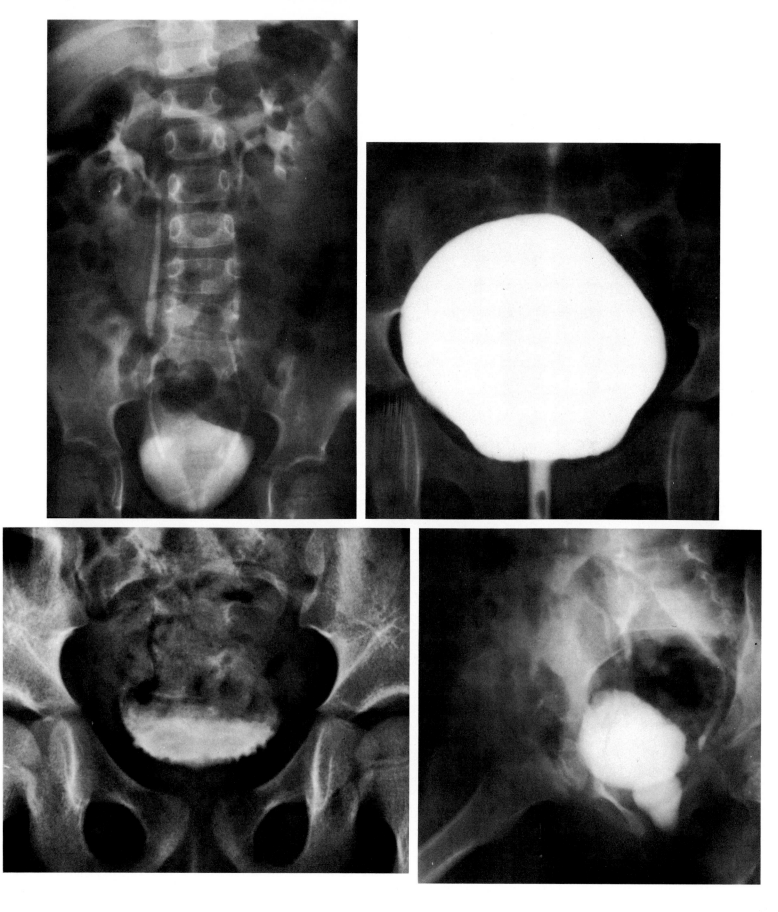

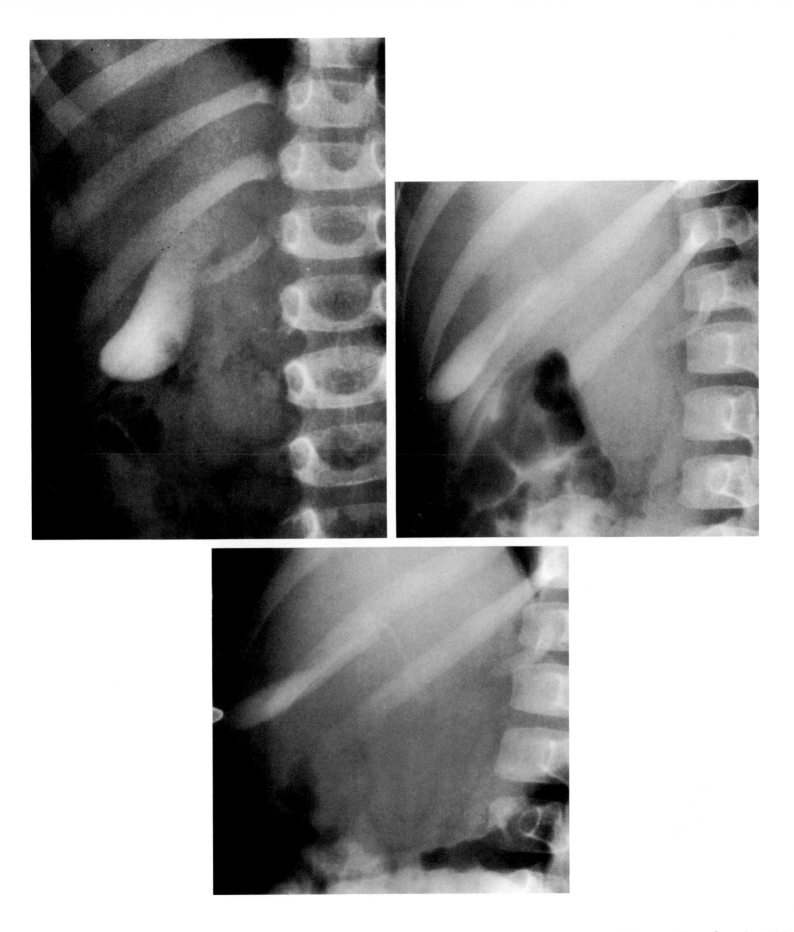

13

5 YEARS

The sphenoid sinus is enlarging. The cervical spinal proportions are now more adult-like. The cervical vertebrae are wedge-shaped. The anterior surfaces of the vertebrae are starting to show a rectangular plateau-like extension with notches above and below the point at which the ring apophyses will appear. Irregularity of the posterior aspect of the distal femoral metaphyses may be evident. The distal femoral epiphysis has a smoother contour and is larger than the metaphysis. This is also true of the distal tibial epiphysis. The intercondylar notch of the distal femur appears. There is an elevation in the adjacent portion of the distal femoral epiphysis. The differences in ossification of the hand and wrist between the male and female are less marked. The capital humeral epiphysis covers the metaphysis. The epiphysis of the radial head appears. The sternal ossification centers are large, but still discrete.

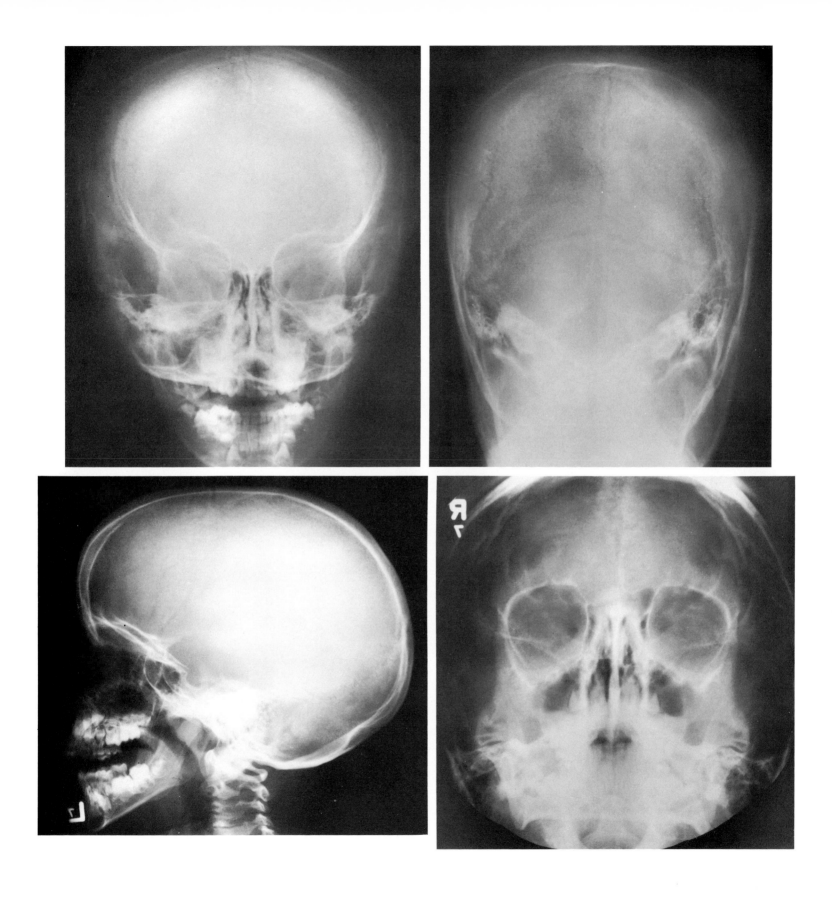

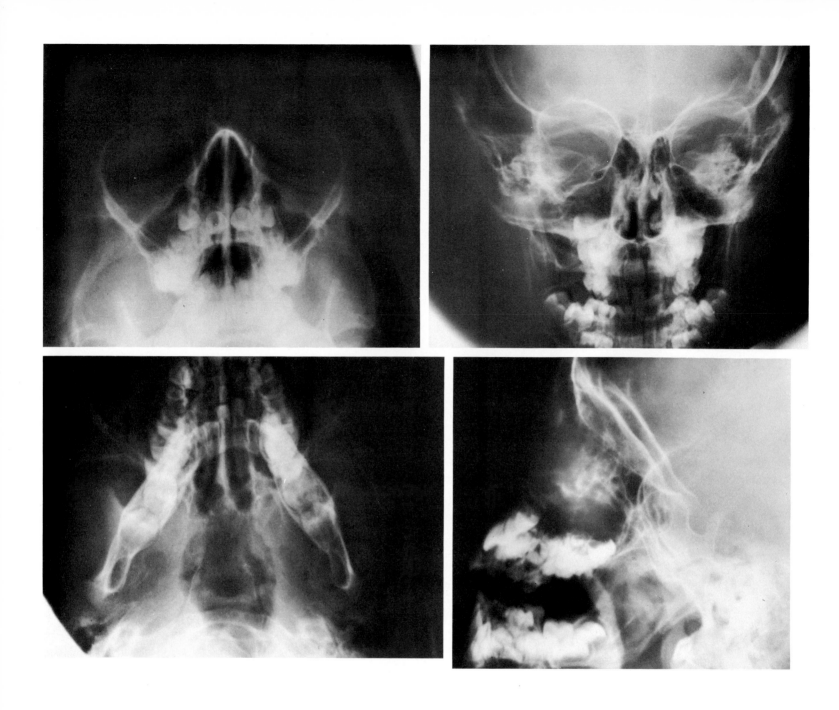

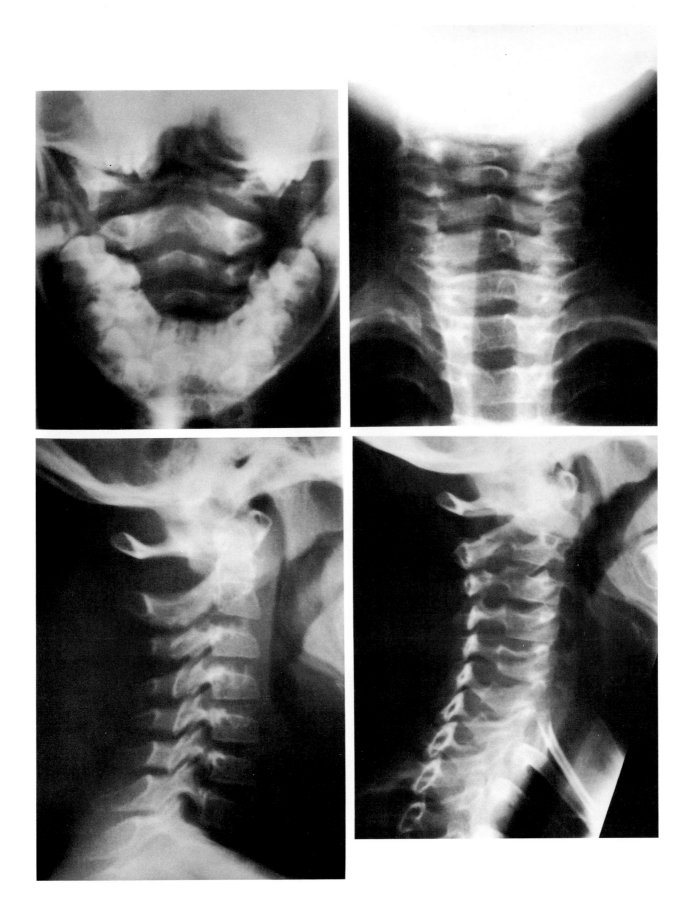

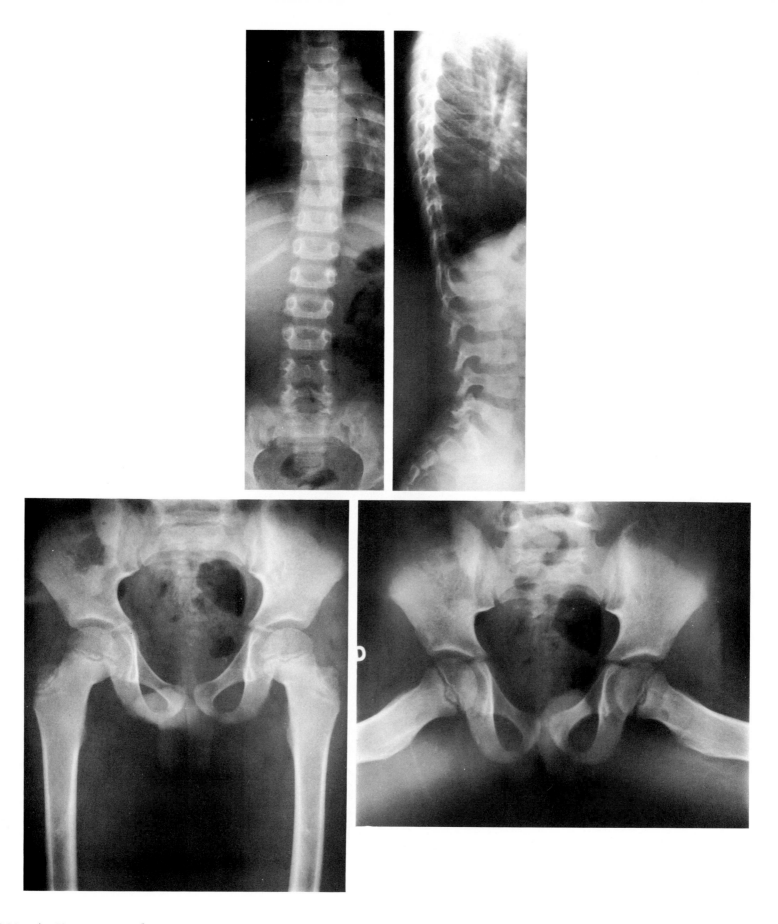

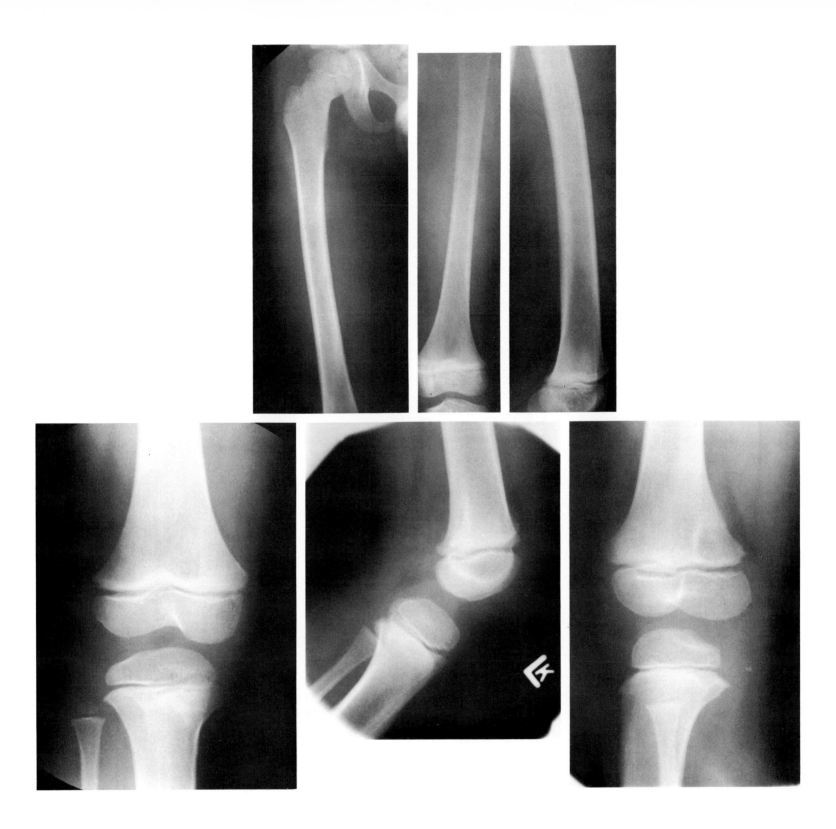

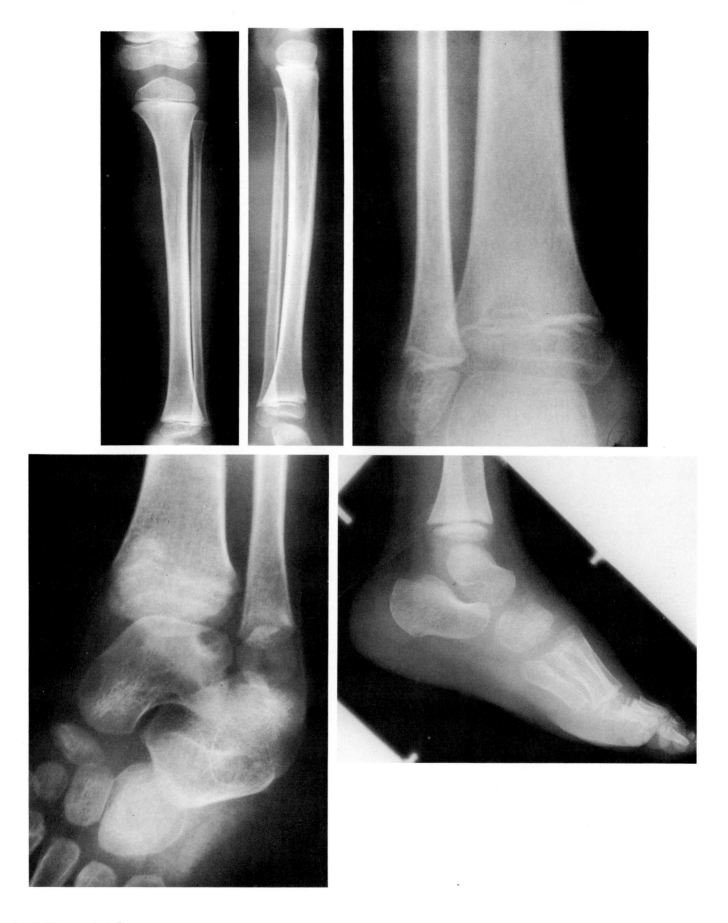

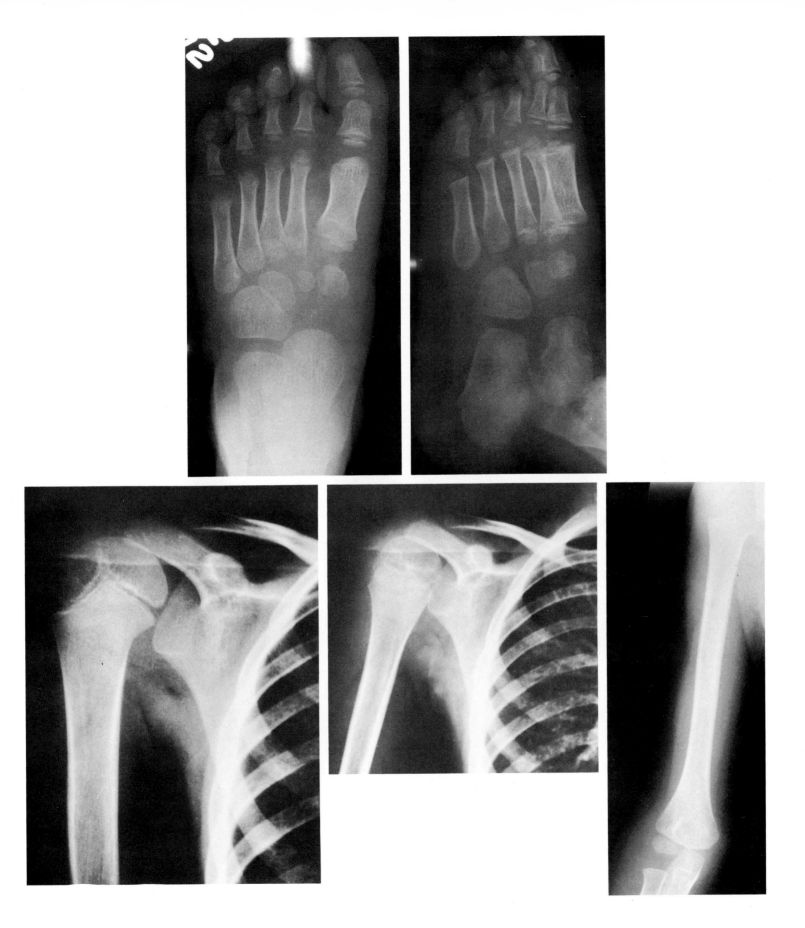

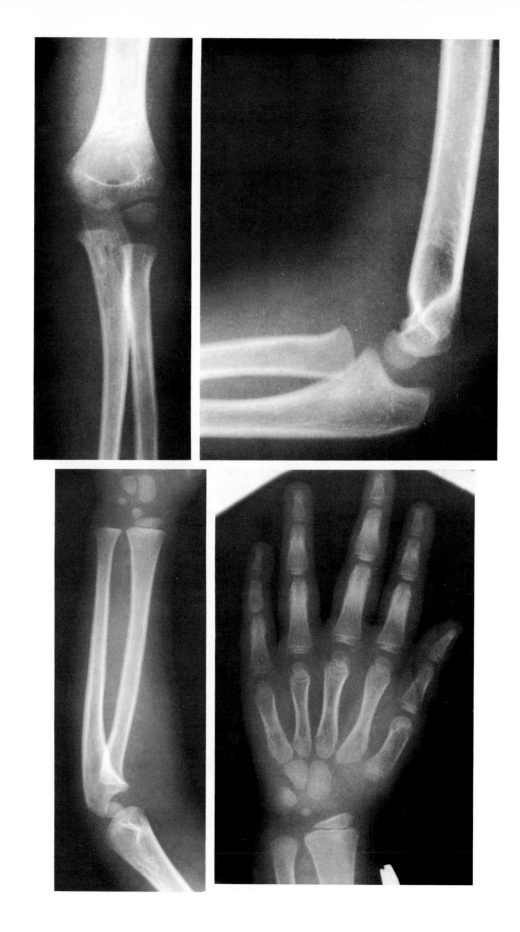

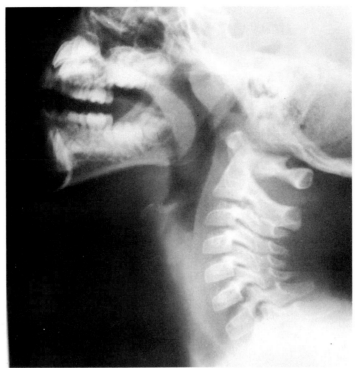

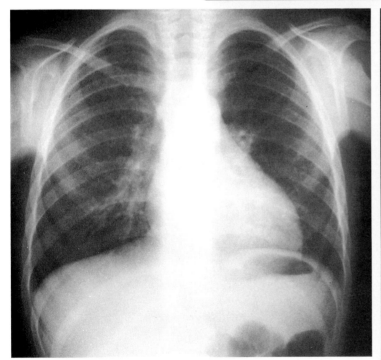

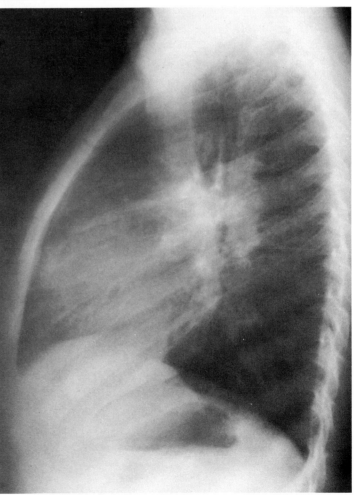

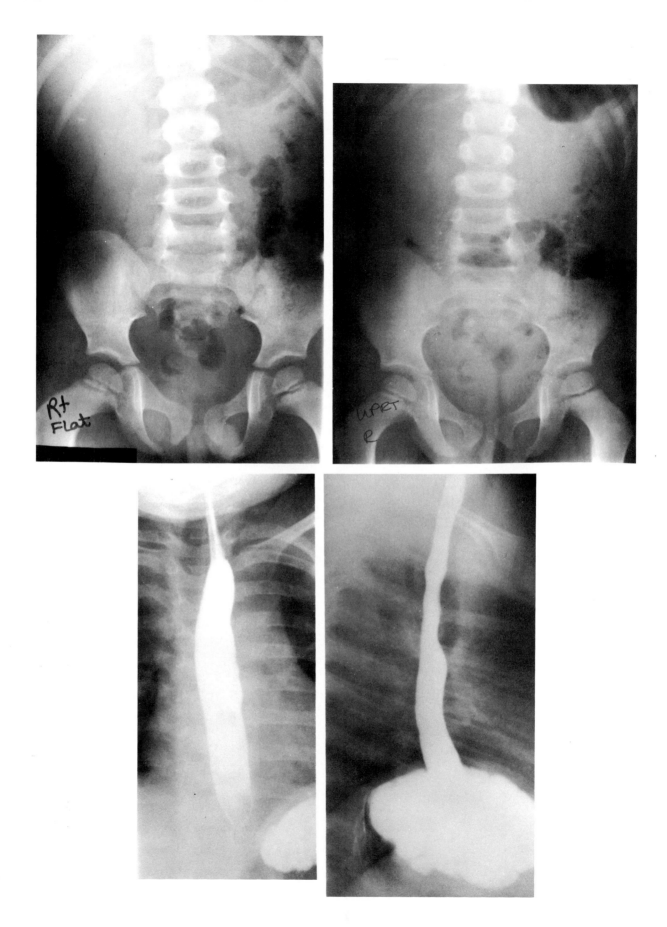

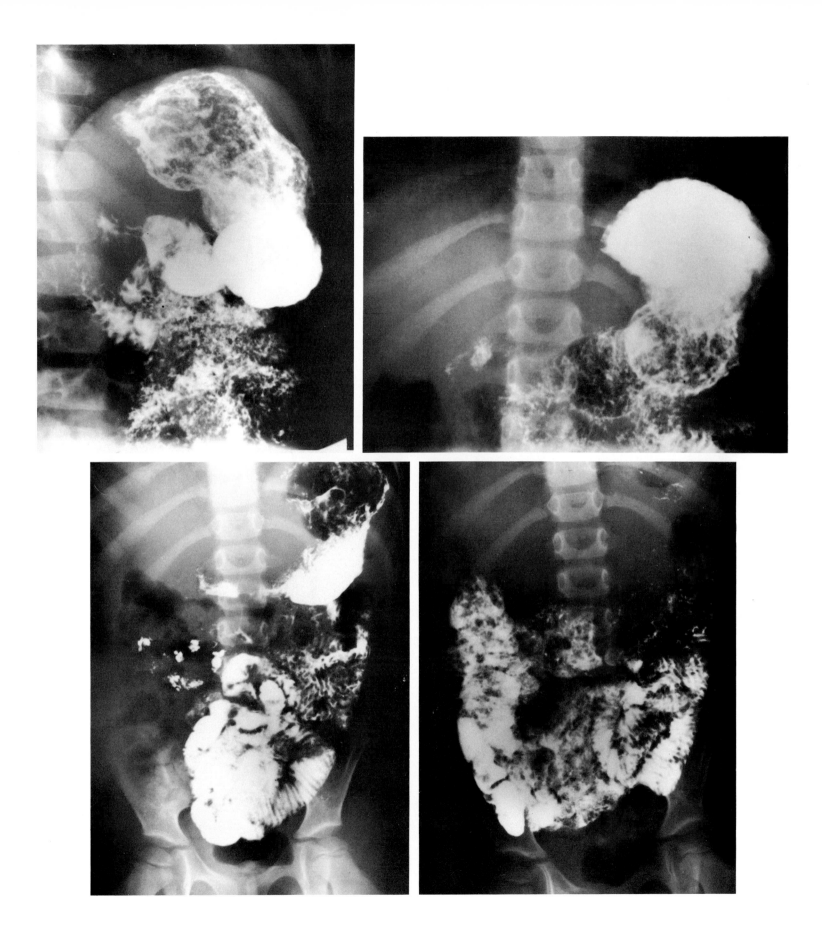

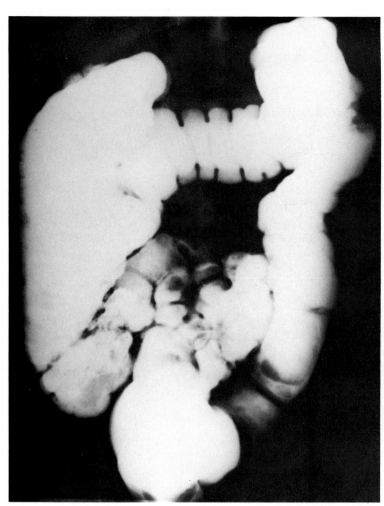 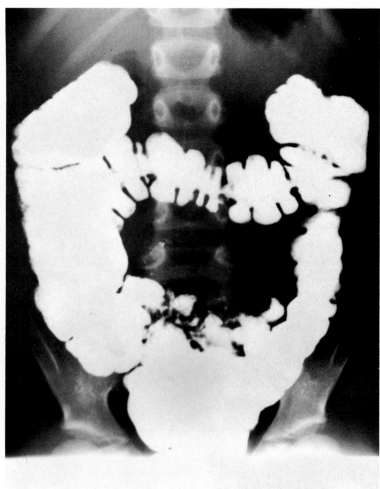

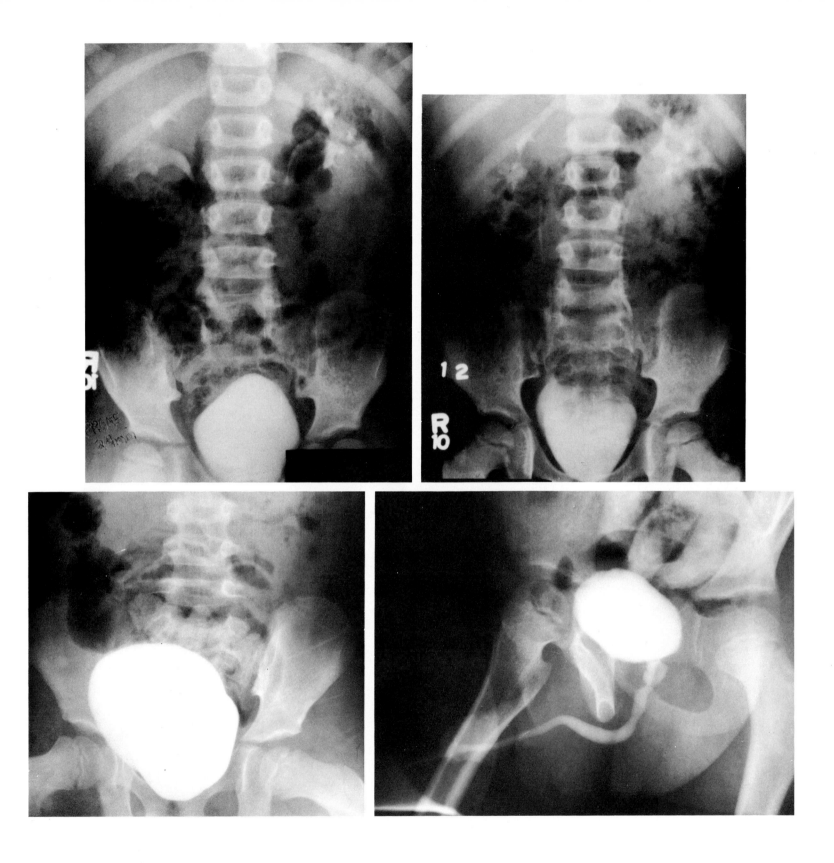

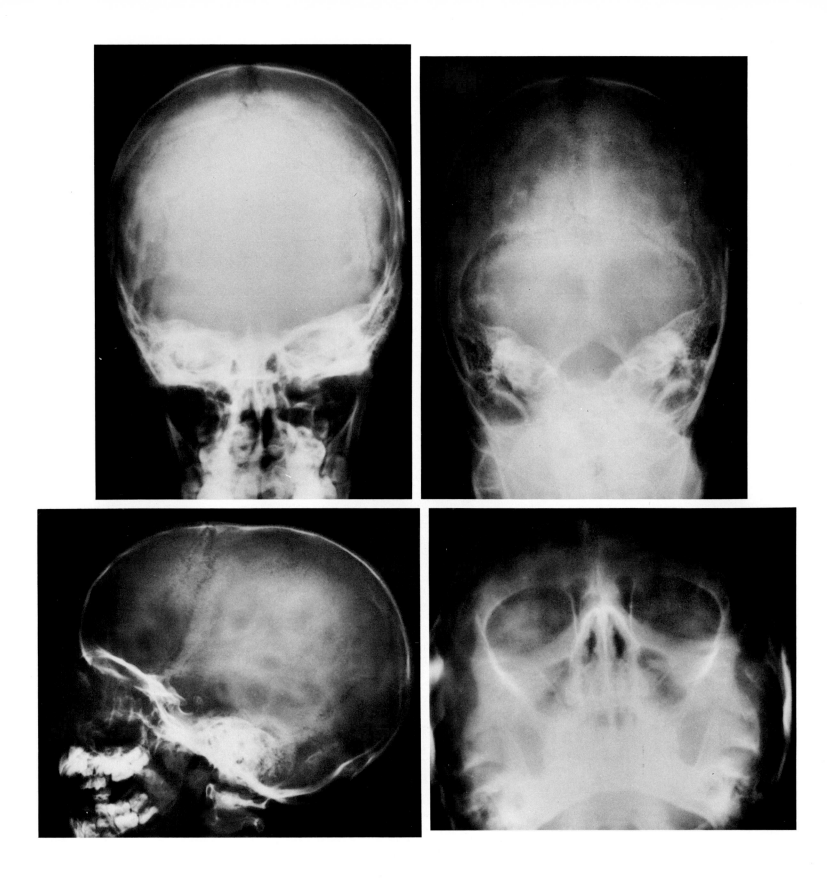

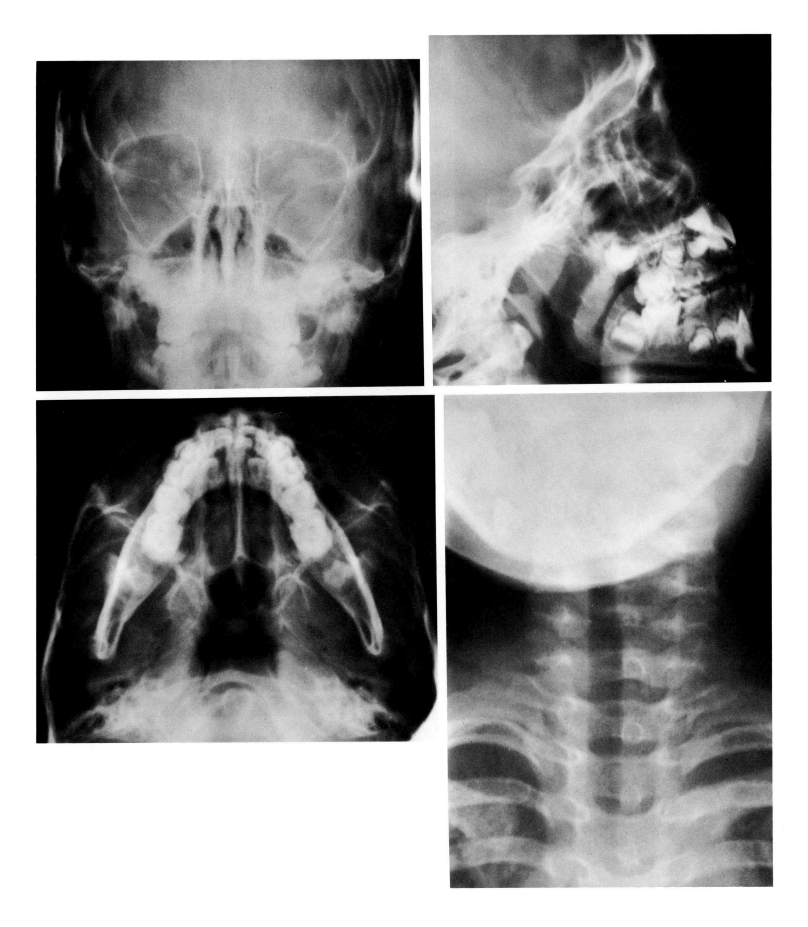

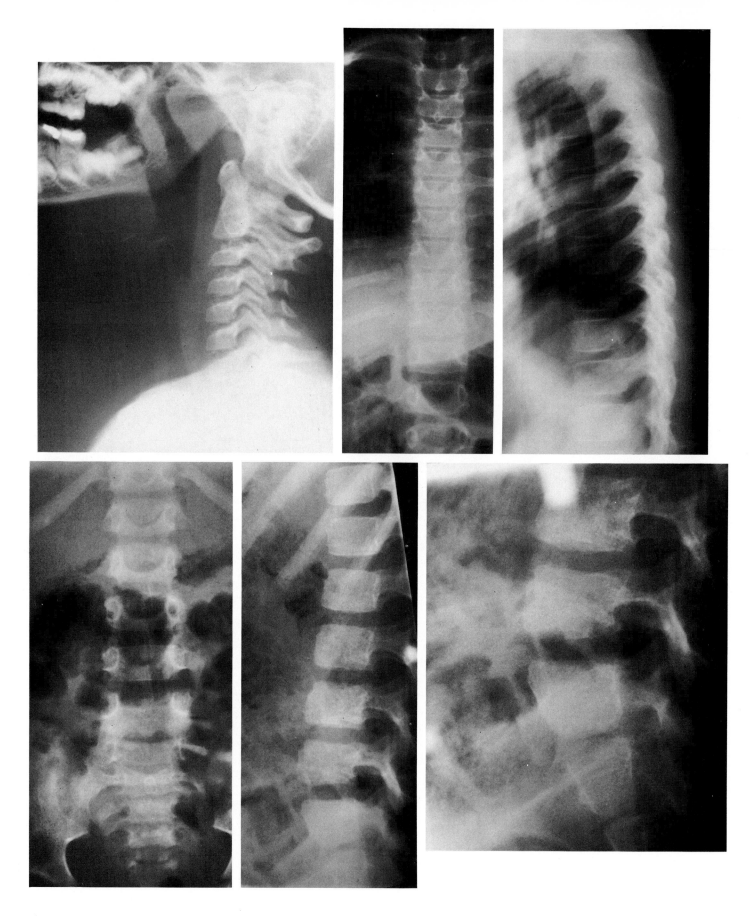

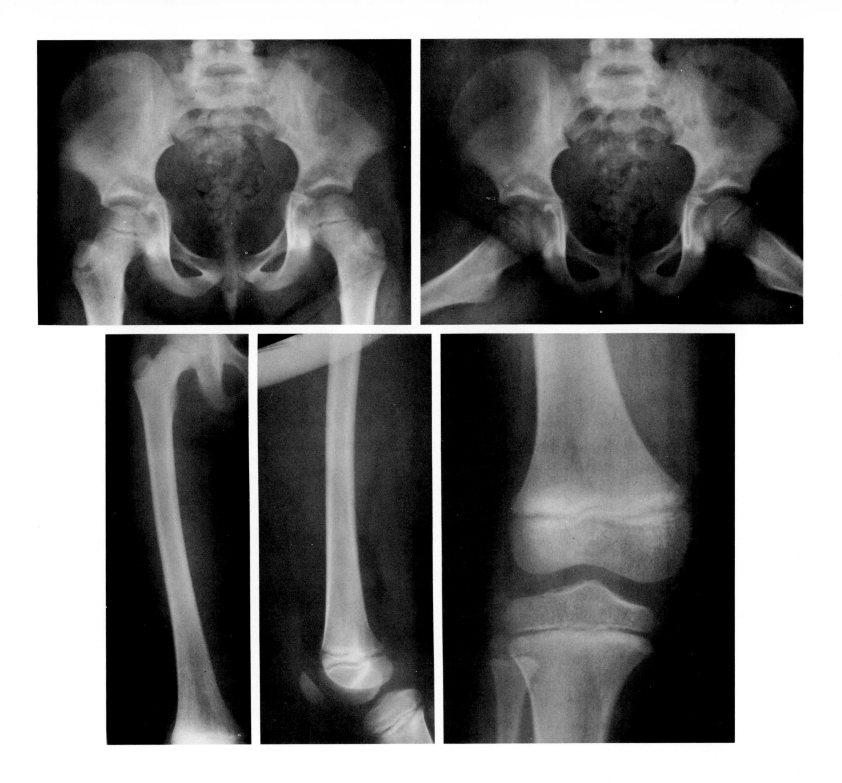

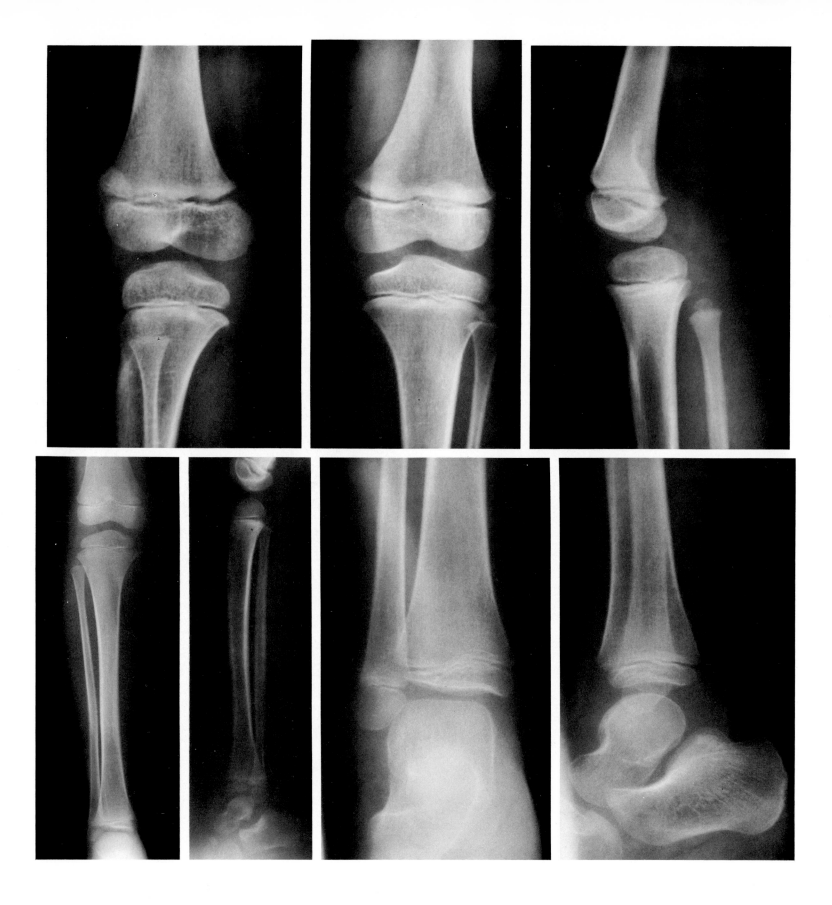

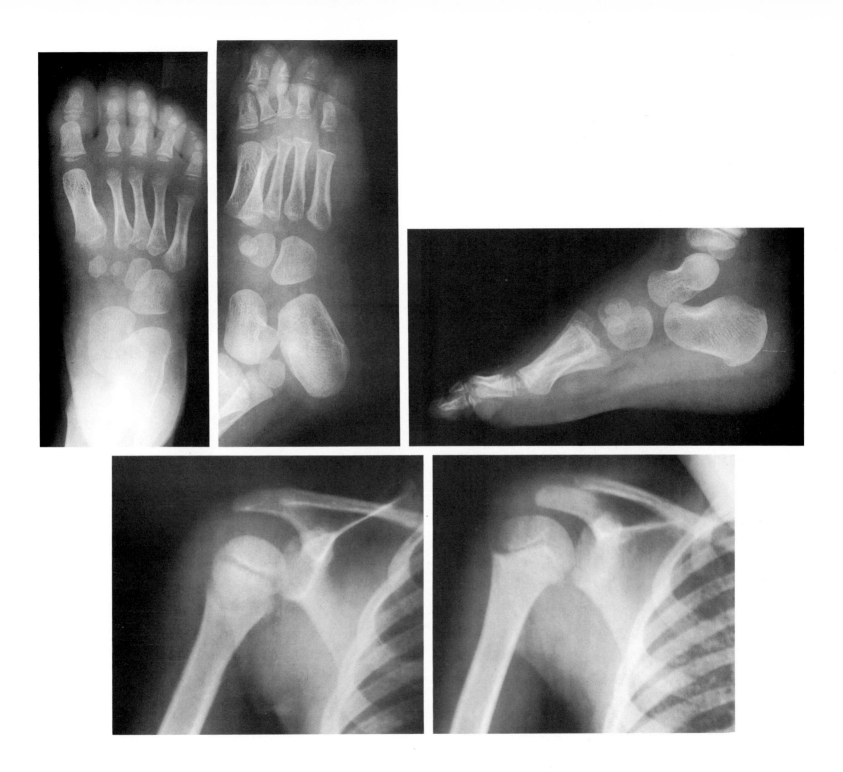

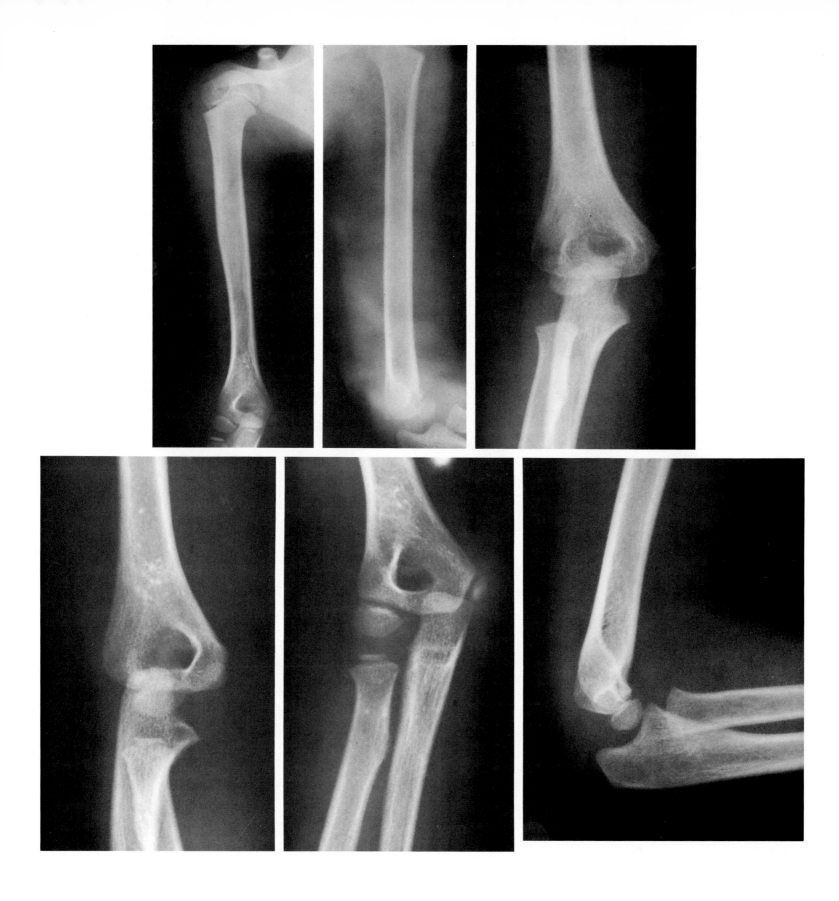

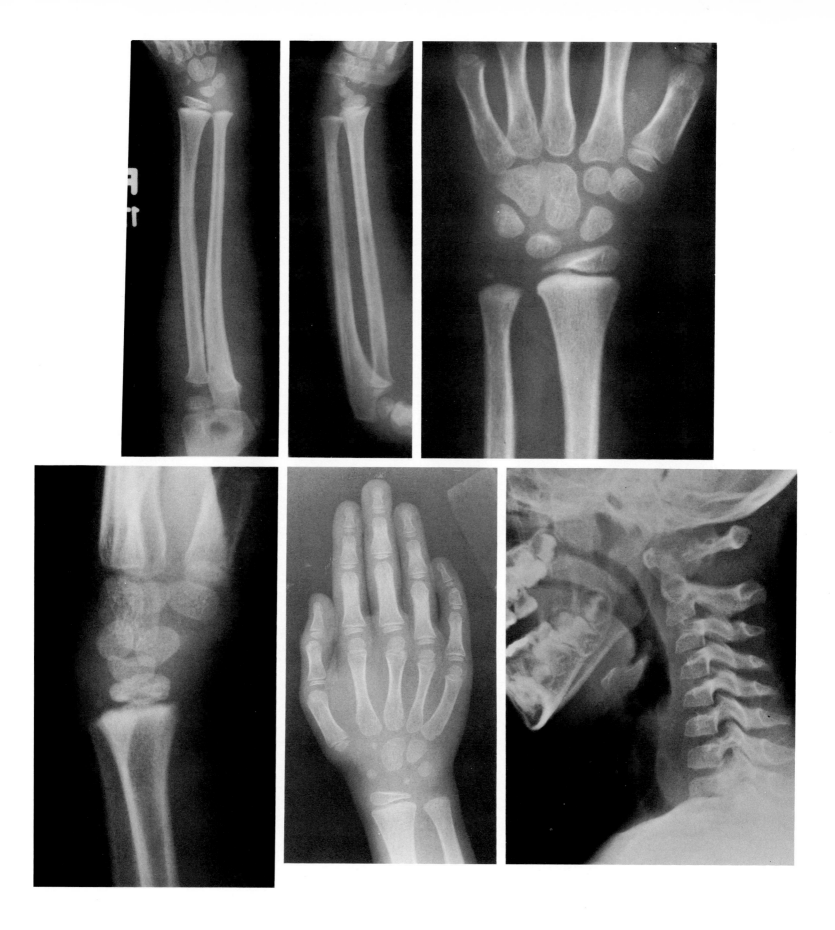

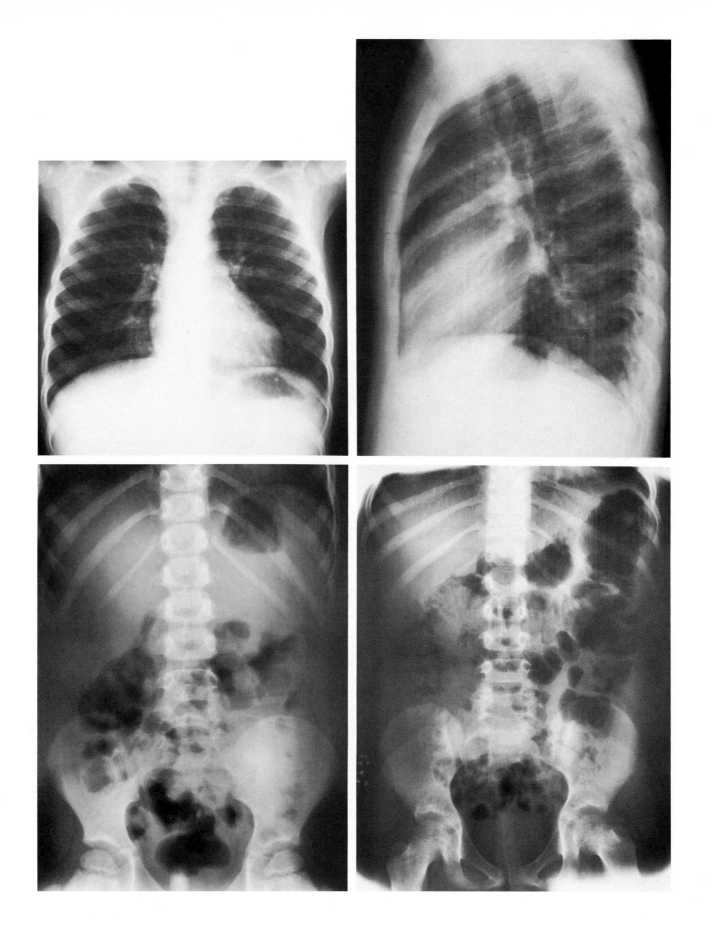

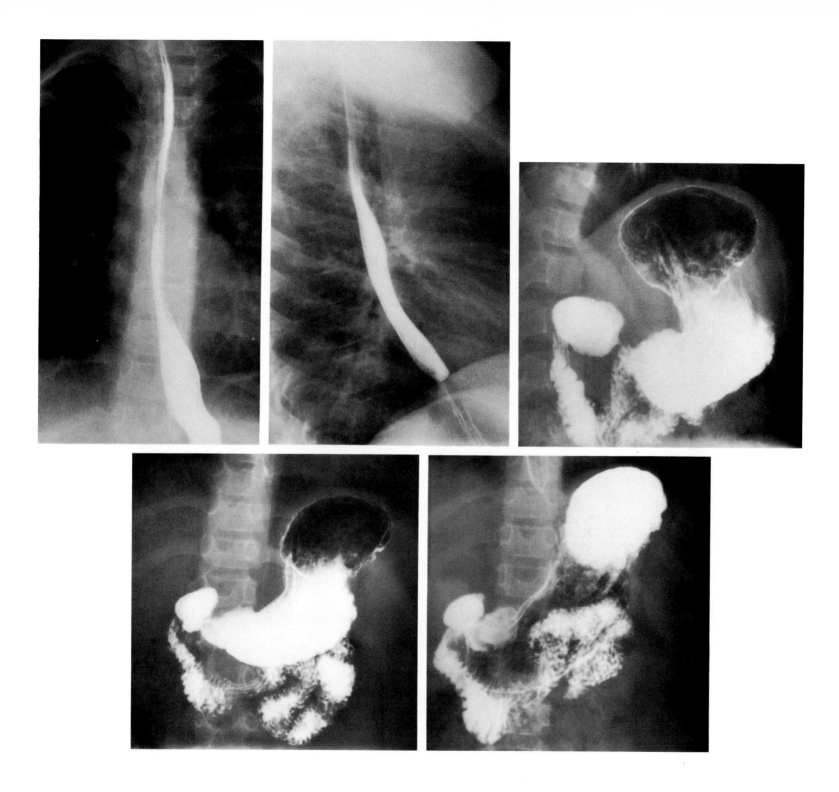

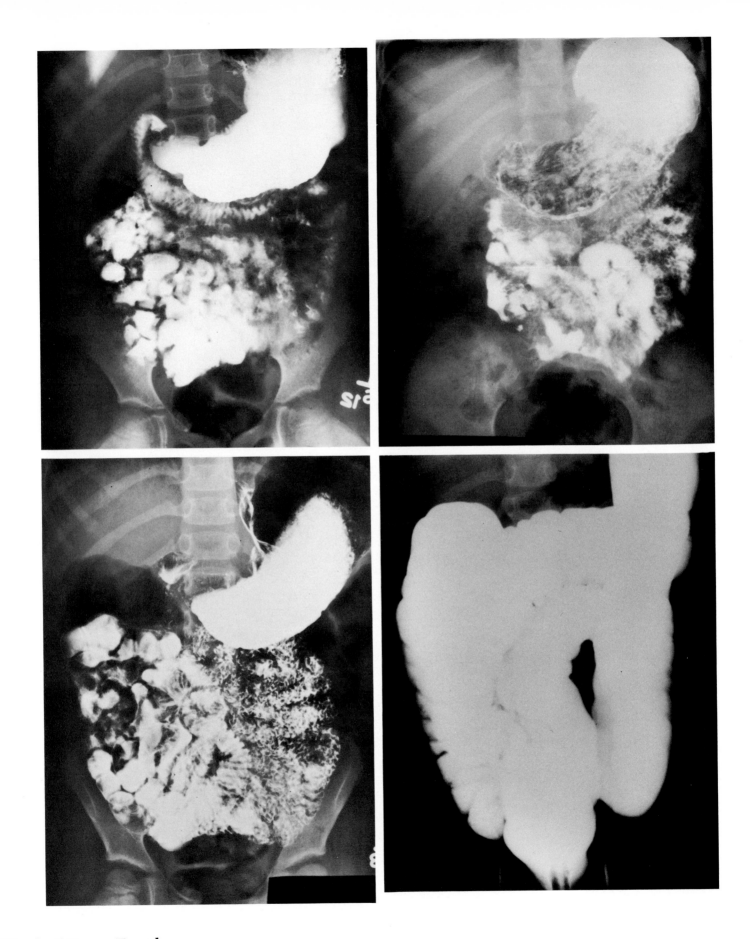

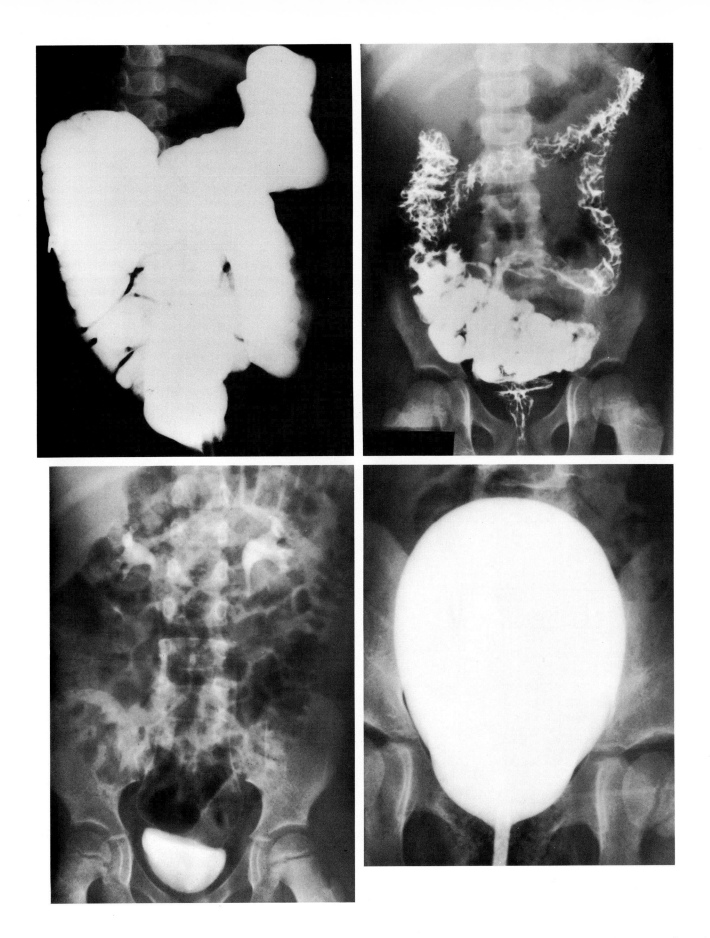

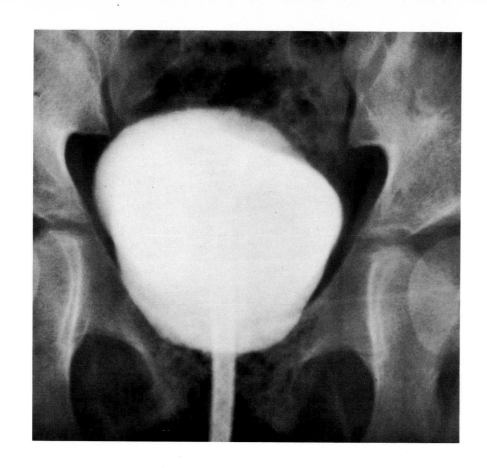

14

6 YEARS

The sphenoid sinus is half pneumatized. The calvariam still shows prominent digital markings. There is an indentation on the superior aspect of the medial surface of the proximal tibial epiphysis that conforms to the enlarging medial condyle of the femurs. The medial malleolus of the tibia is not well formed. The capital humeral epiphysis is ball-shaped and is longer than the metaphysis. The hyoid bone is evident.

The cervical vertebrae appear less wedge-shaped. The prominences on the anterior surfaces of the vertebrae are more evident. The ischiopubic synchondroses are still open. The distal femoral metaphyseal irregularities are less apparent.

The distended urinary bladder does not extend beyond the bony pelvis at this age.

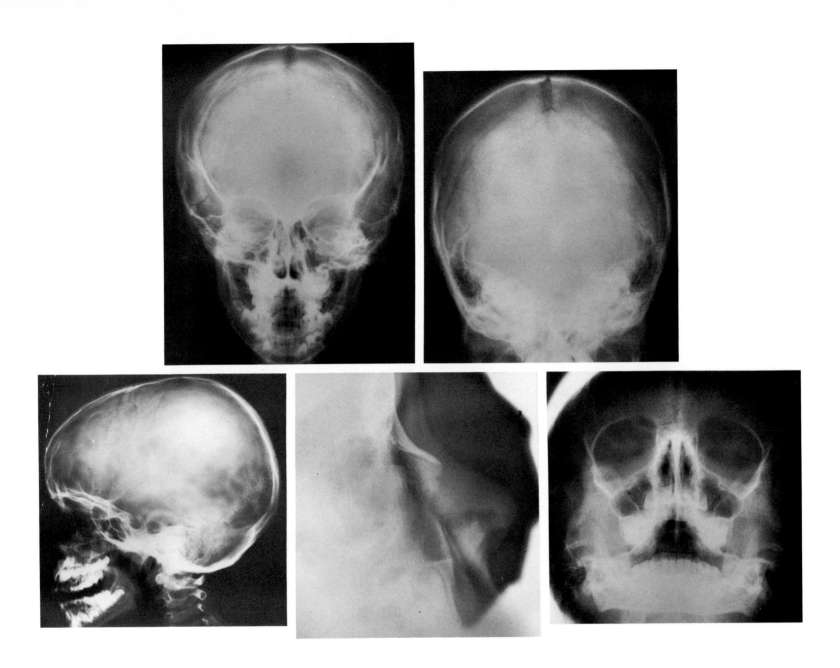

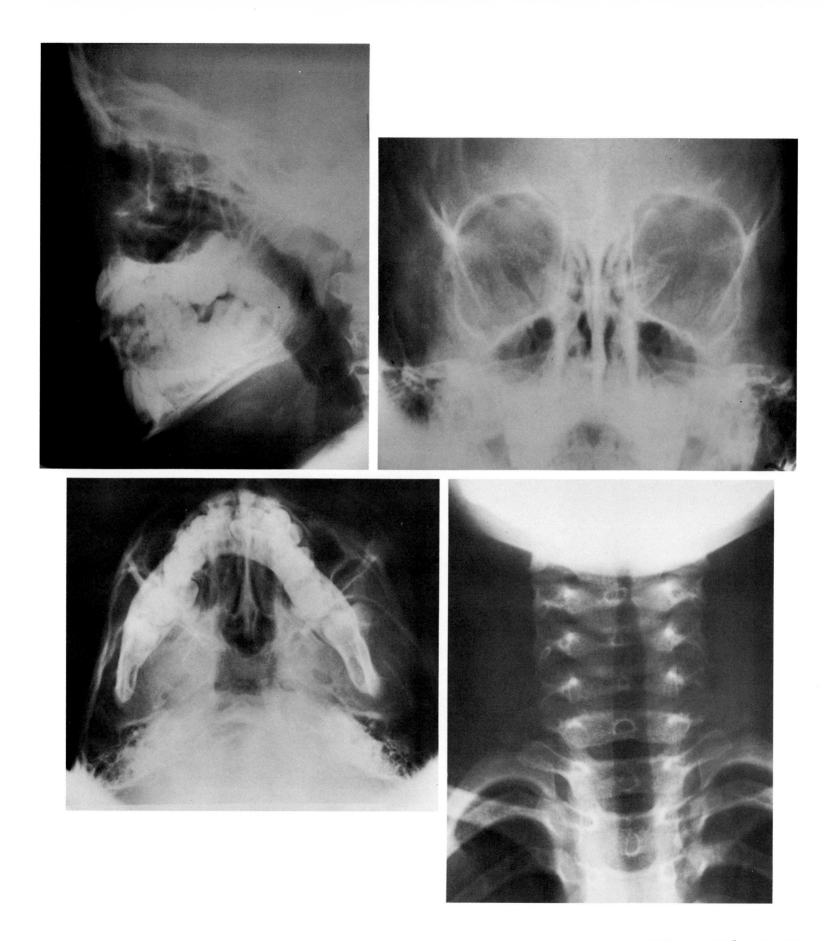

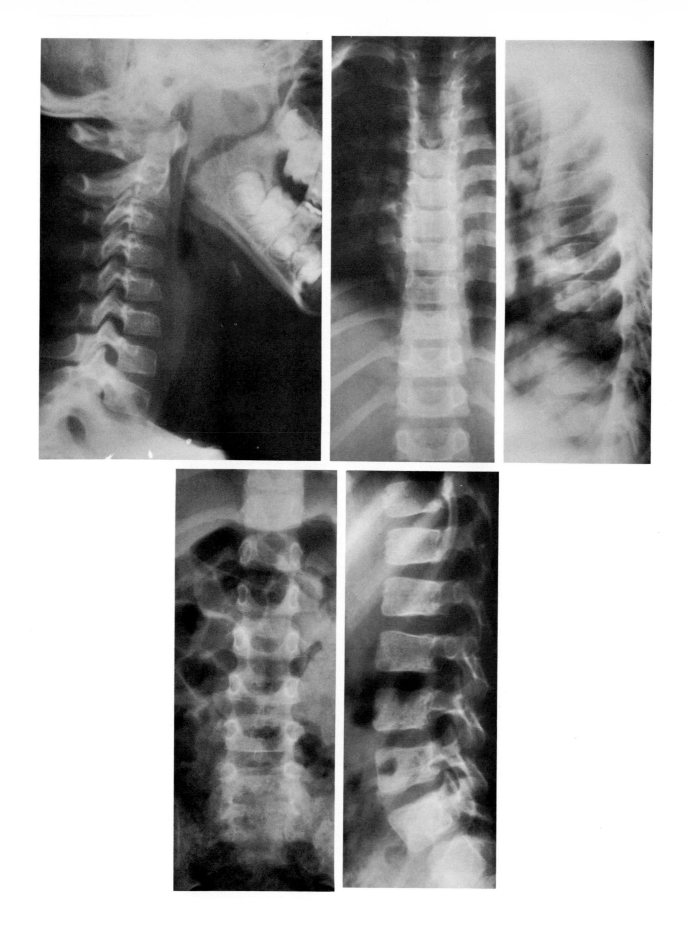

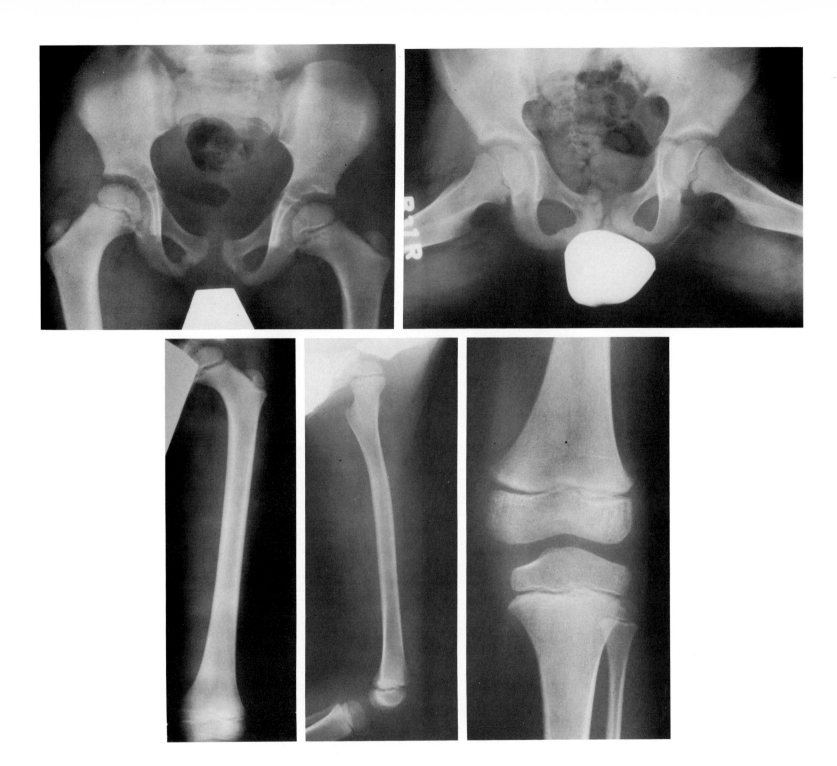

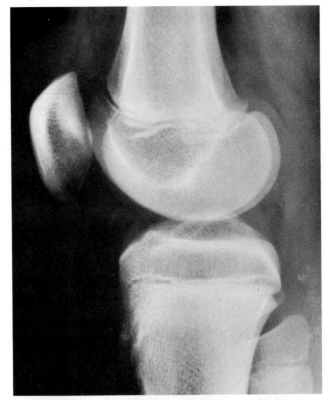

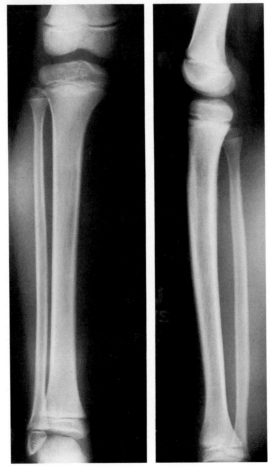

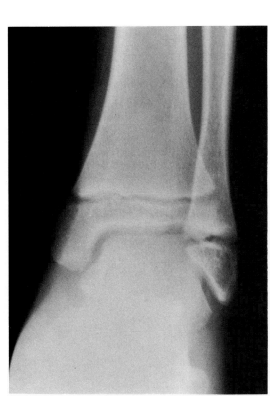
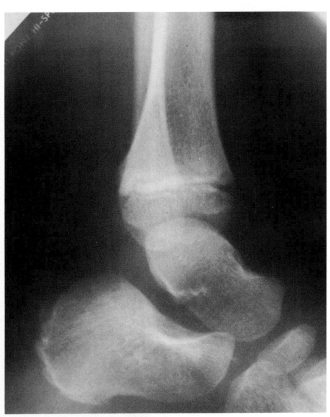
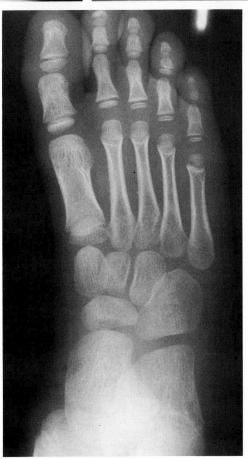

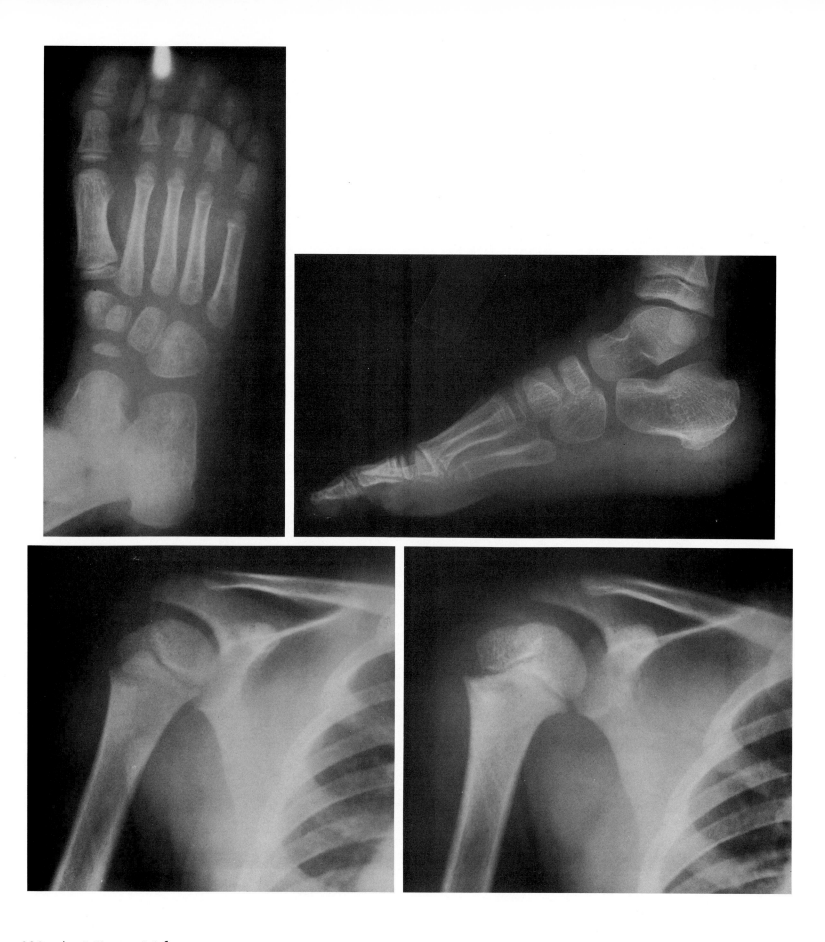

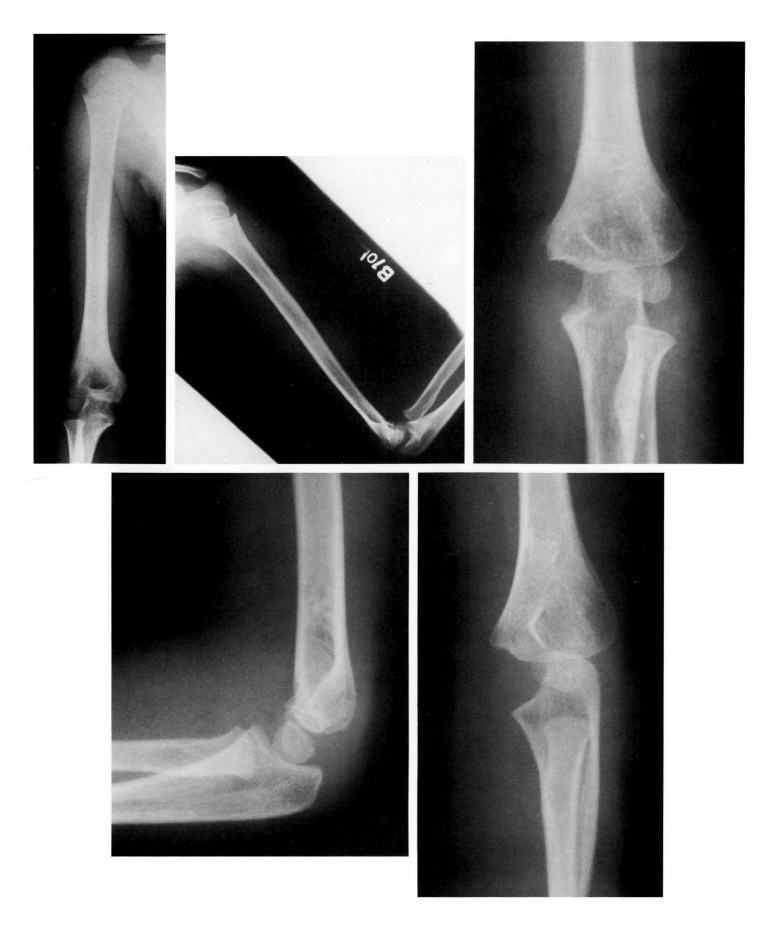

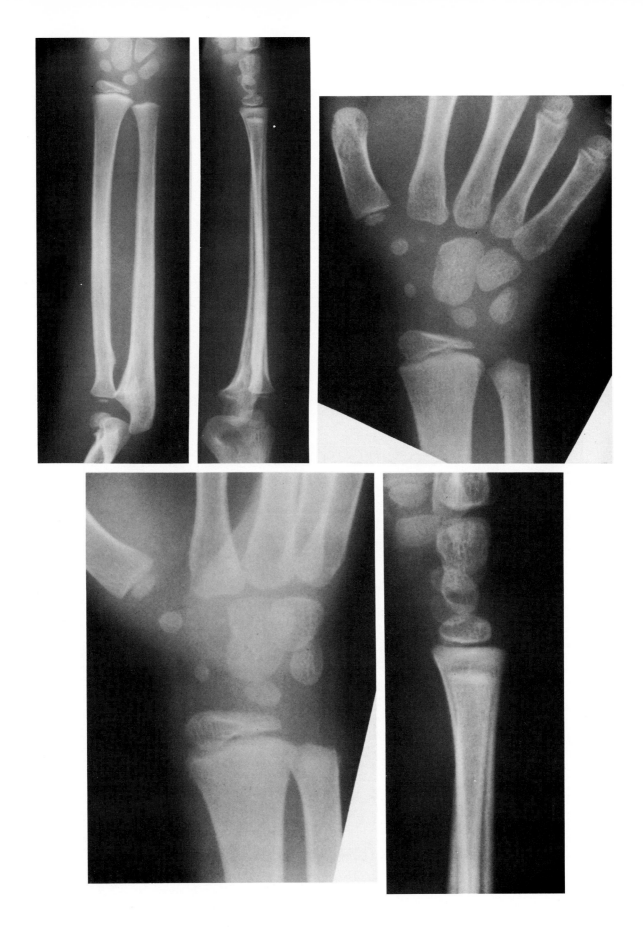

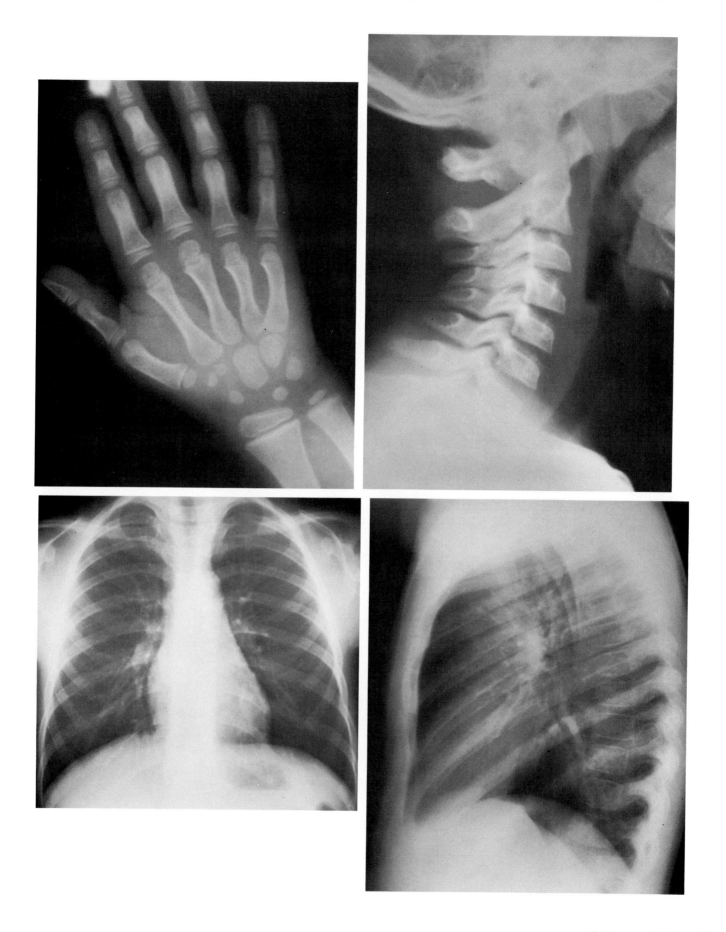

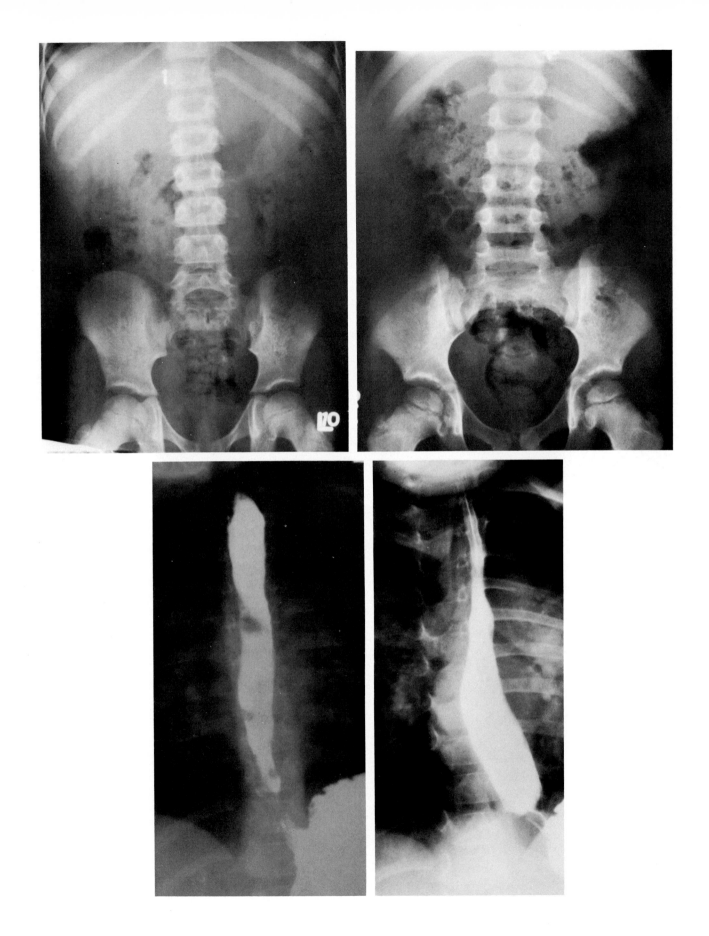

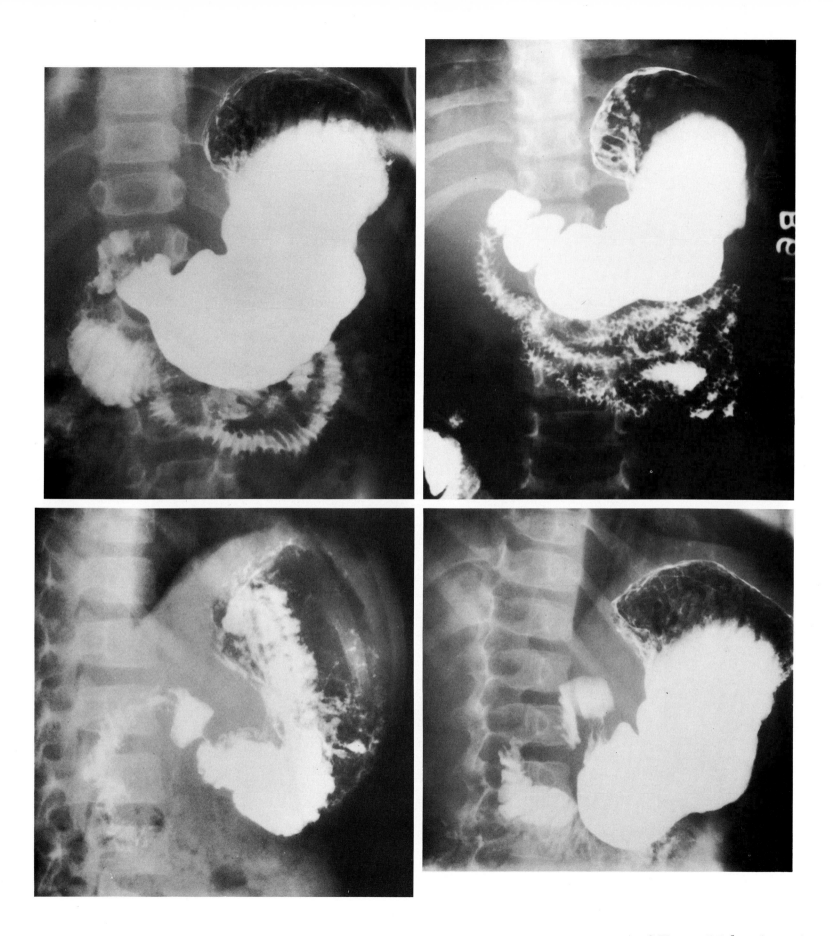

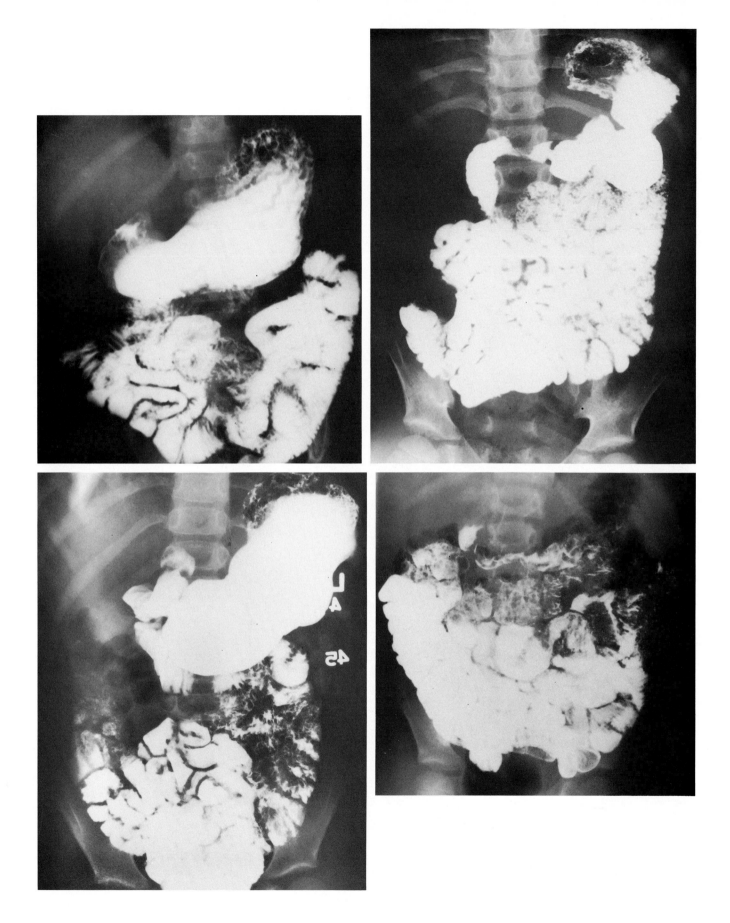

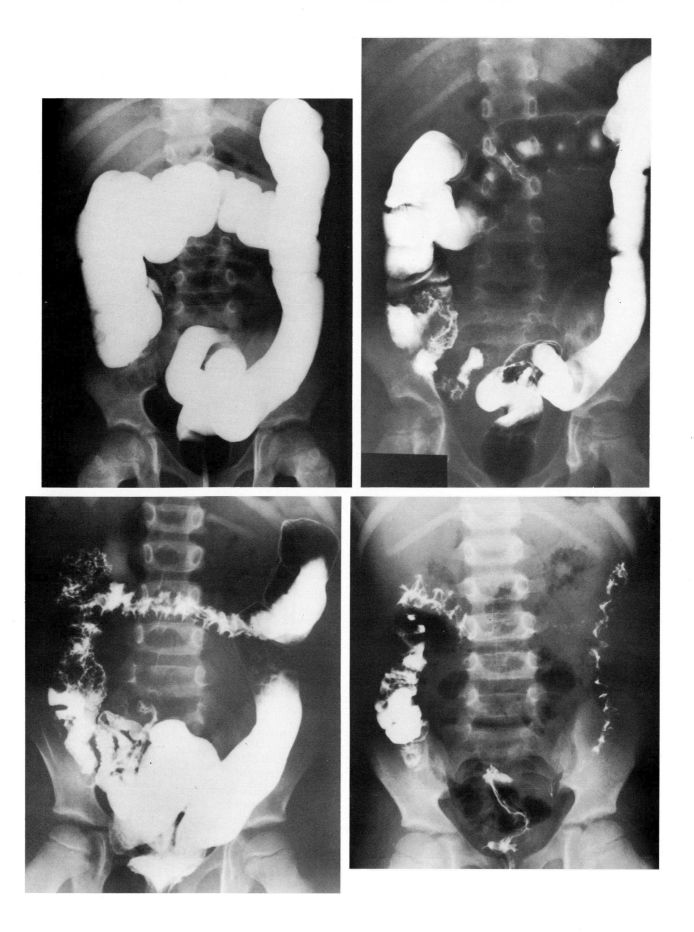

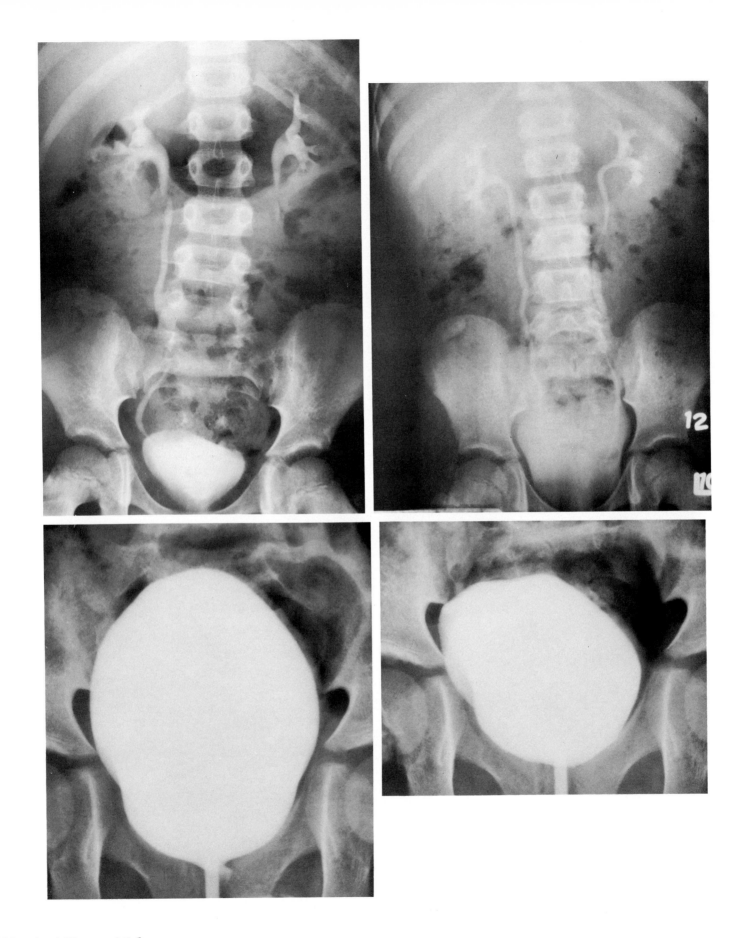

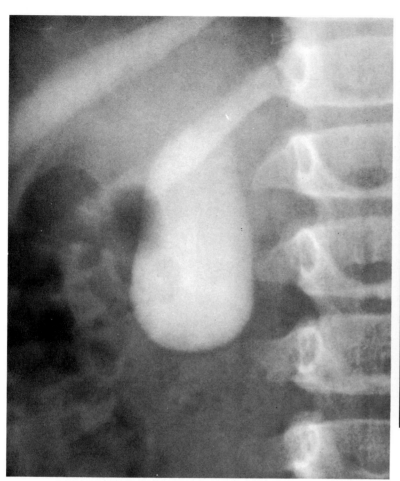
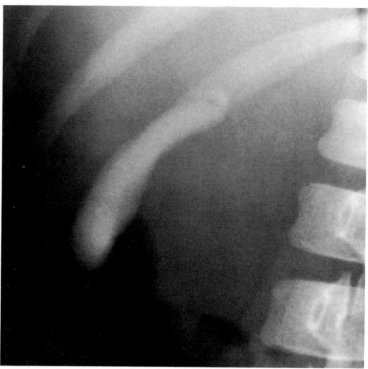

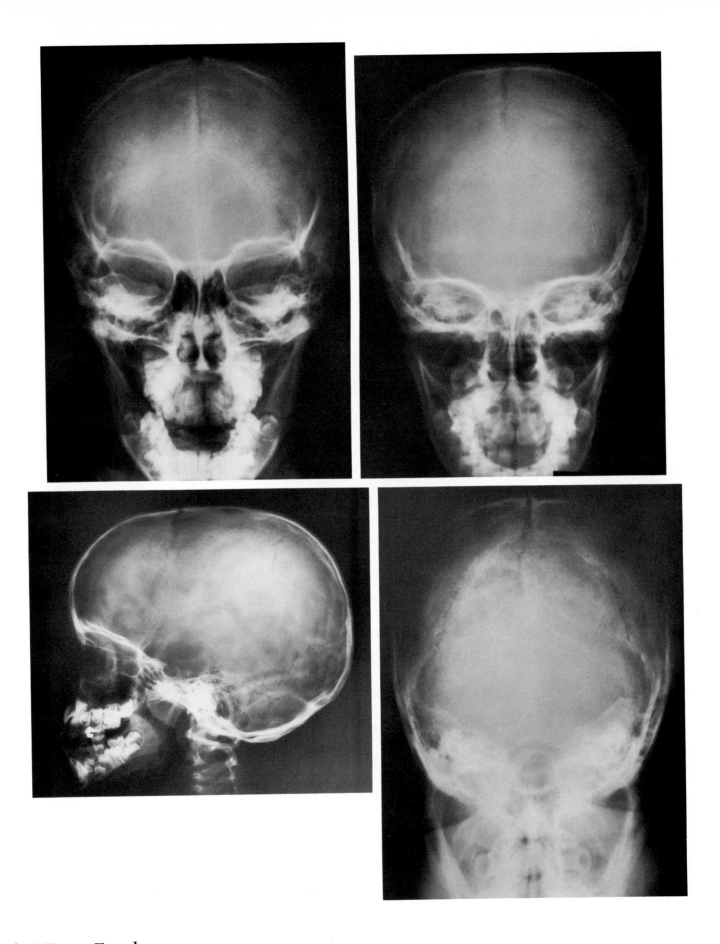

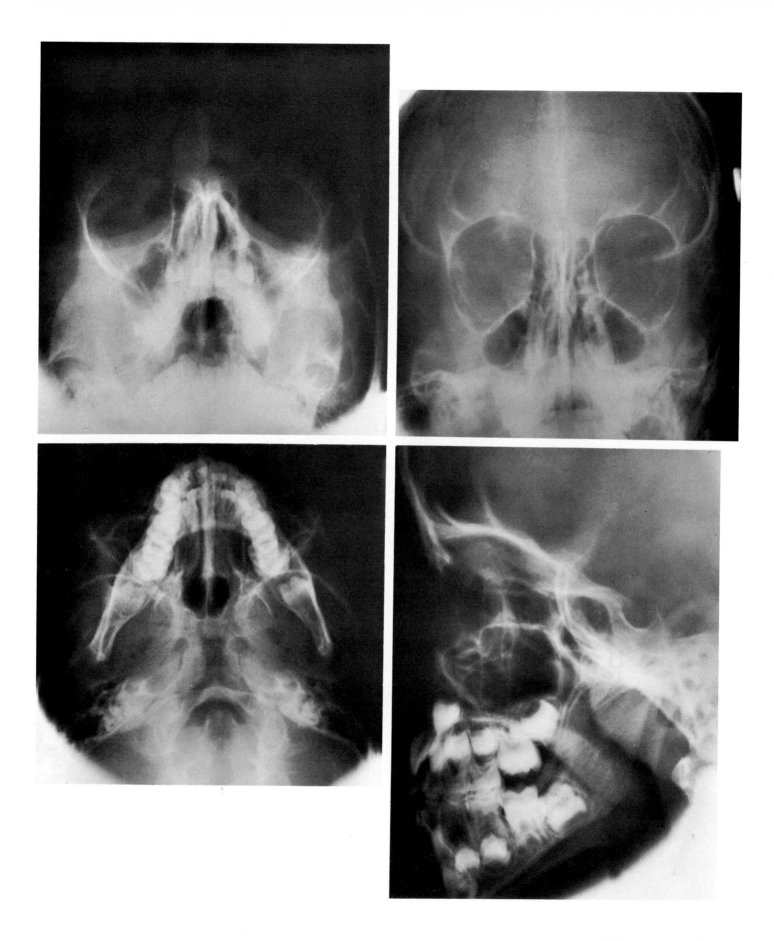

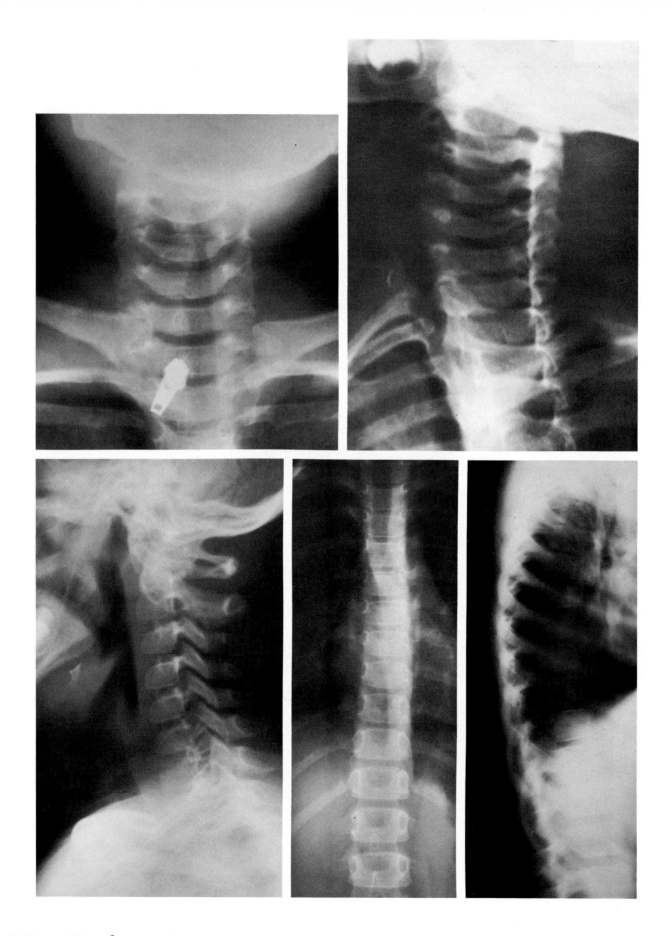

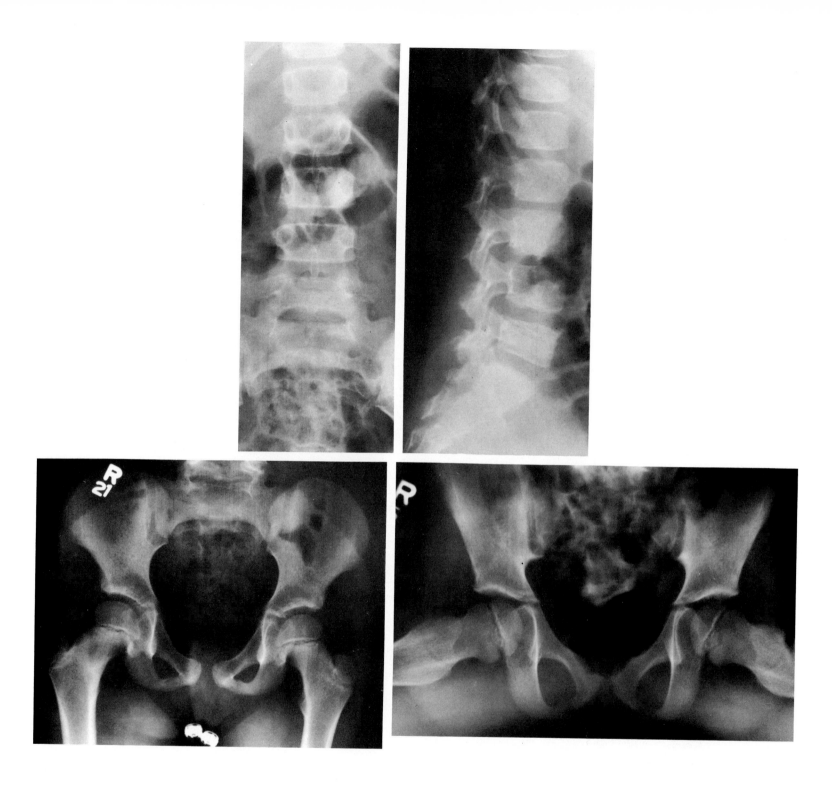

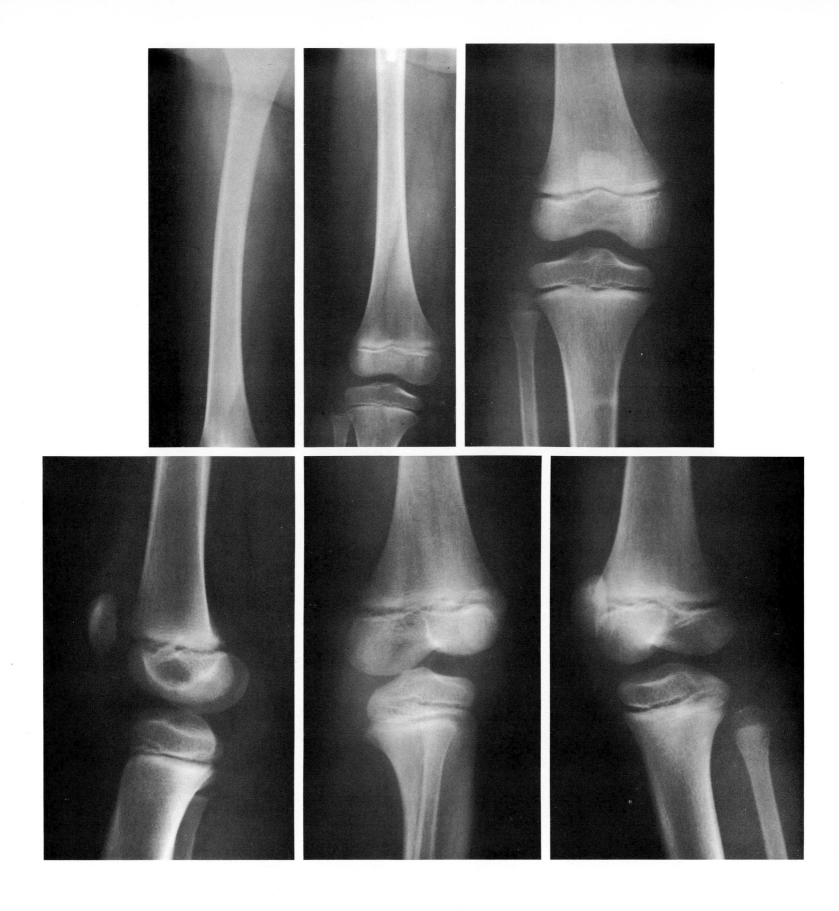

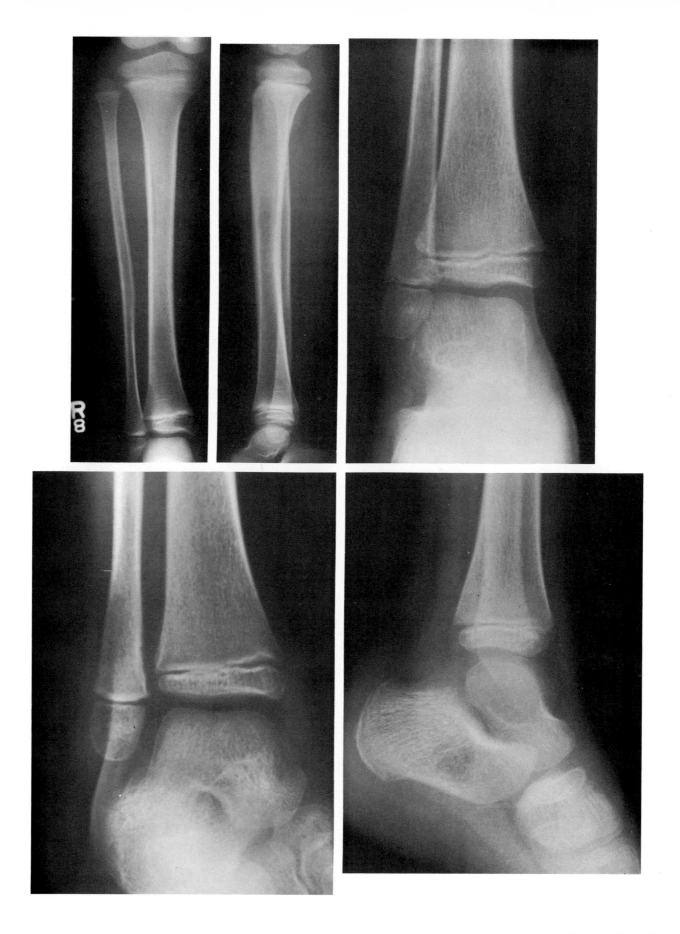

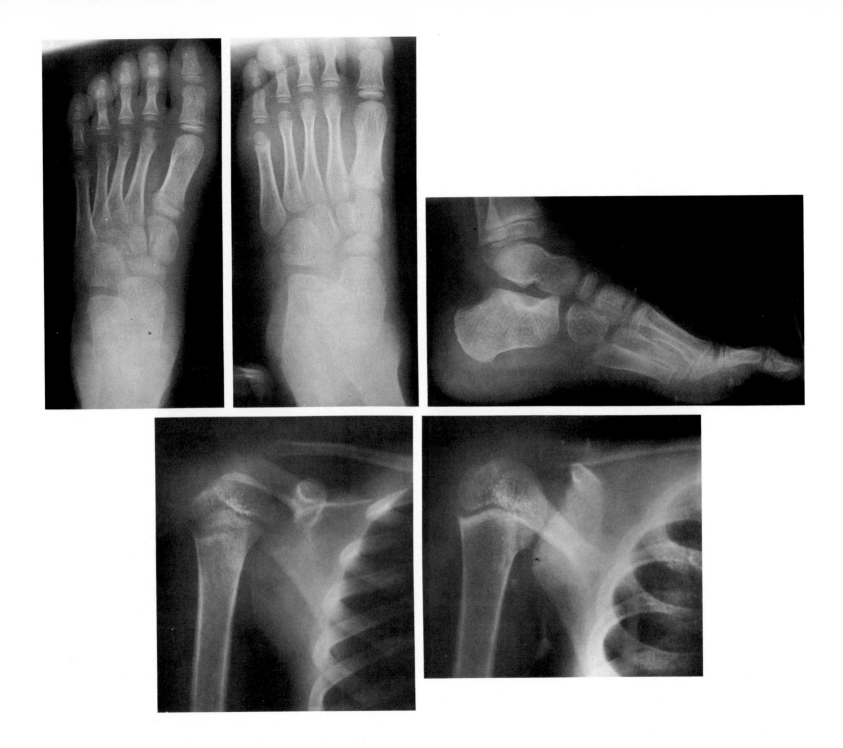

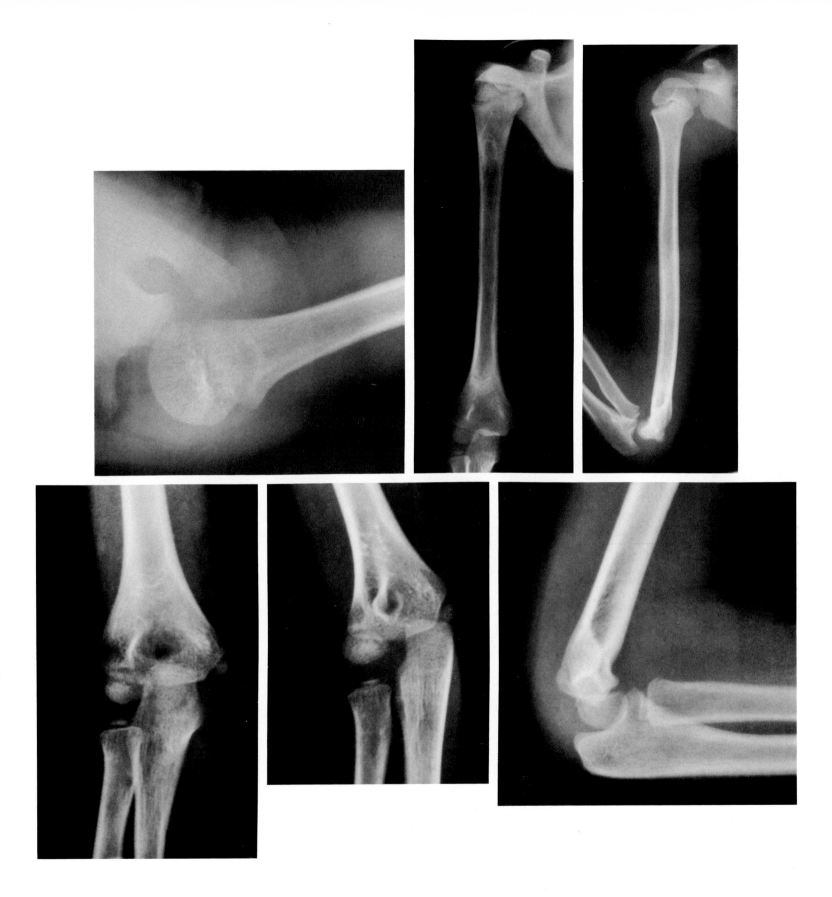

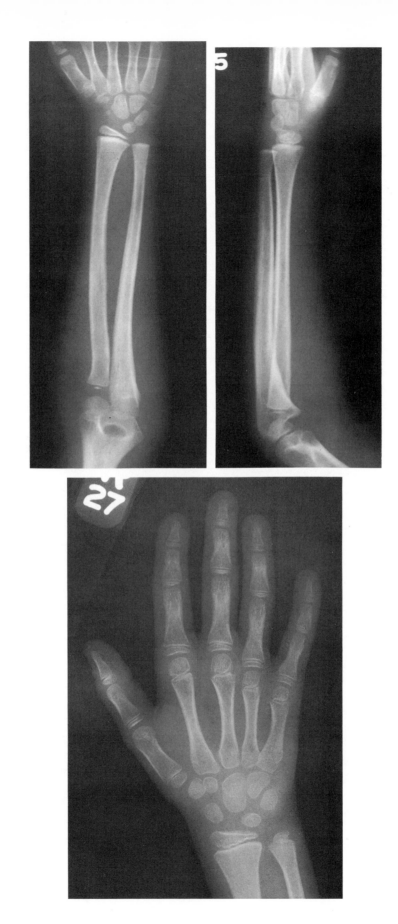

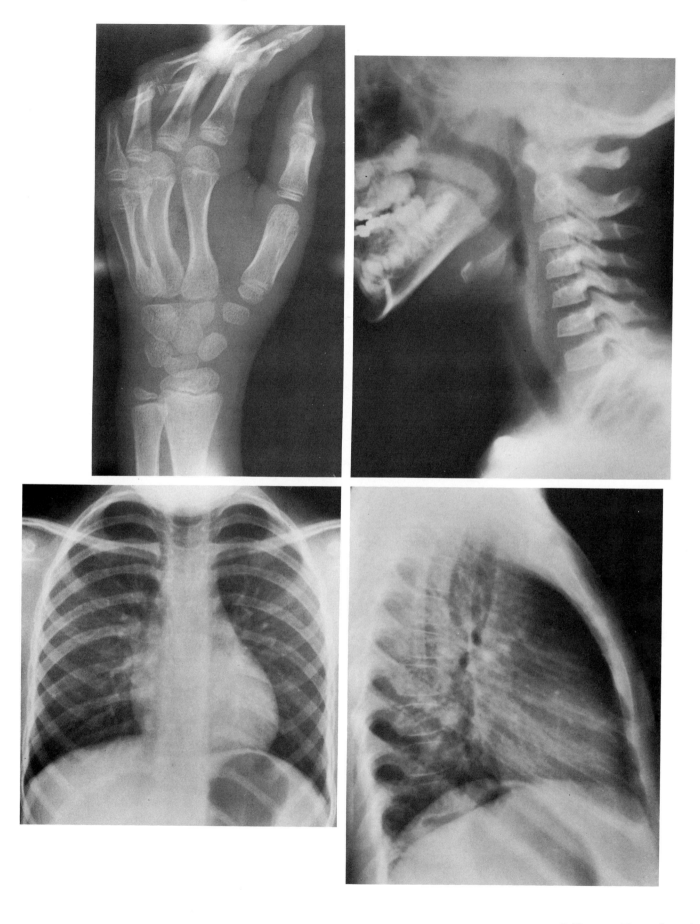

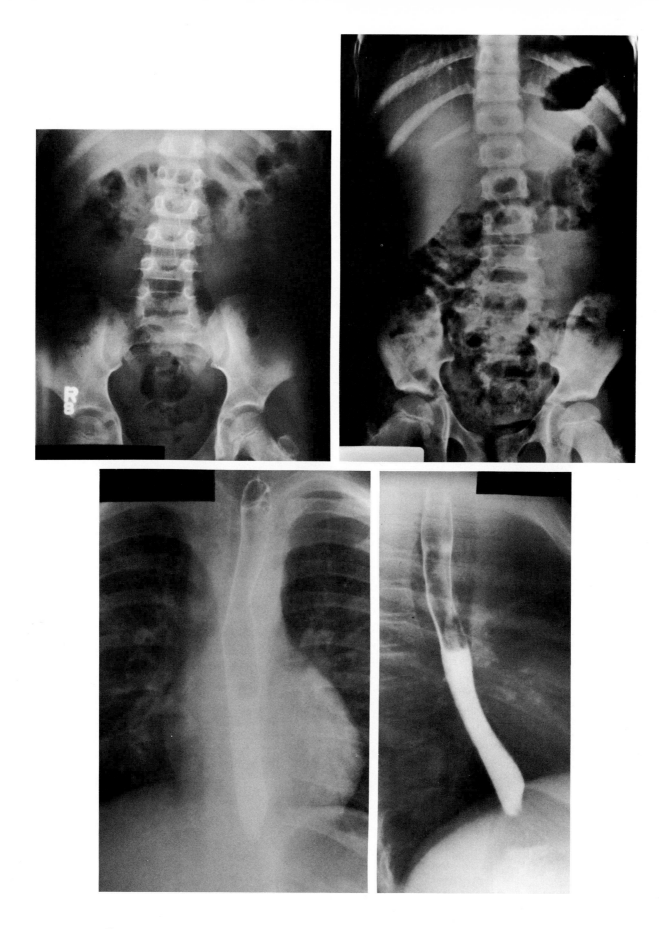

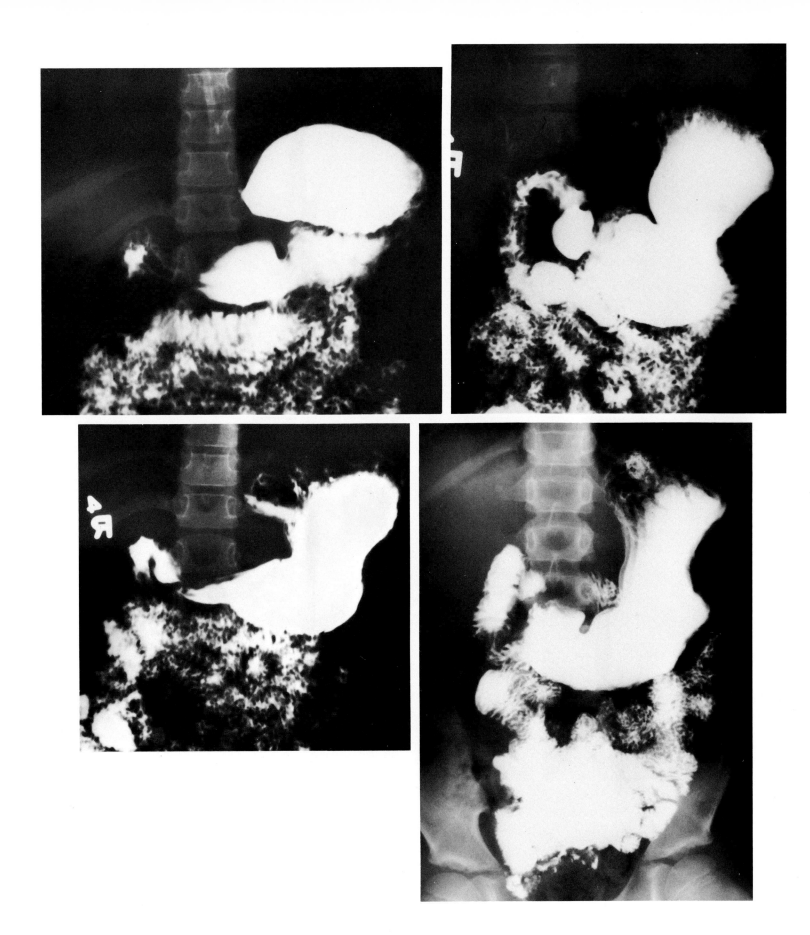

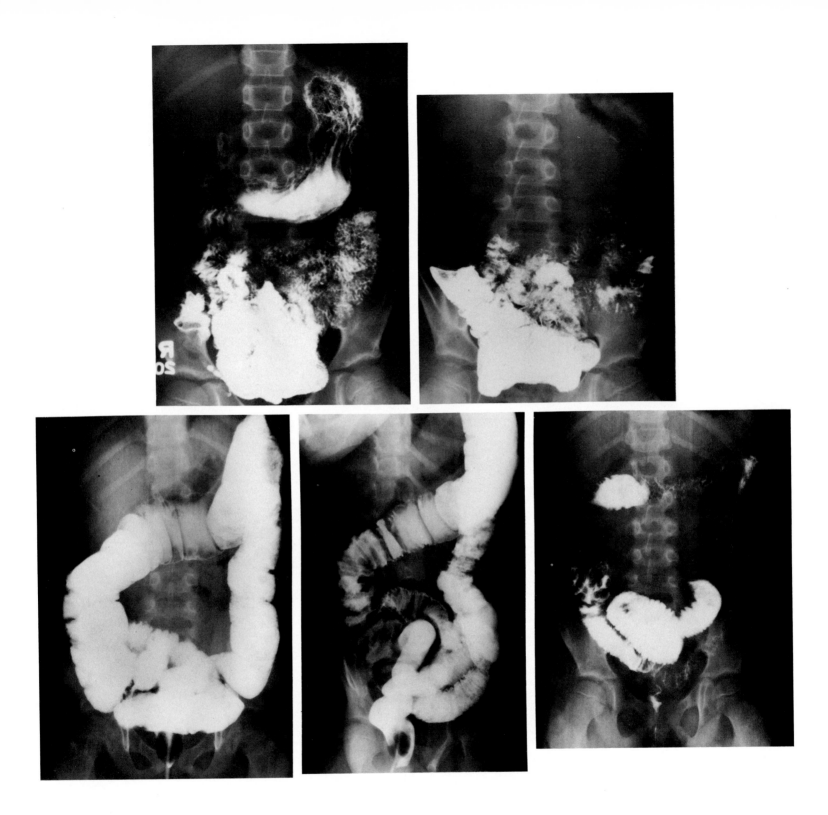

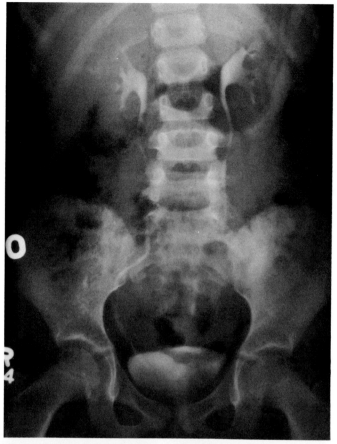

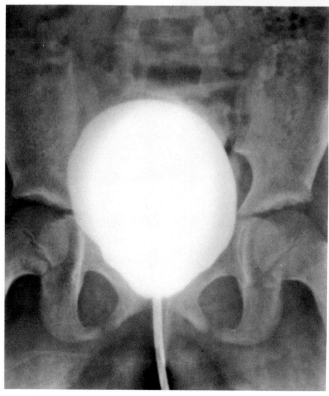

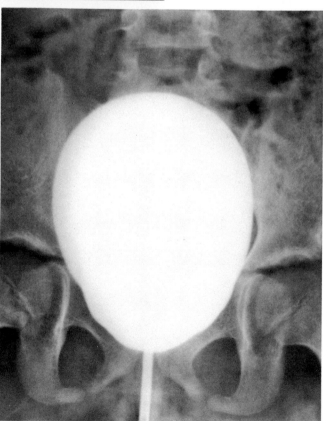

15

7 YEARS

The calvarial digital markings are less prominent. The adenoids remain large. The upper cervical vertebrae are wedge-shaped, more so than the lower. Posterior scalloping of the lumbar vertebrae is still apparent. The ischiopubic synchondroses may still be open. The slight overlap of the shadow of the anterior aspect of the distal tibial epiphysis onto the adjacent metaphysis is now visible and produces an apparent discontinuity of the epiphyseal plate in the frontal plane. The capitellum is enlarging.

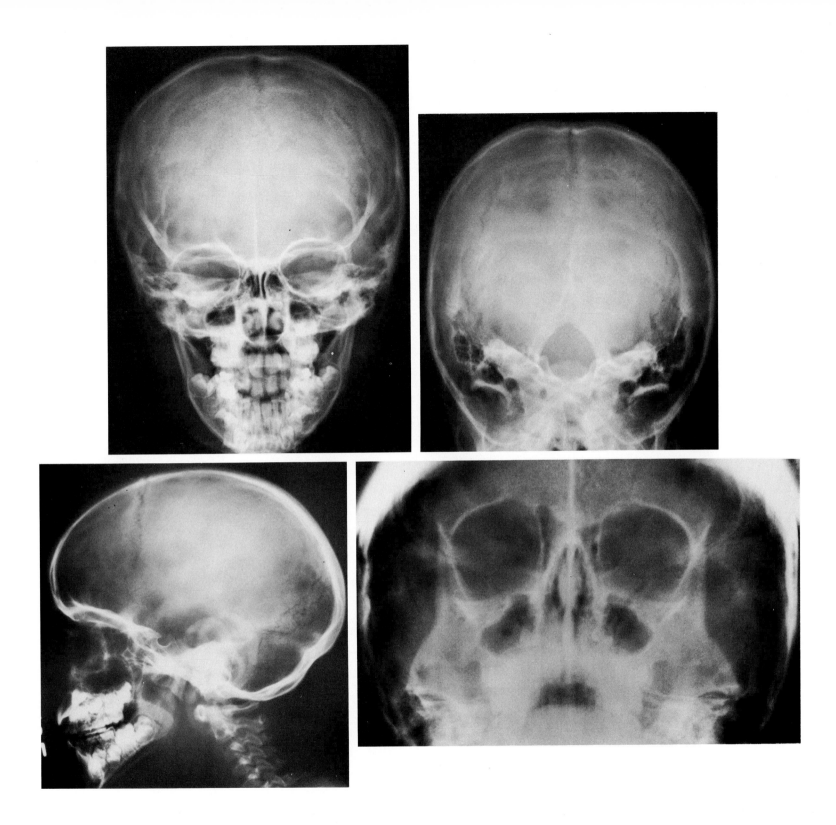

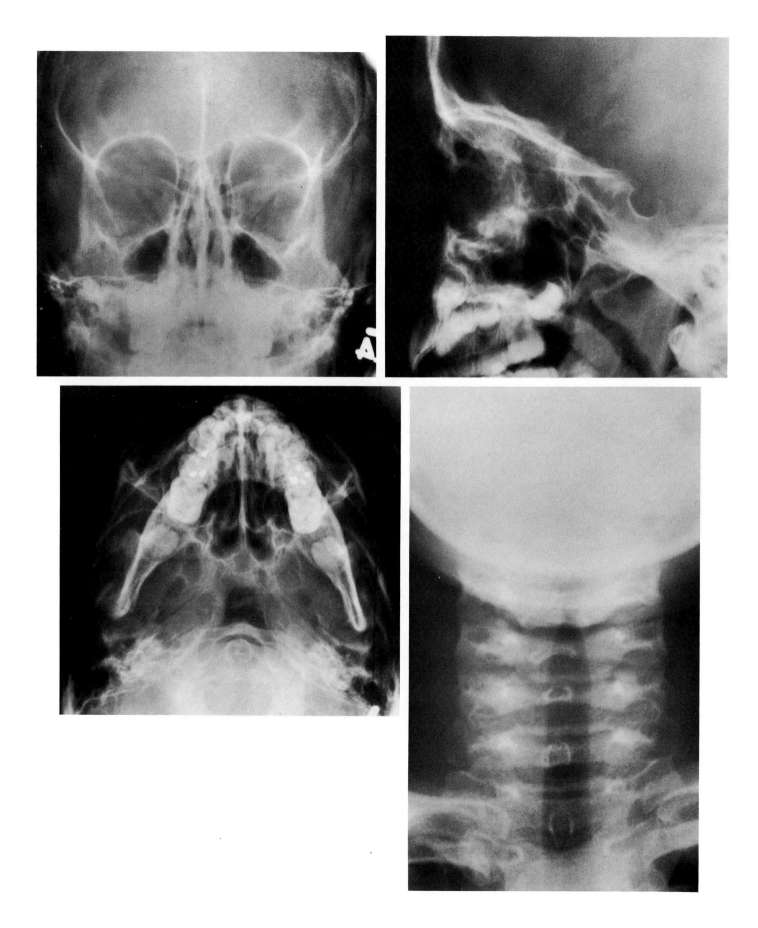

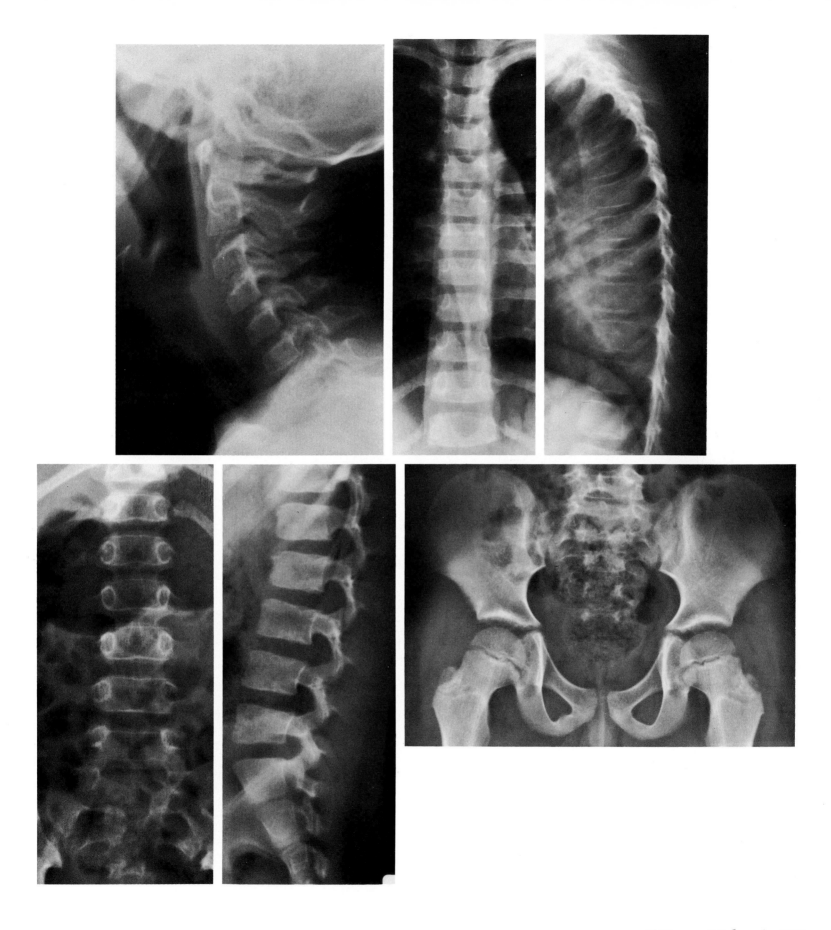

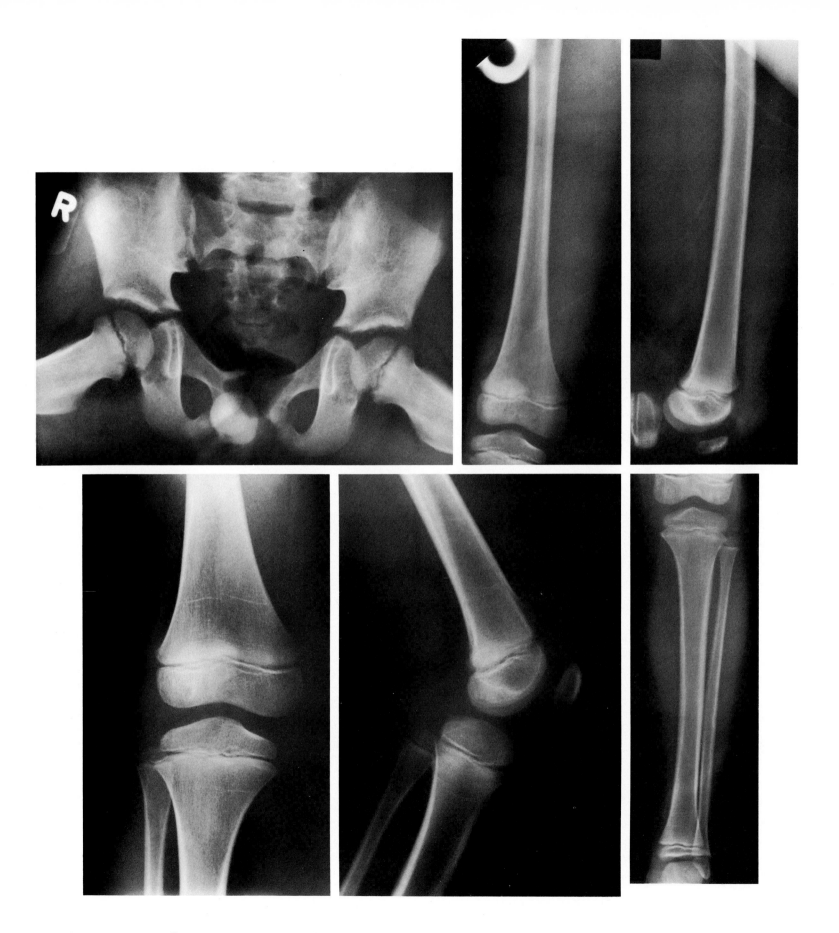

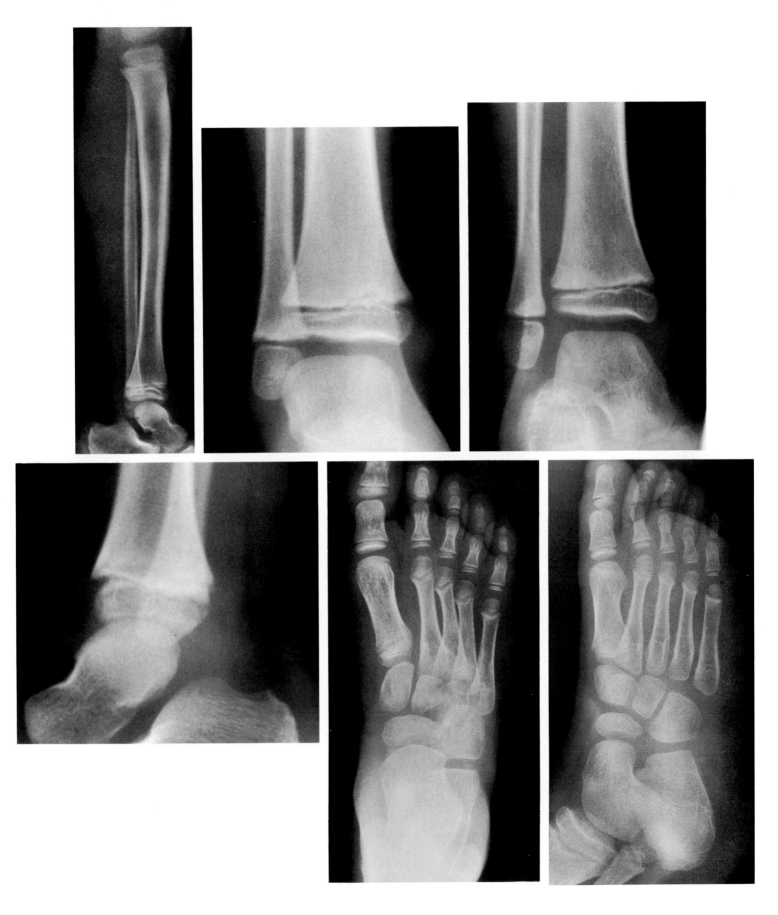

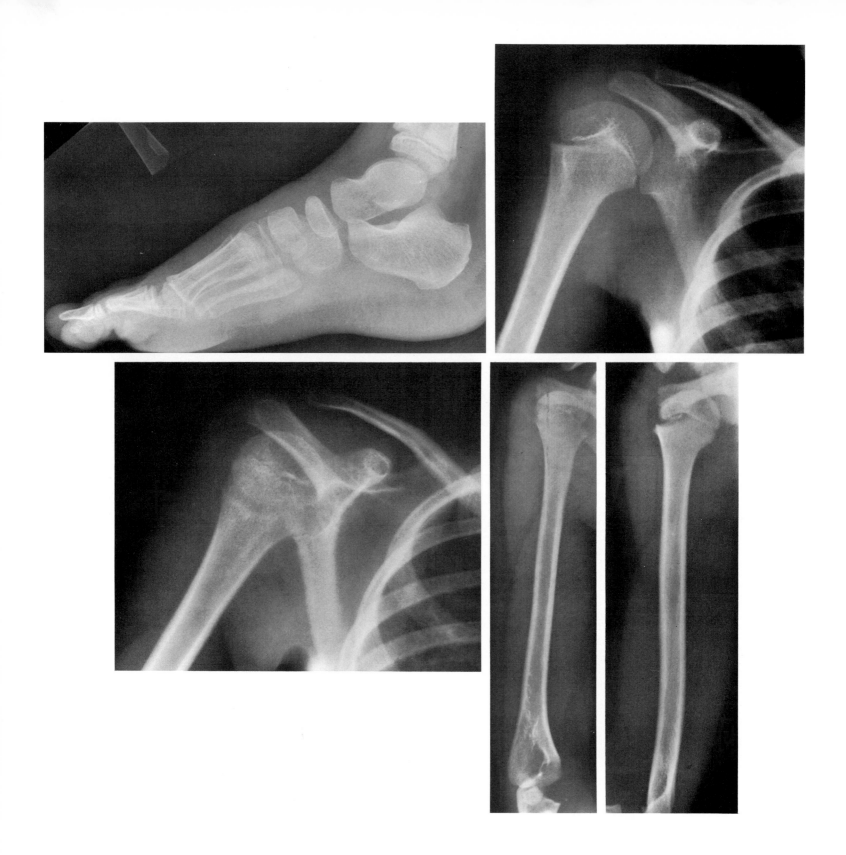

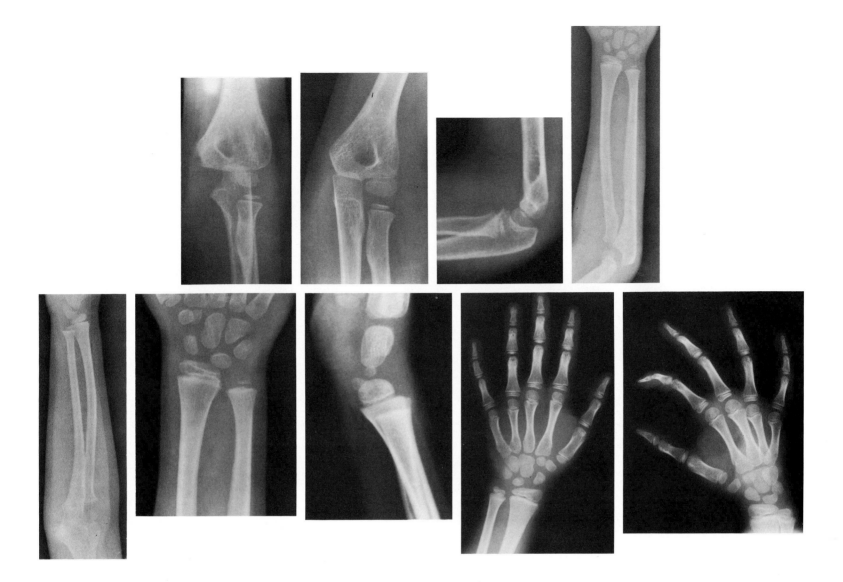

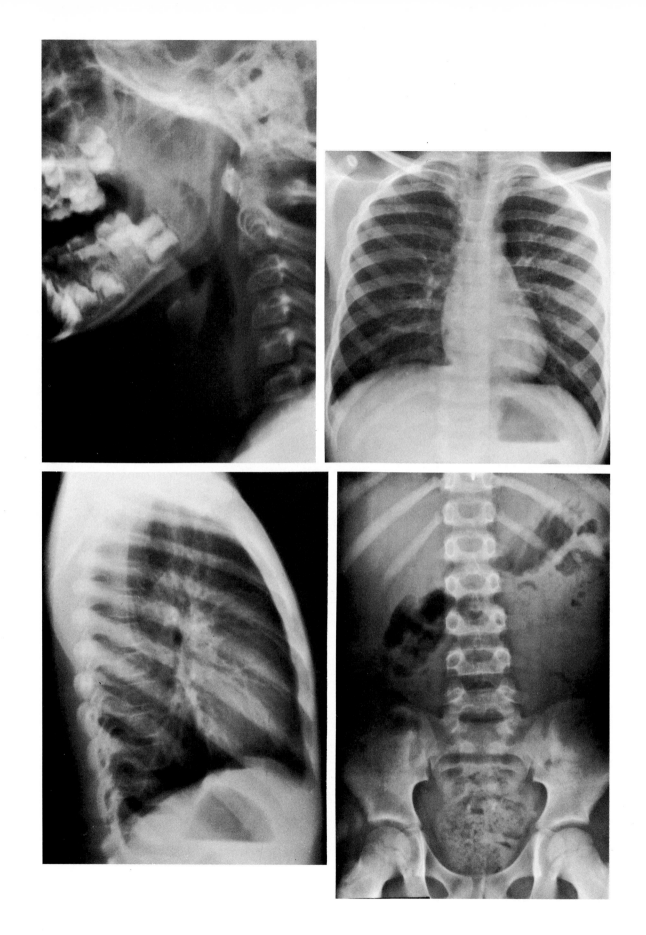

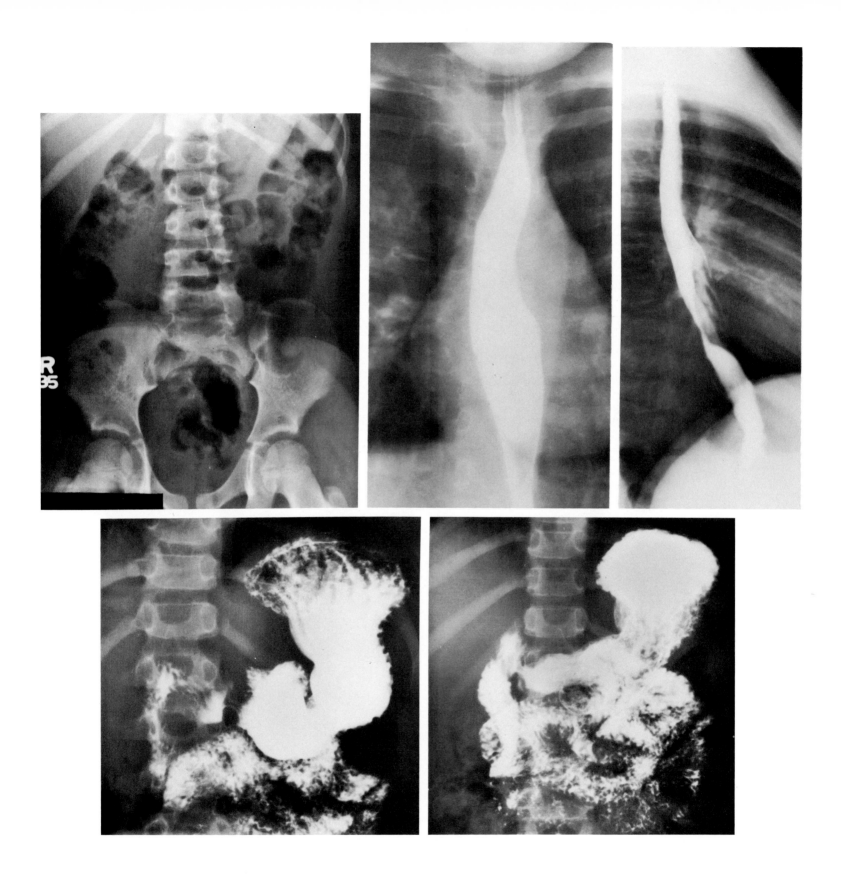

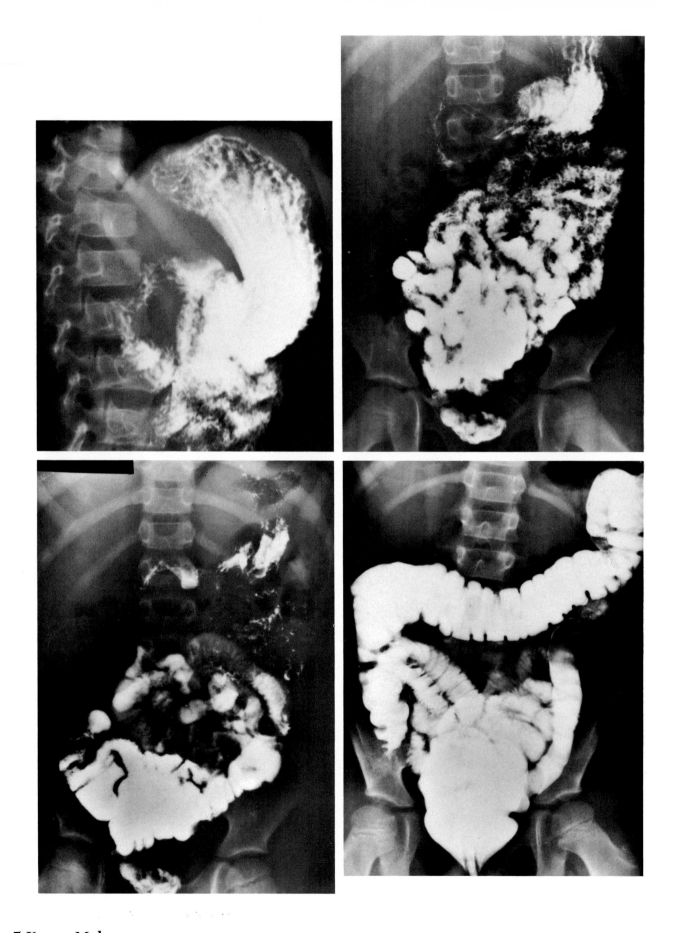

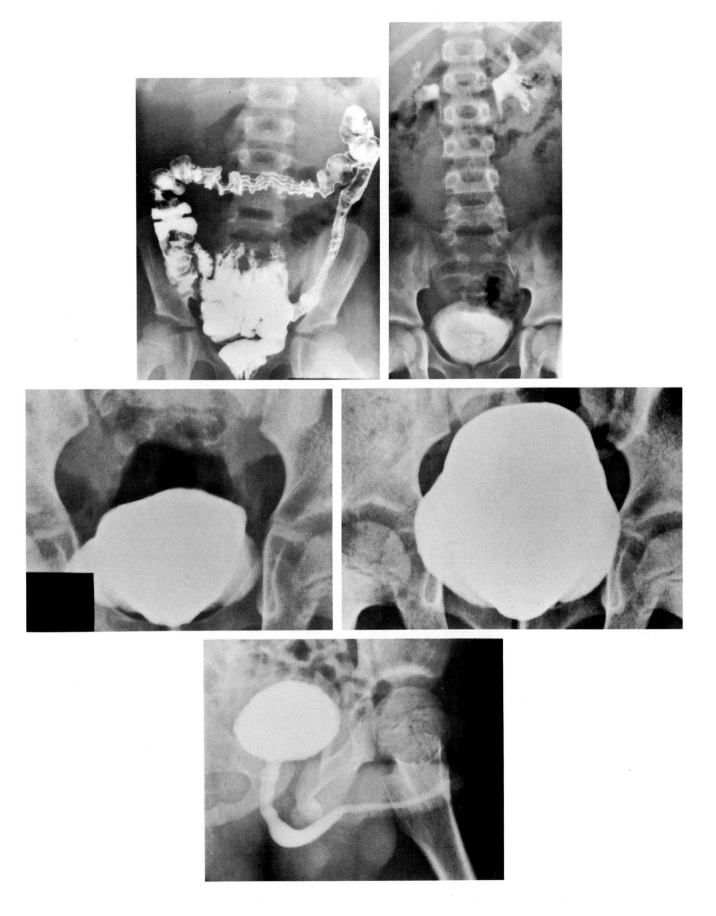

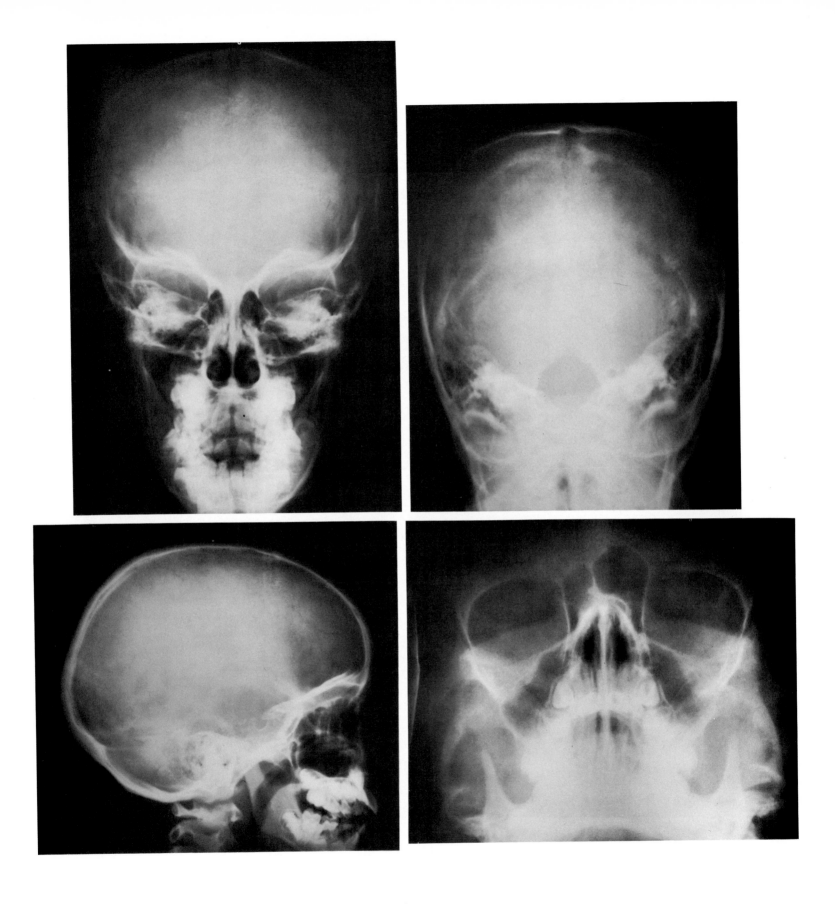

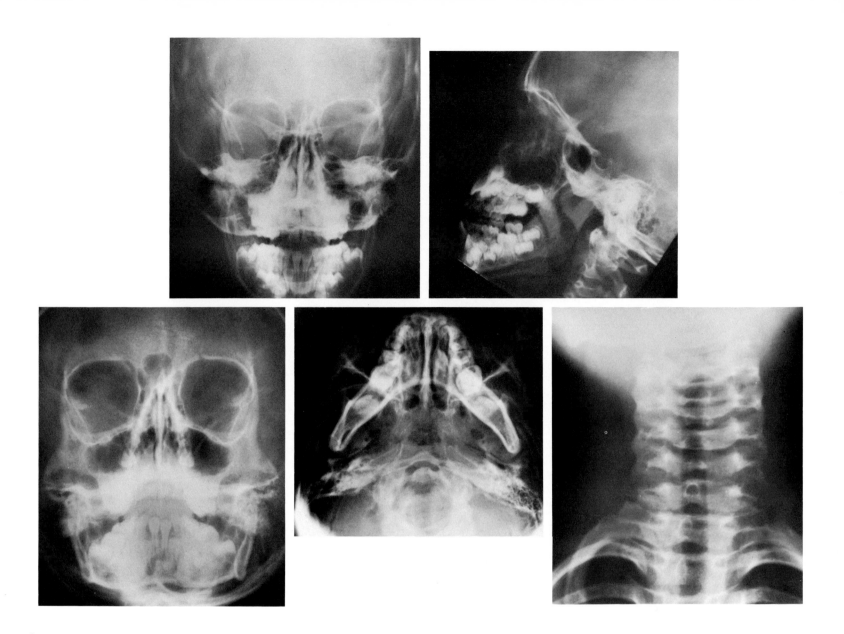

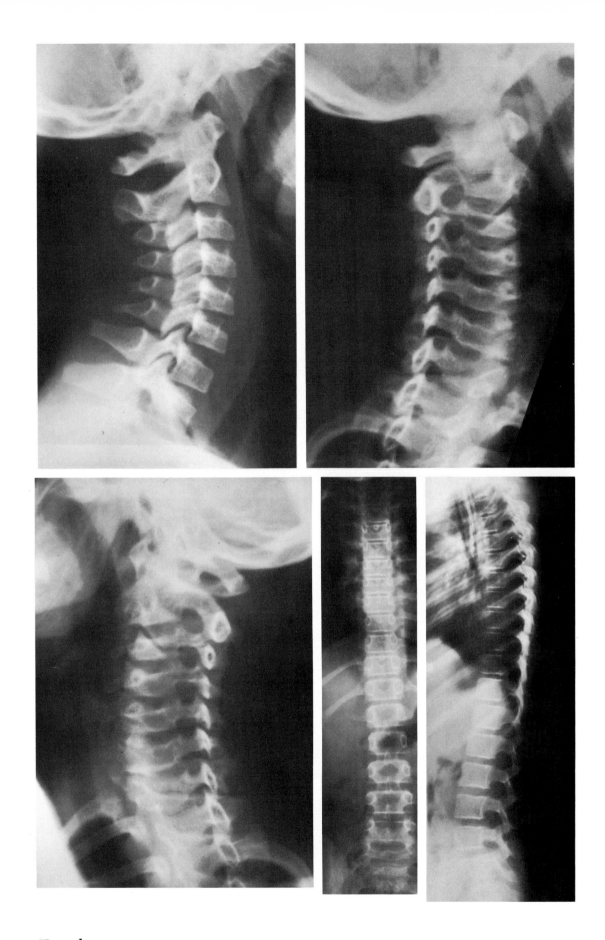

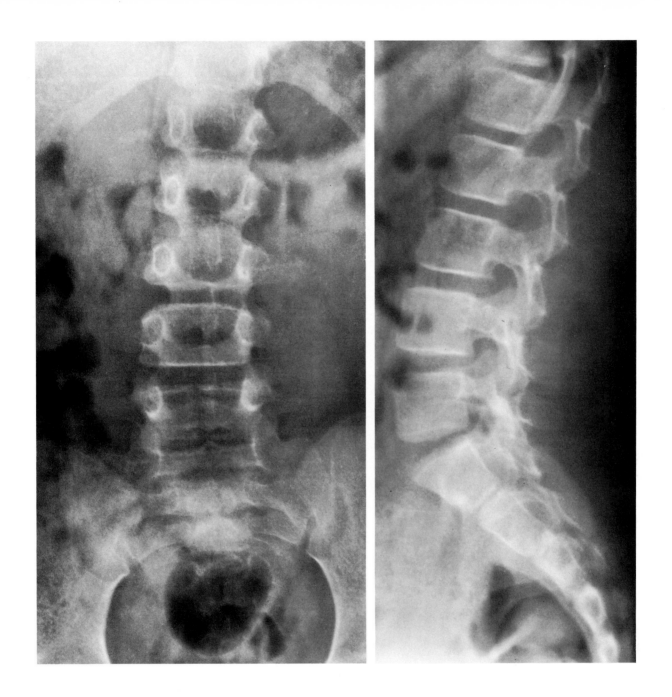

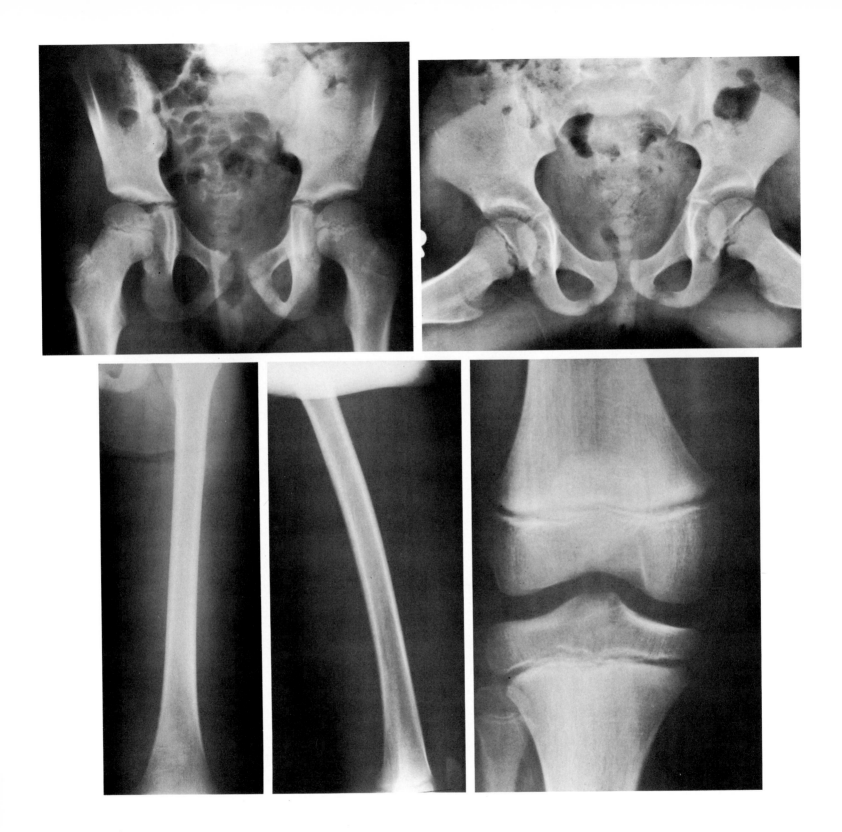

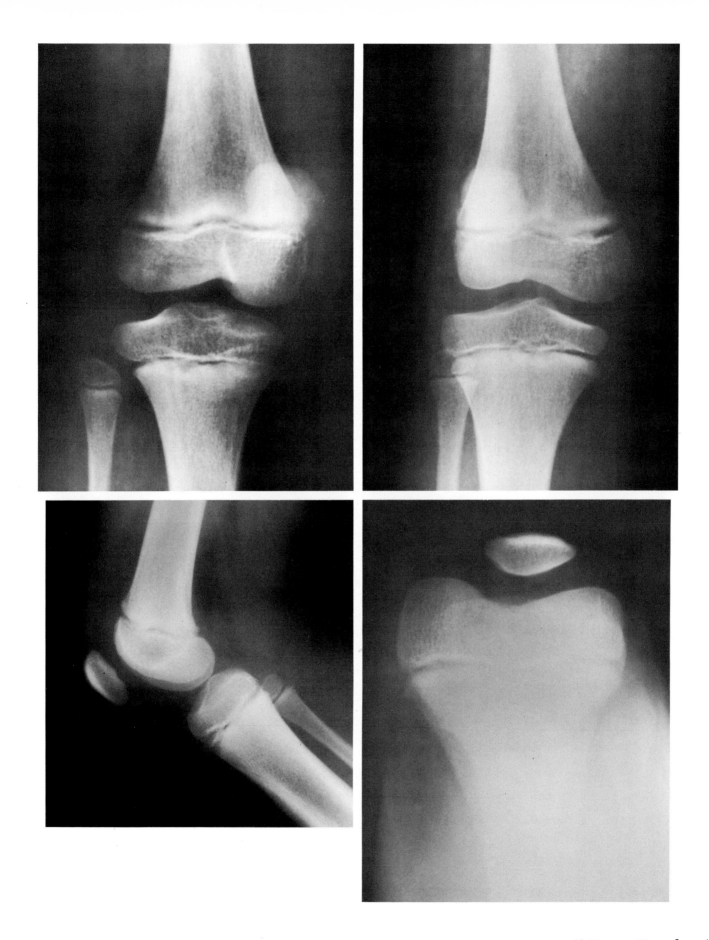

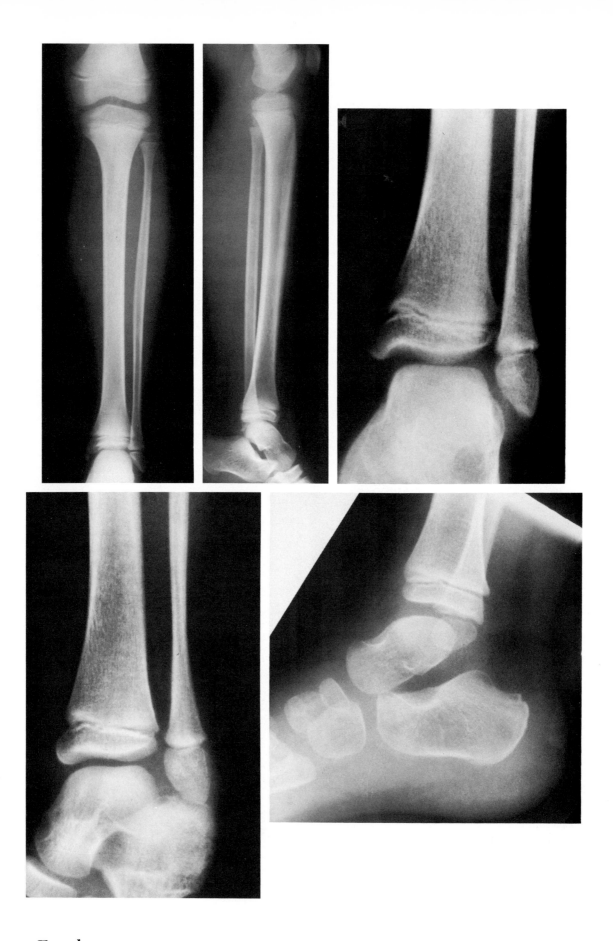

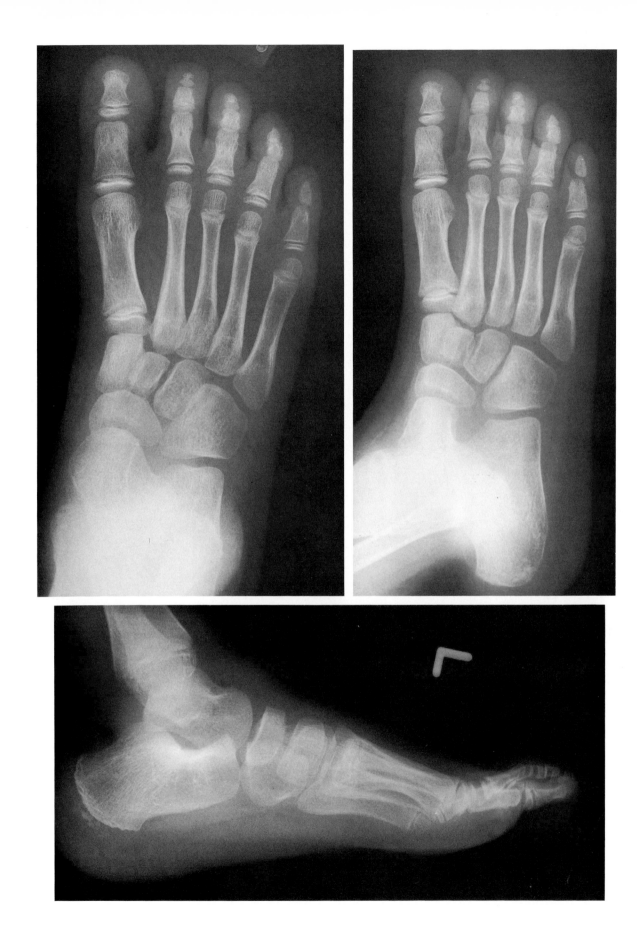

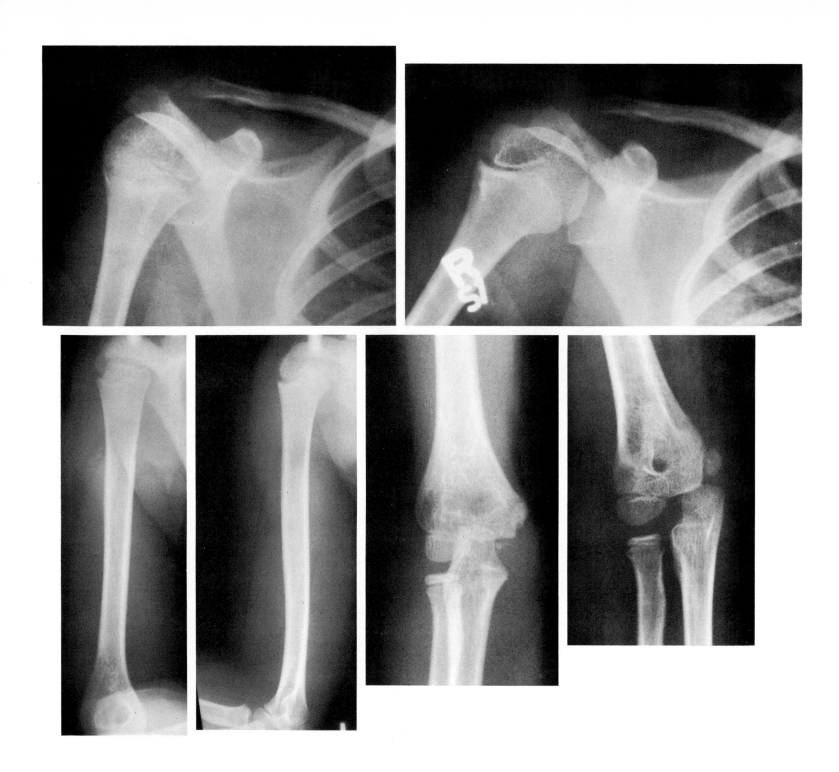

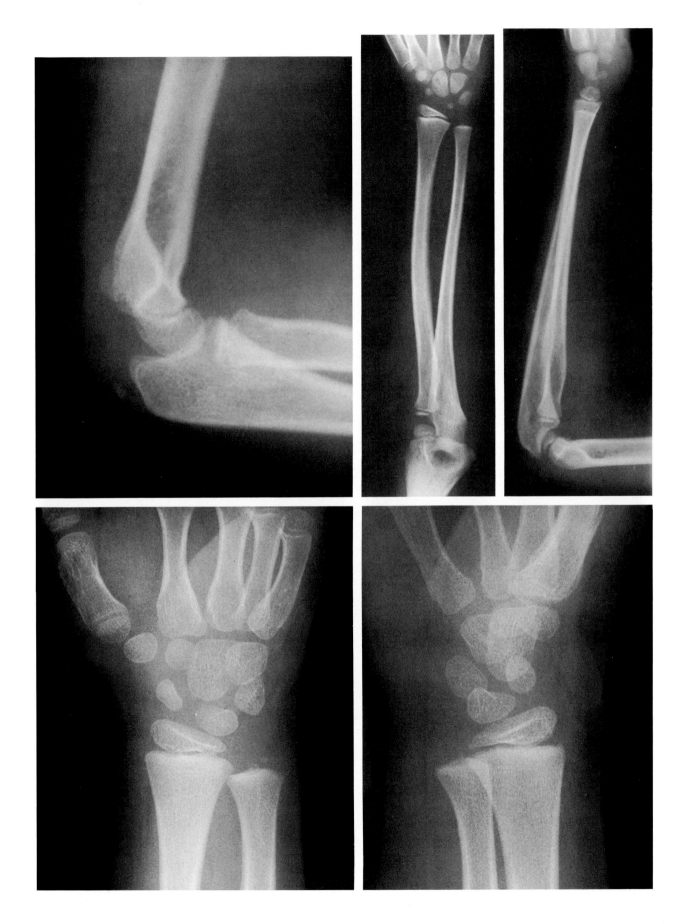

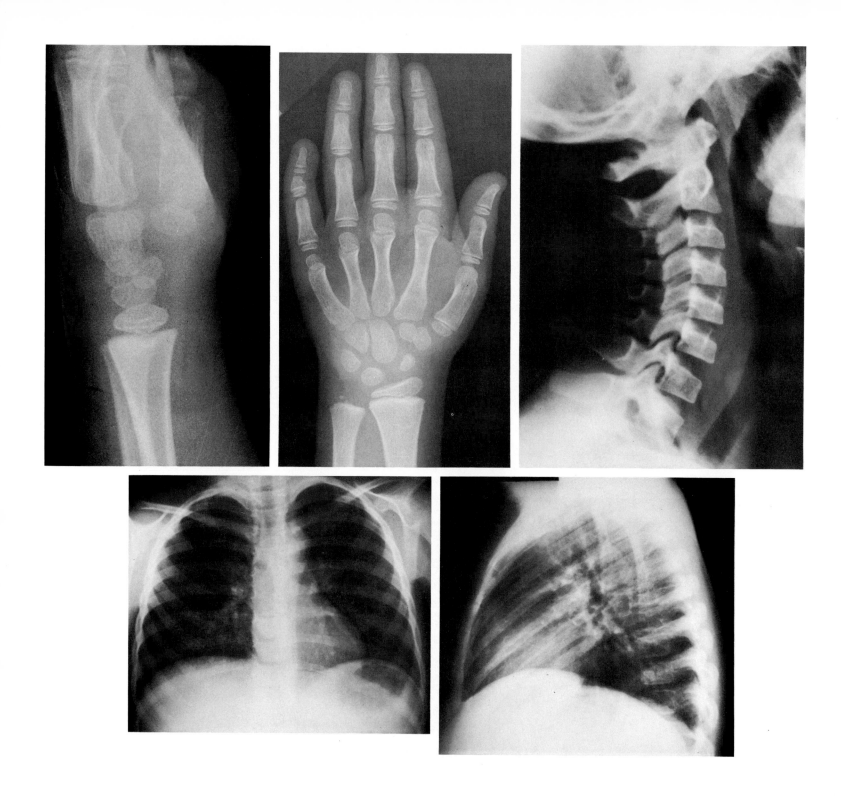

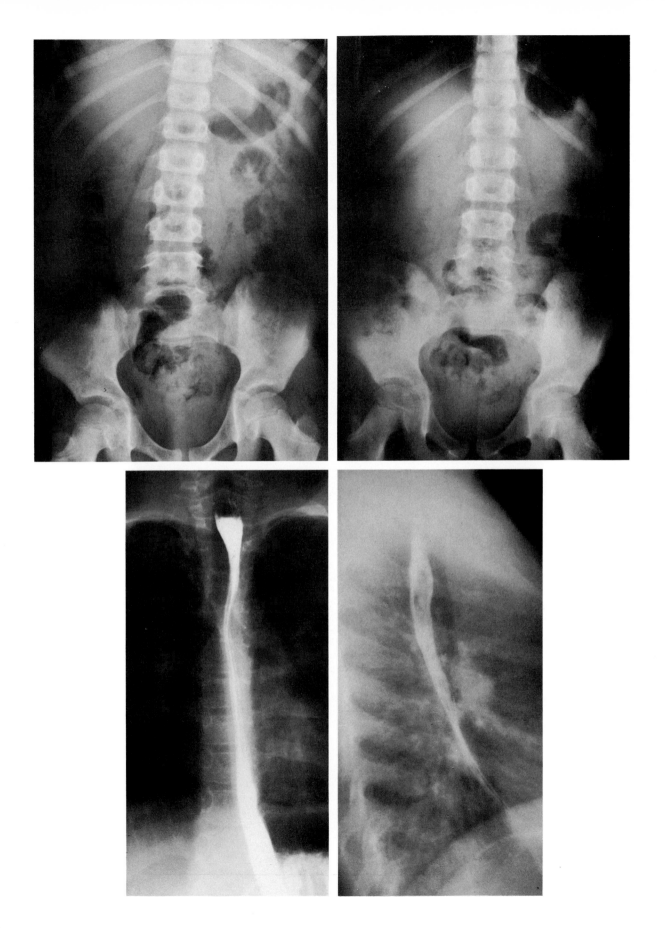

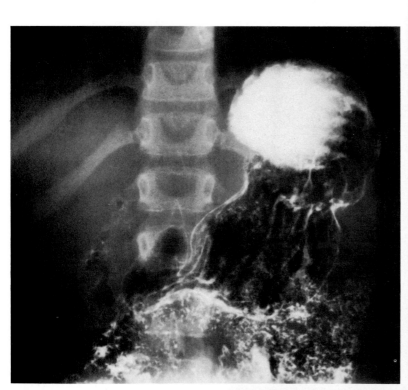

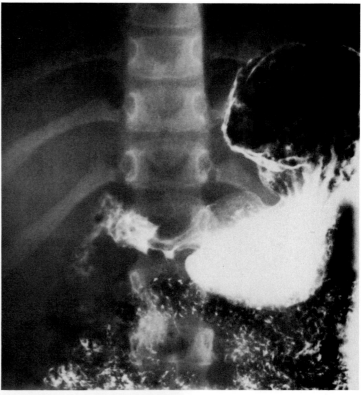

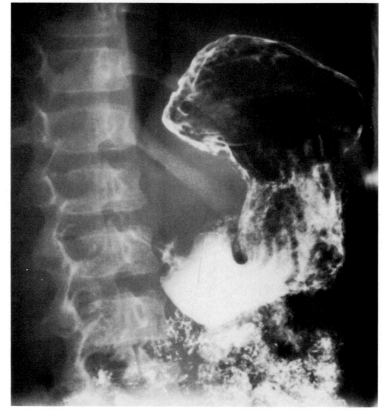

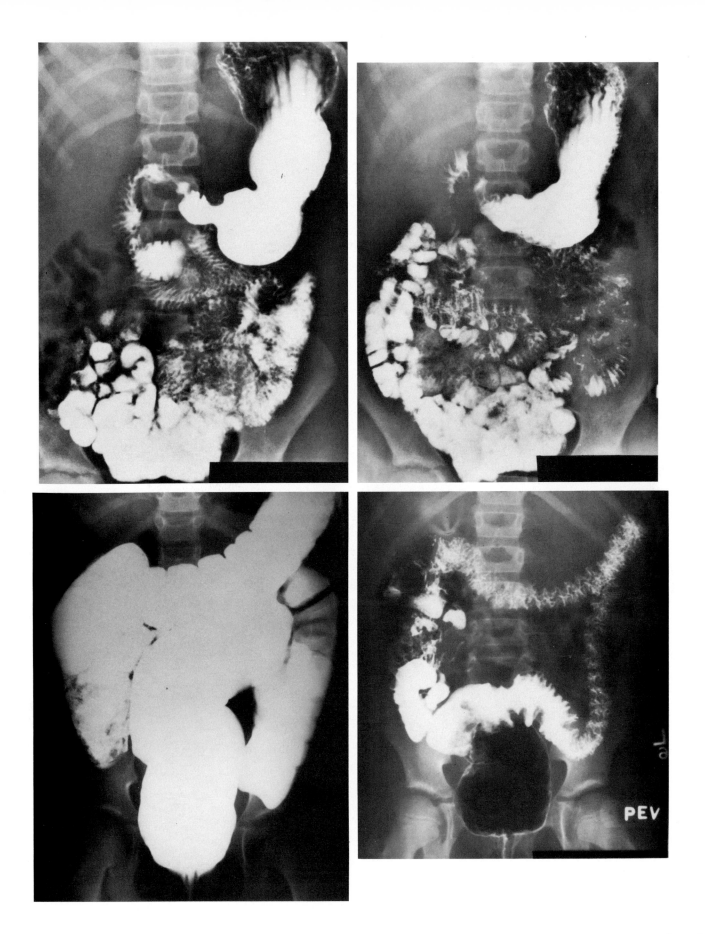

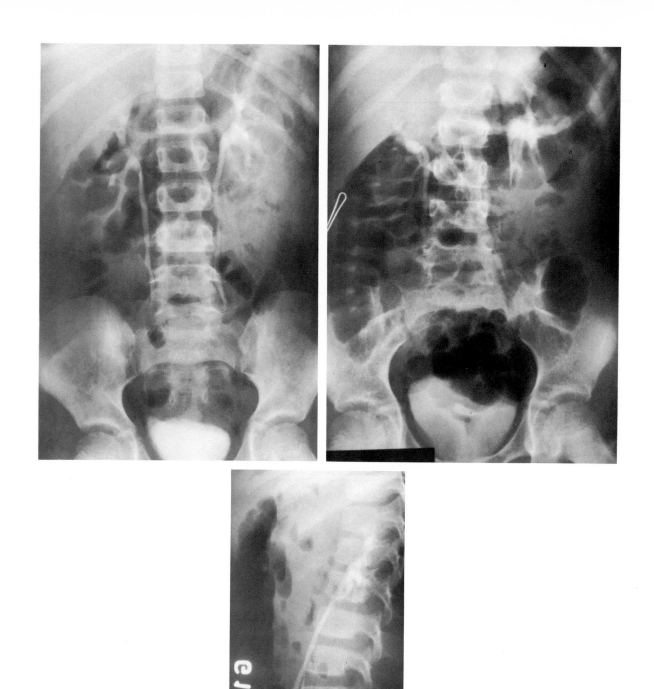

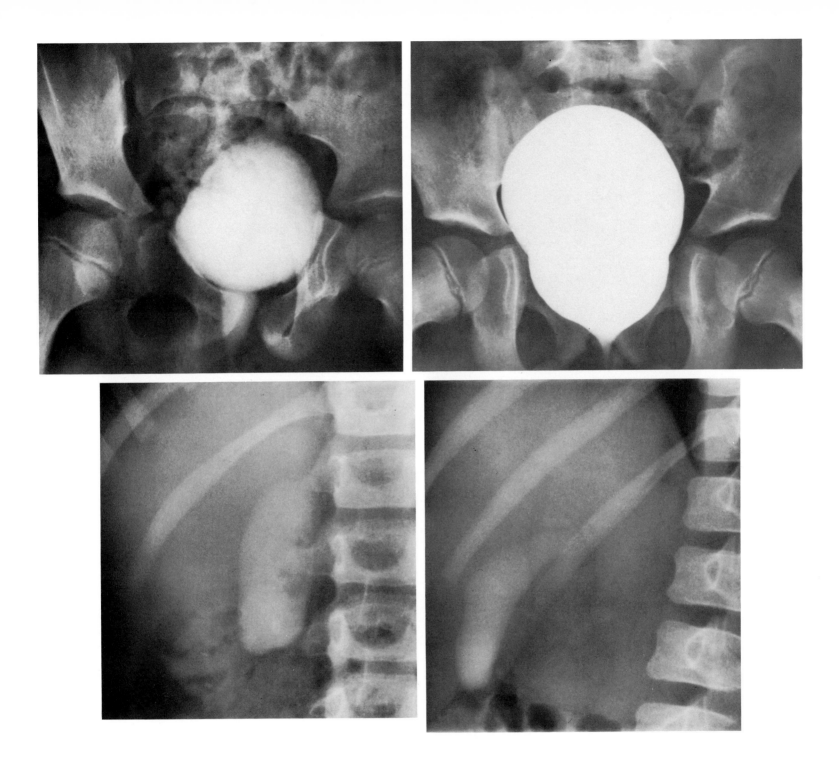

16

8 YEARS

The tip of the odontoid may still be clefted superiorly with the secondary ossification center. The ischiopubic synchondroses may still be open or closed at this age. The discontinuity of the distal tibial epiphyseal plate, first seen in the 7-year-old, is evident. The calcaneal apophysis appears and may be fragmented. The ossification center for the trochlea appears. The epiphysis of the radial head may be quite dense, as is the calcaneal apophysis and the epiphysis of the proximal phalanx of the great toe.

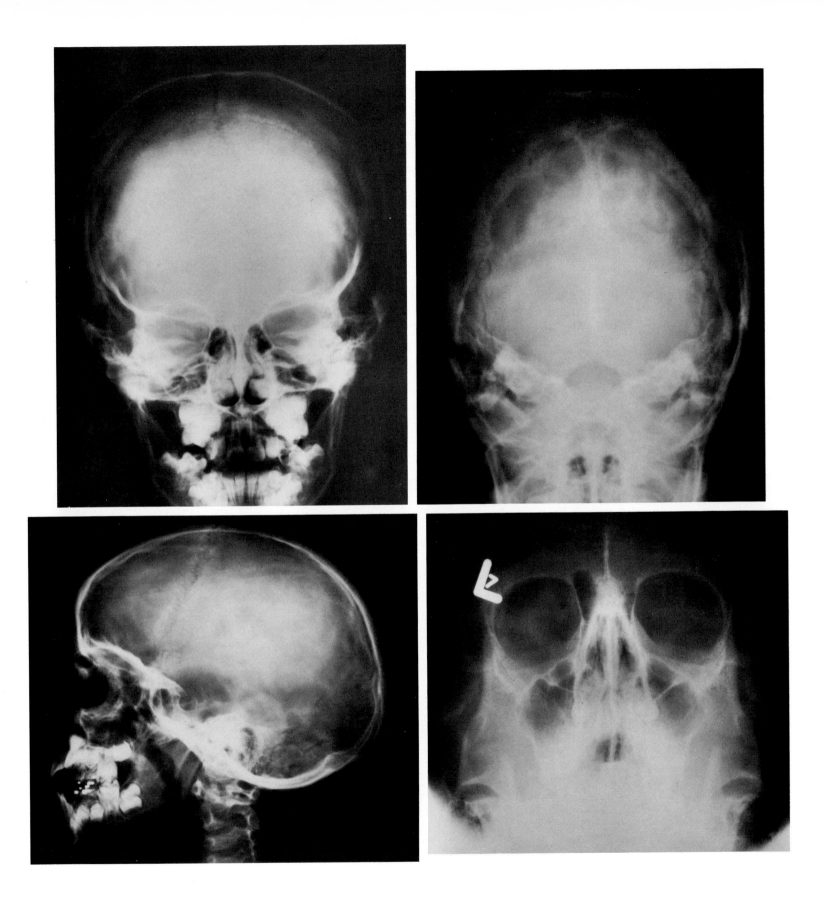

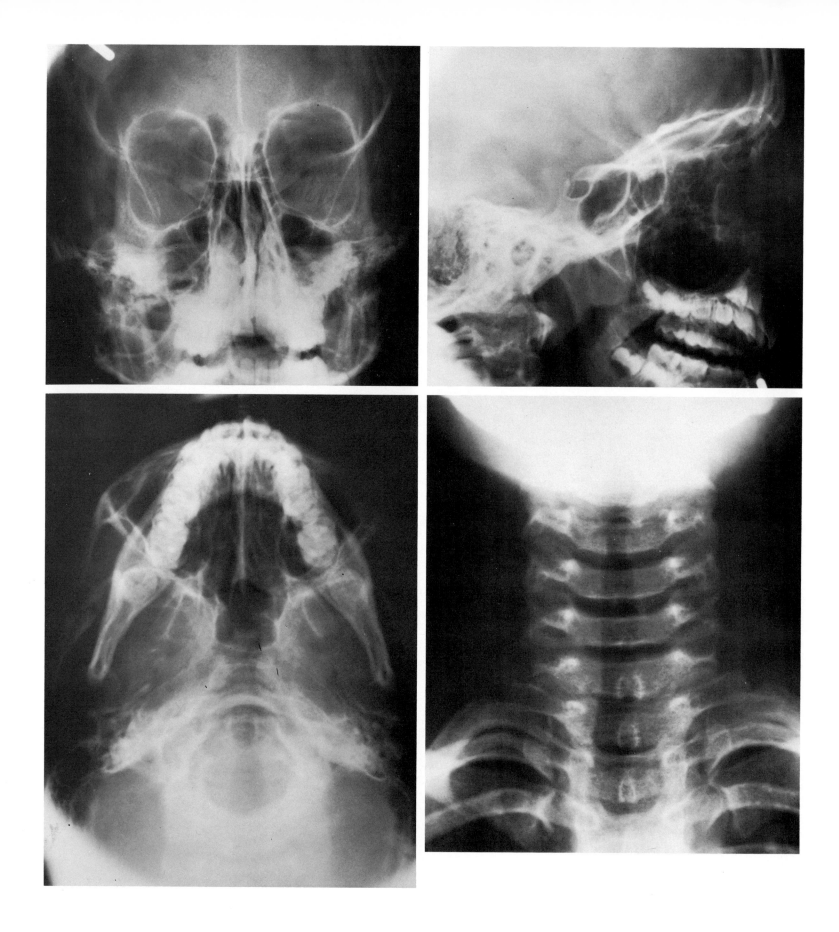

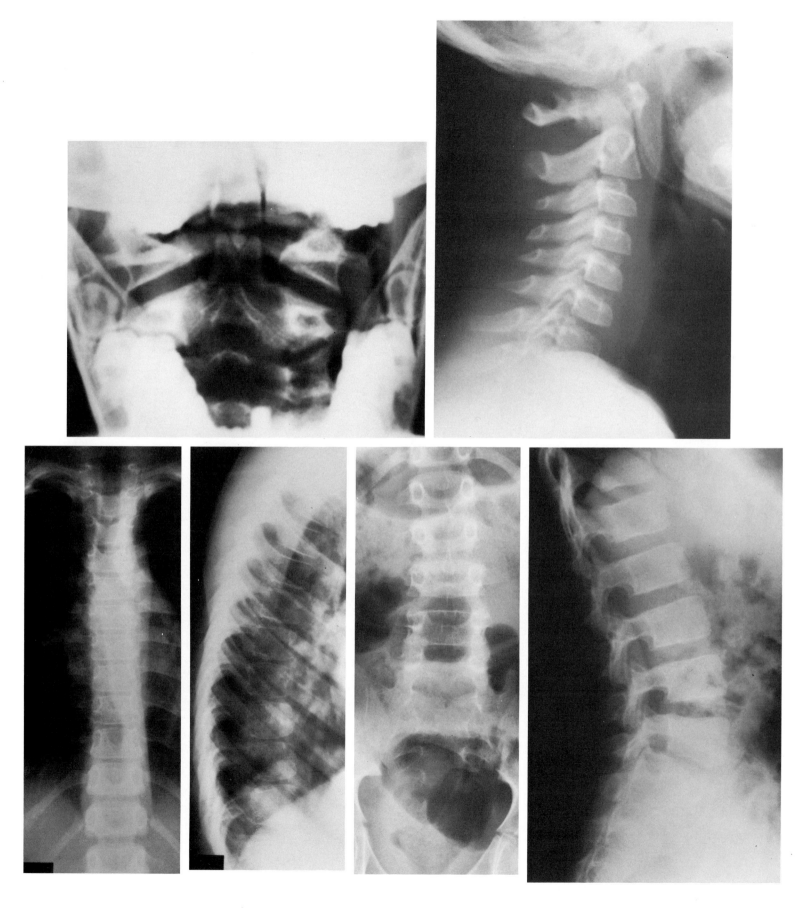

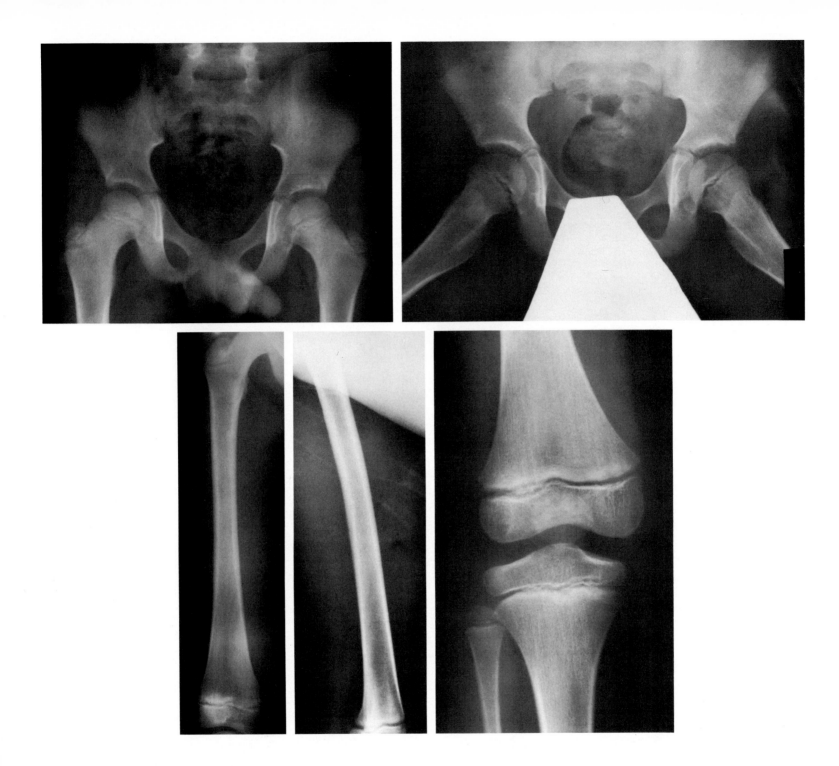

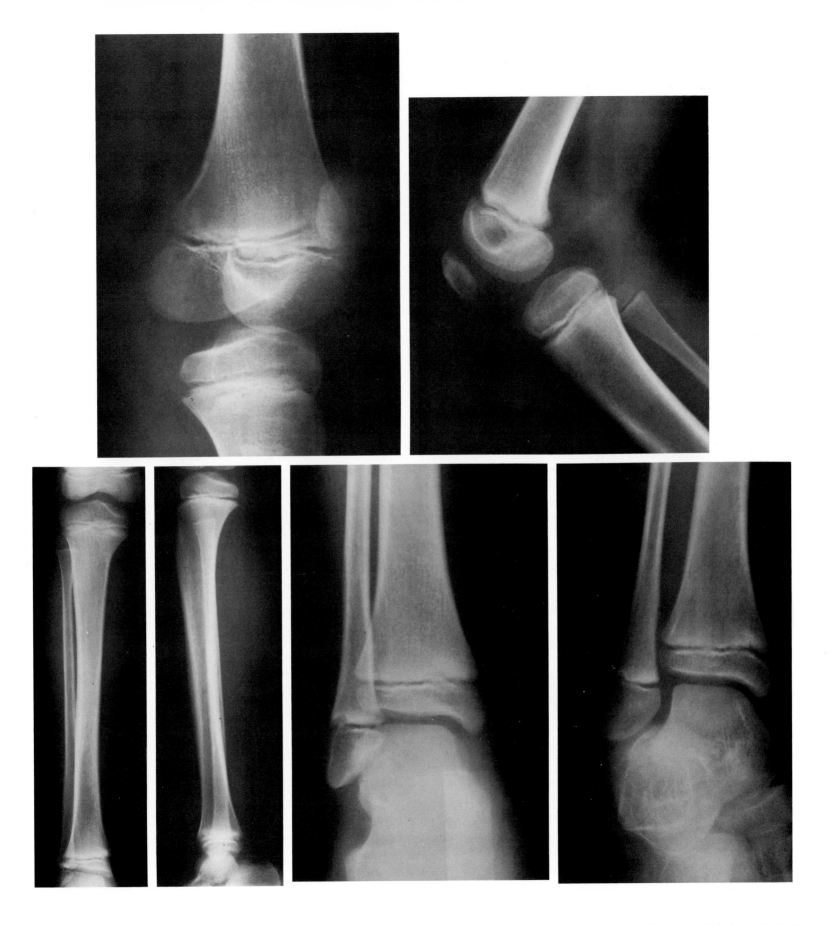

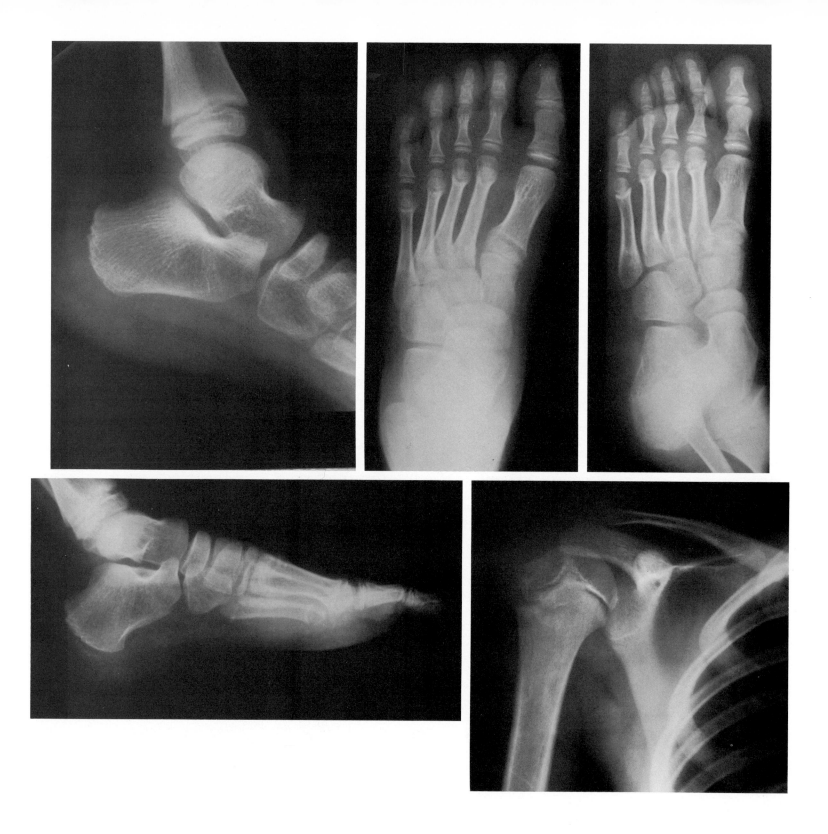

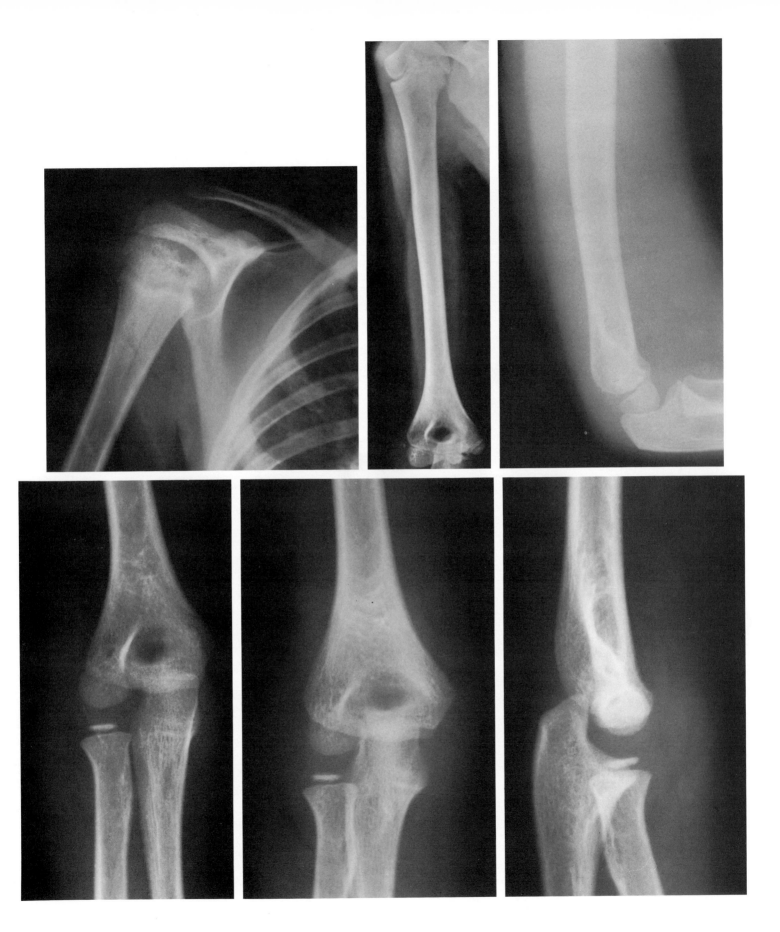

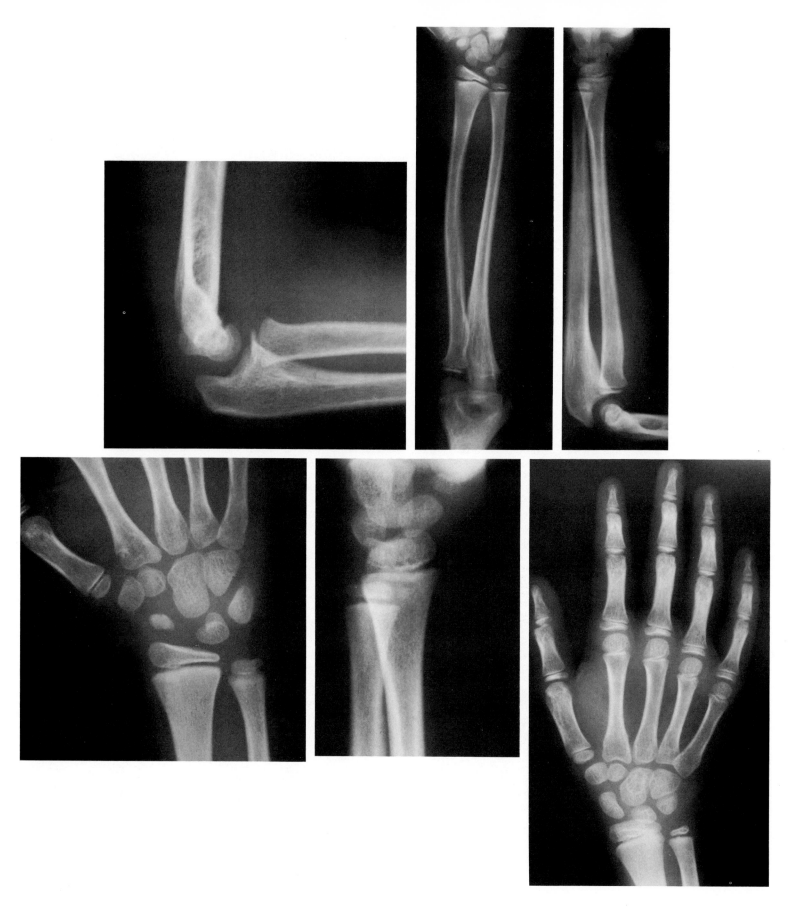

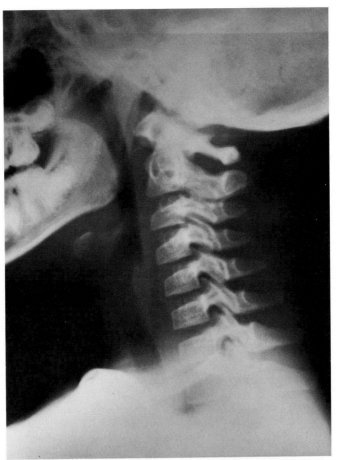

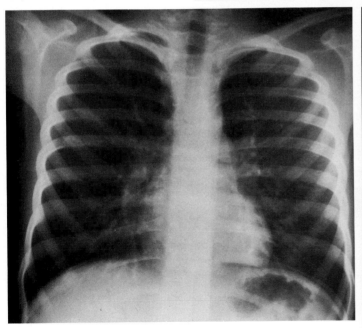

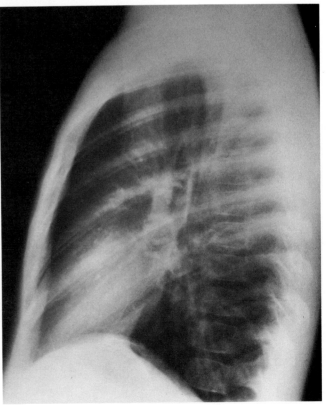

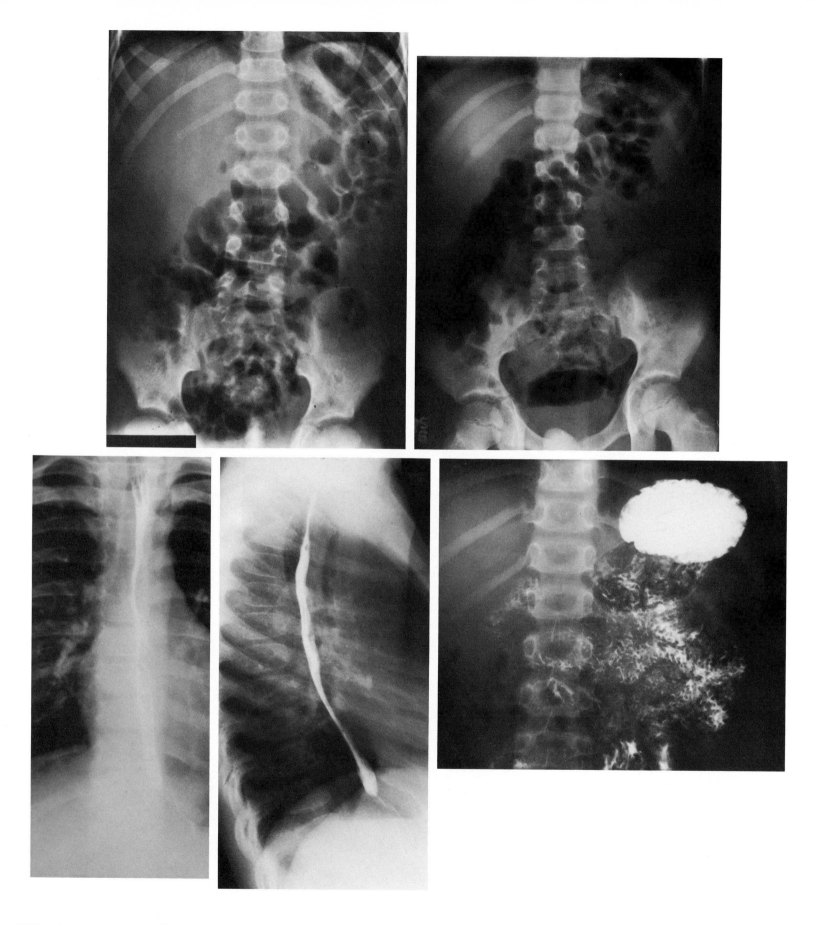

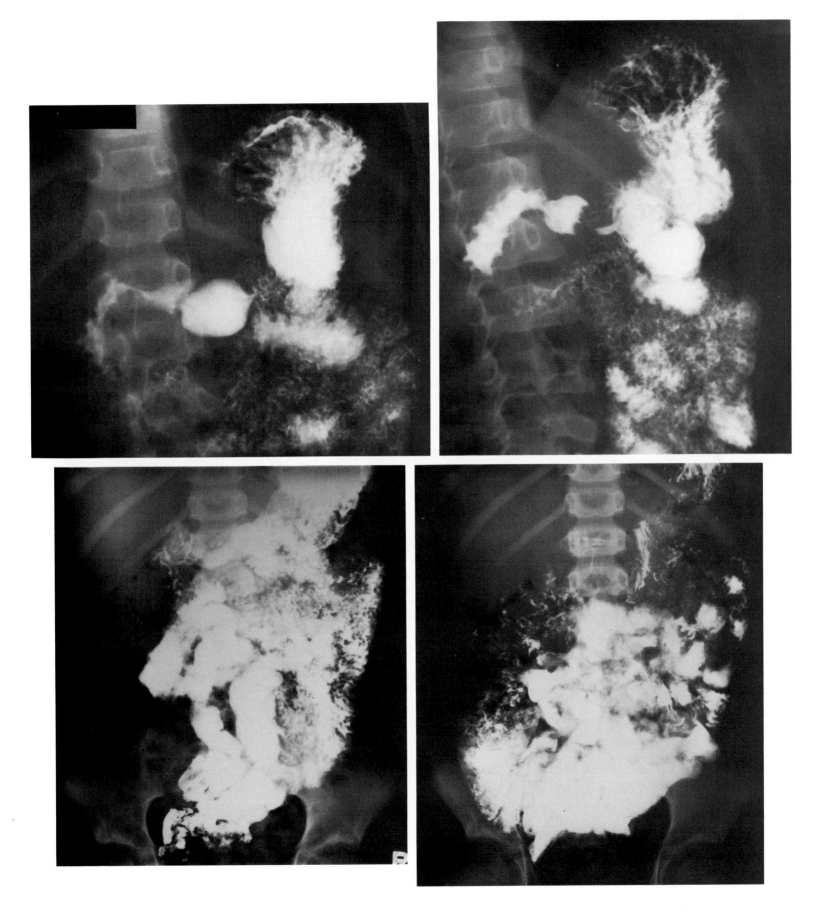

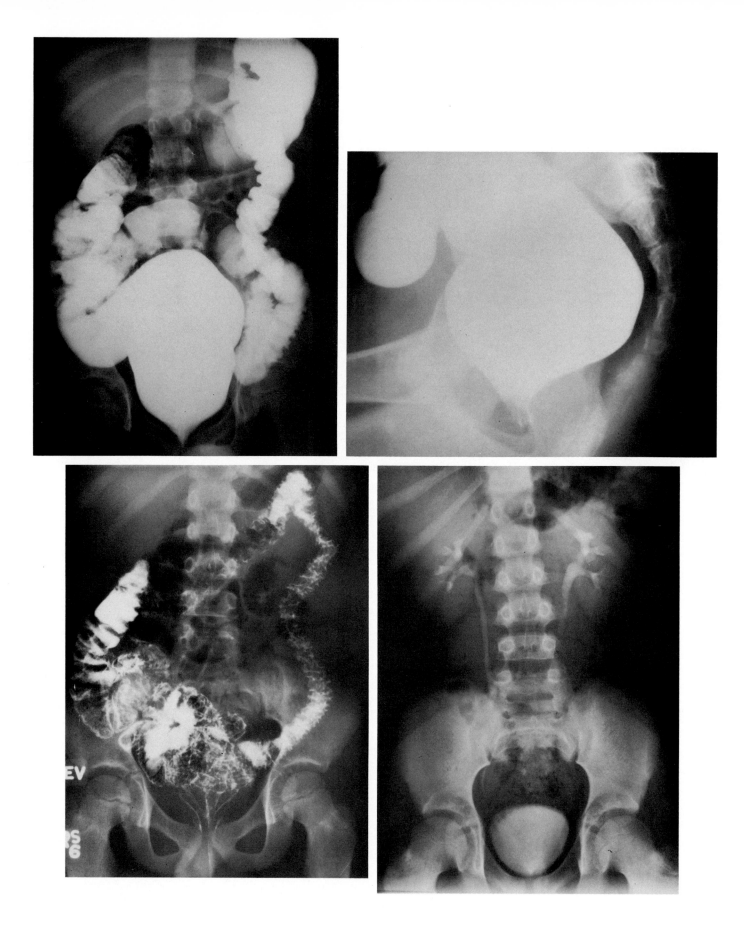

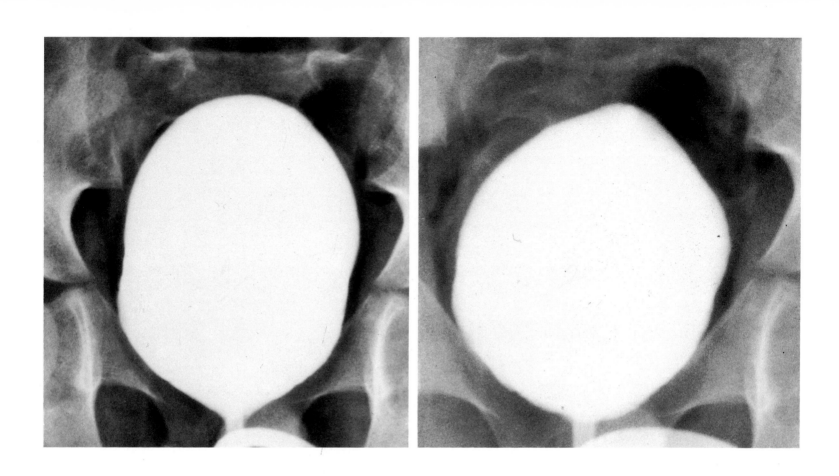

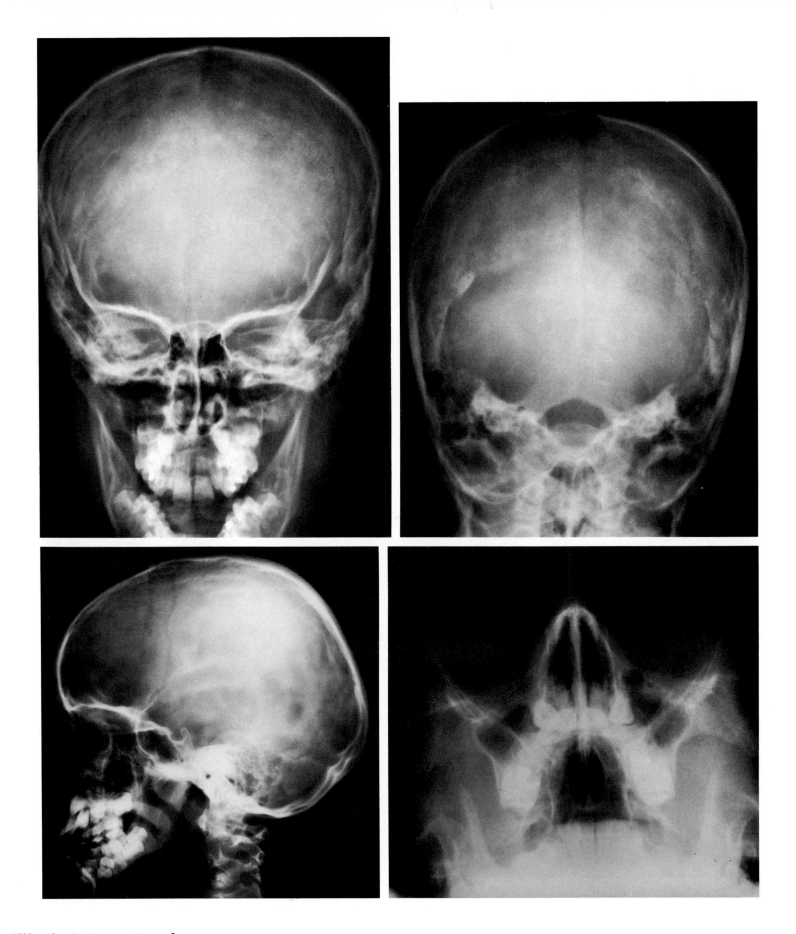

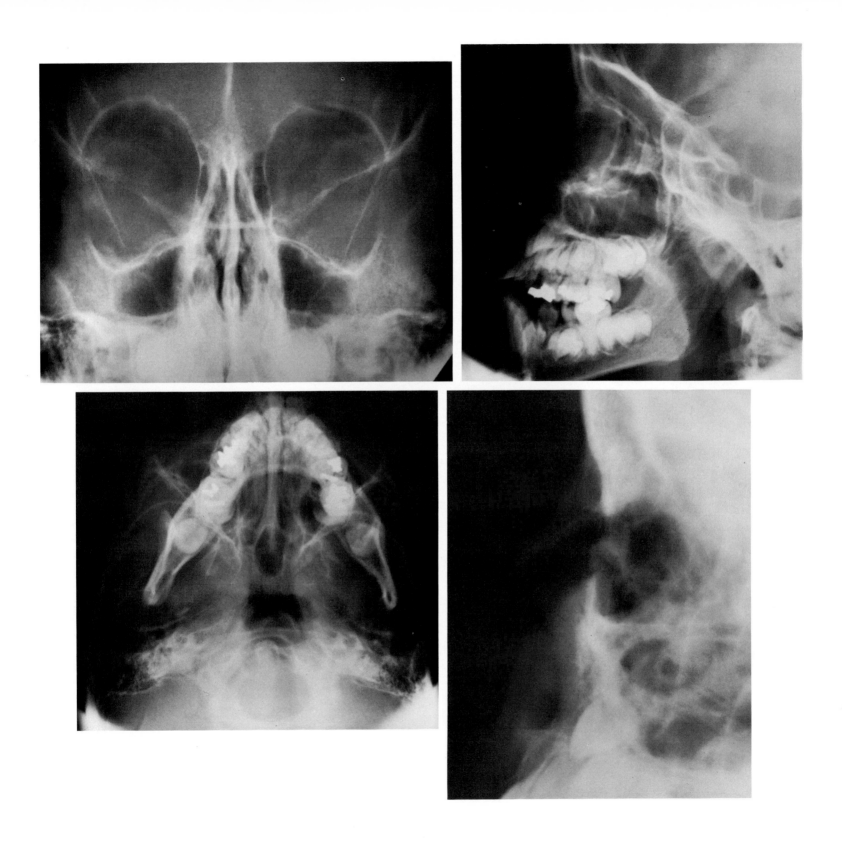

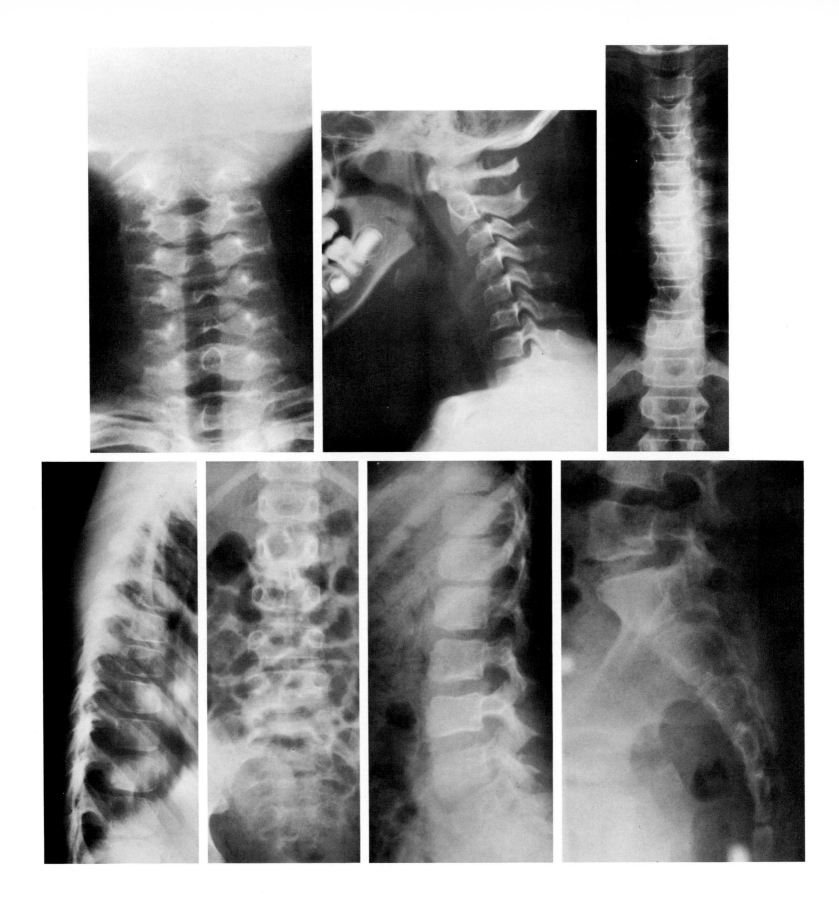

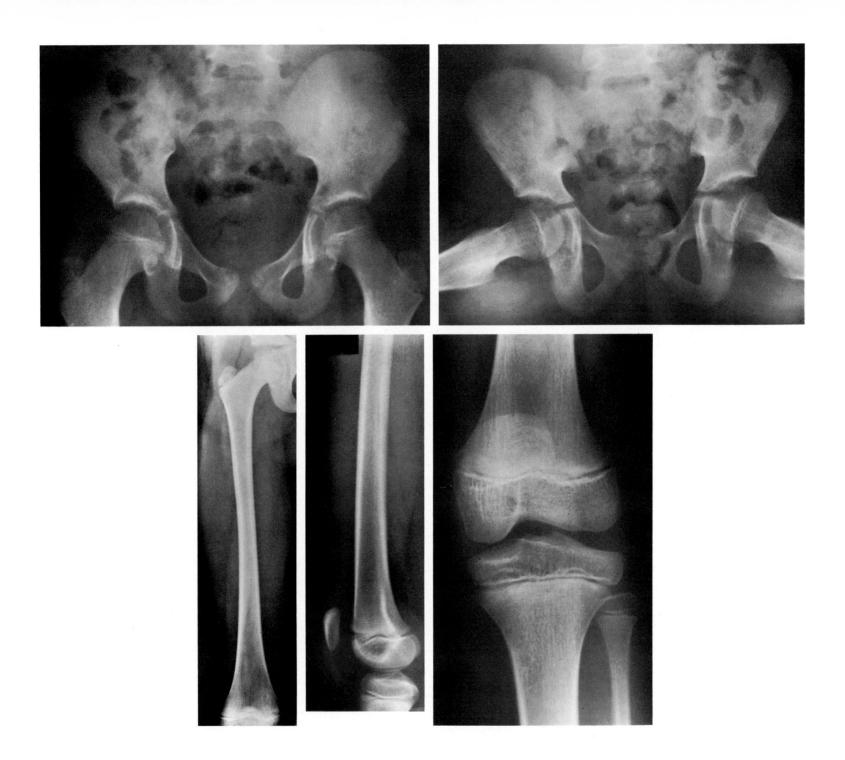

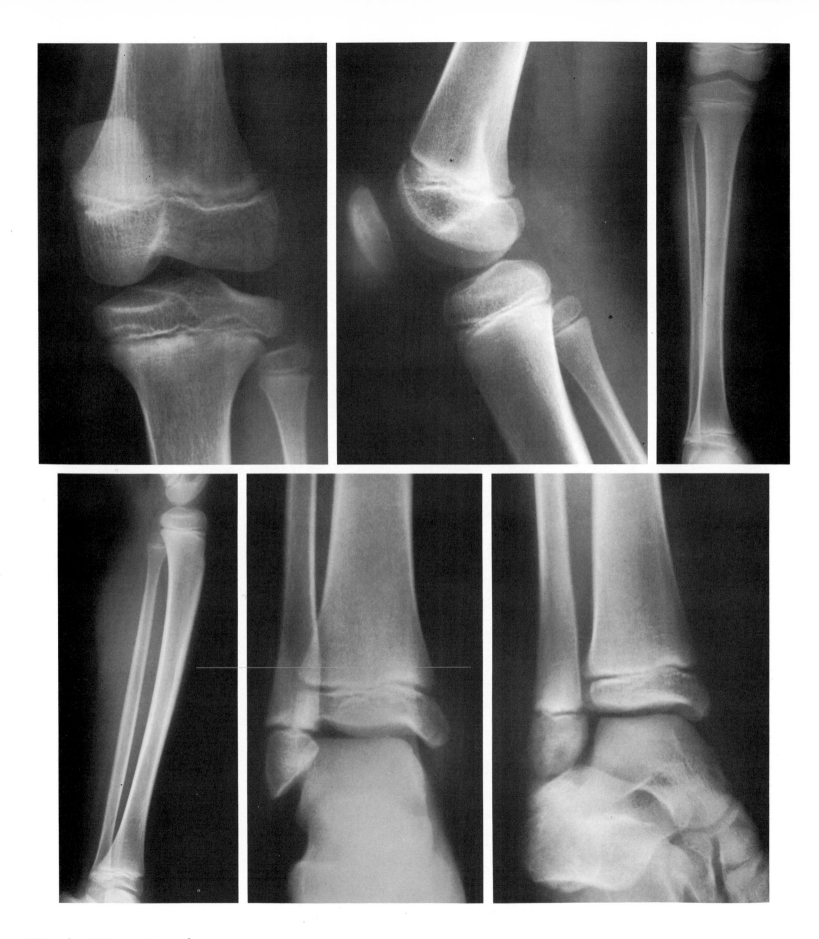

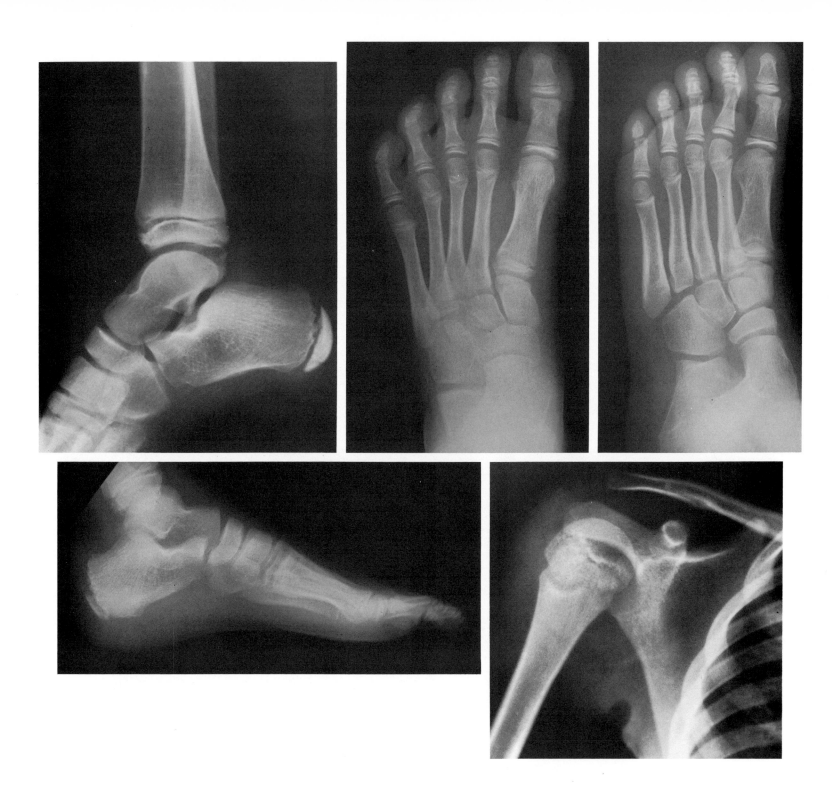

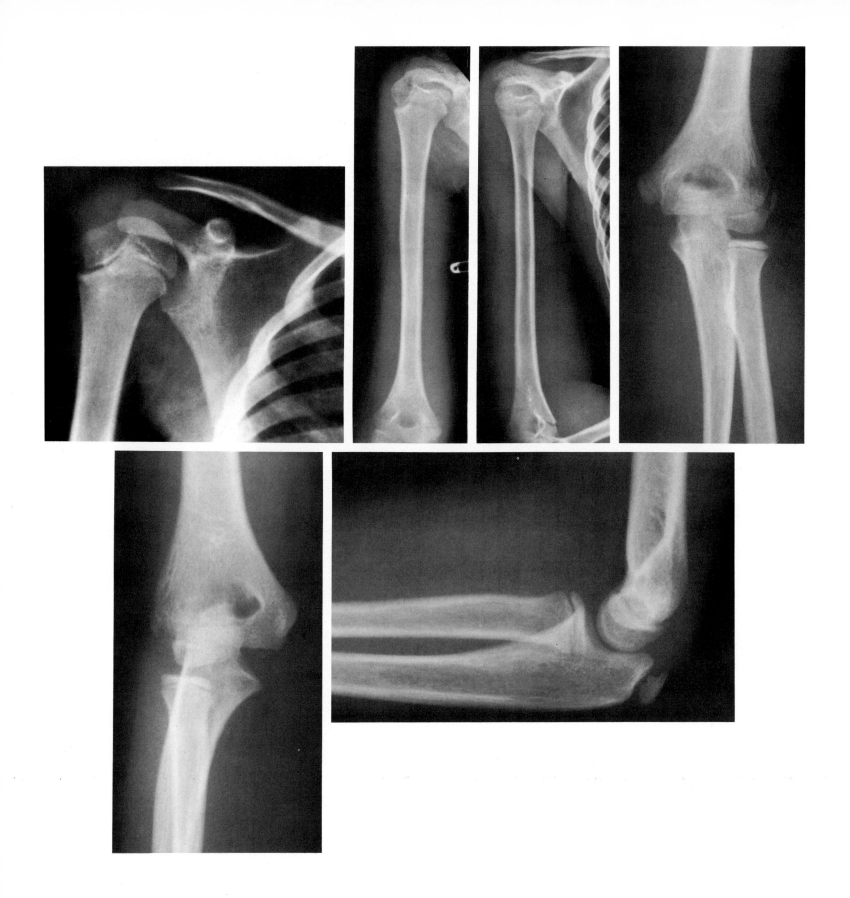

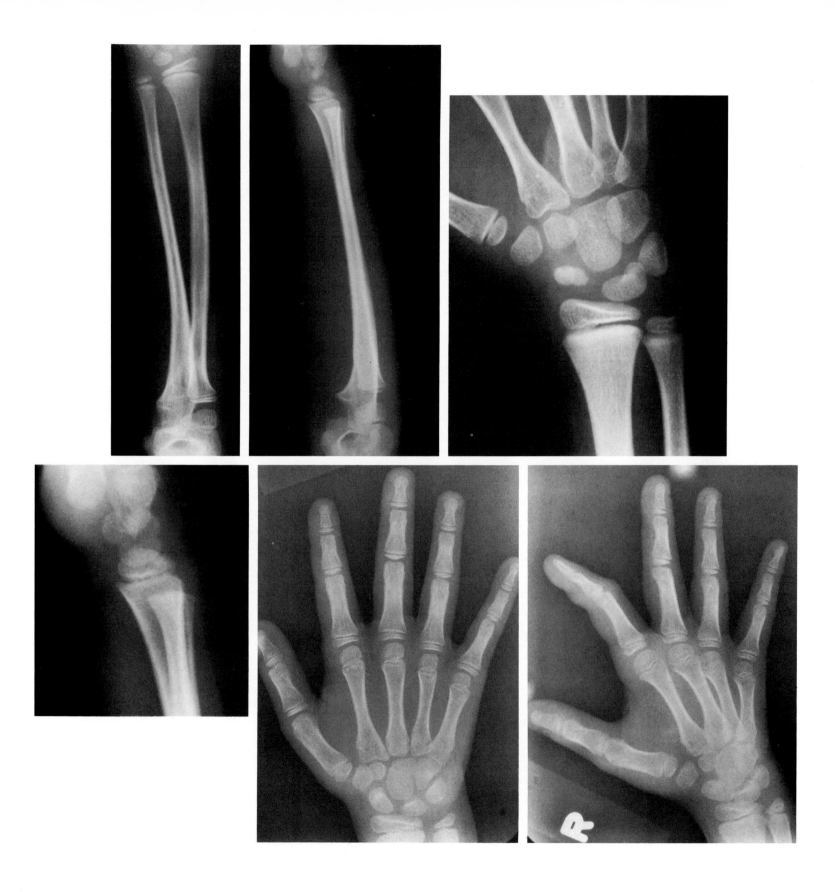

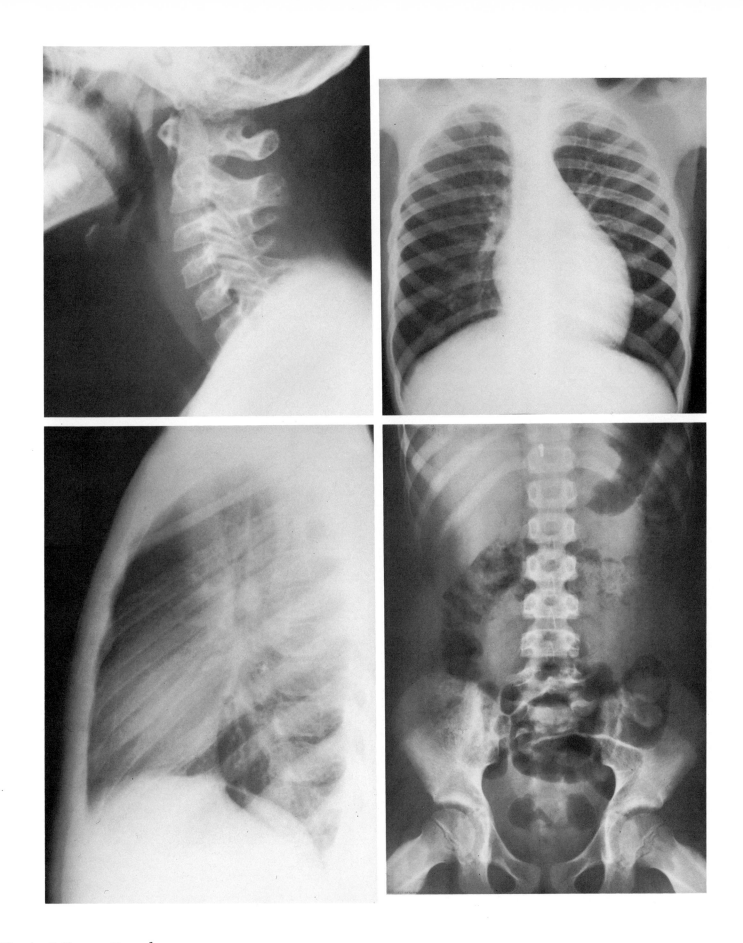

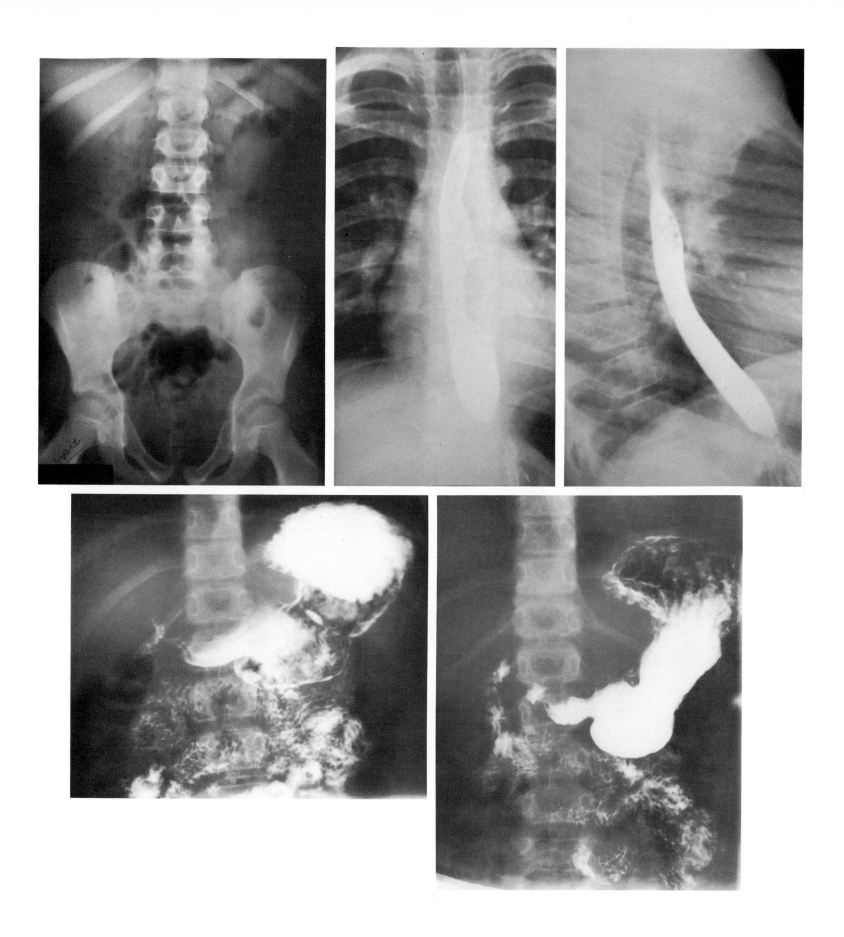

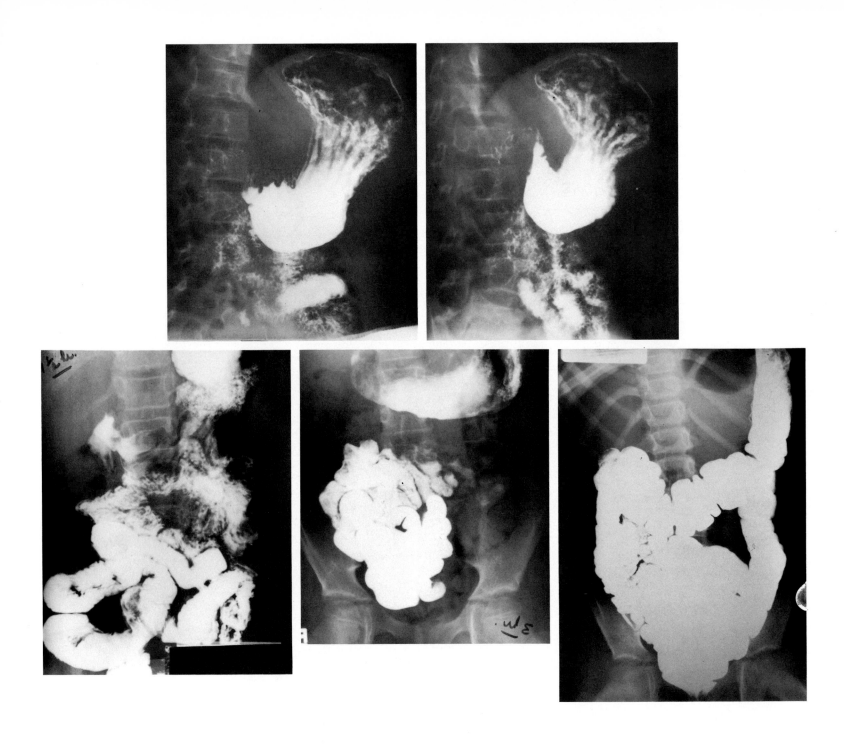

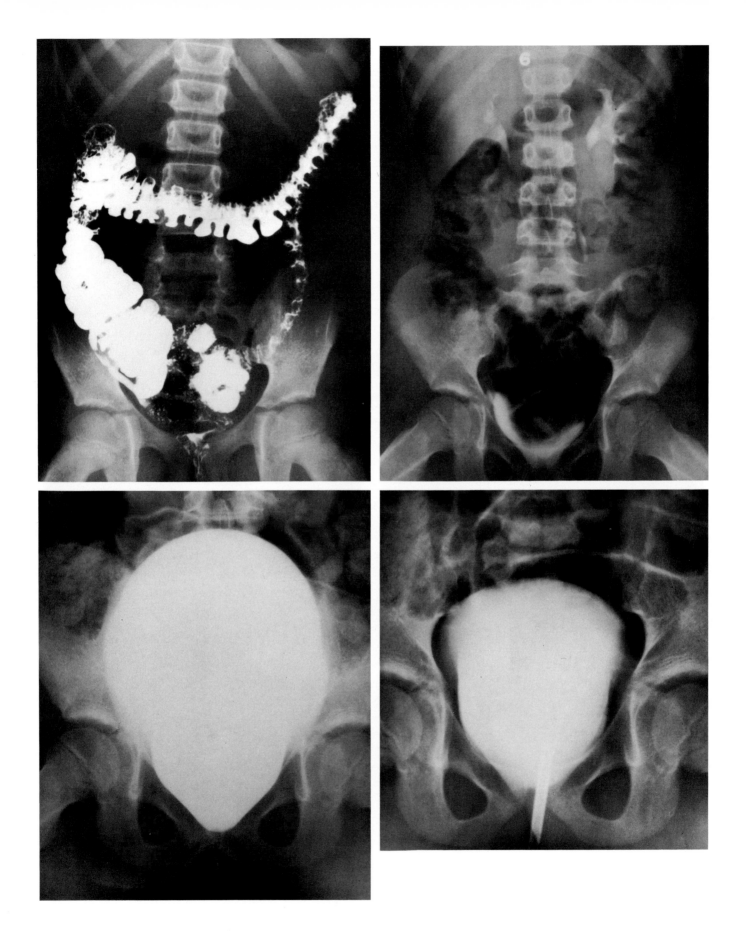

17

9 YEARS

The frontal sinuses are pneumatizing. Digital marking of the calvaria may still be quite prominent. The adenoids are still large. The vertebrae are now rectangular, with notching in the areas of development of the ring apophyses. The ischiopubic synchondroses may still be open. The sacroiliac joints are wide. The patella has an adult configuration. The feet are now adult-like in configuration. The calcaneal apophysis may be very dense. The epiphyses of the distal humerus may ossify from many foci, producing a fragmented appearance. The ossification center for the olecranon process appears.

The pulmonary artery may be prominent in some individuals.

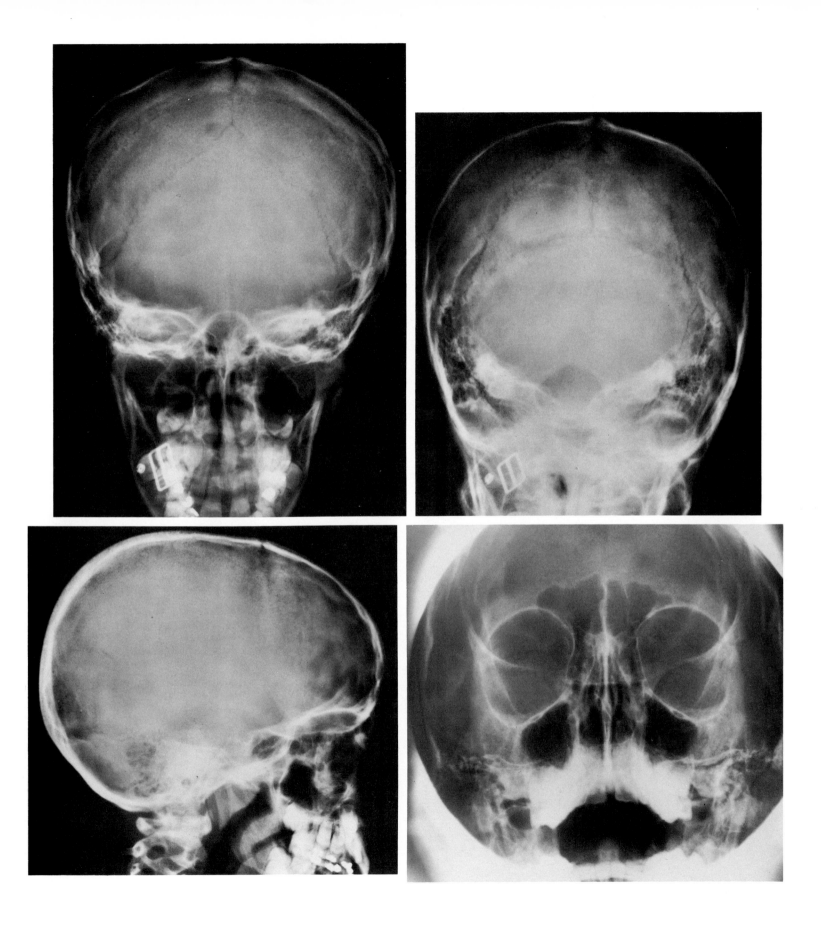

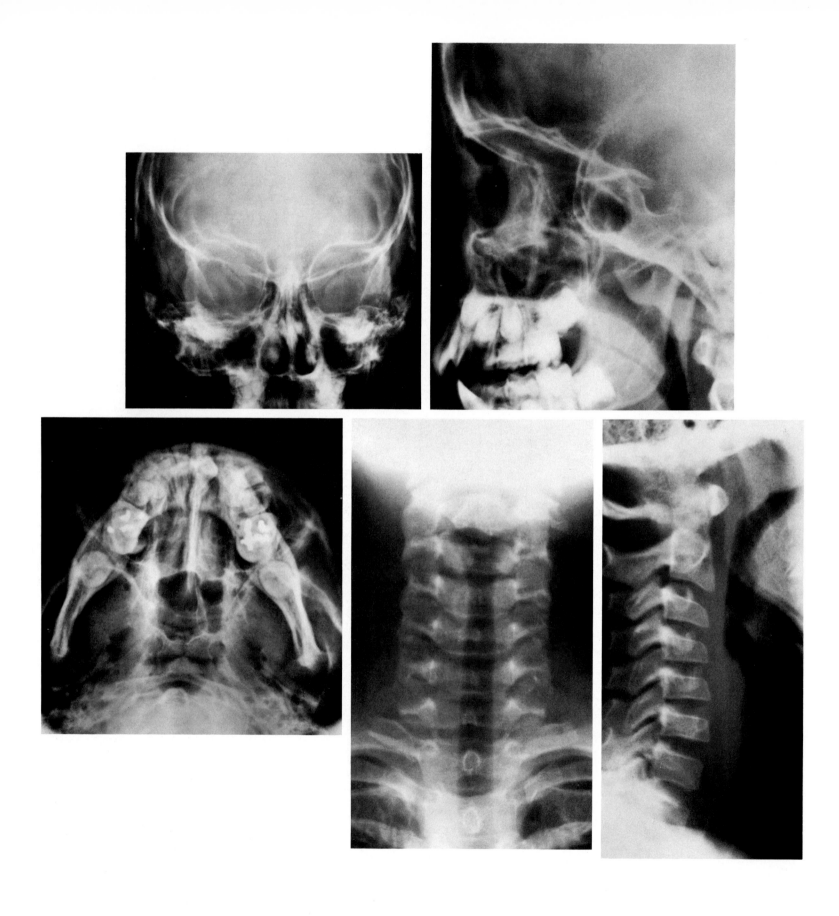

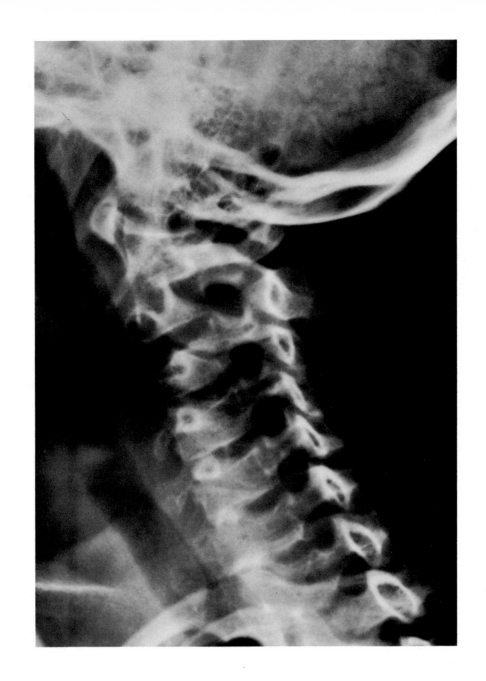

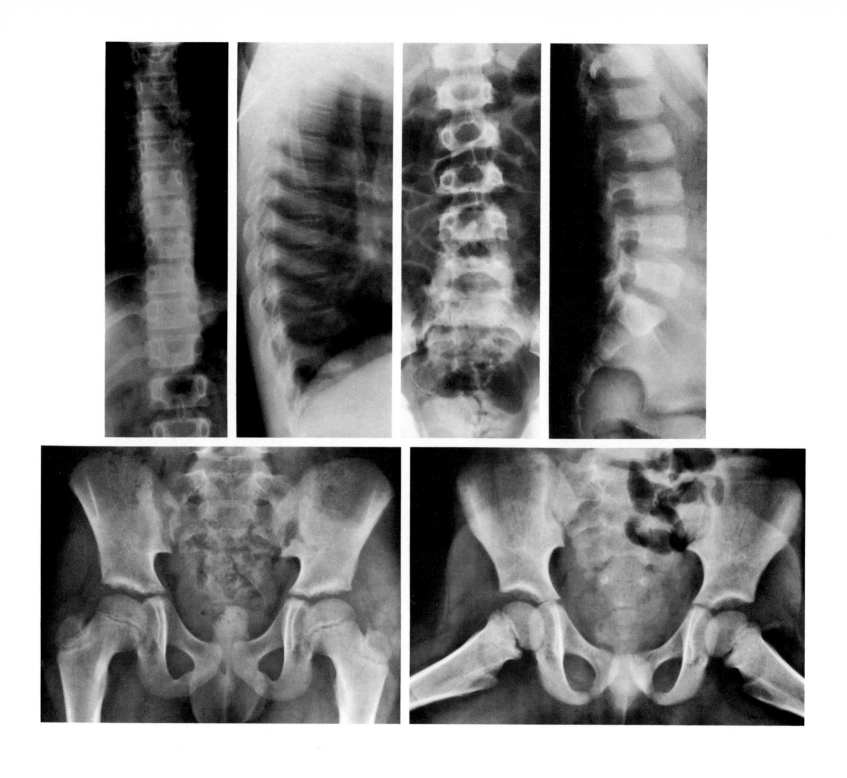

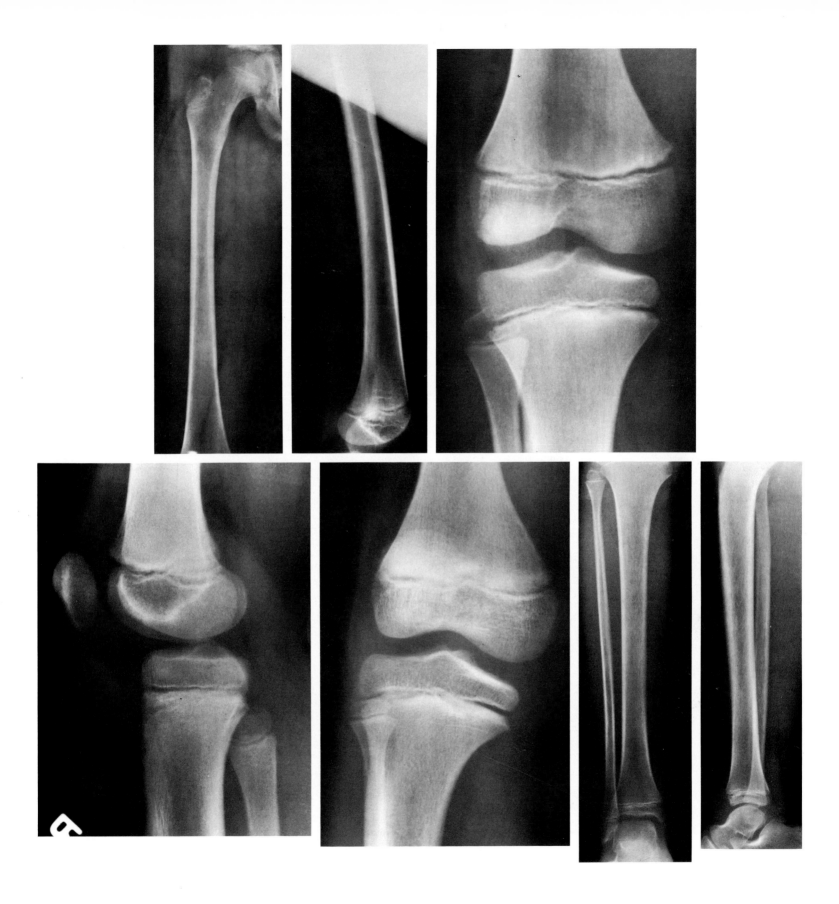

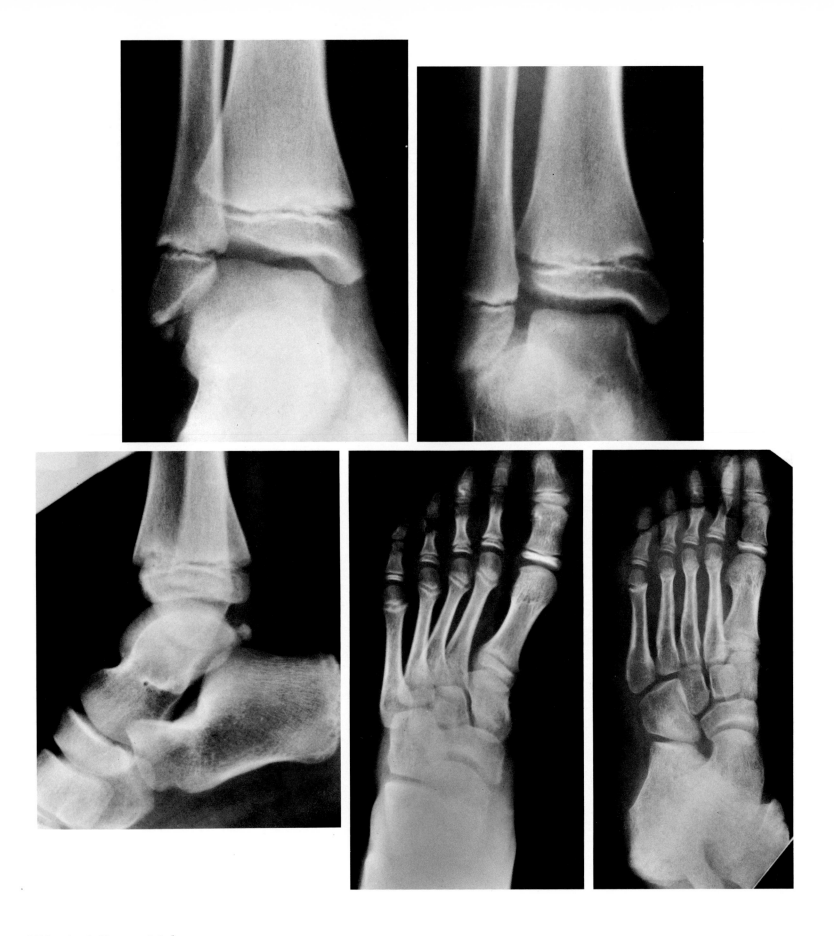

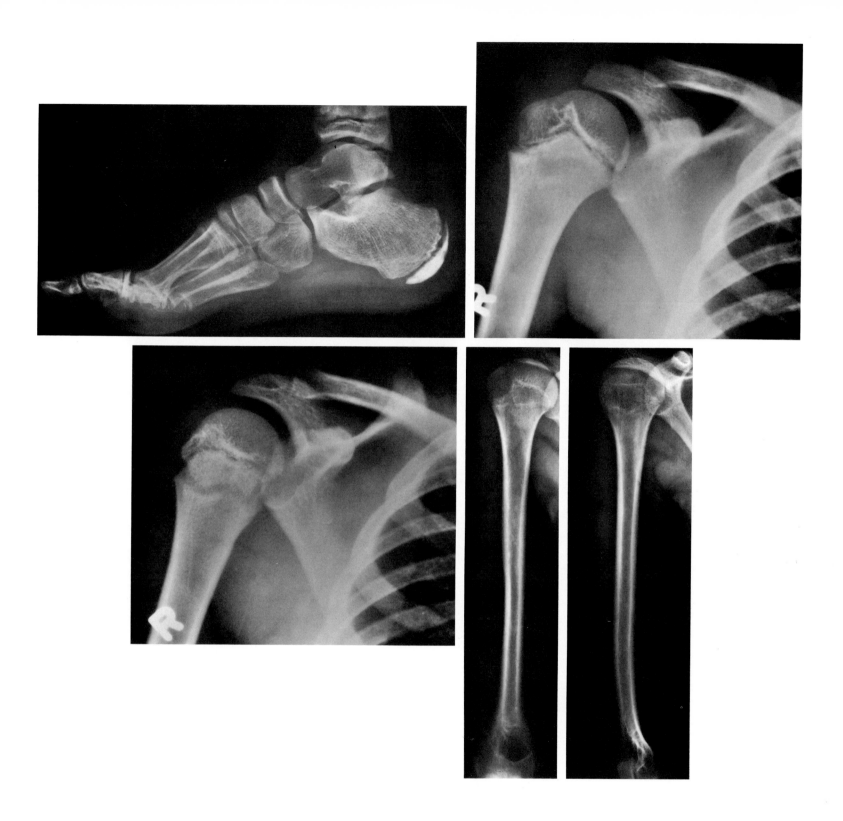

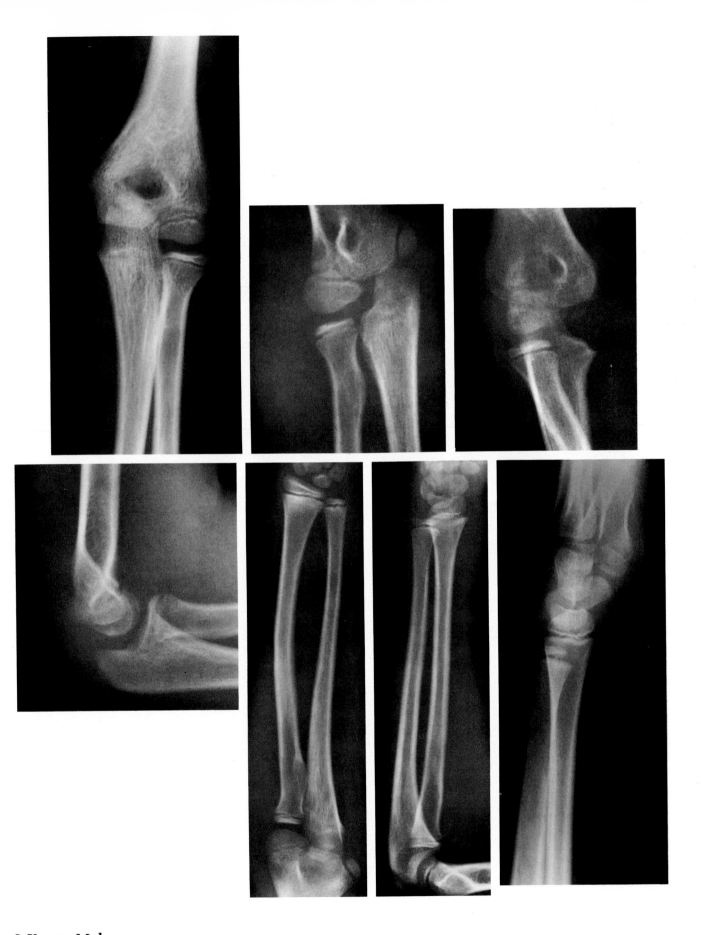

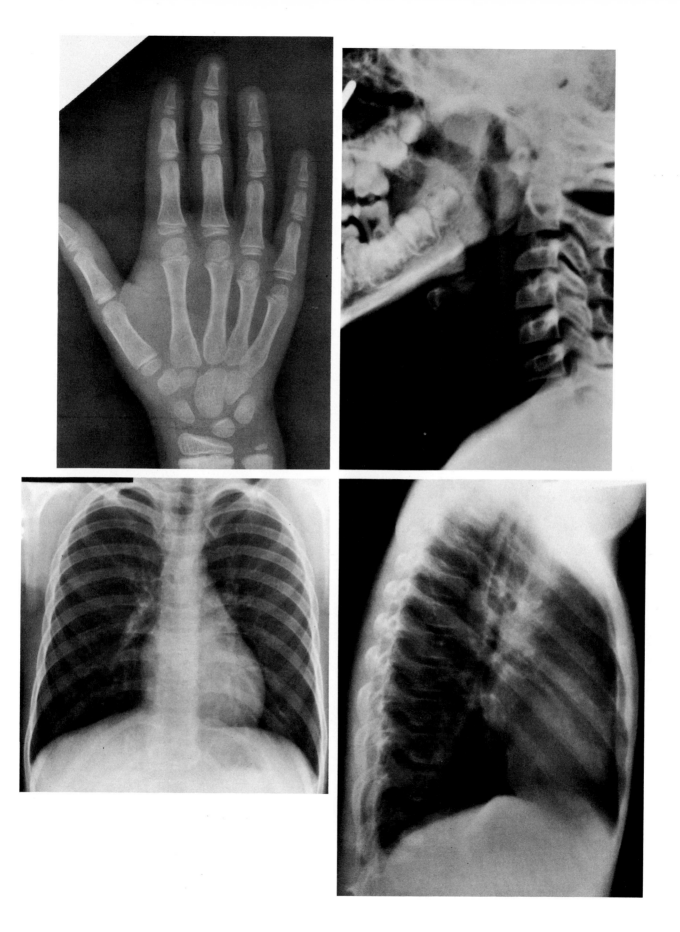

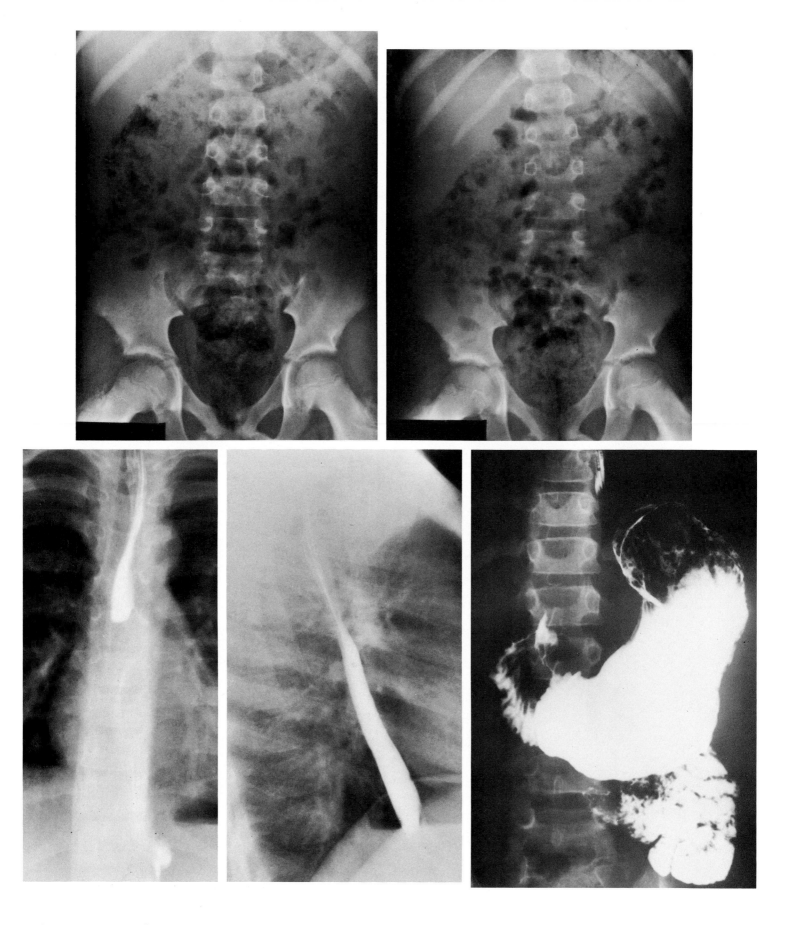

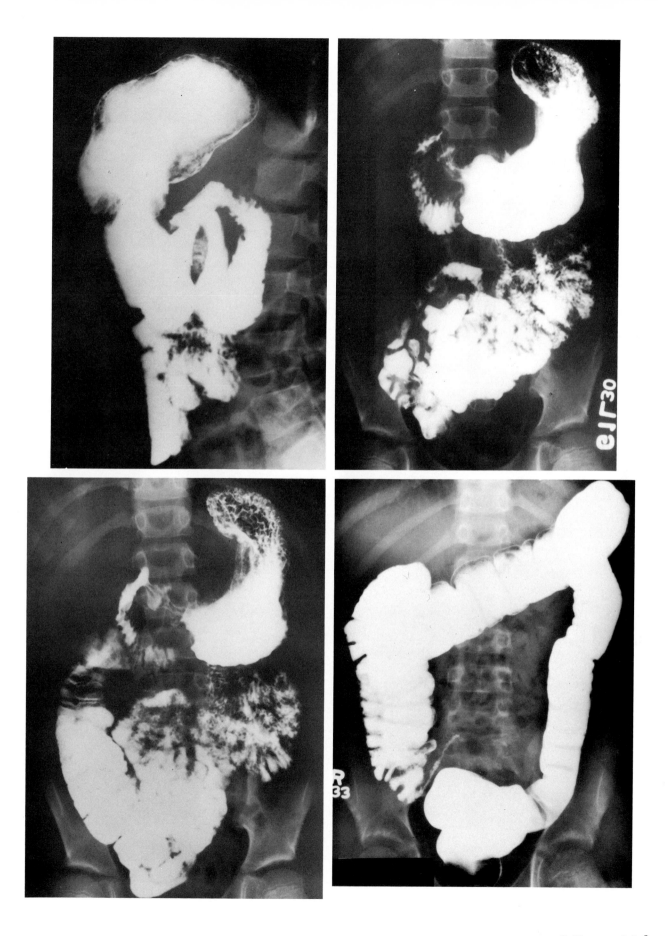

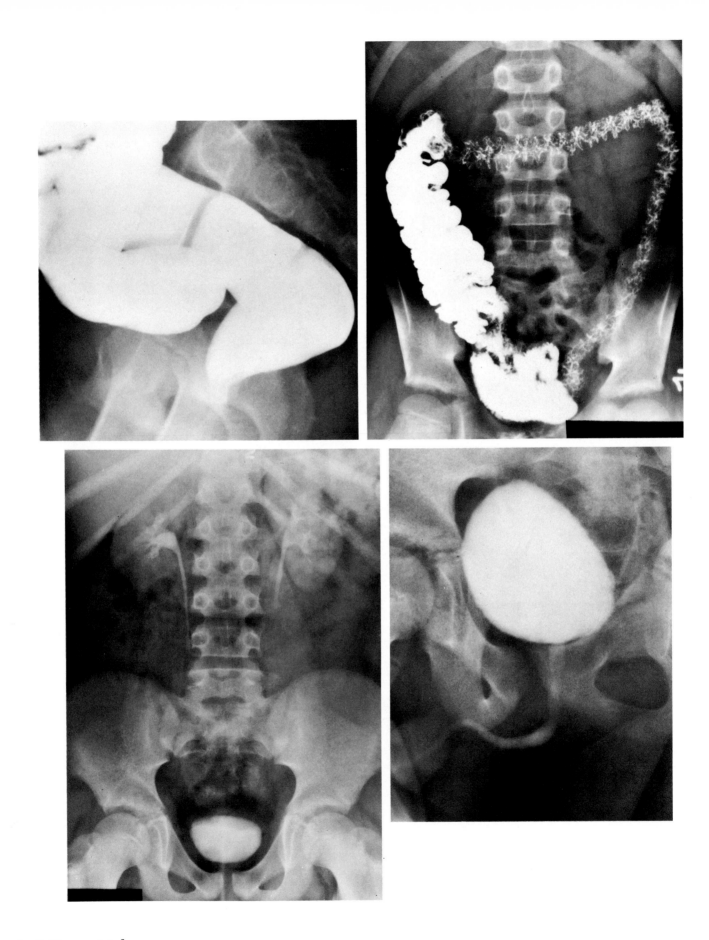

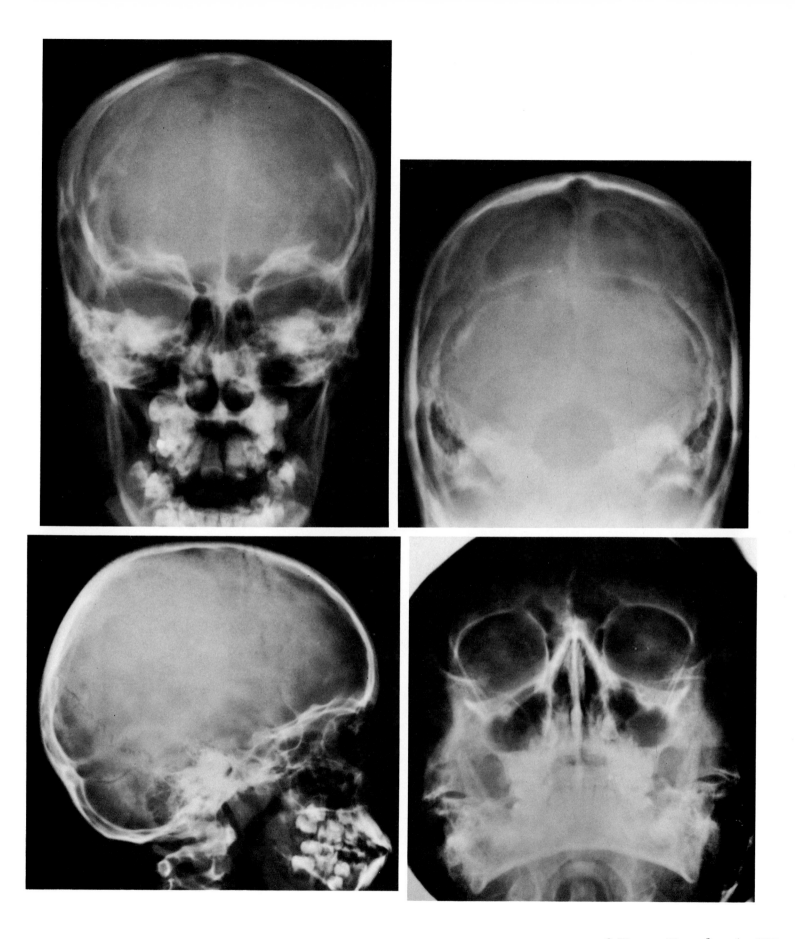

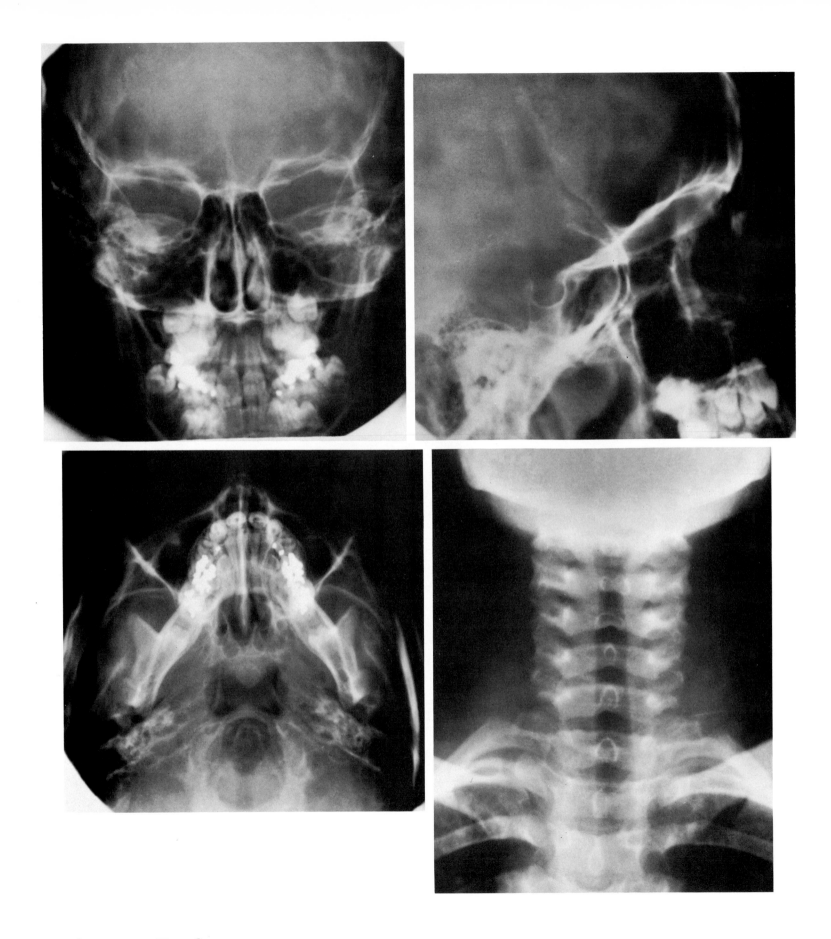

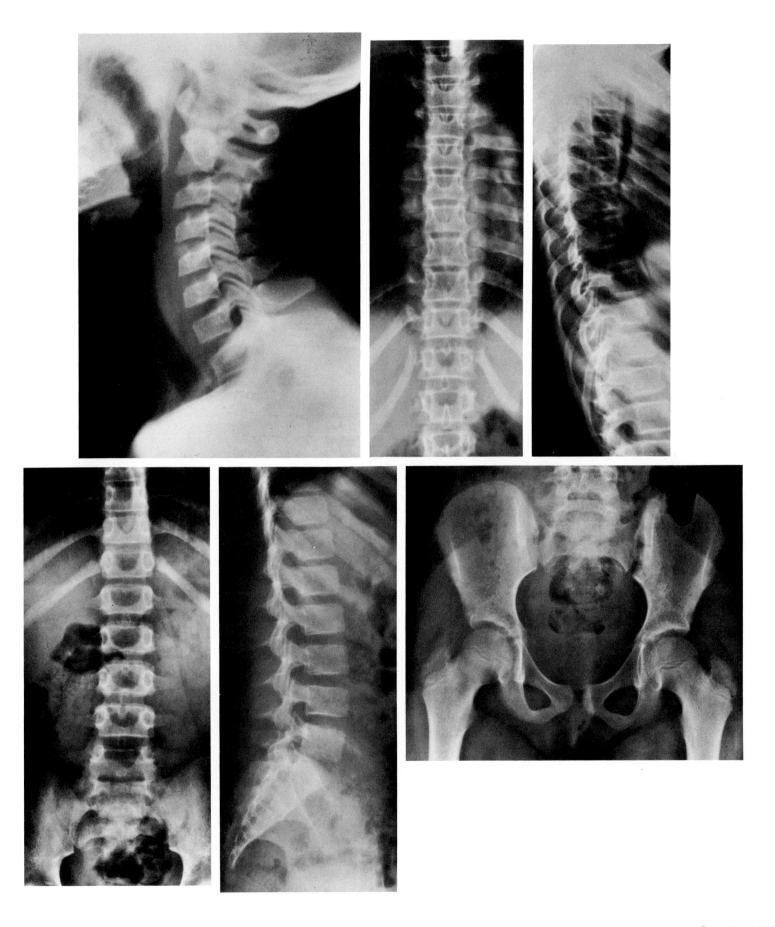

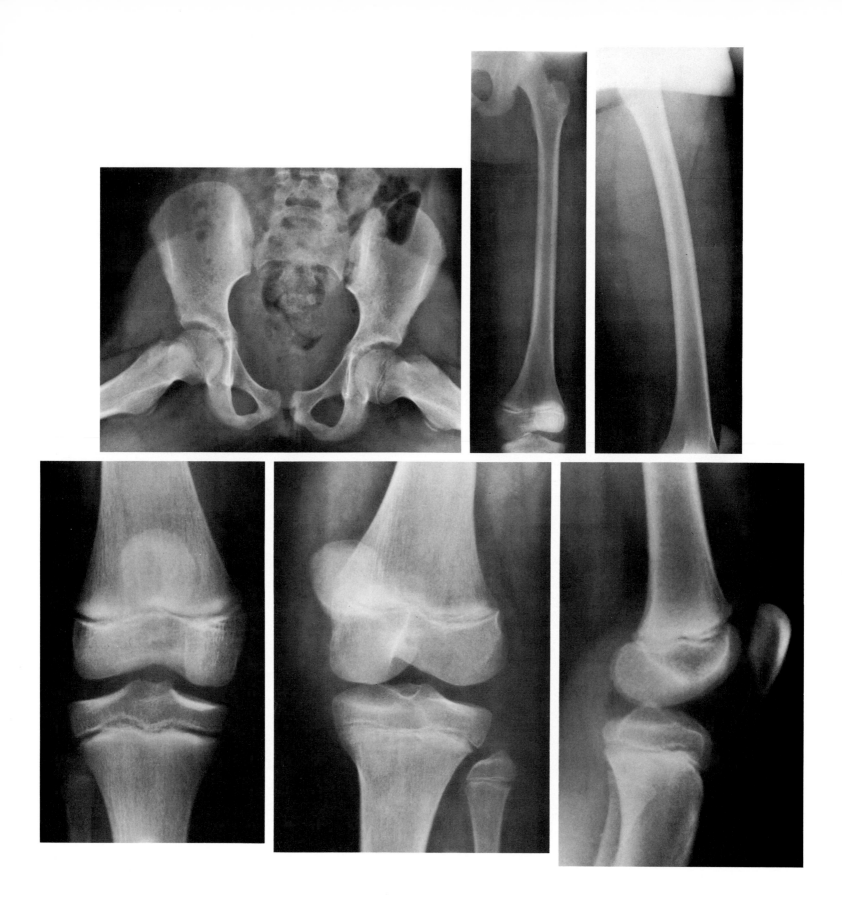

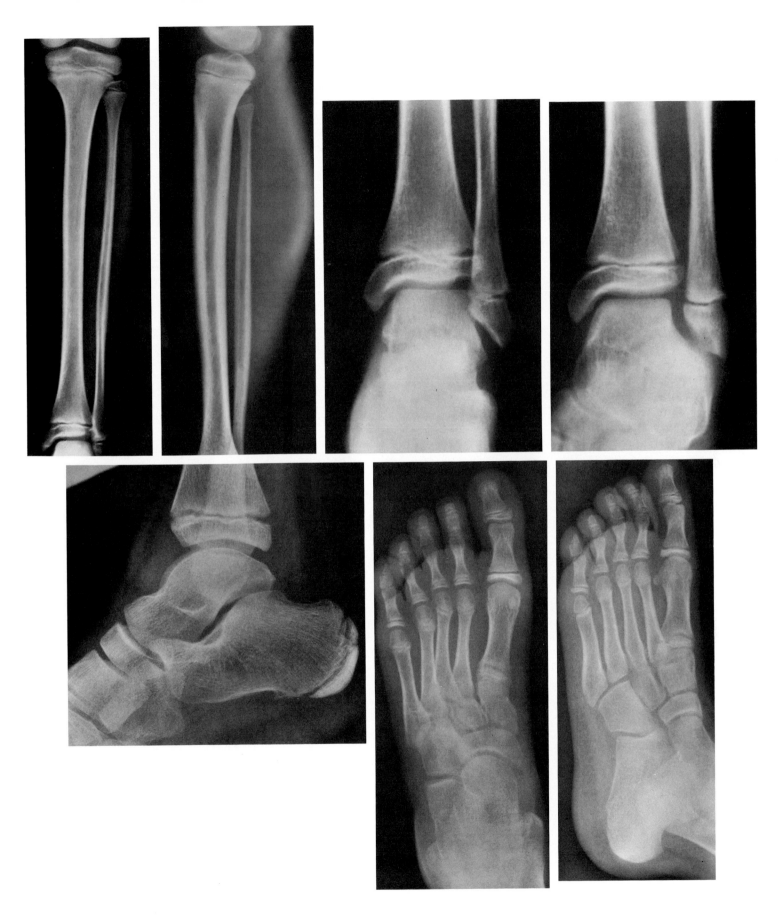

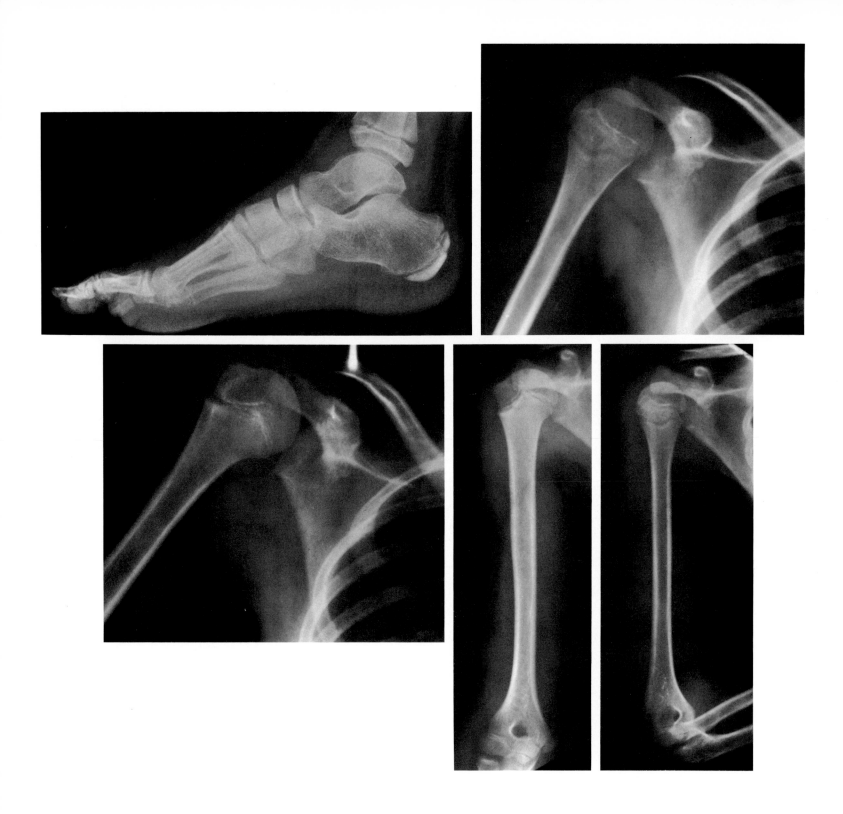

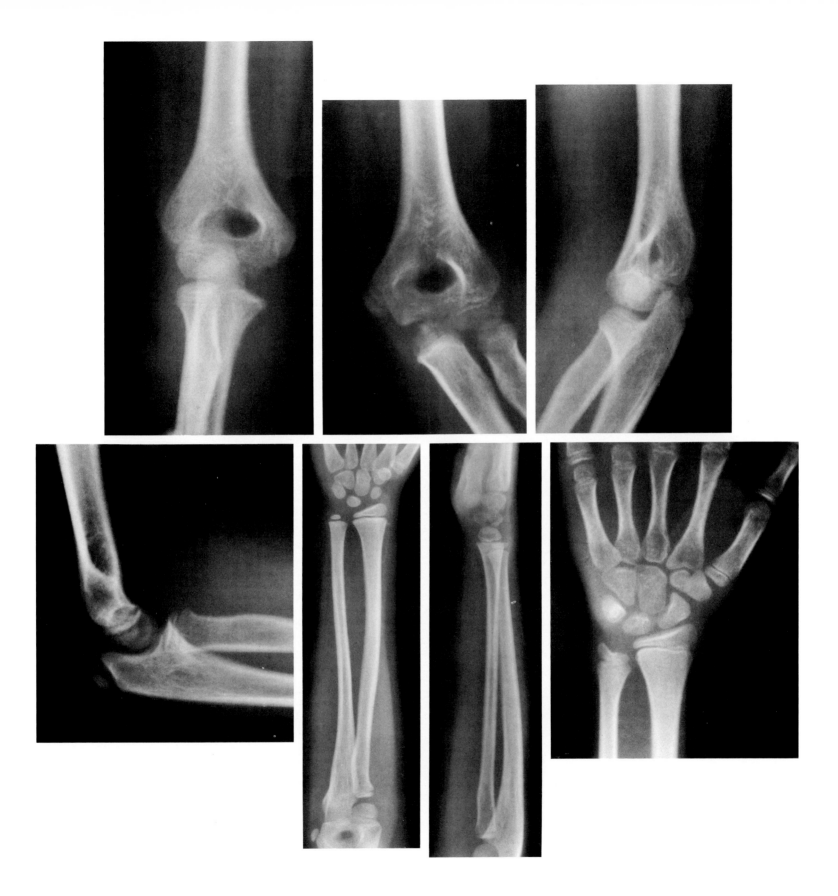

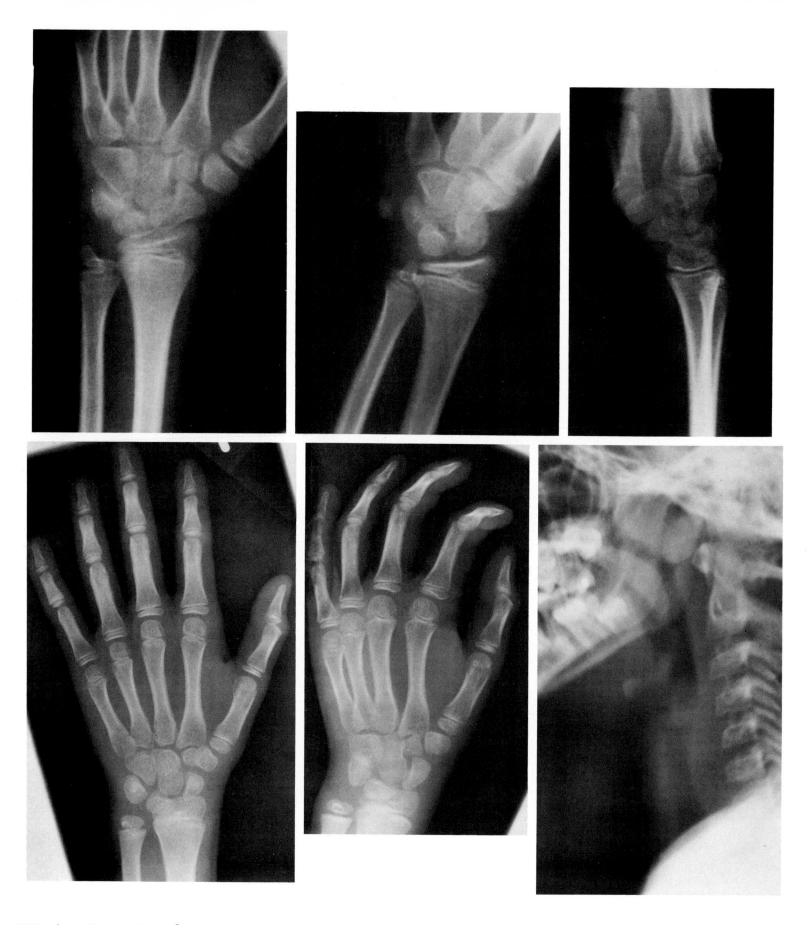

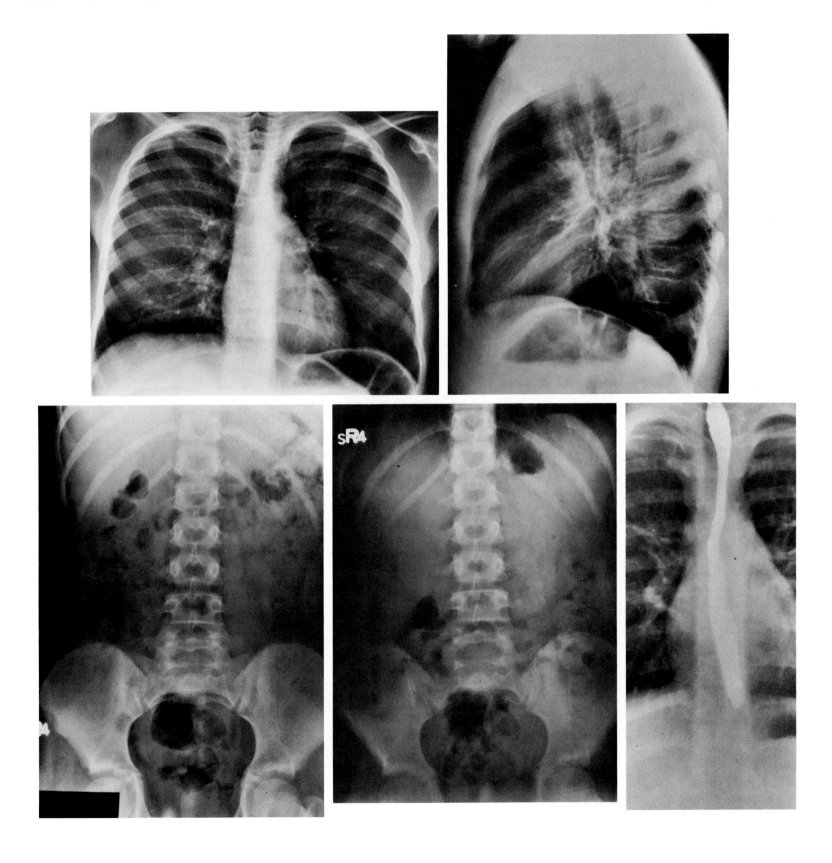

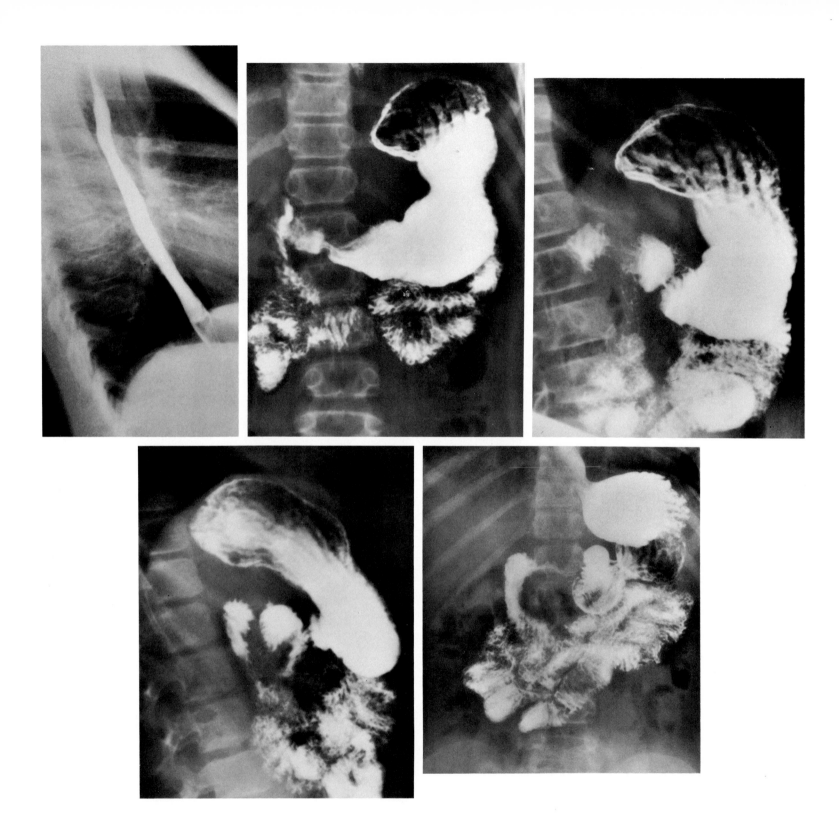

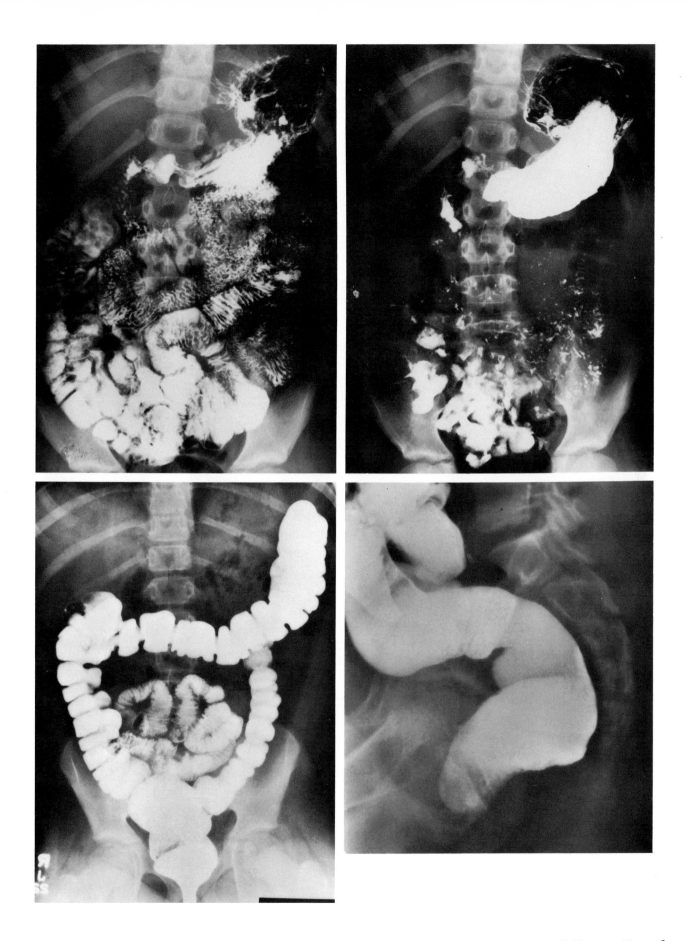

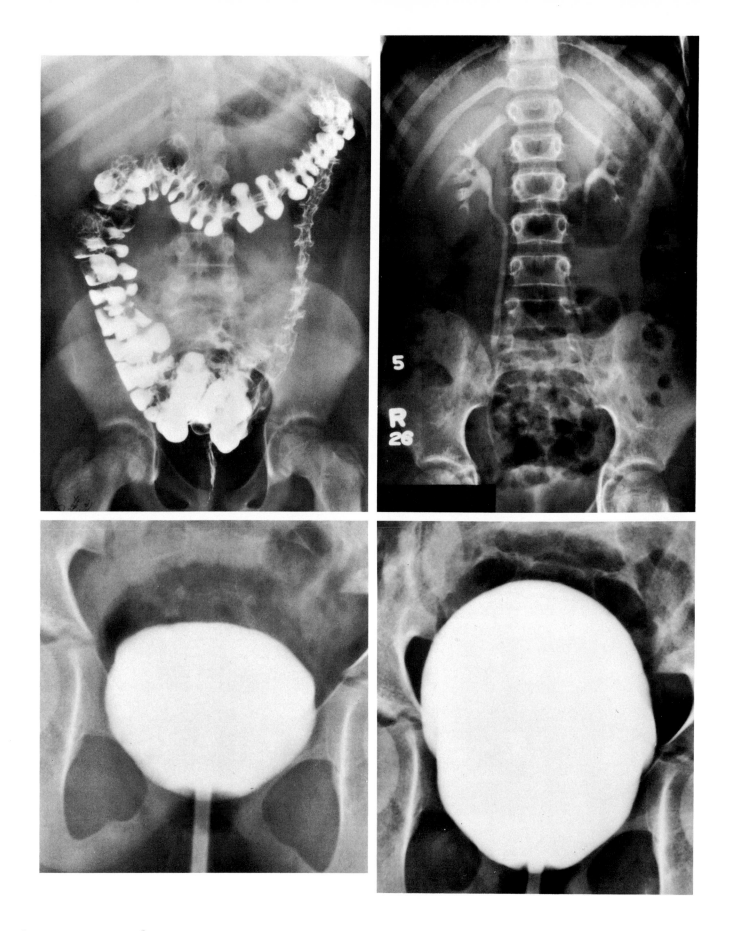

18

10 YEARS

Pneumatization of the frontal and sphenoid sinuses continues. Calvarial digital markings may still be prominent. The cervical vertebral bodies are still wedge-shaped. The development of the odontoid process may be complete at this age. The ilia are wider than previously, as are the ischia and pubes. The ischiopubic synchondroses are closing. The apparent discontinuity of the distal tibial epiphyseal plate persists. The ossification center for the lateral epicondyle appears. The epiphysis for the trochlea at the elbow remains irregular. The apophysis of the calcaneal tuberosity is still dense, as is the epiphysis of the base of the proximal phalanx of the great toe.

The epiglottis may appear quite elongated at this age. Breast shadows are becoming evident.

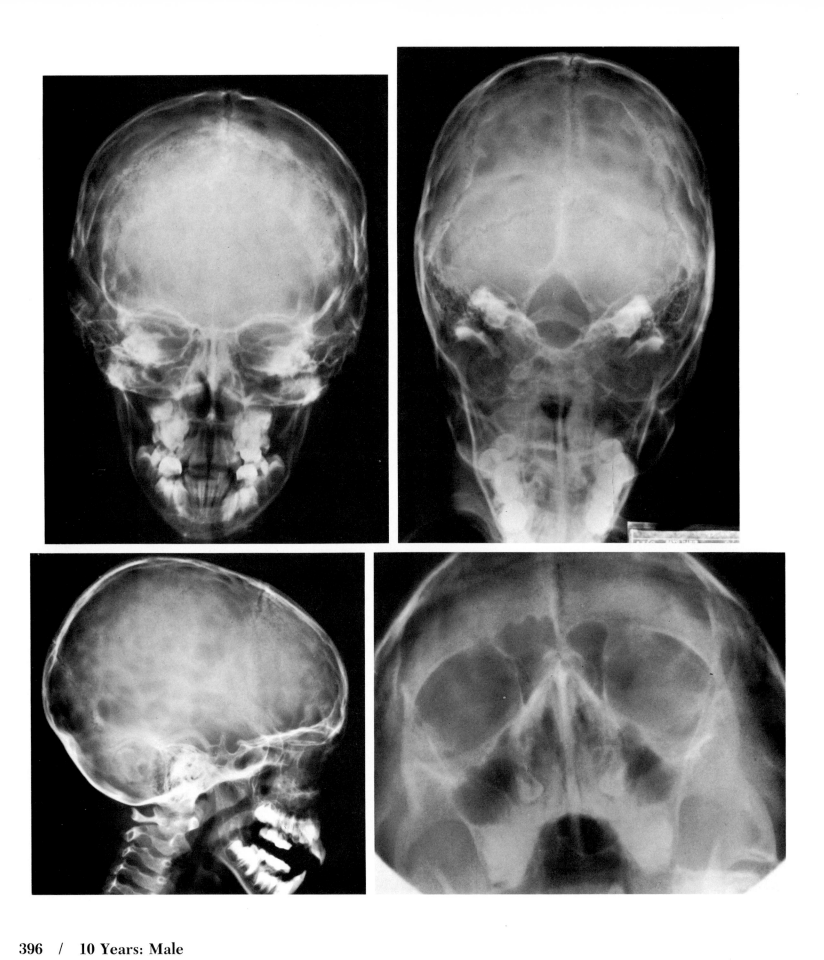

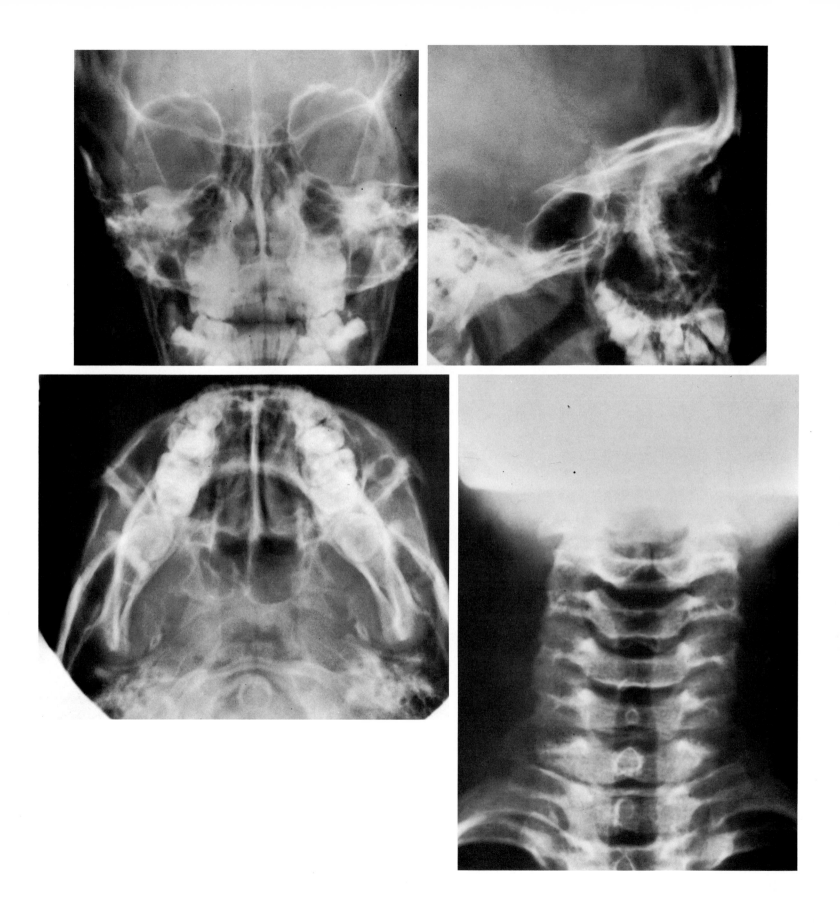

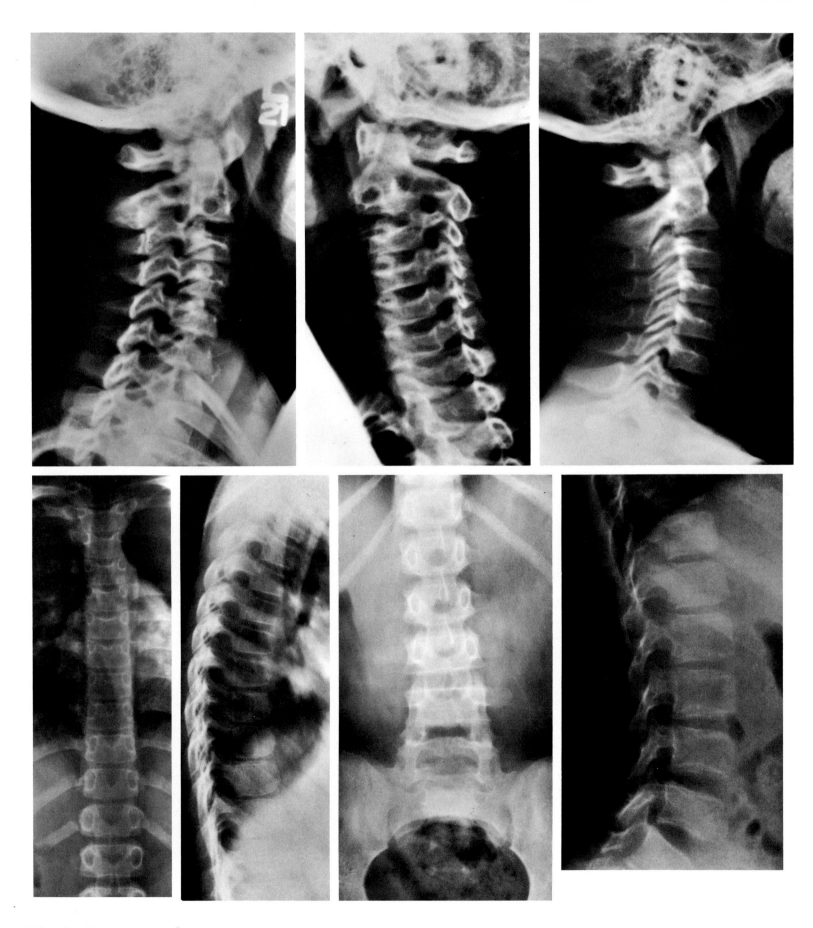

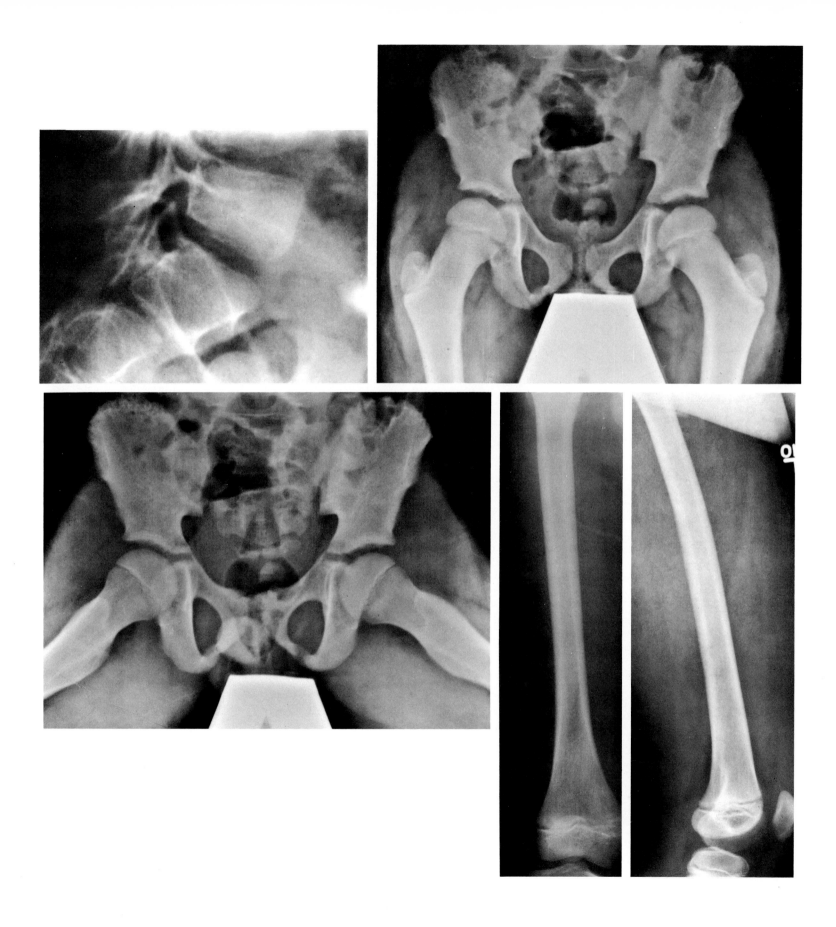

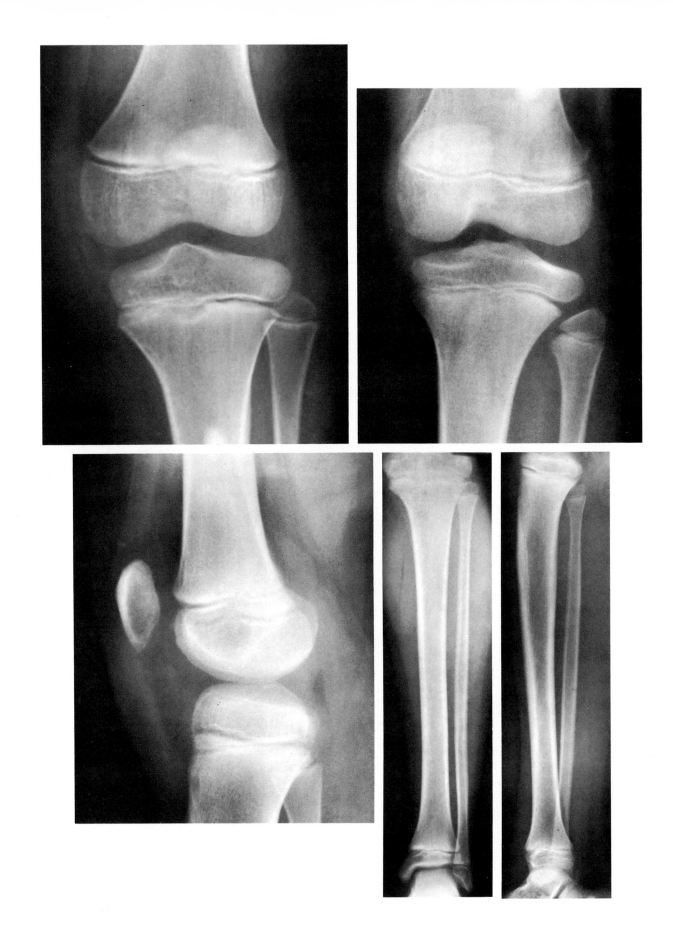

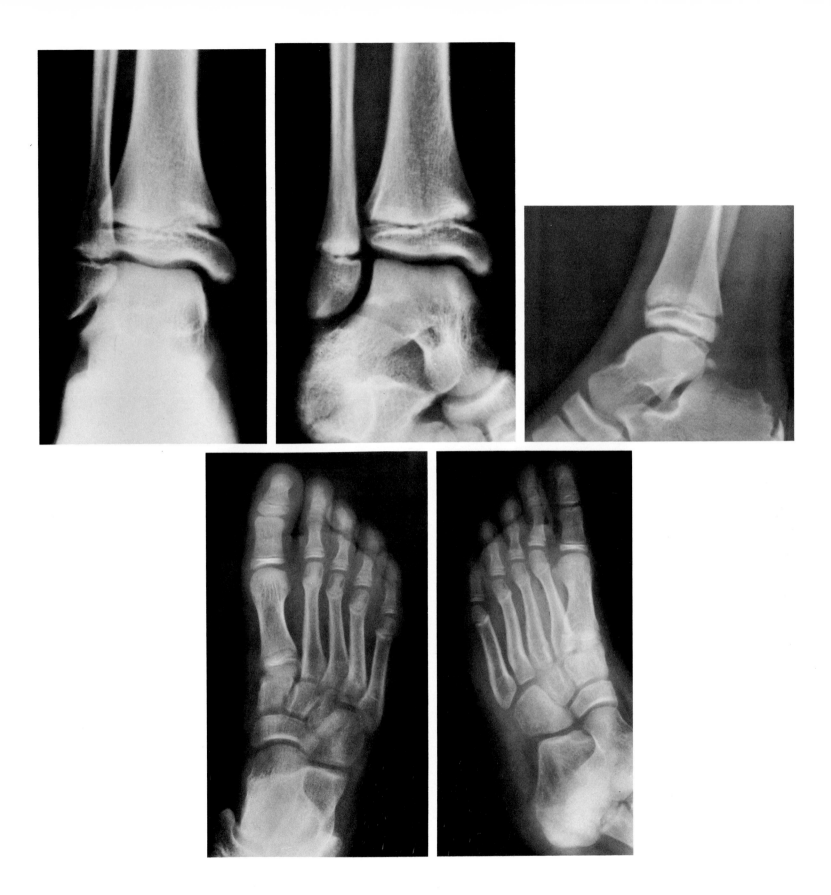

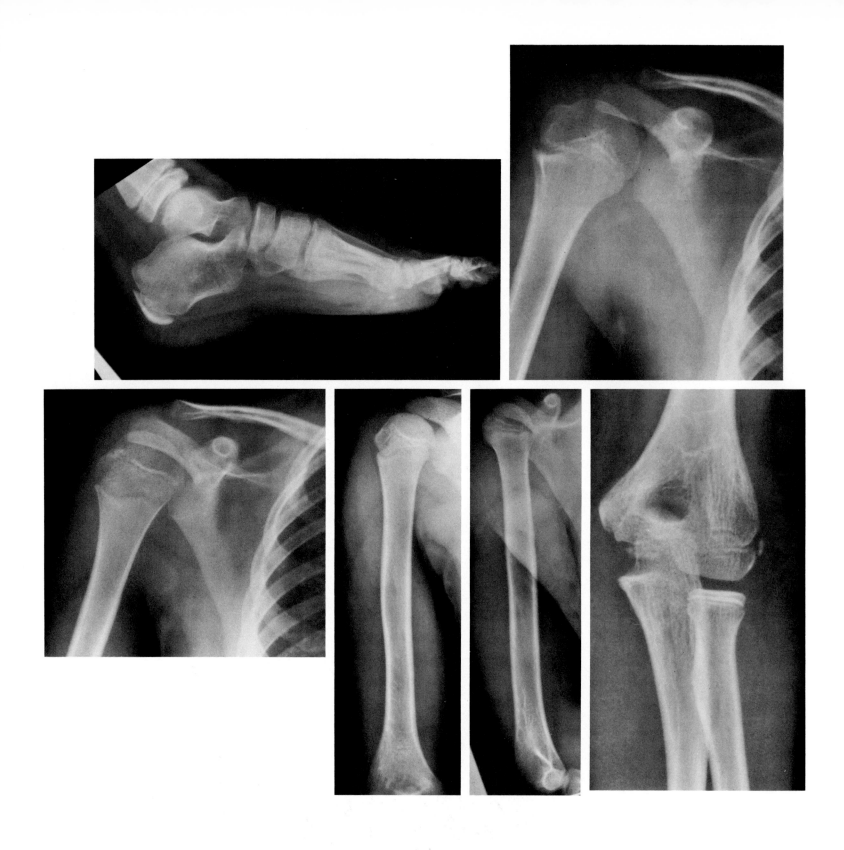

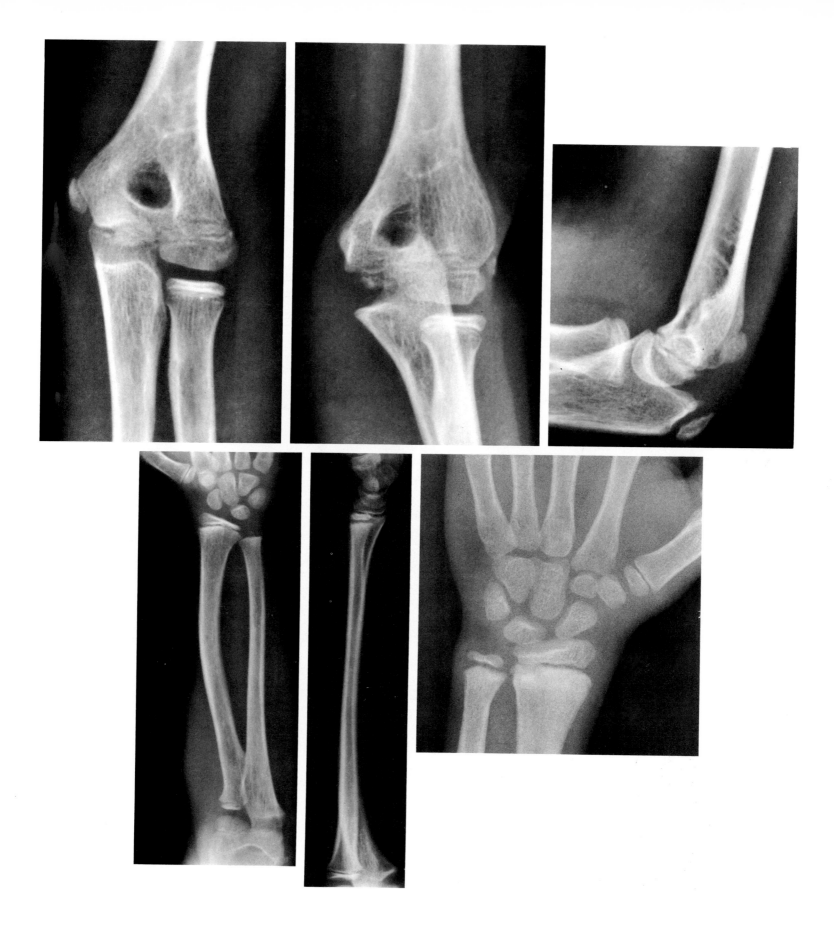

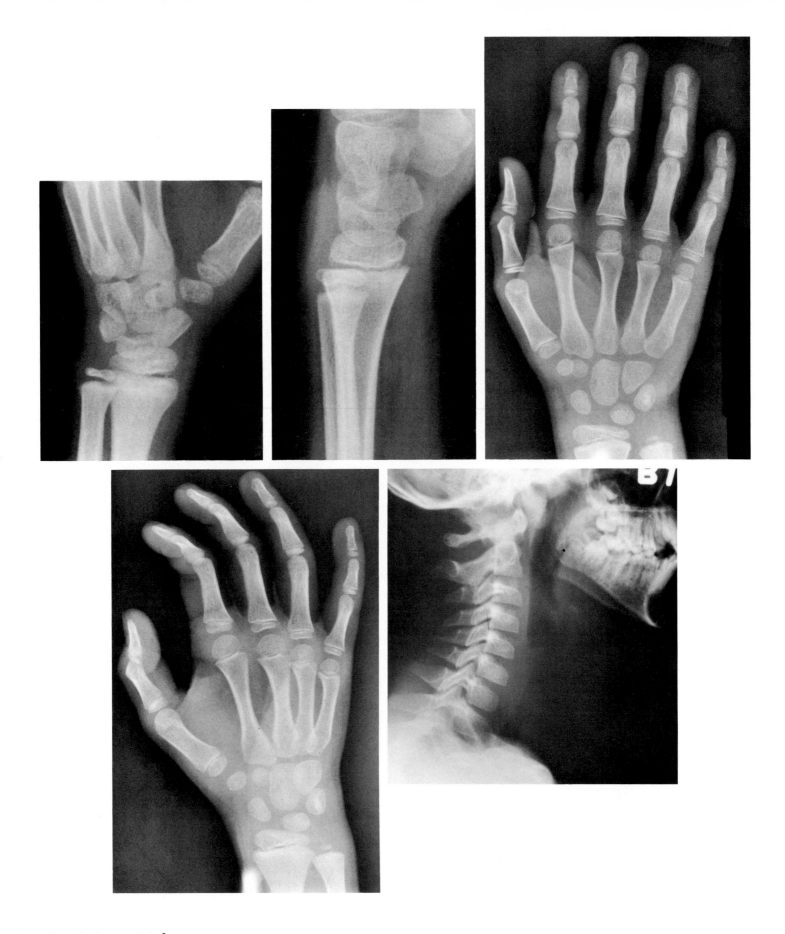

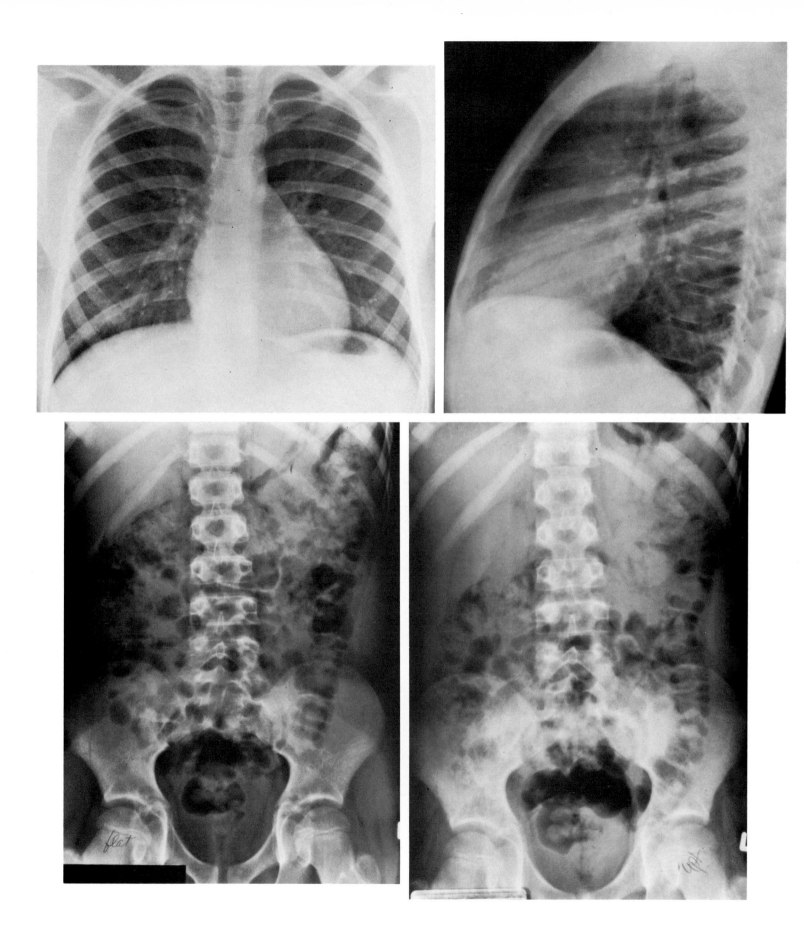

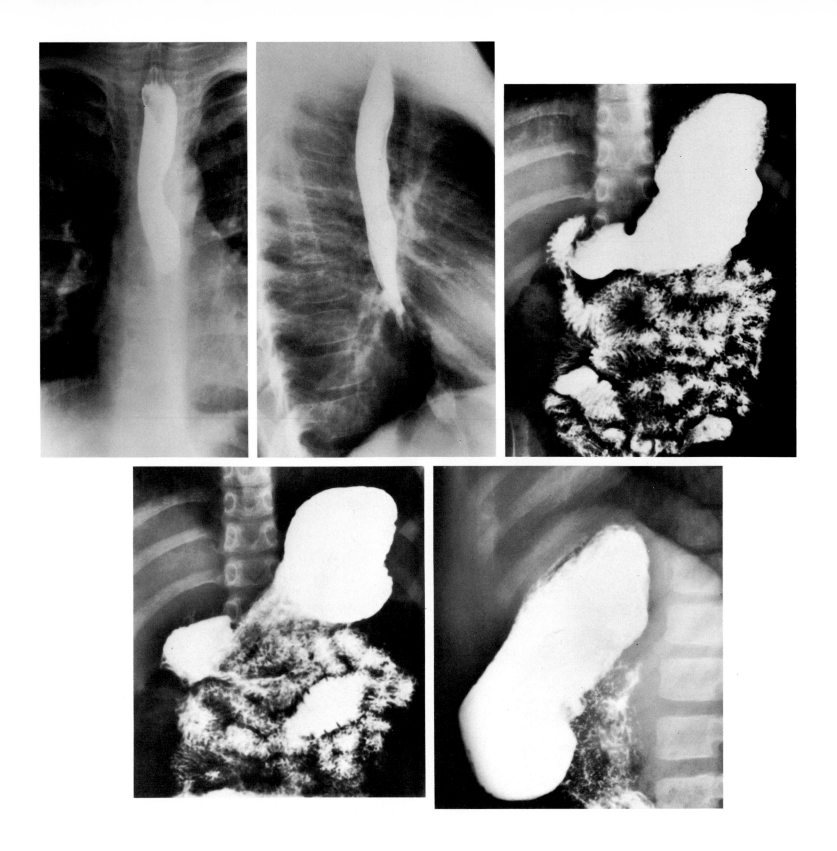

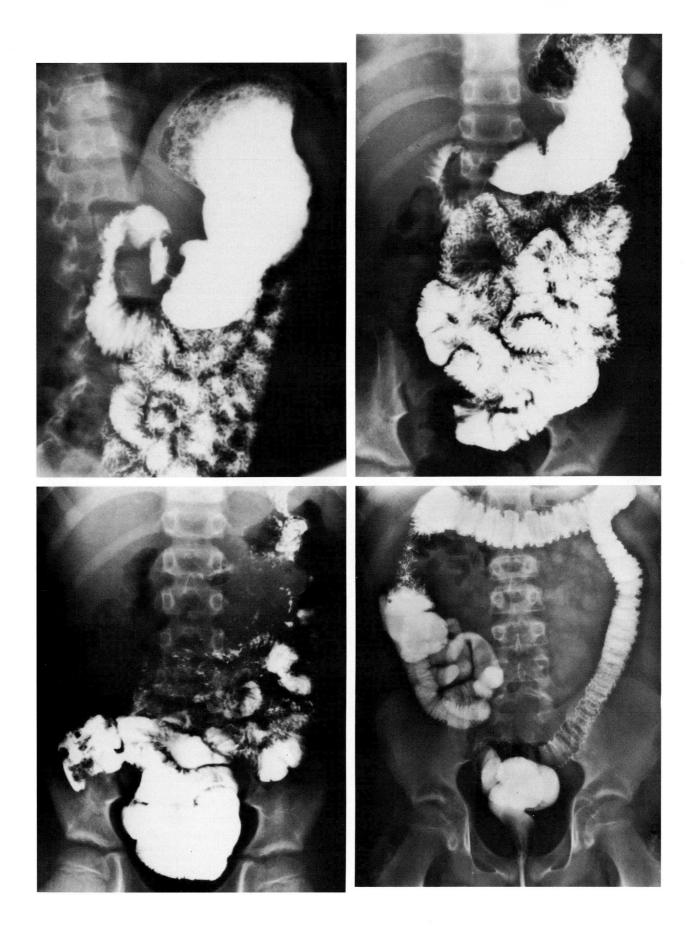

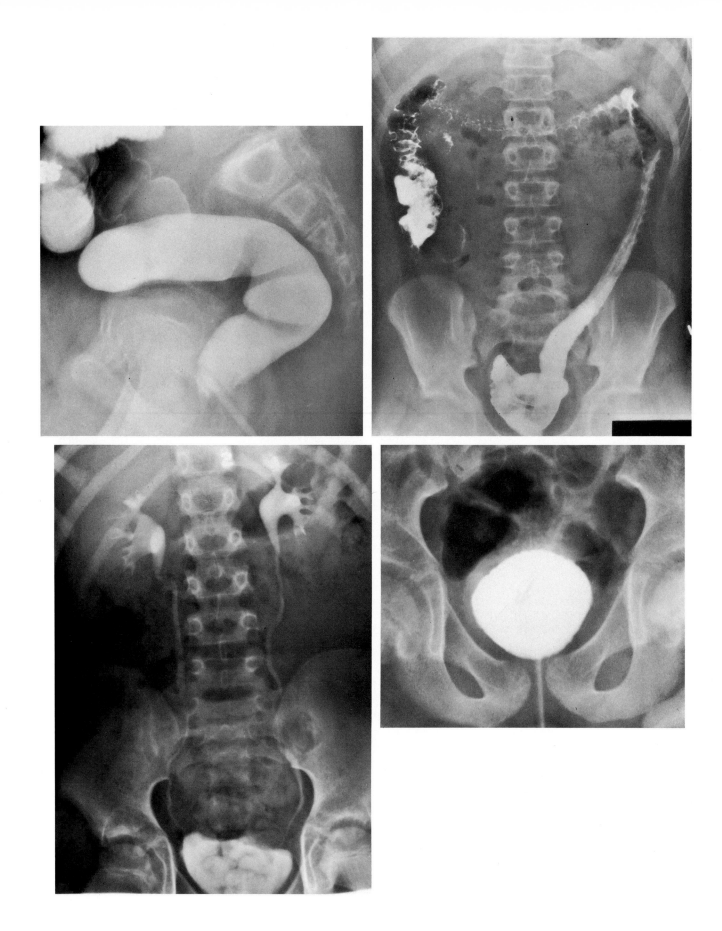

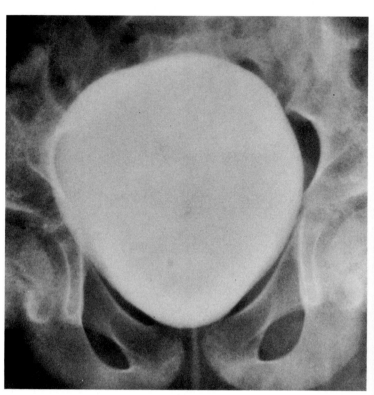

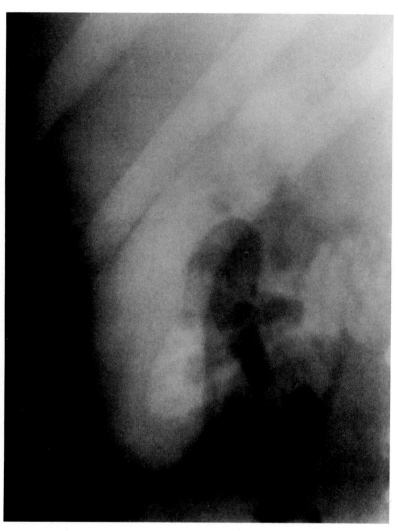

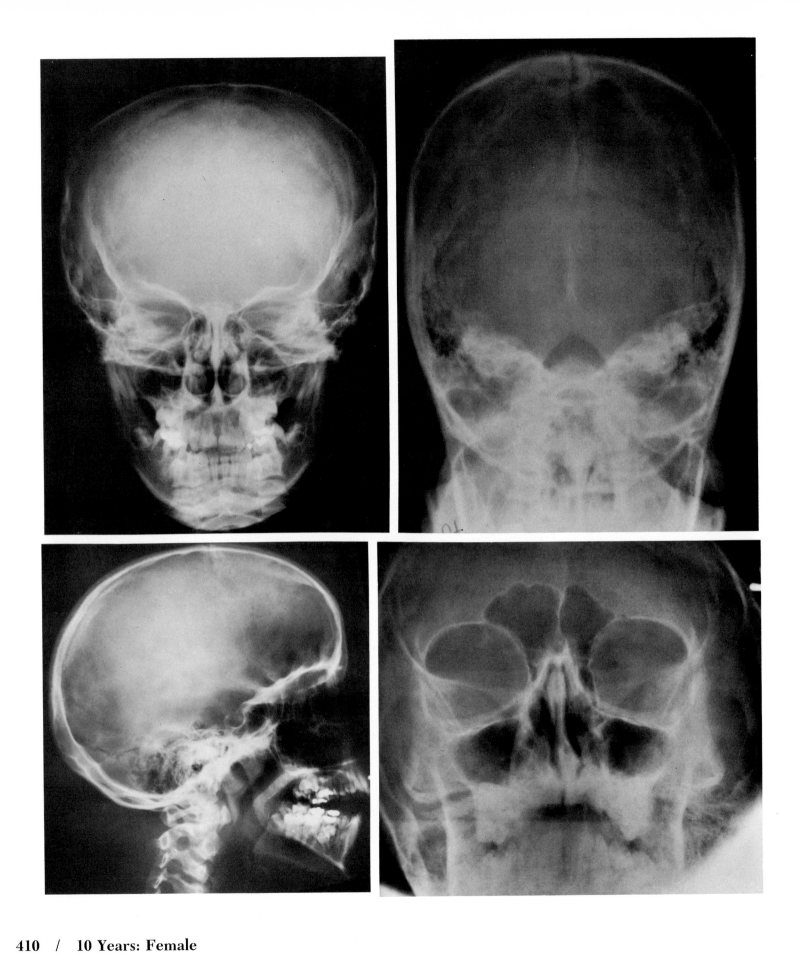

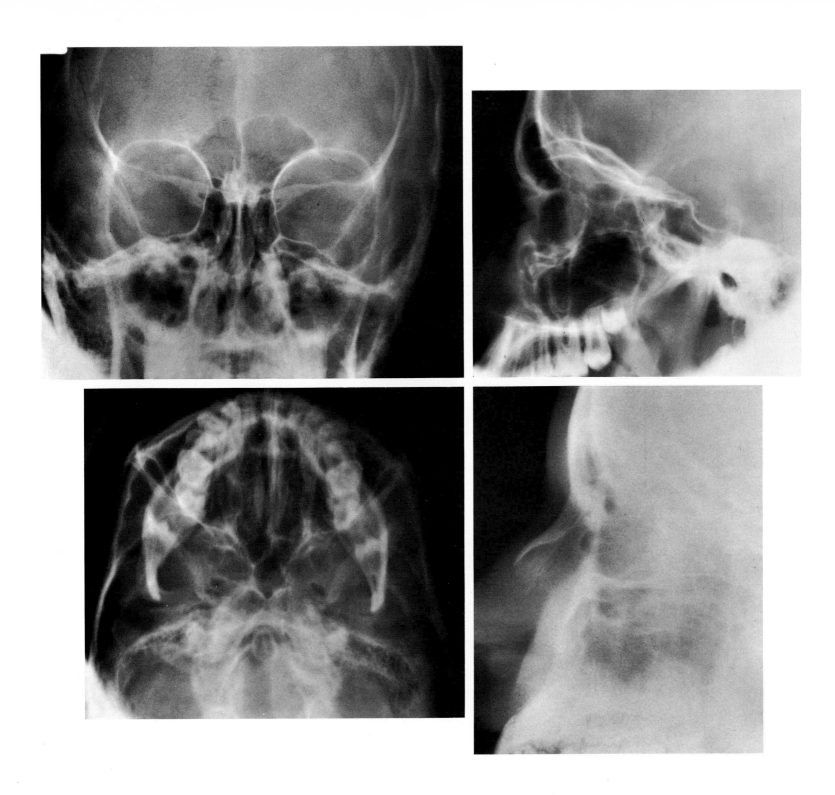

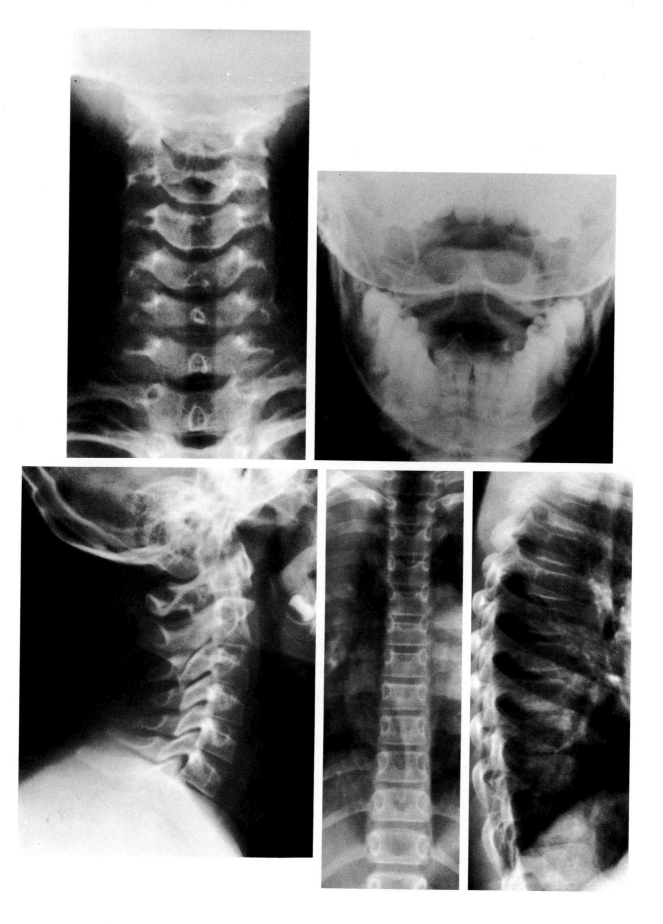

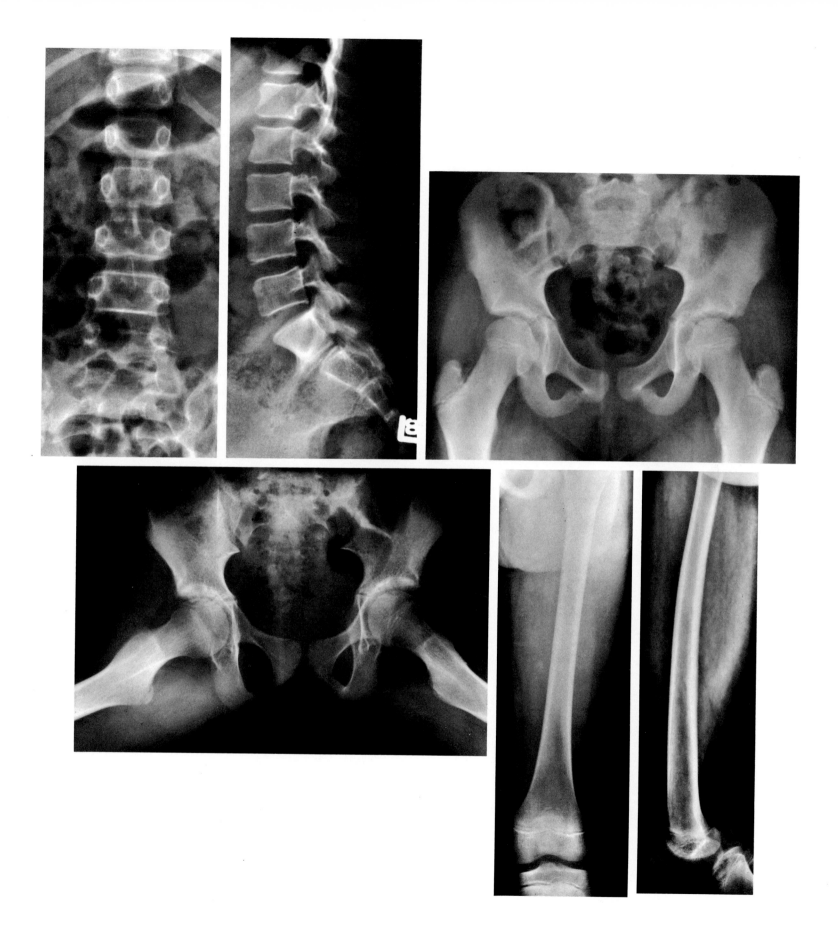

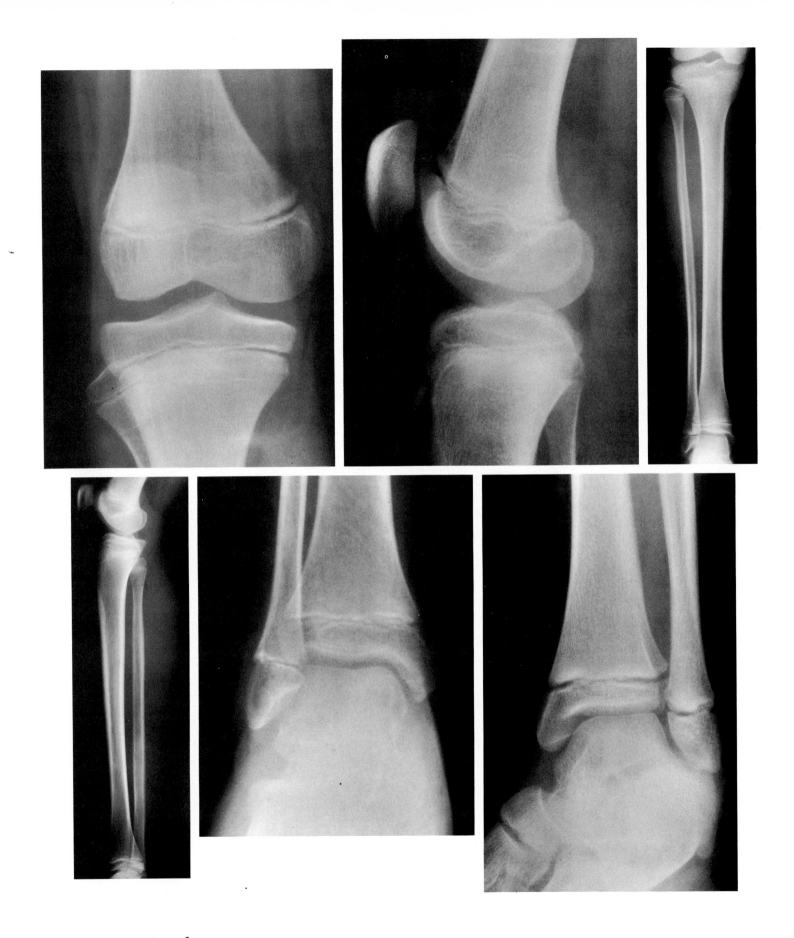

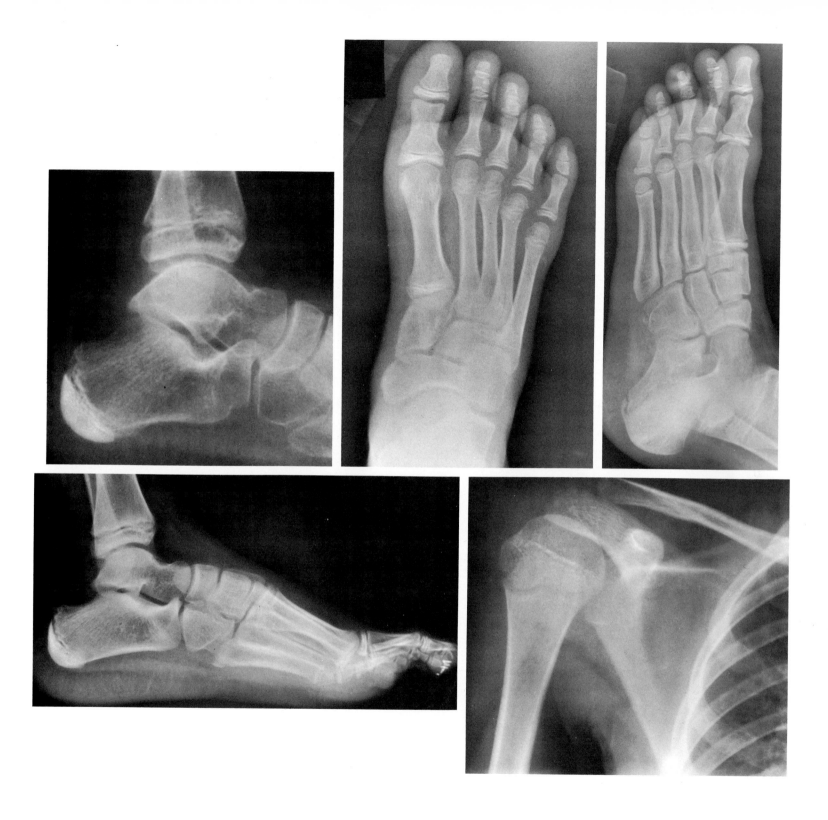

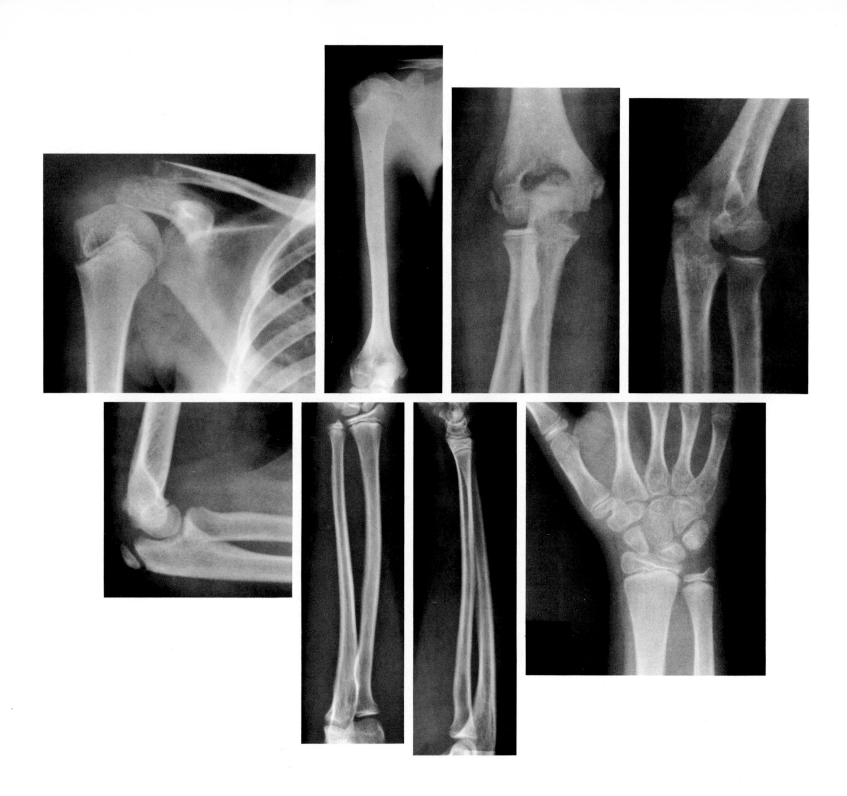

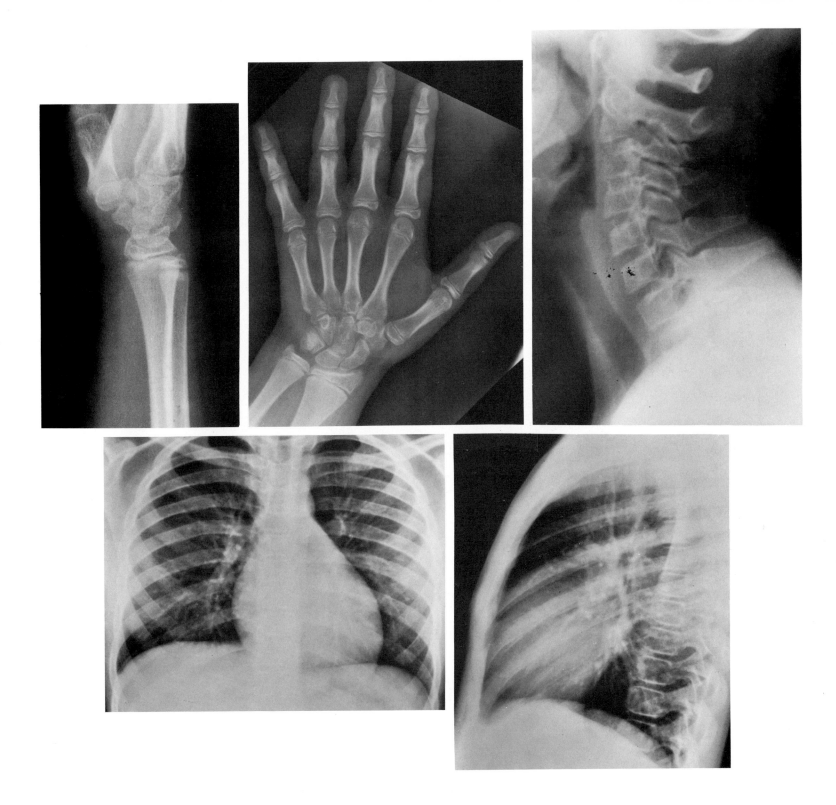

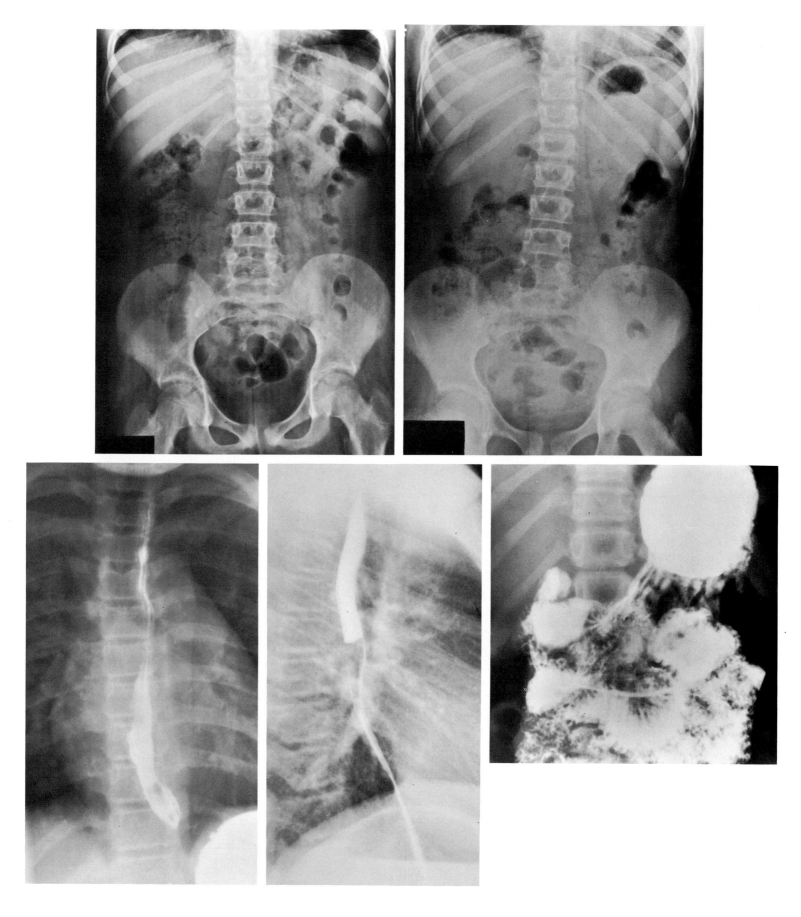

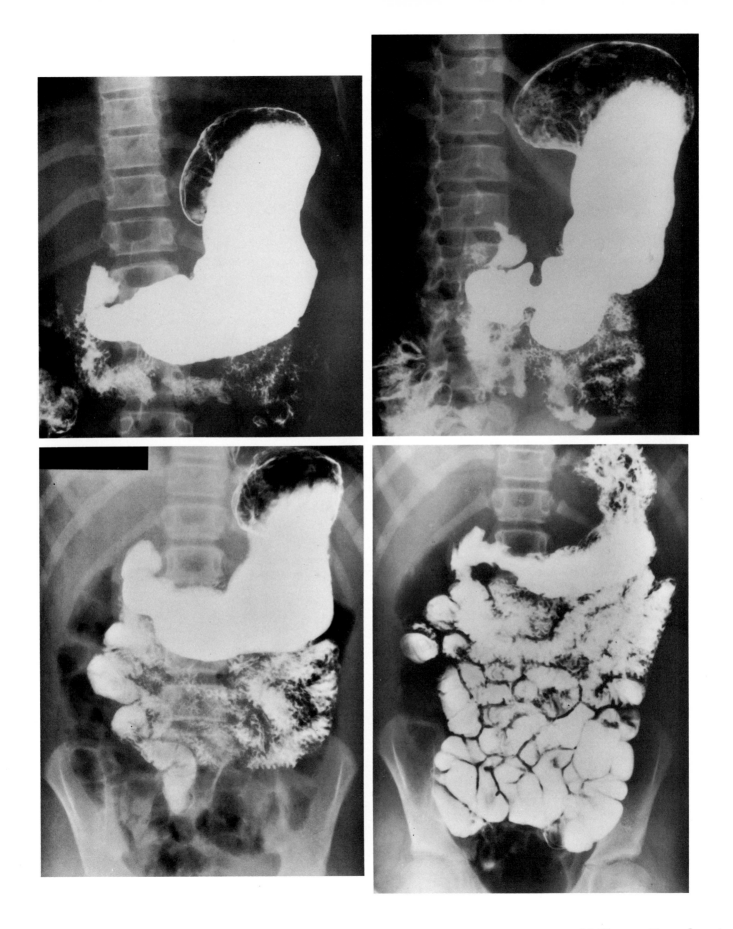

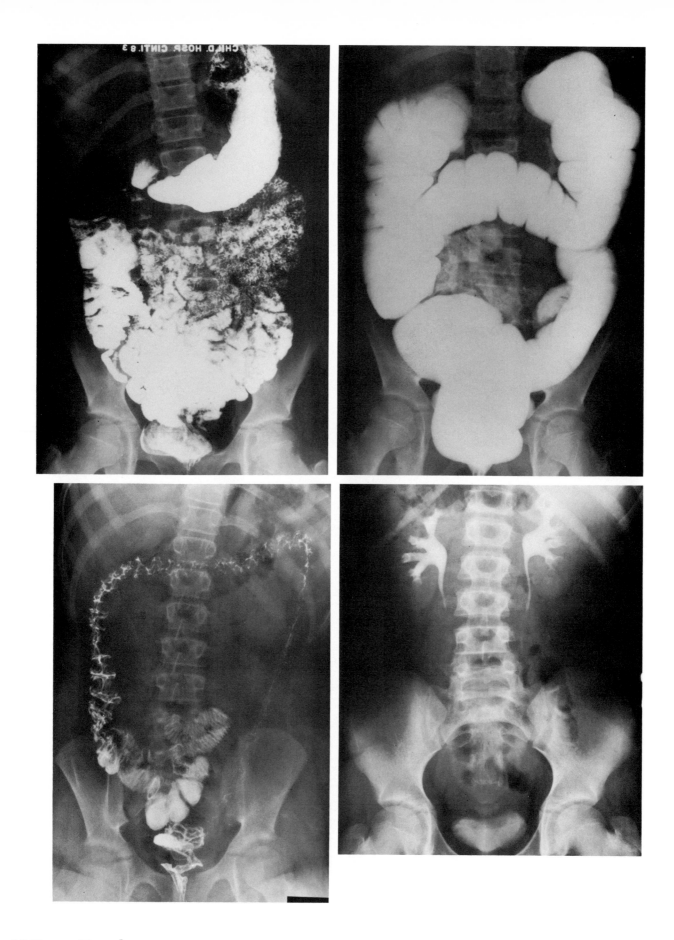

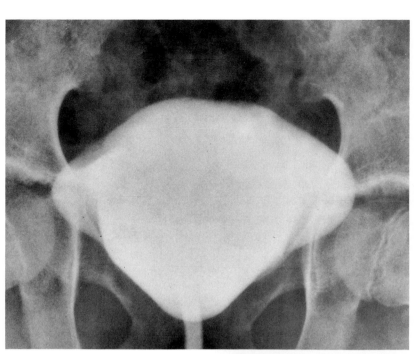

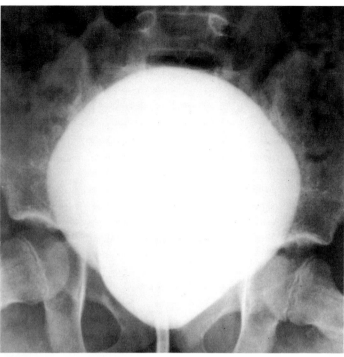

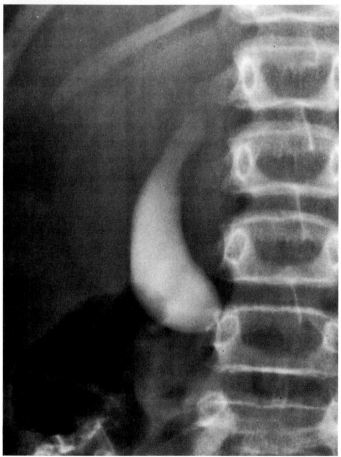

19

11 YEARS

The adenoids are now less prominent. The cervical vertebral bodies remain variably wedge-shaped. The notches for the ring apophyses of the vertebrae are quite marked. The physiologic protrusio acetabula, which were only slightly visible previously, are now quite prominent. The beaking of the anterior aspect of the distal tibial epiphysis is very striking. The medial malleolus is now well developed. The epiphyses of the elbow are now more regular in outline. The ulnar styloid process is forming.

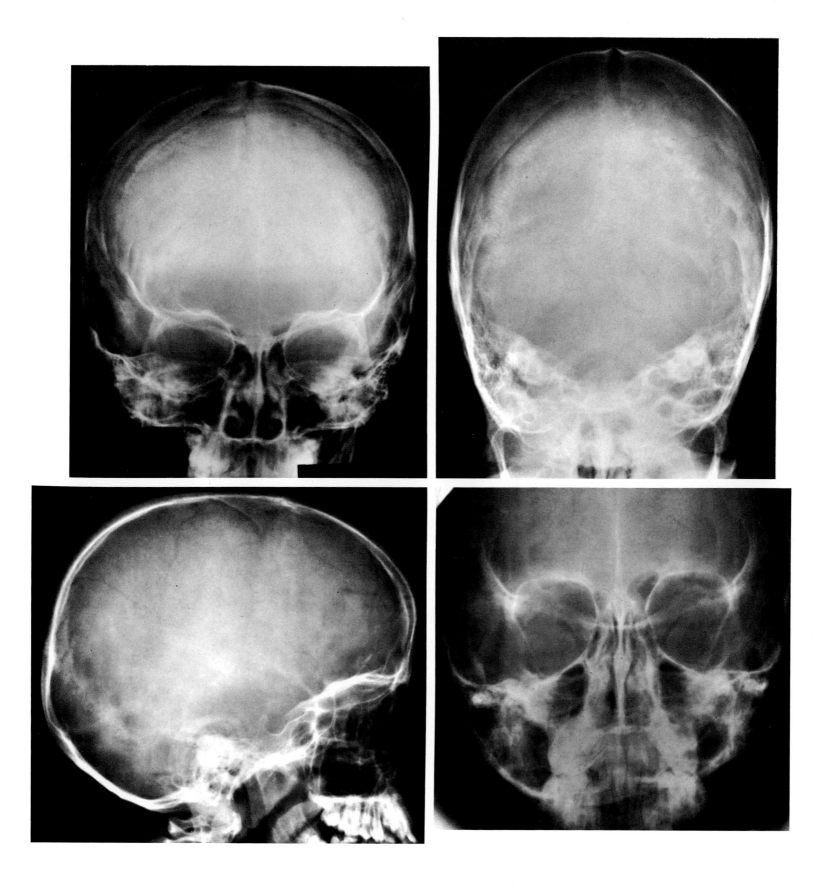

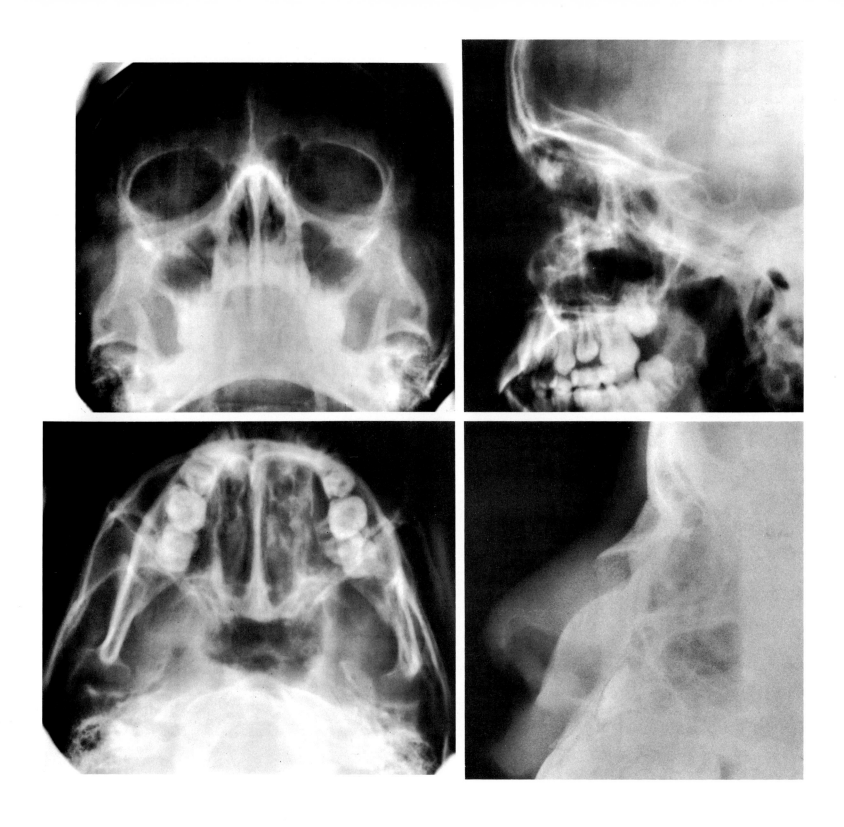

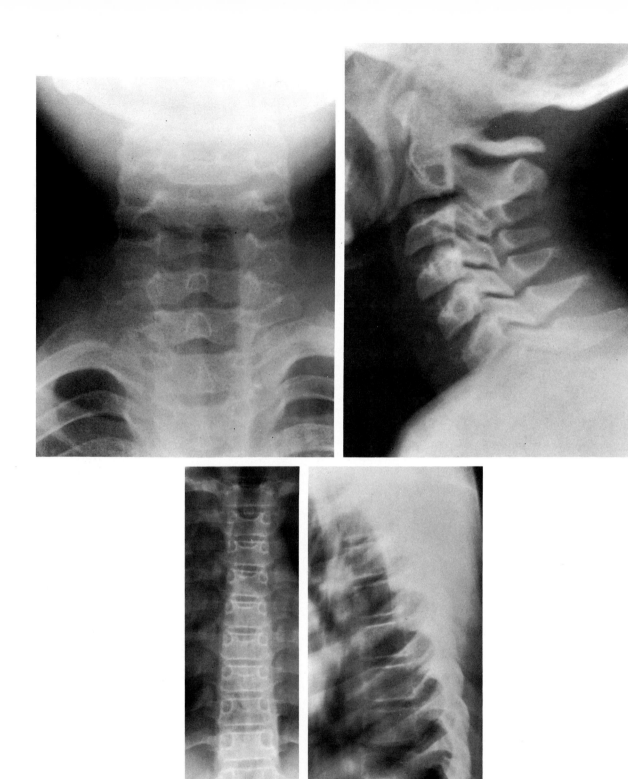

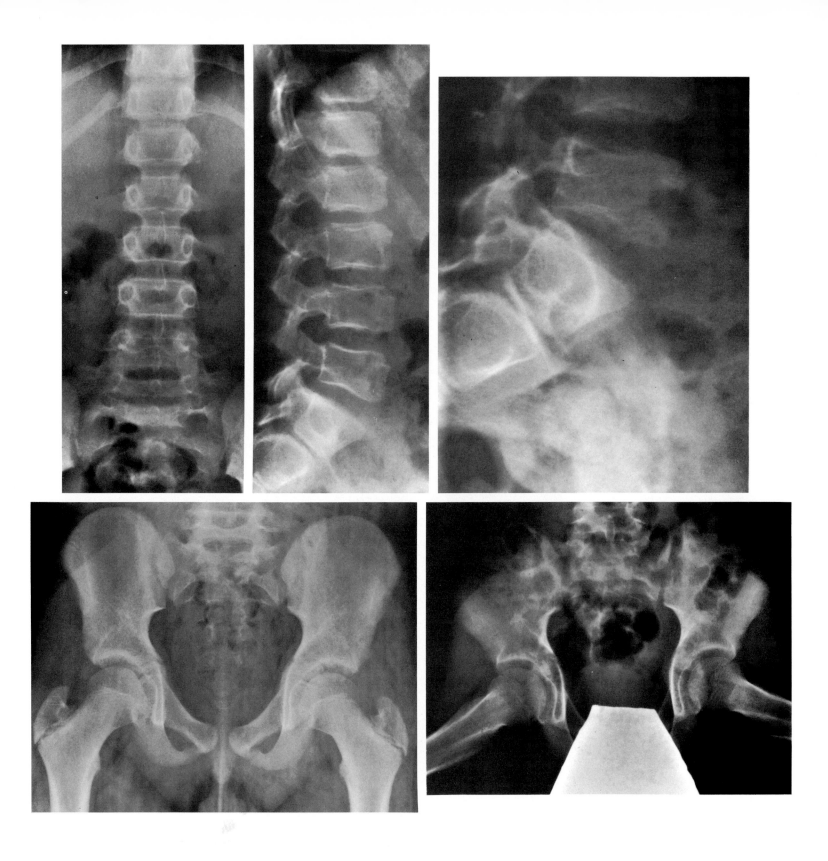

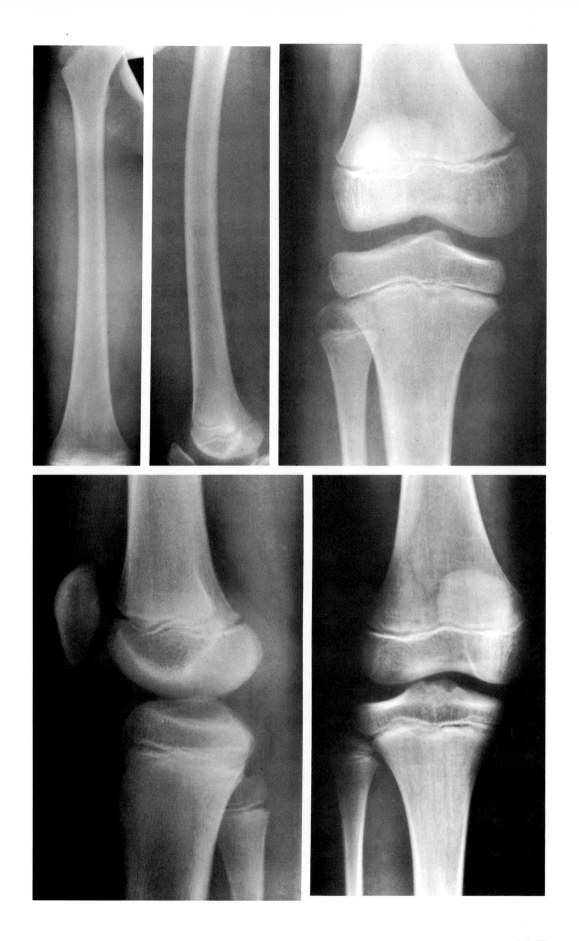

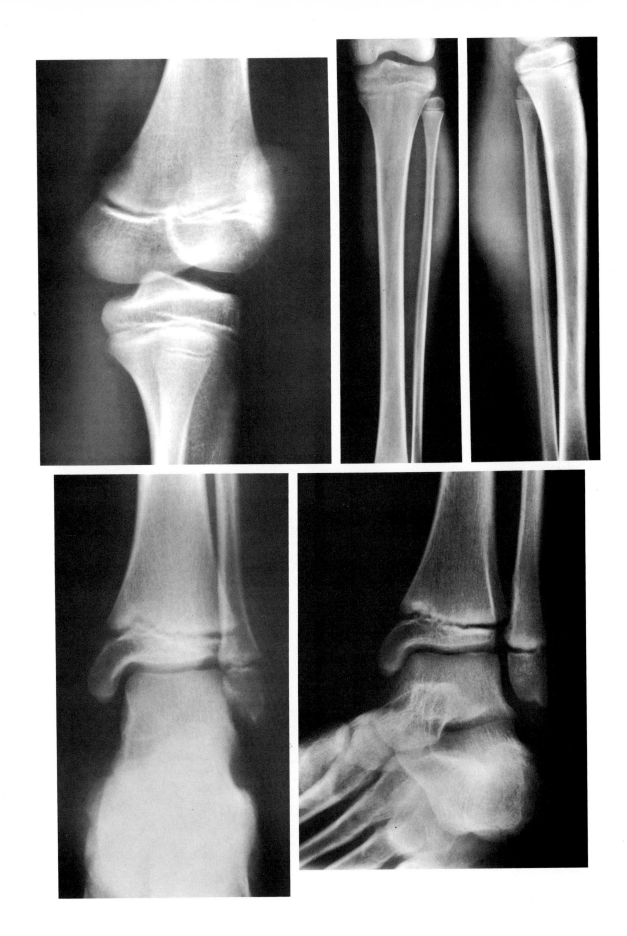

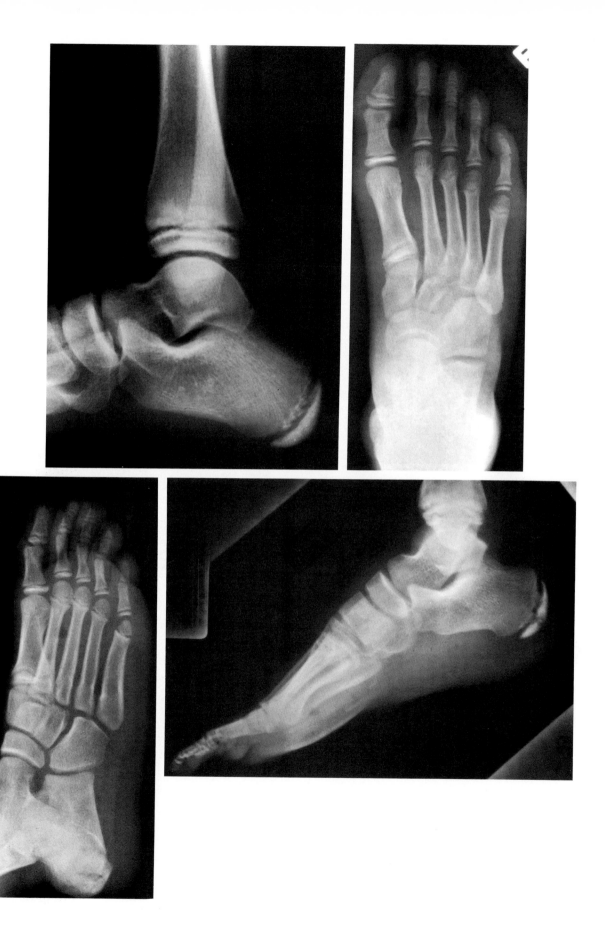

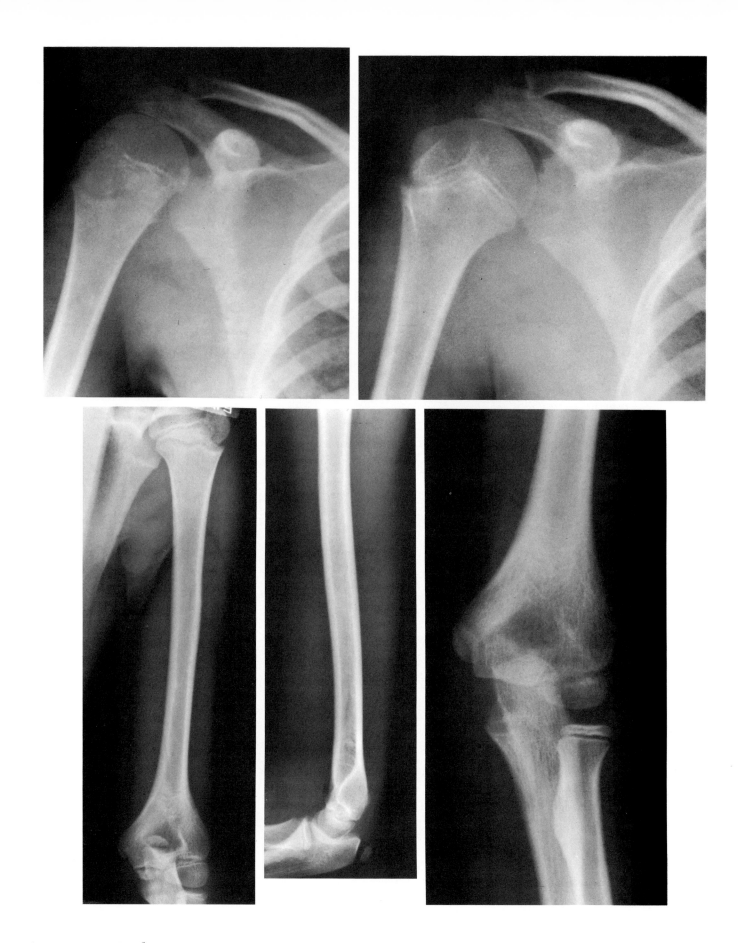

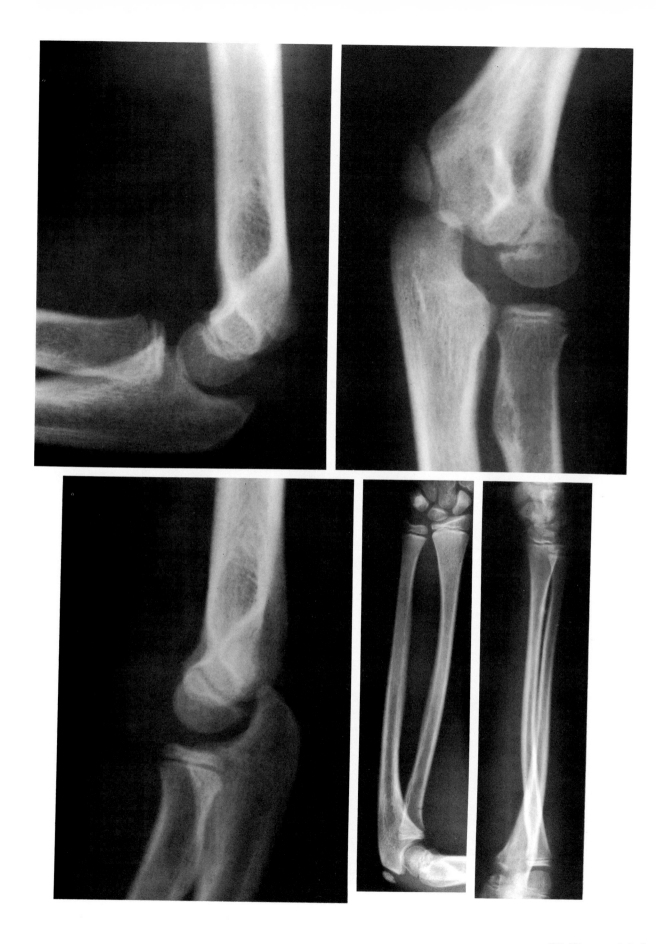

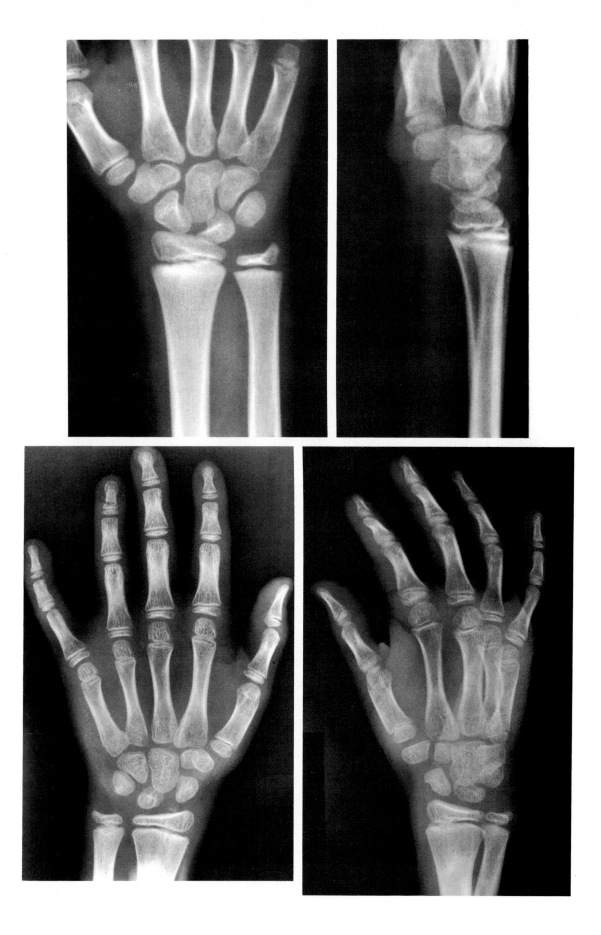

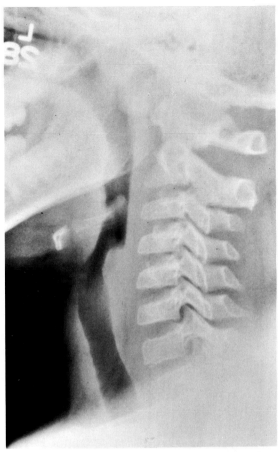

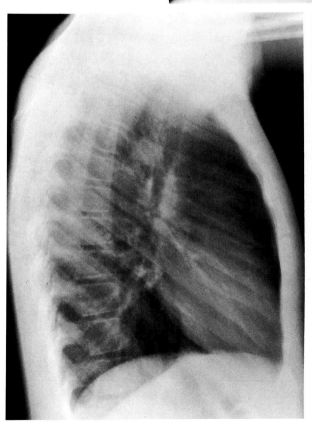

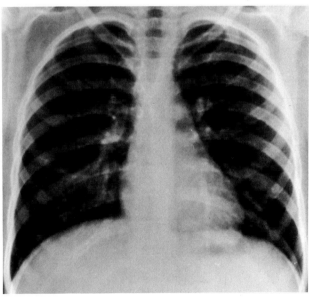

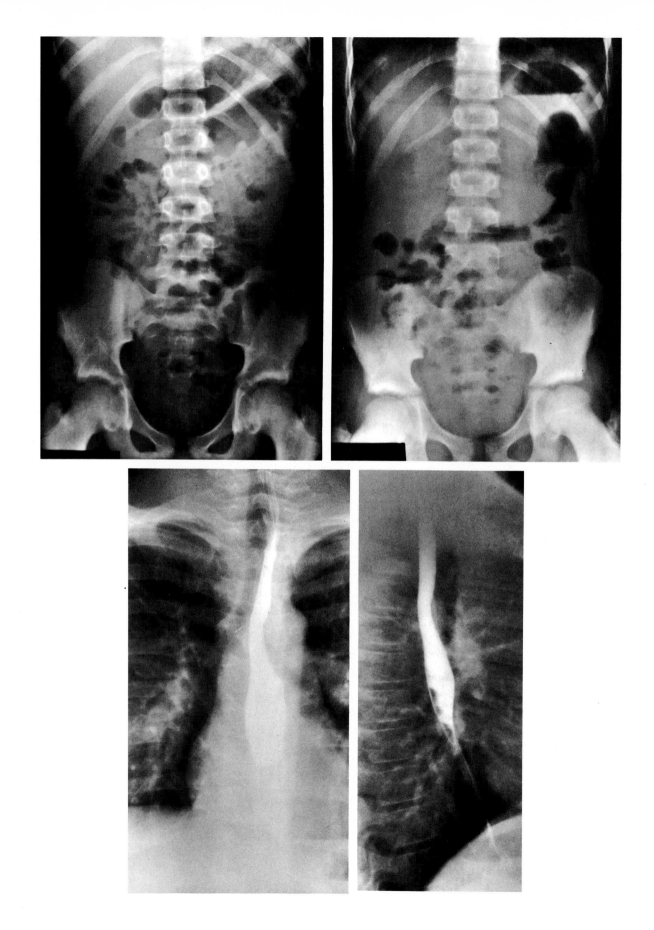

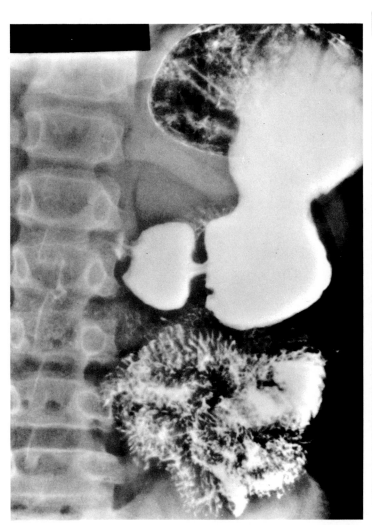
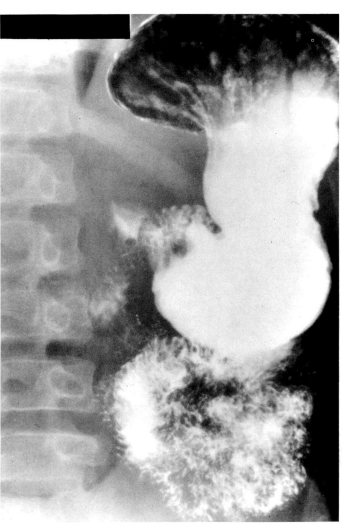
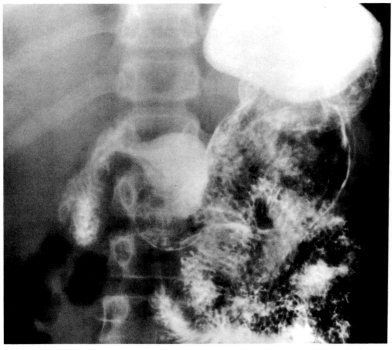

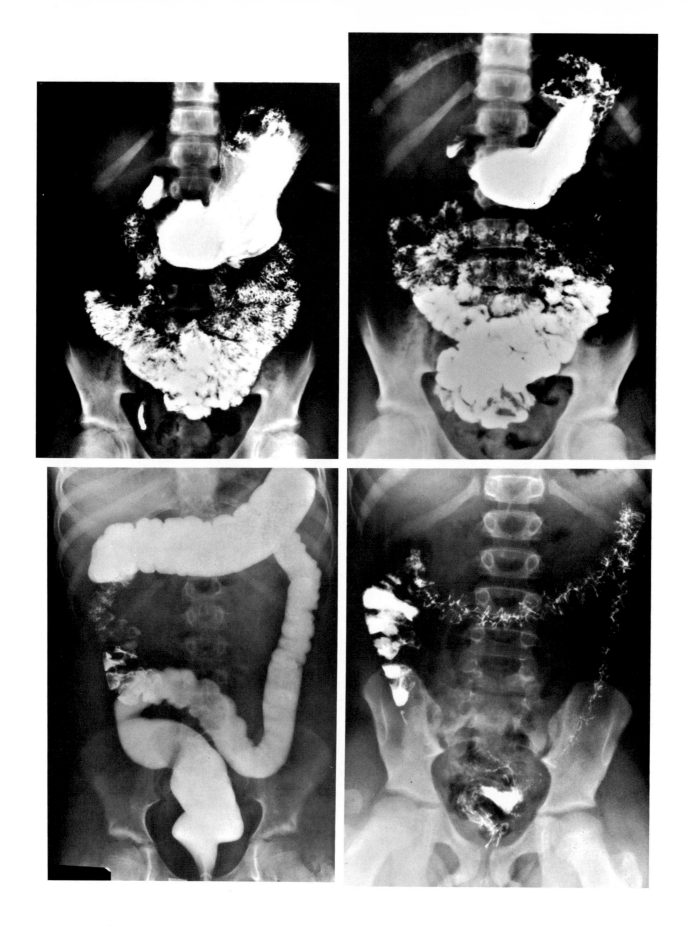

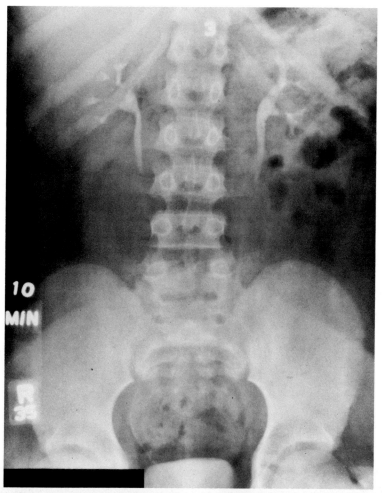

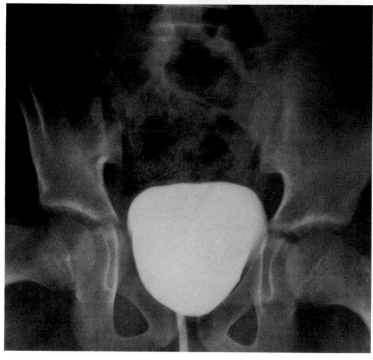

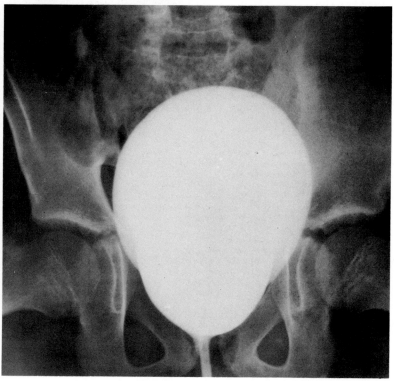

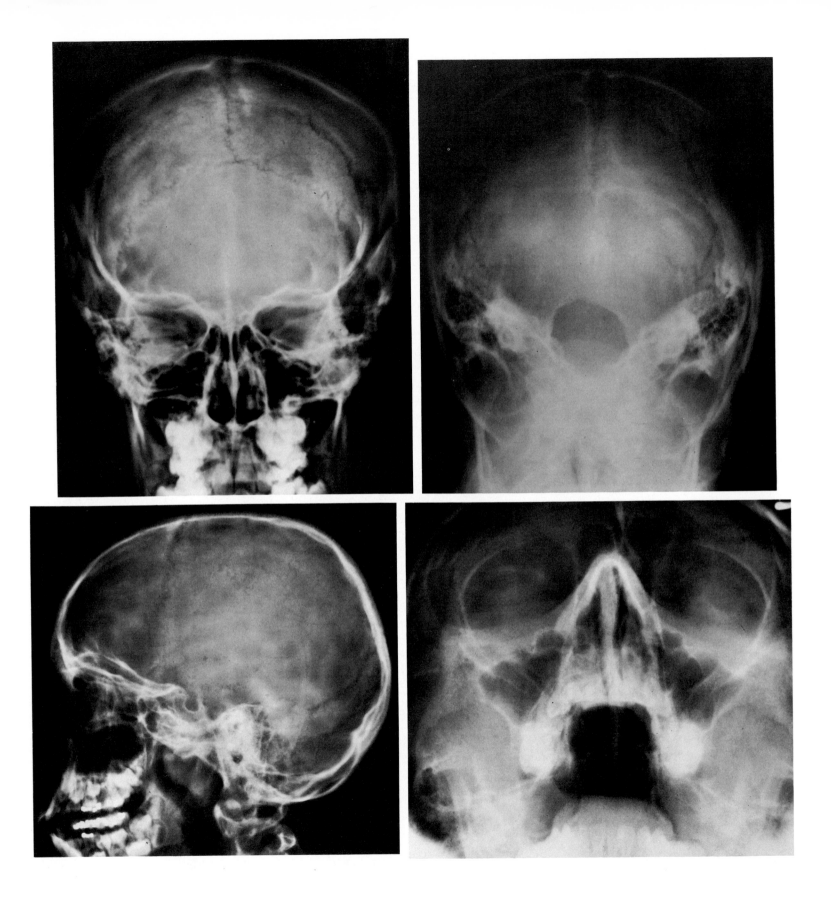

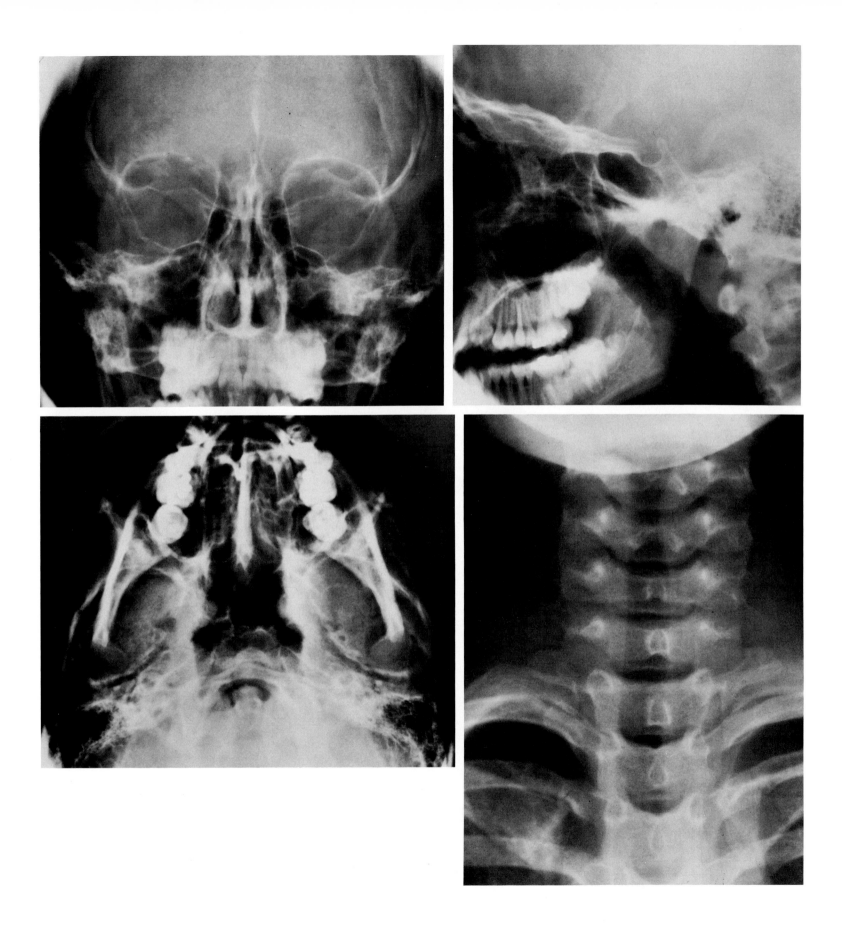

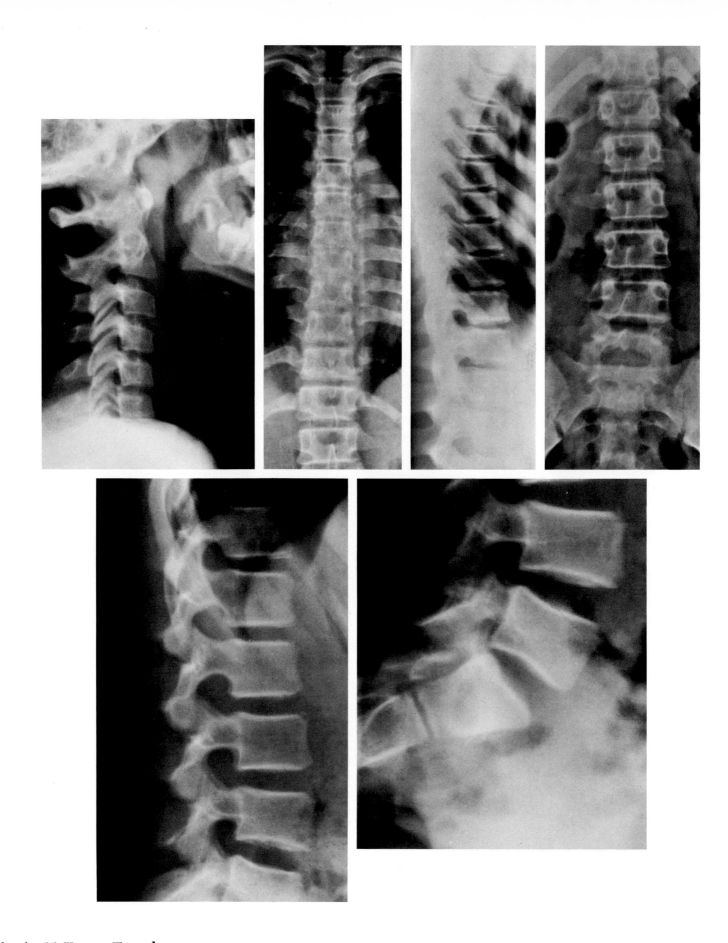

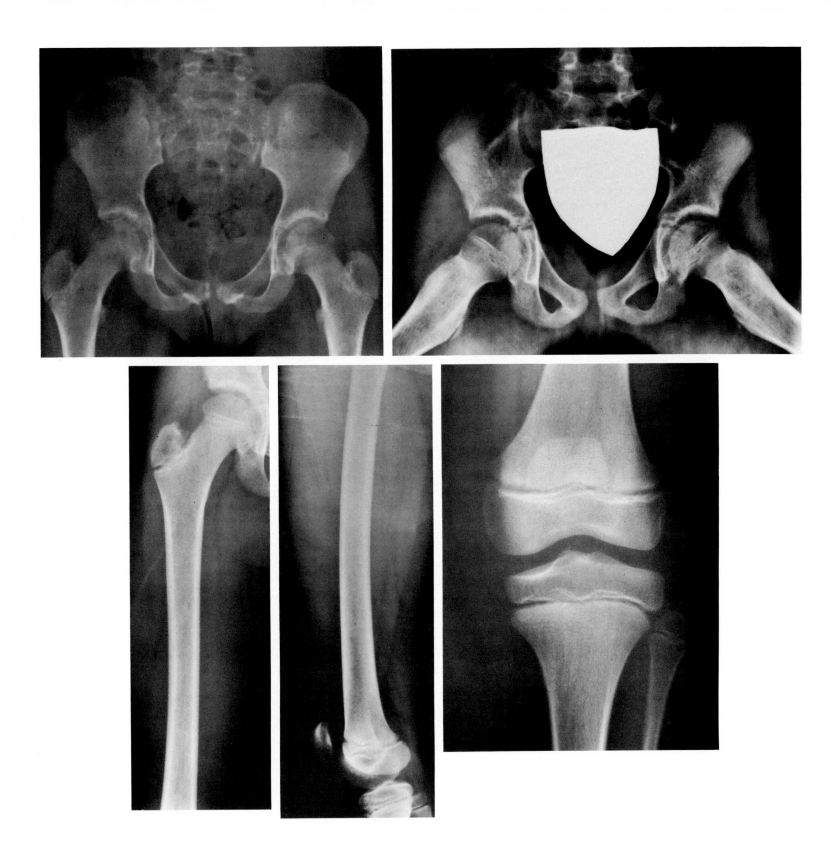

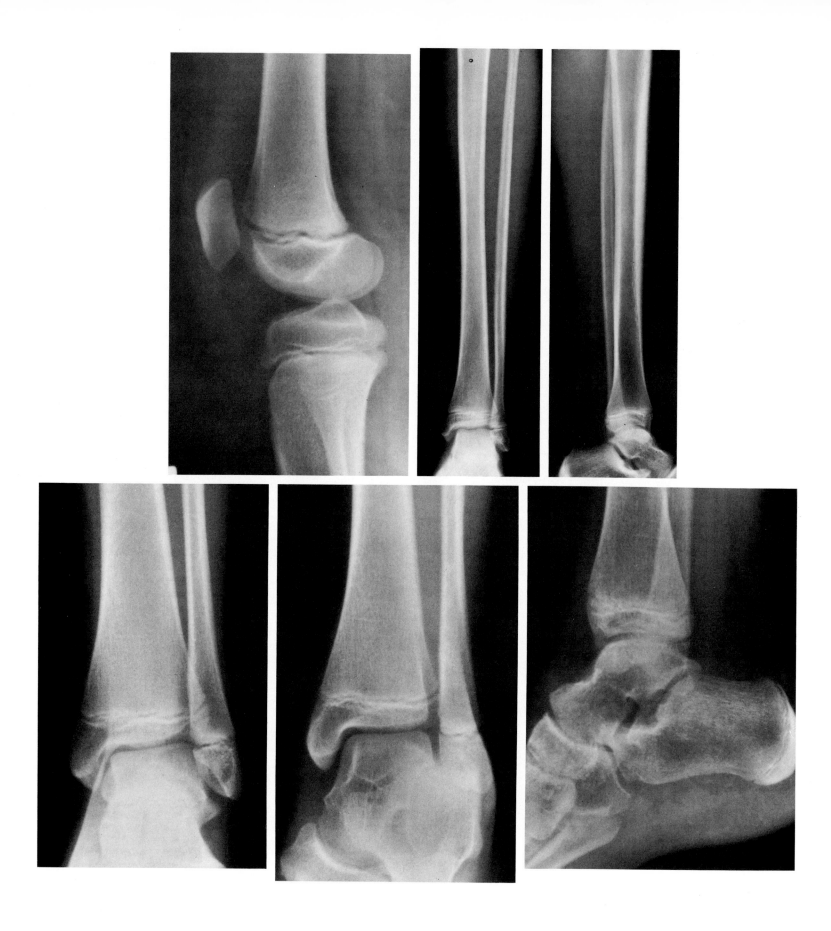

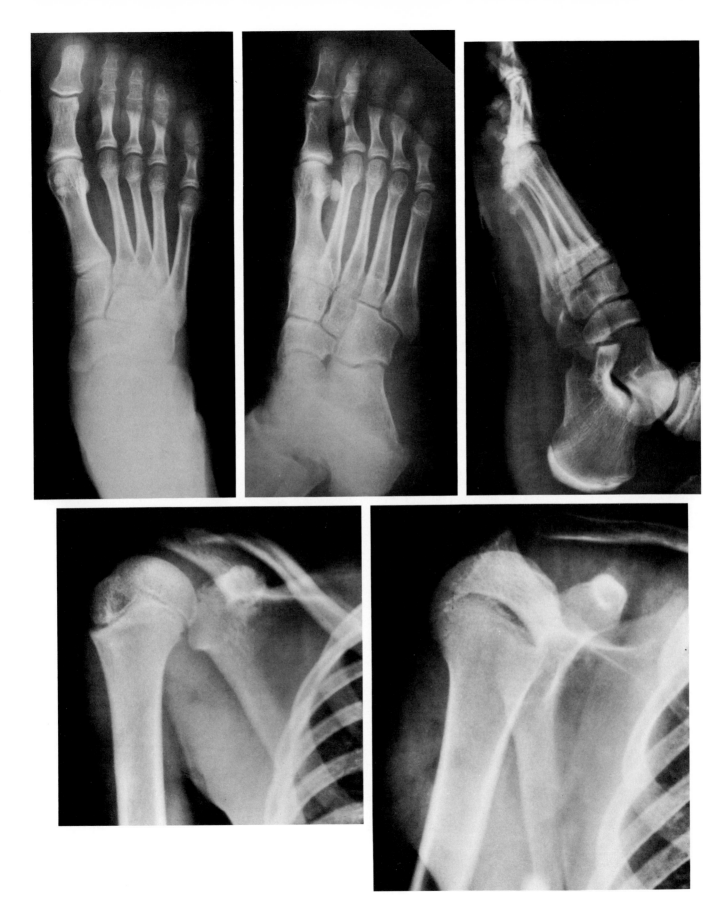

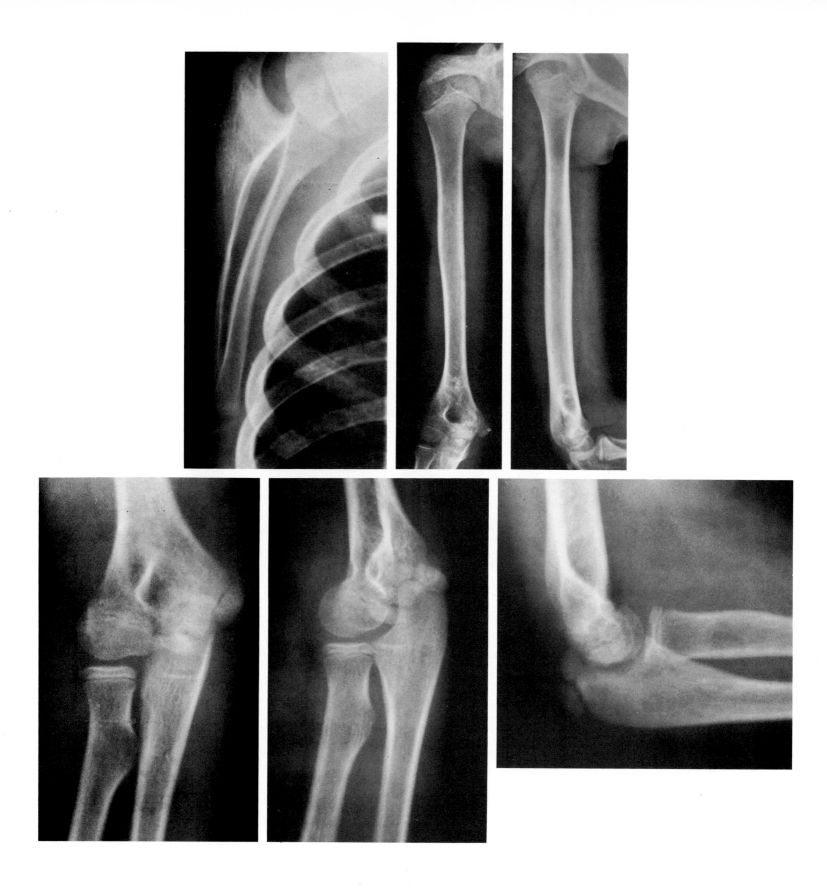

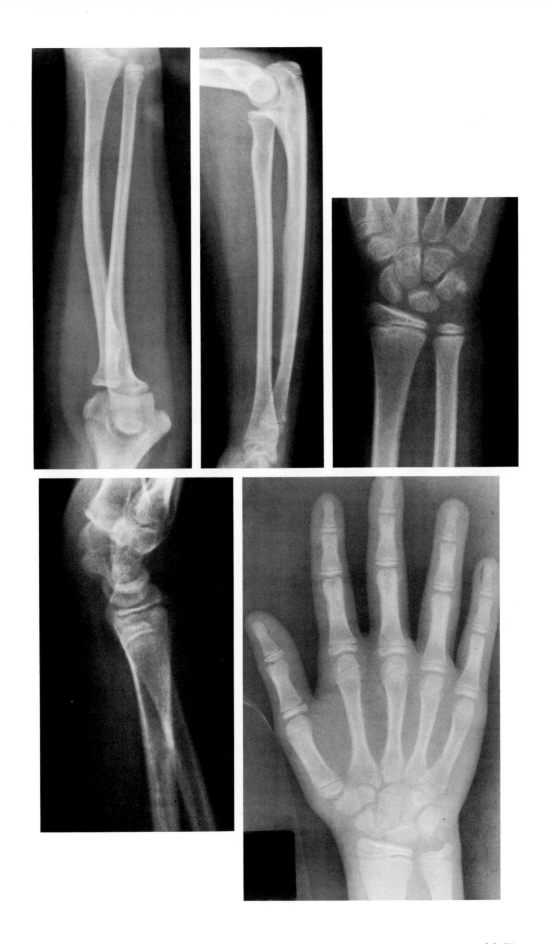

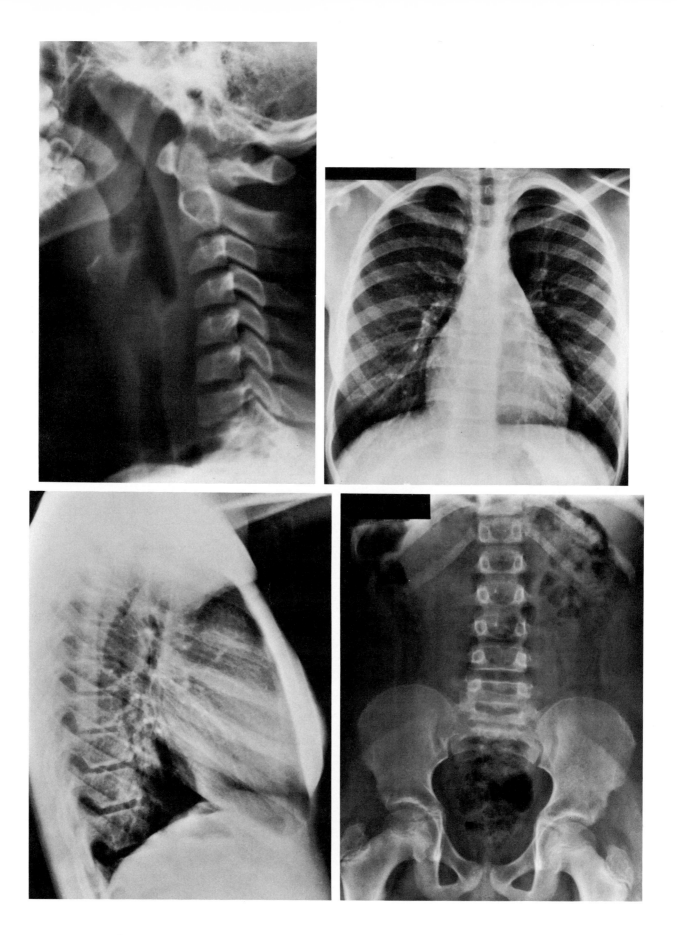

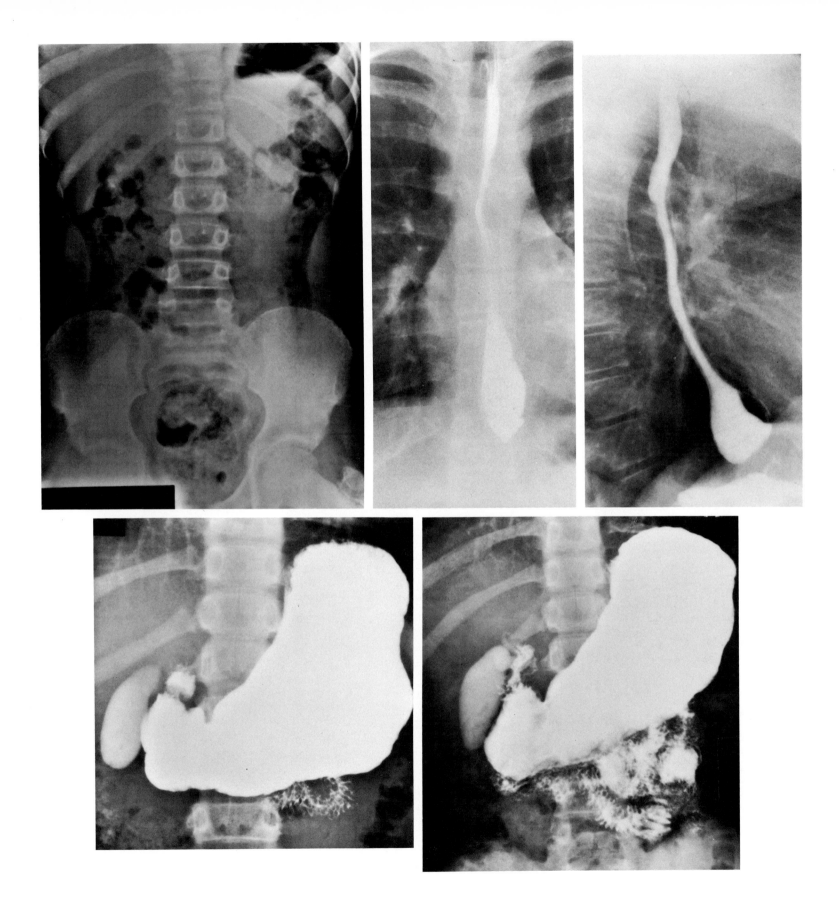

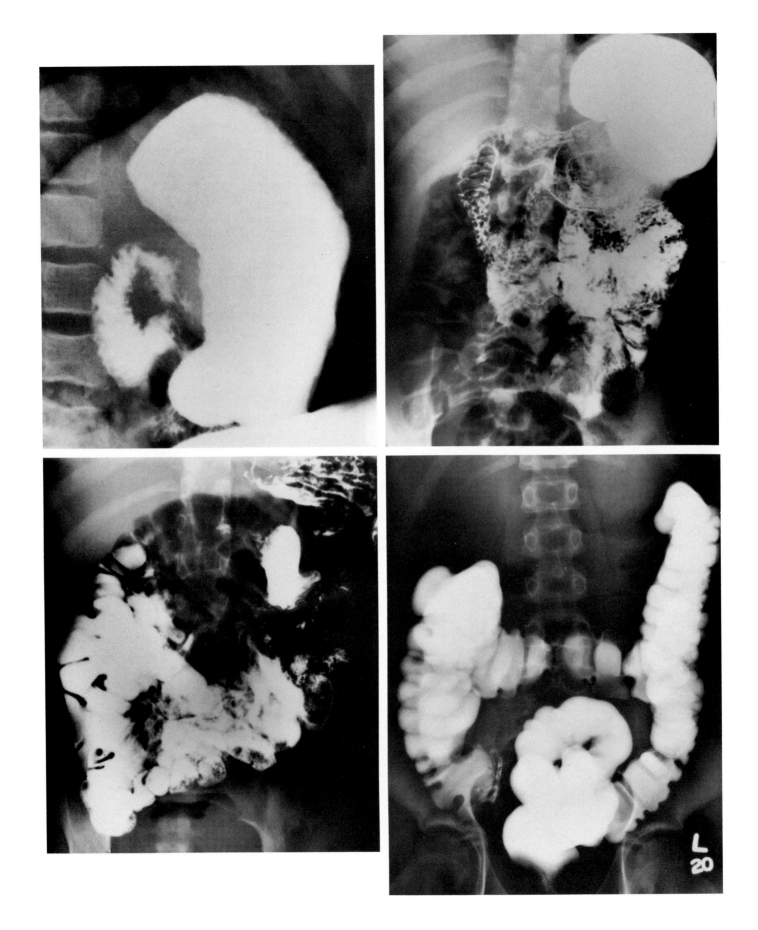

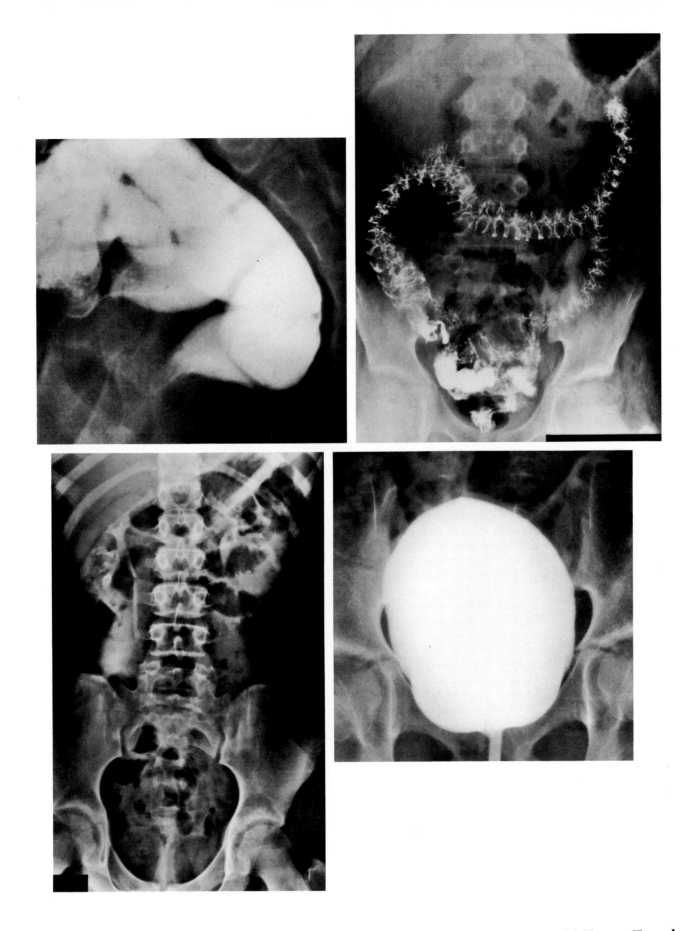

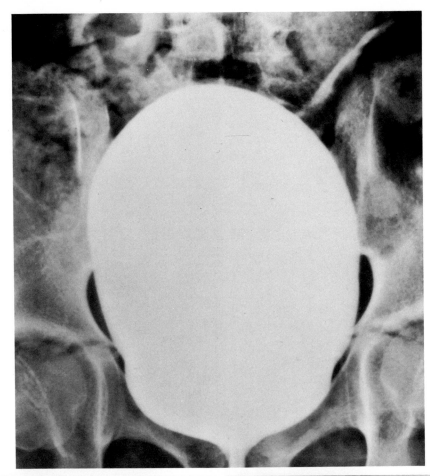

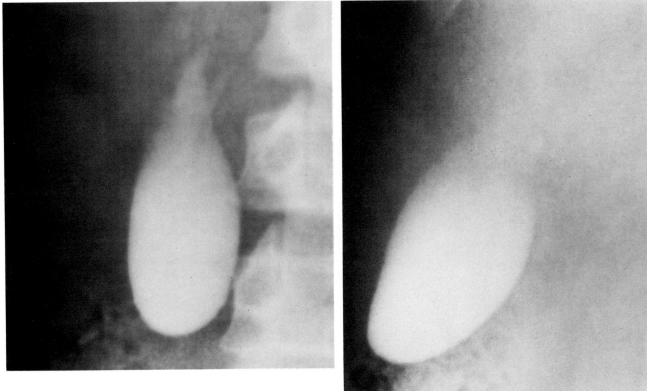

20

12 YEARS

The frontal sinuses vary in size. The sphenoid sinus is over half pneumatized. Calvarial digital markings may still be prominent. The wedge-shaped configuration of the cervical vertebral bodies is less marked than previously, and the notches of the ring apophyses of the lumbar vertebrae are less apparent. The ischiopubic synchondroses are closed.

The ischial apophyses are now evident. The pelvis has an adult configuration, and the sacroiliac joints are narrower than before.

The epiphysis for the calcaneal tuberosity is closed, but remains dense, as does the epiphysis of the base of the proximal phalanx of the great toe. The capitellum is fusing, and the radial head now conforms to the capitellum. The bones of the hands and wrists are approaching adult size, but the epiphyses are still open.

The small bowel patterns have a more "feathery" appearance than before.

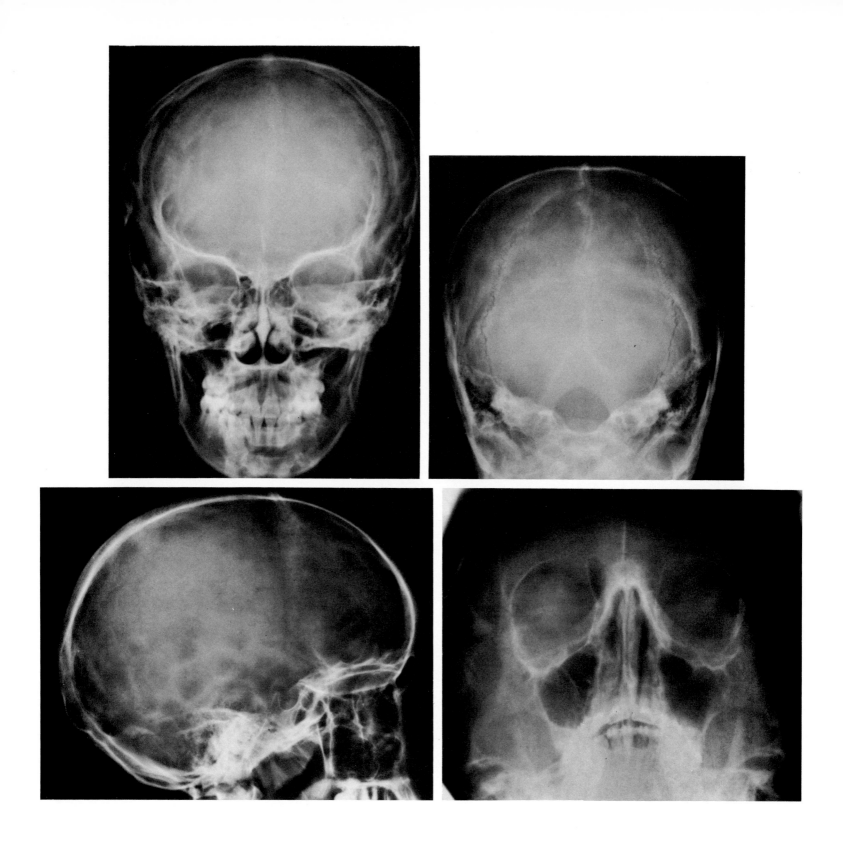

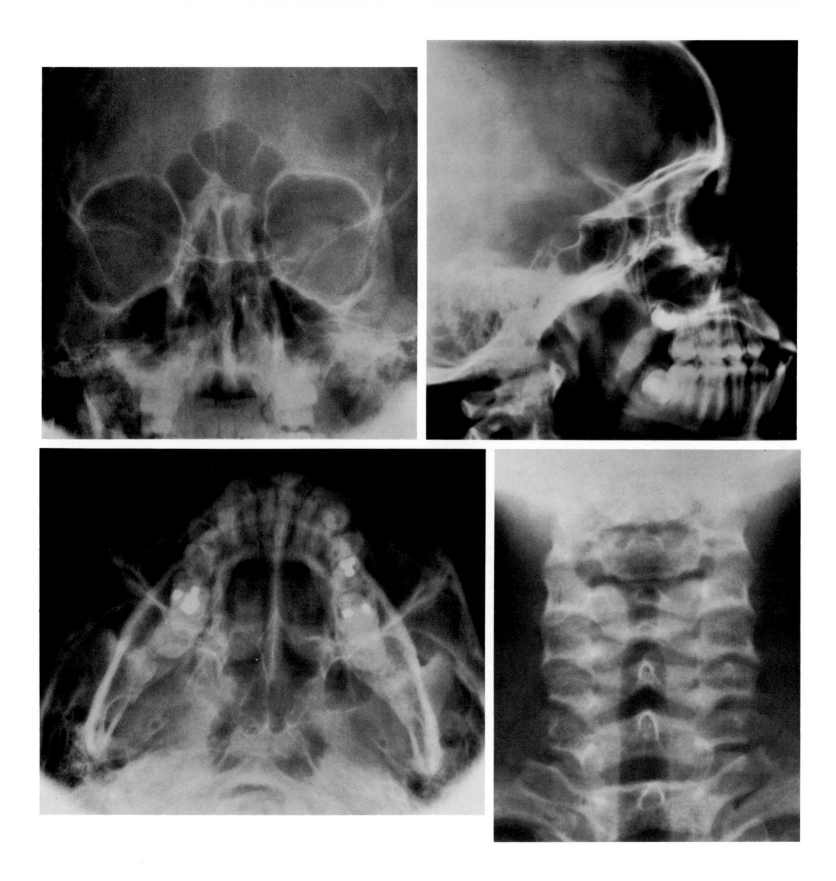

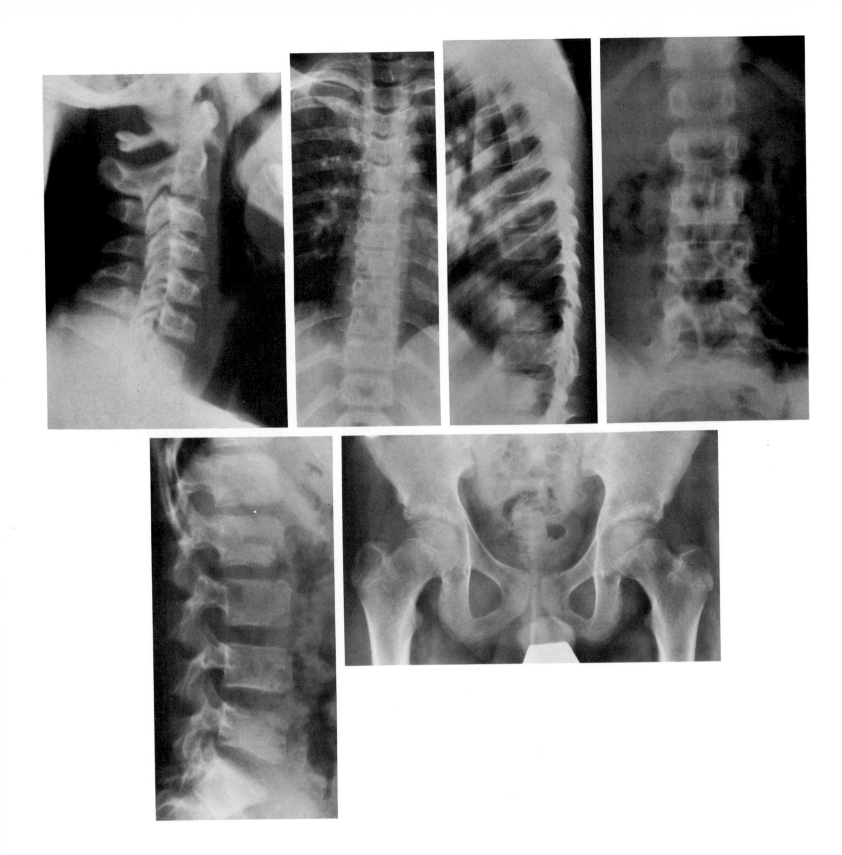

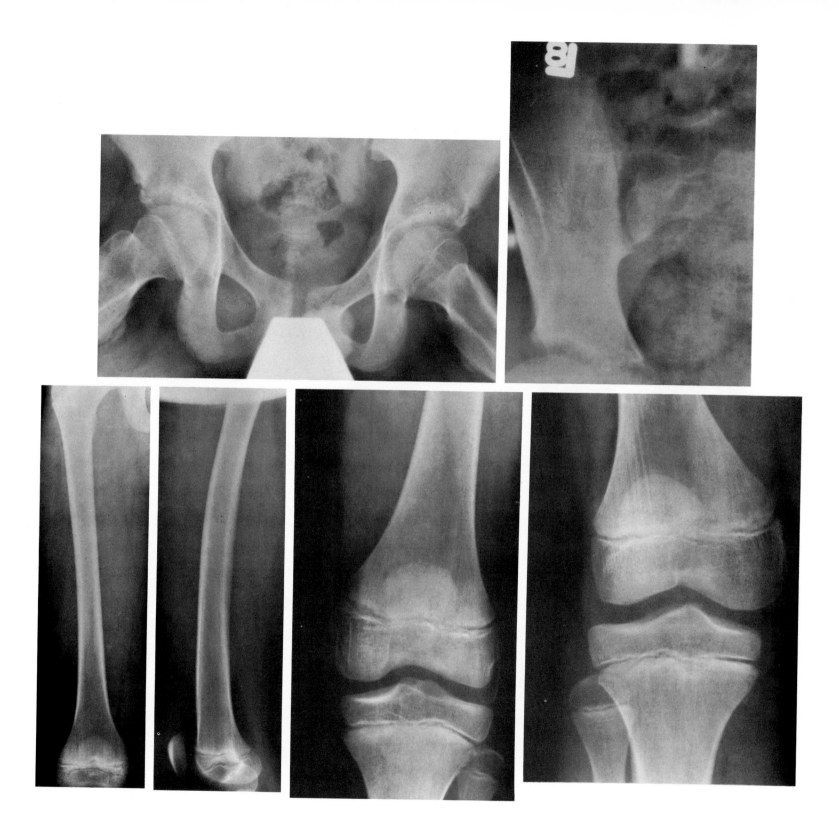

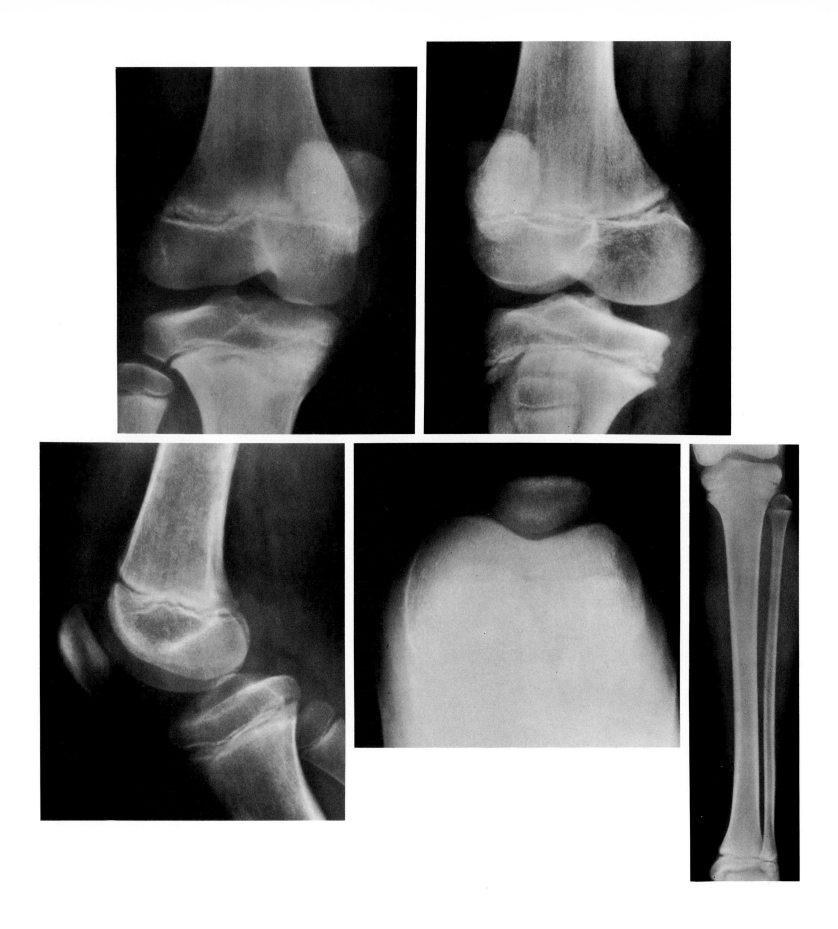

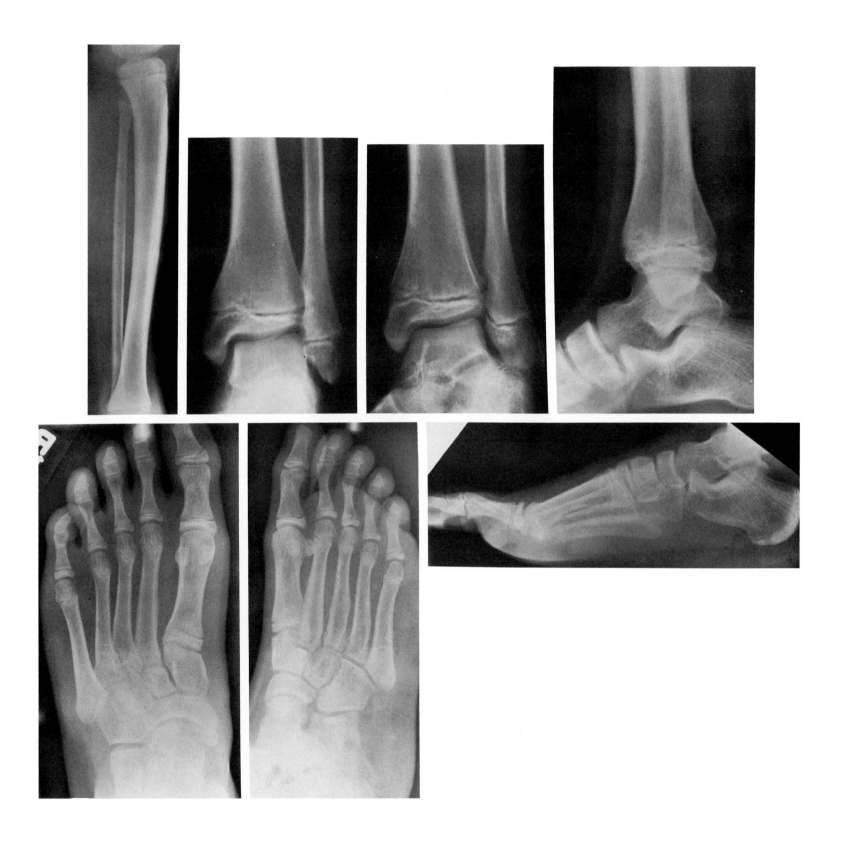

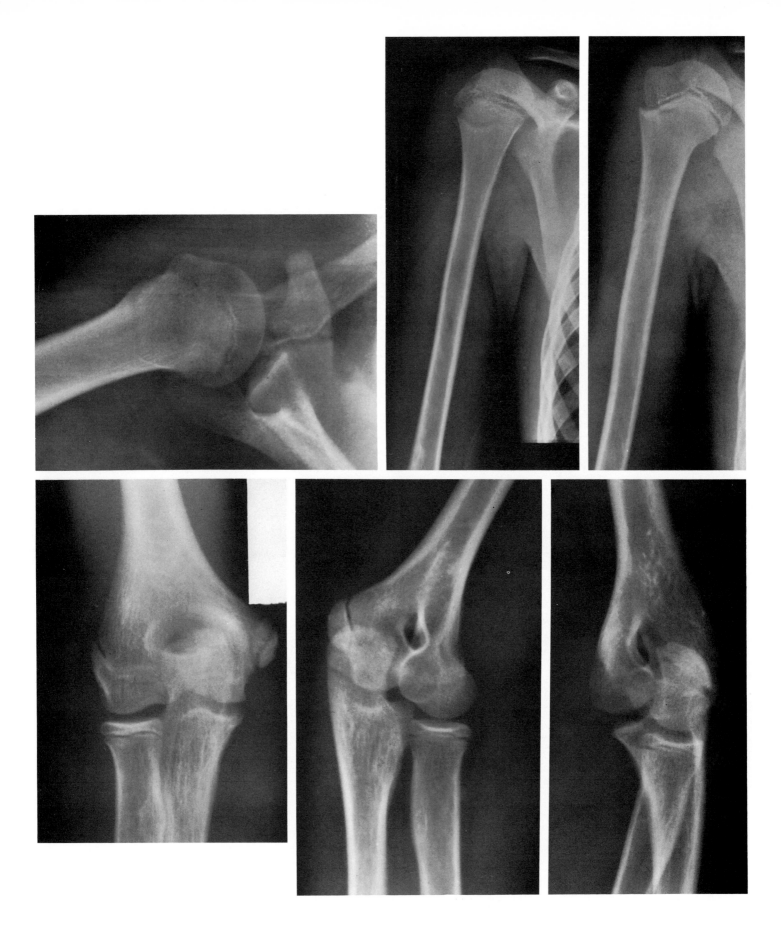

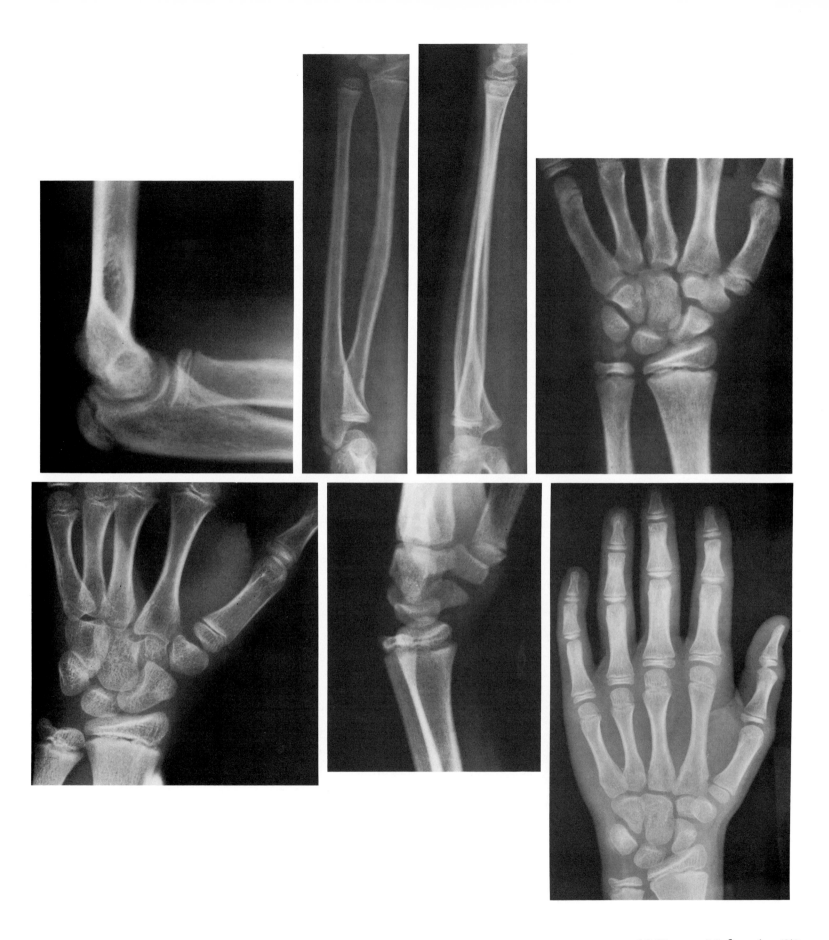

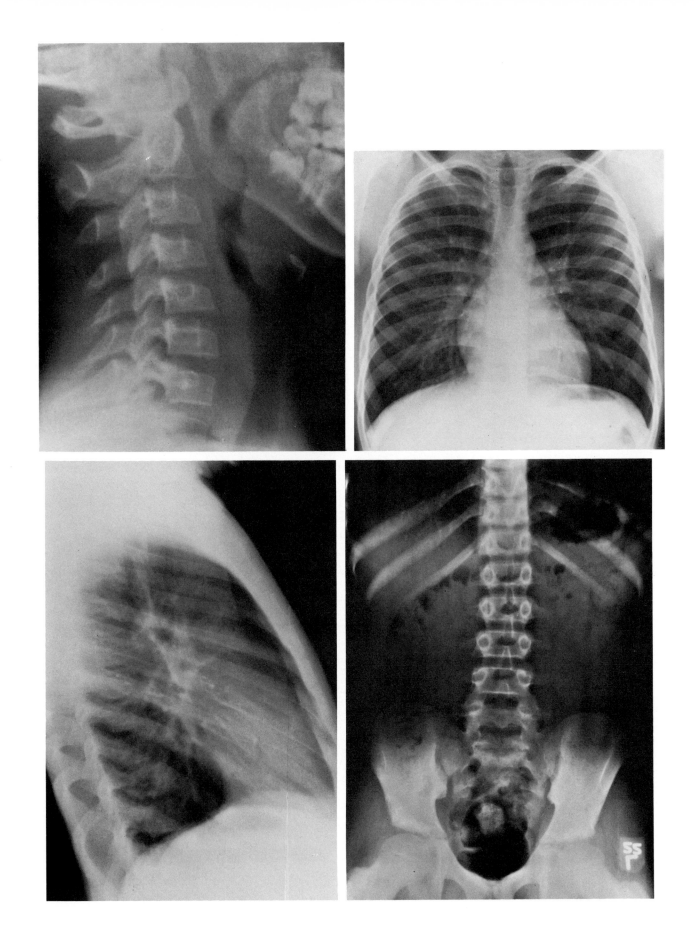

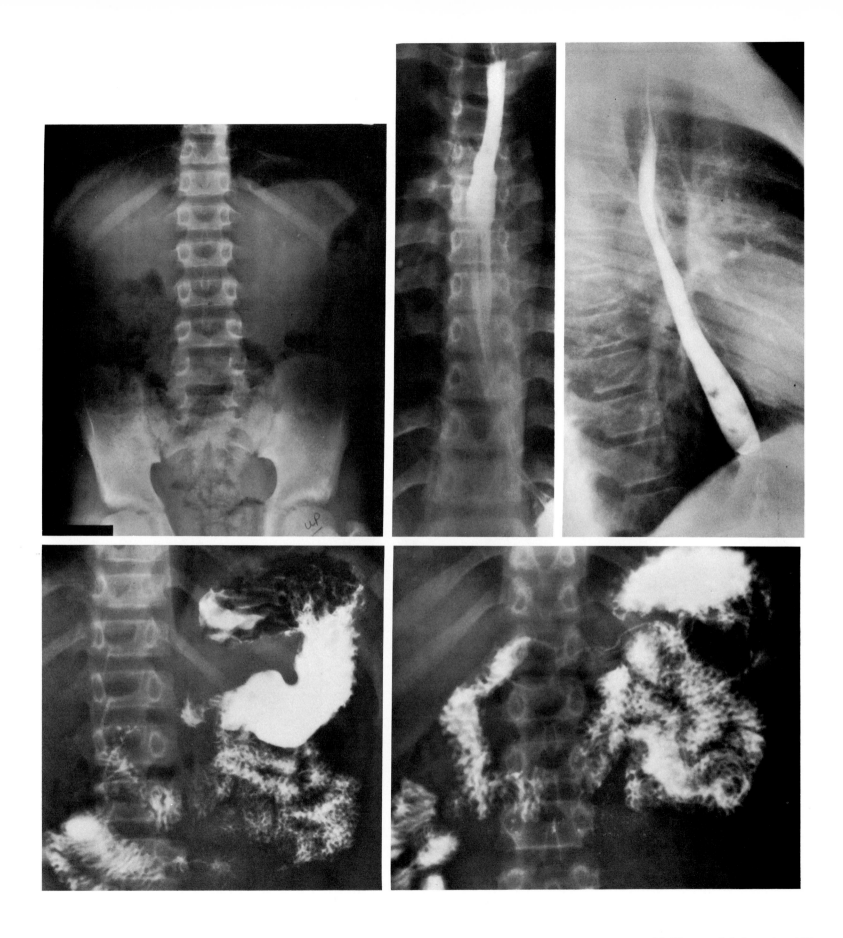

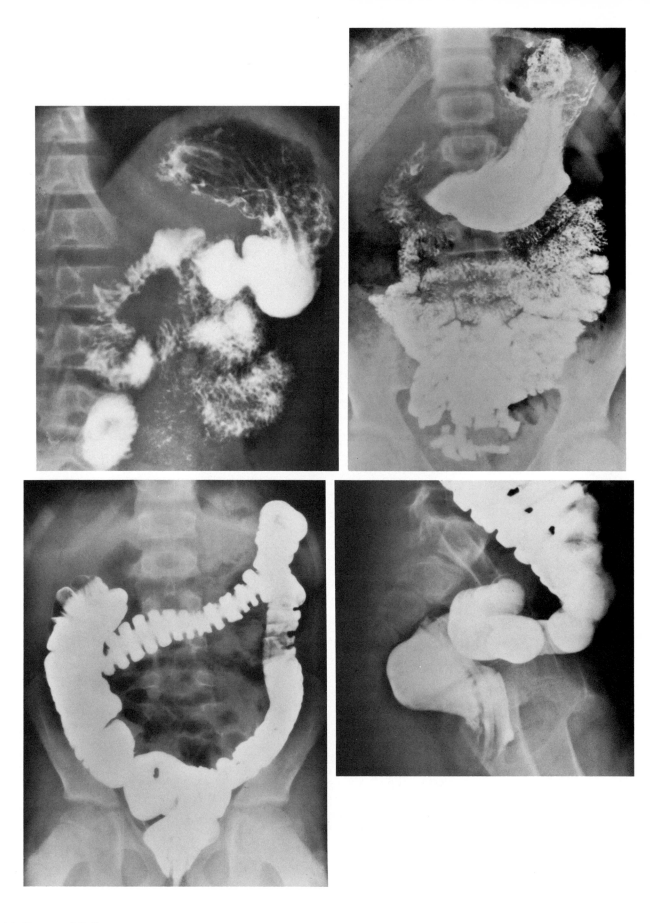

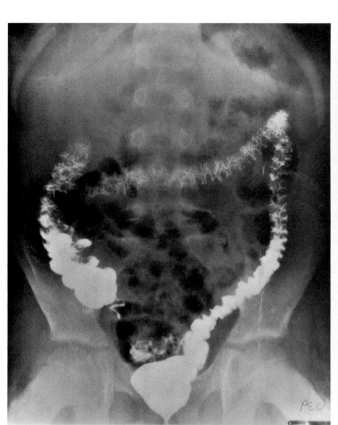

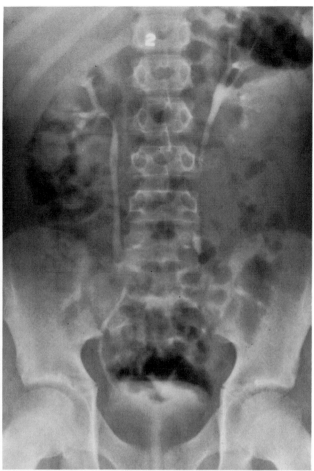

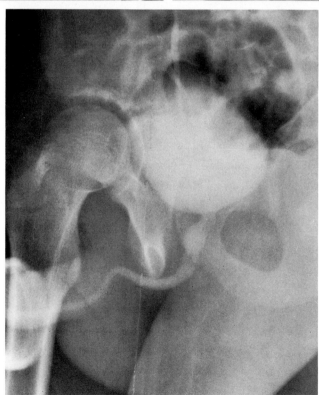

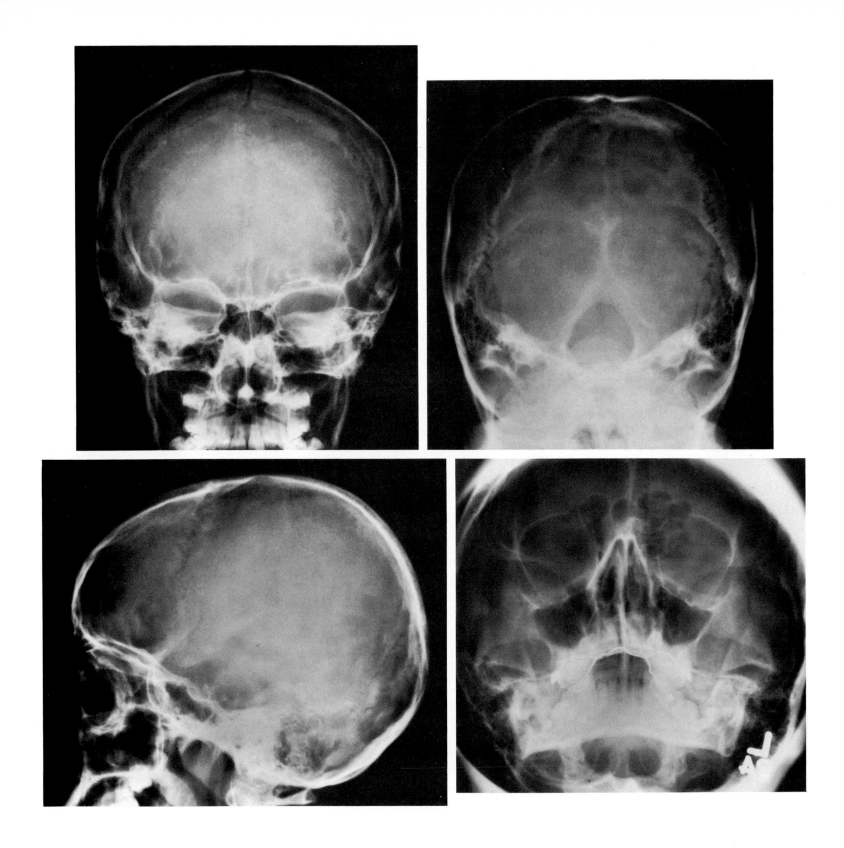

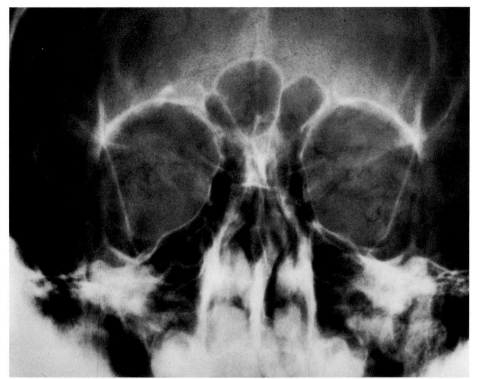

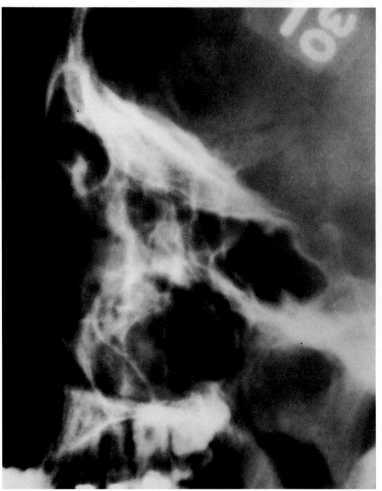

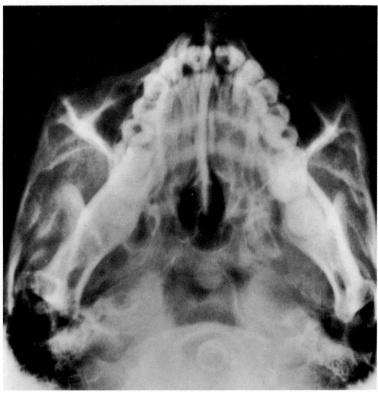

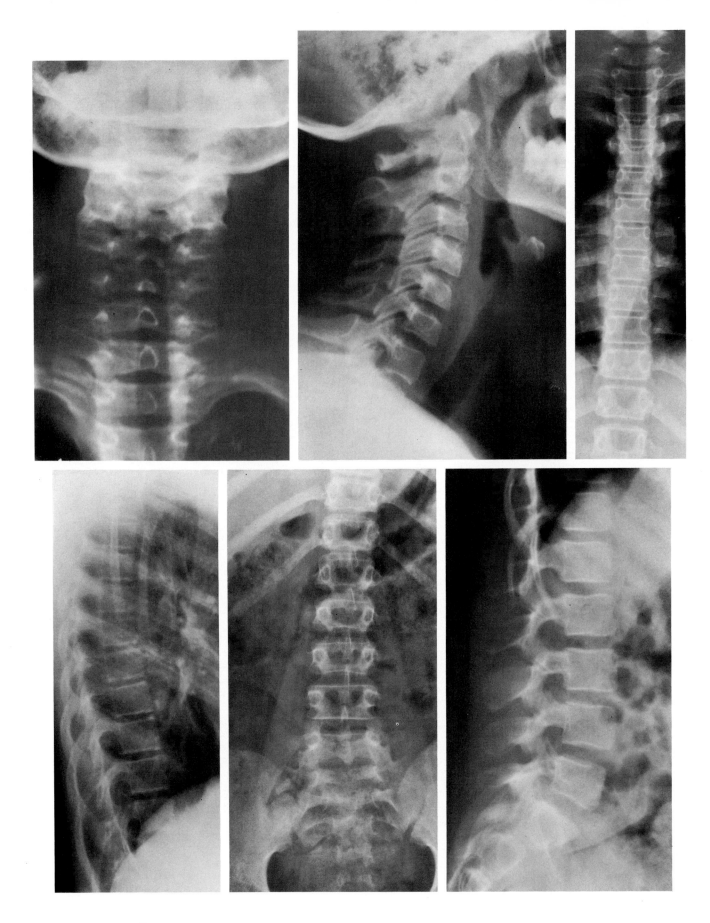

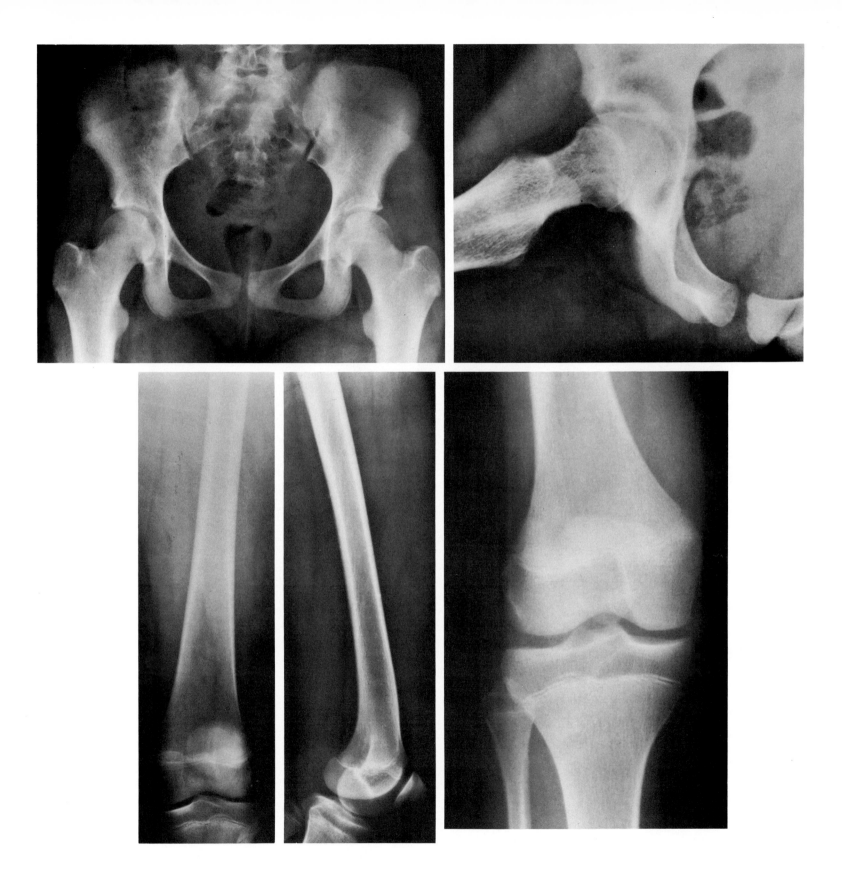

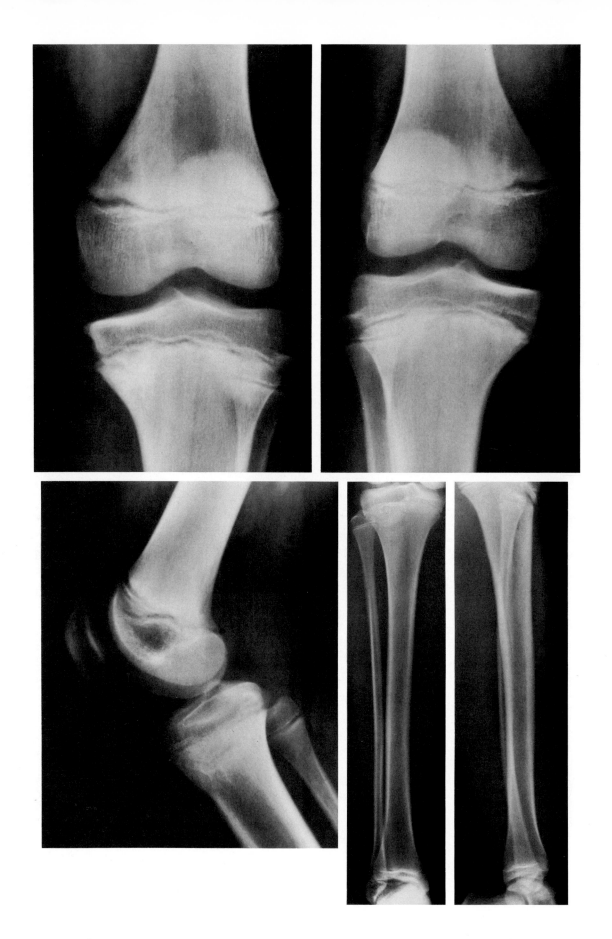

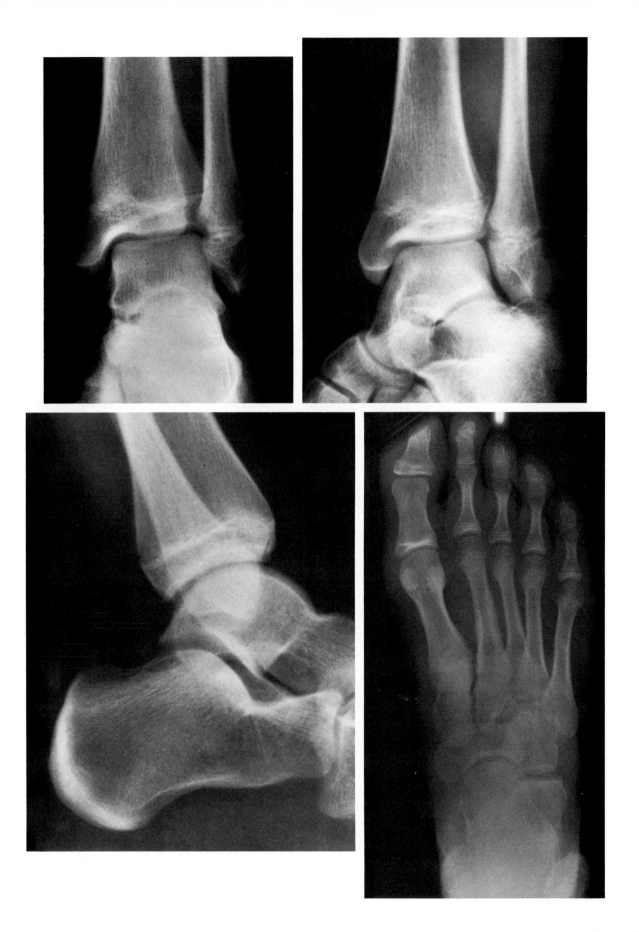

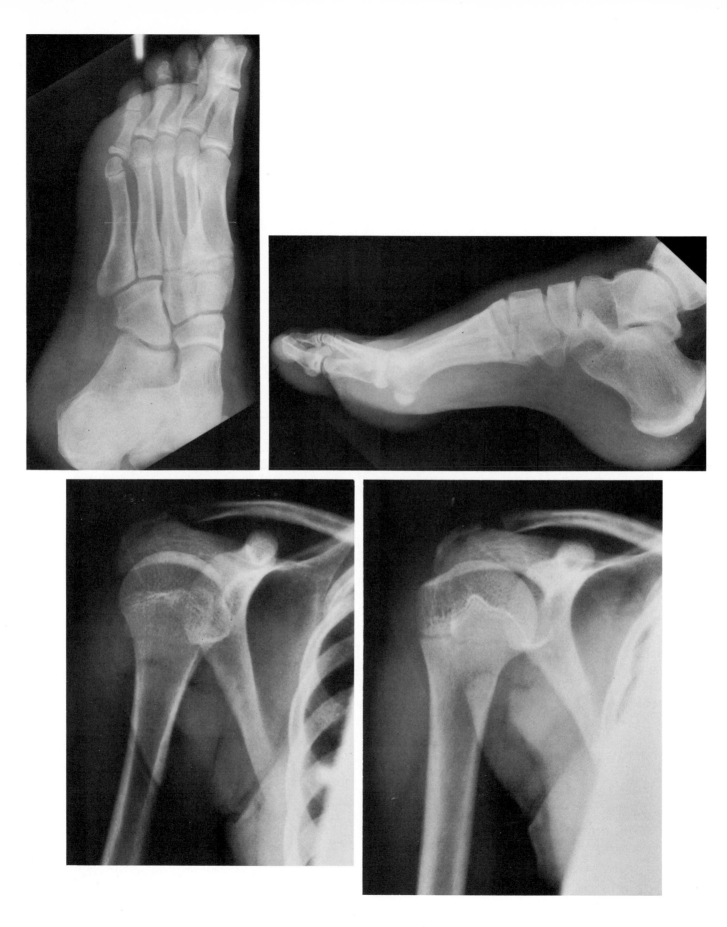

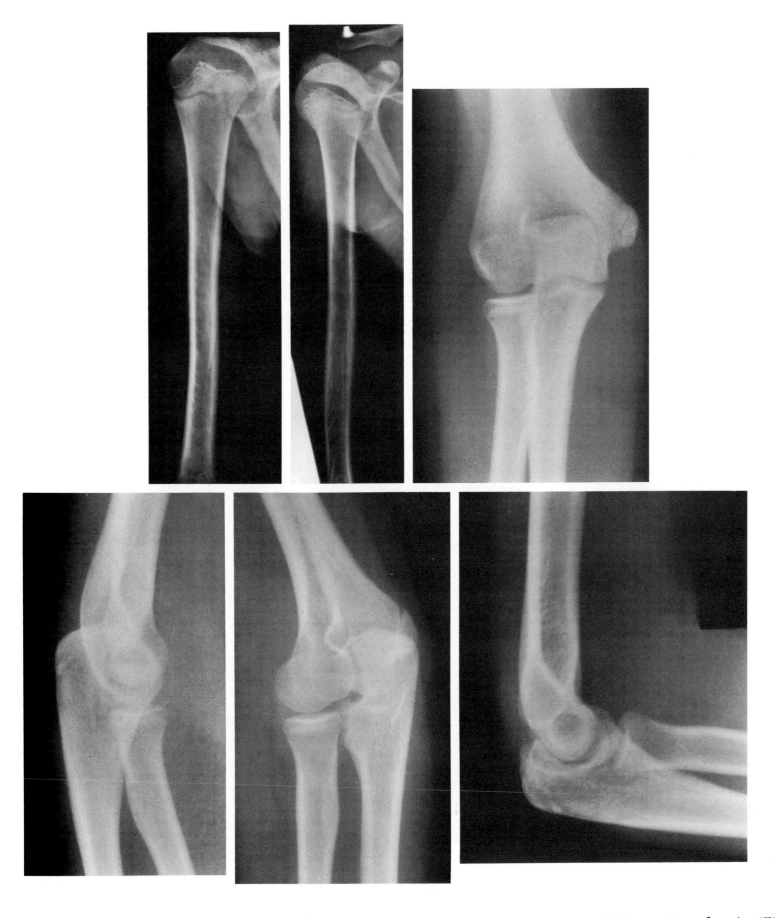

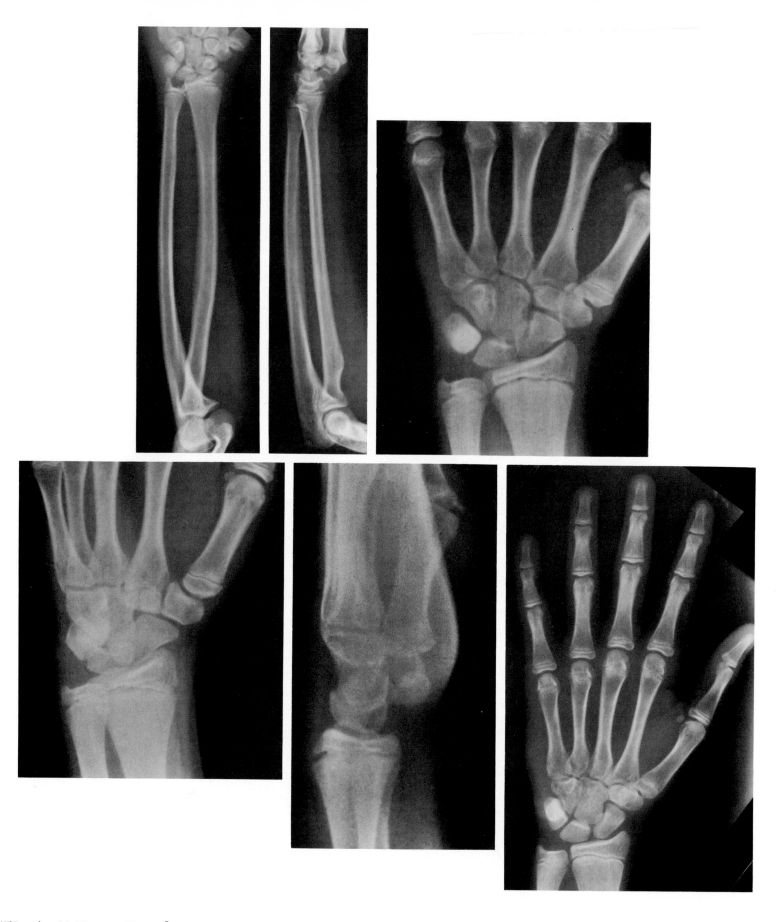

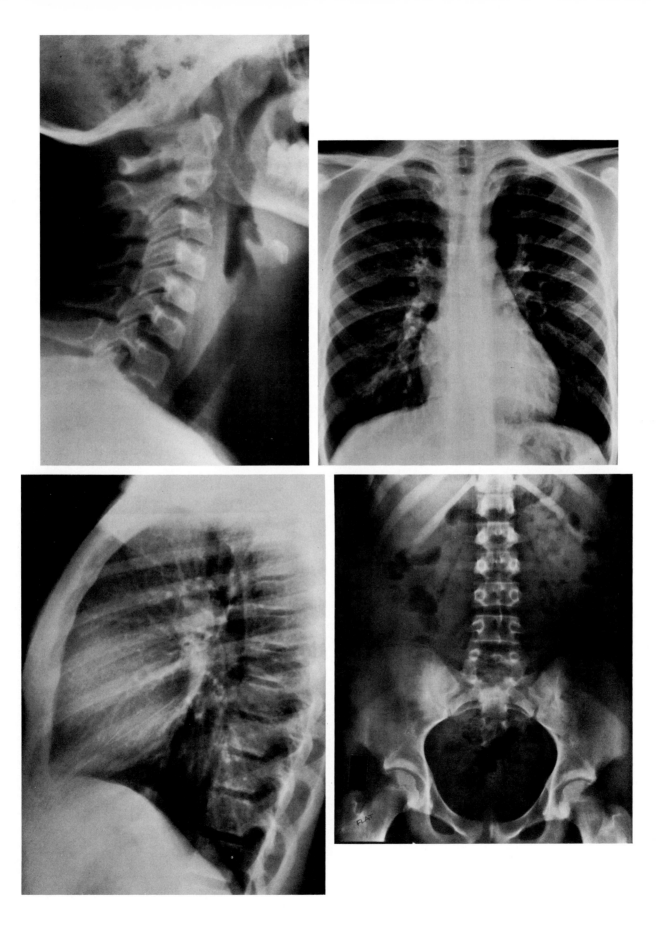

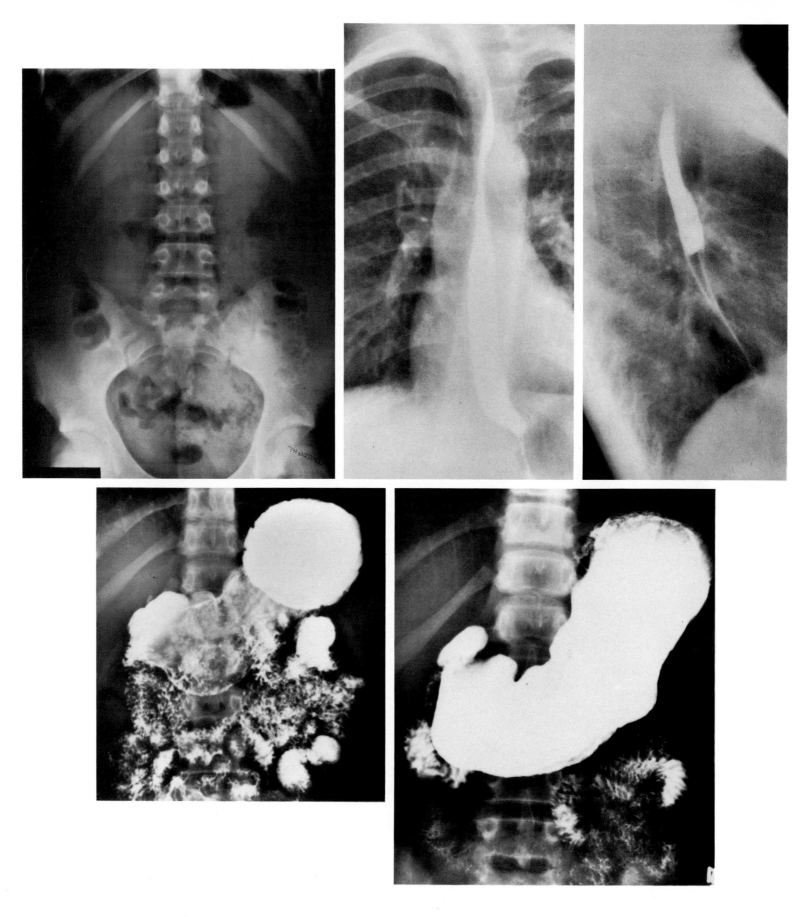

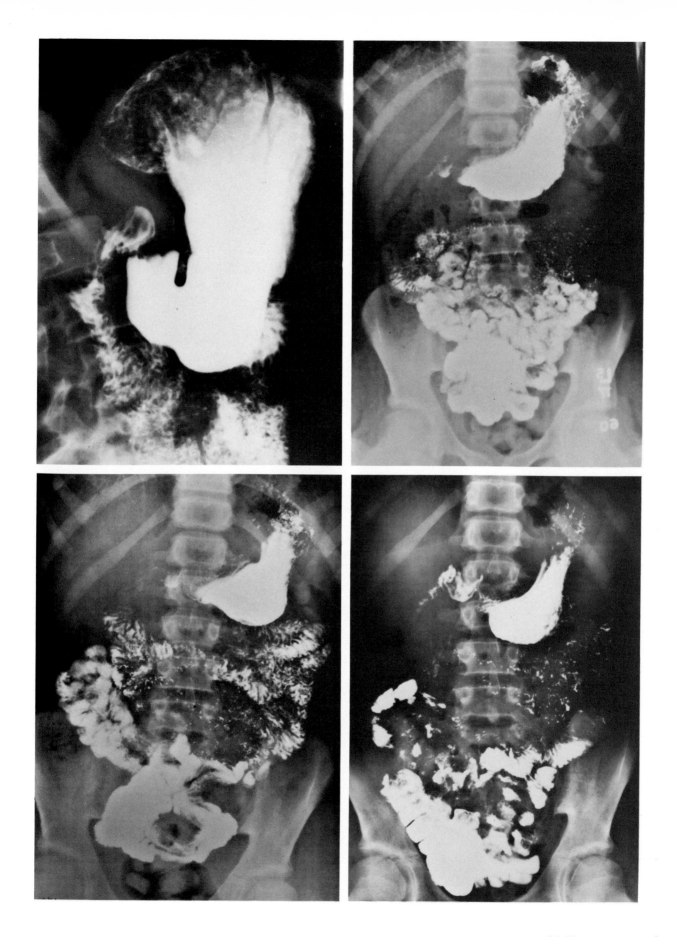

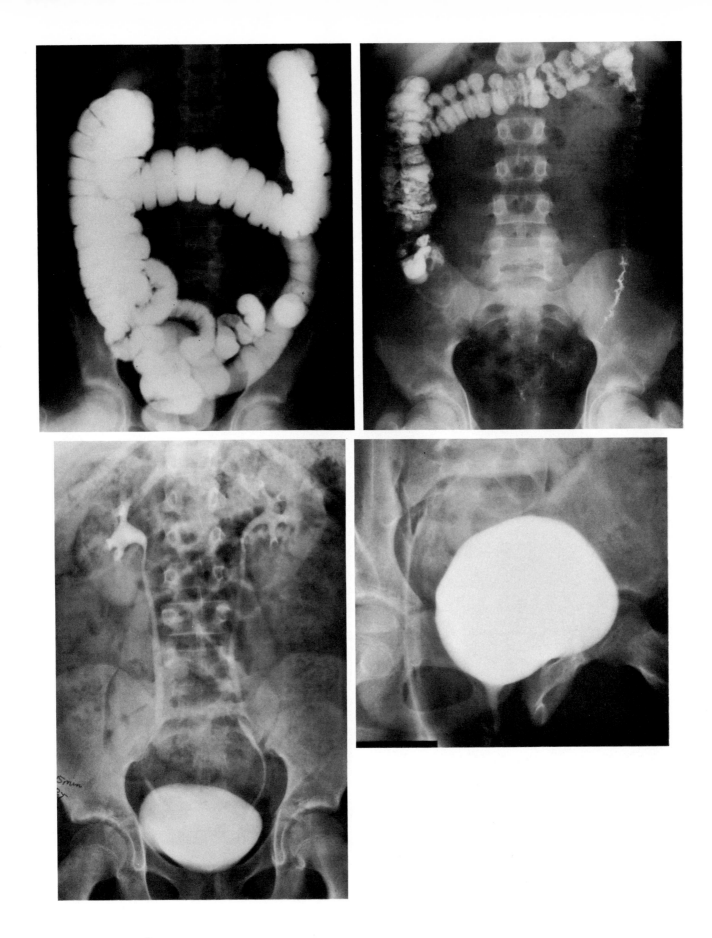

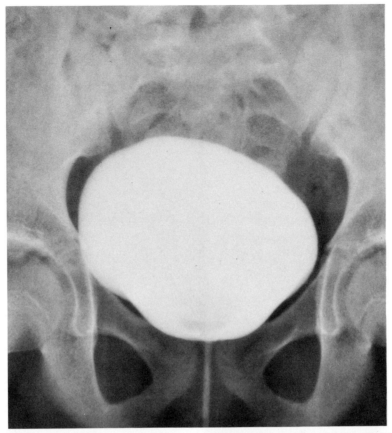

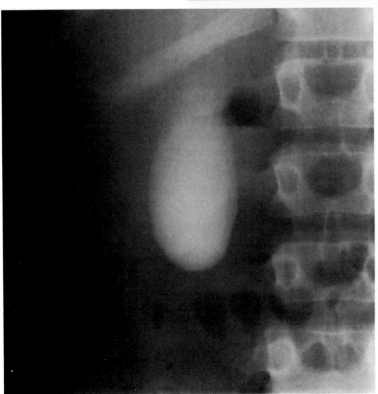

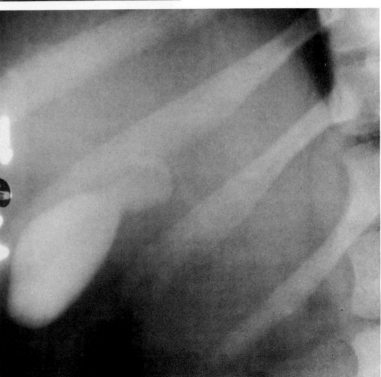

21

13 YEARS

The skull is adult in its proportions. Calvarial digital markings are minimal, but inner table impressions are evident. Some sutural sclerosis is present. The cervical vertebral bodies may retain some wedging, but the dorsal and lumbar vertebrae are adult-like in configuration. The end plates may have an undulating contour.

The physiologic protrusio acetabuli are less marked. The fossa of the fovea capitis is seen. The iliac apophyses are visible.

The airway and chest are adult in configuration. The pulmonary artery prominence persists in some individuals.

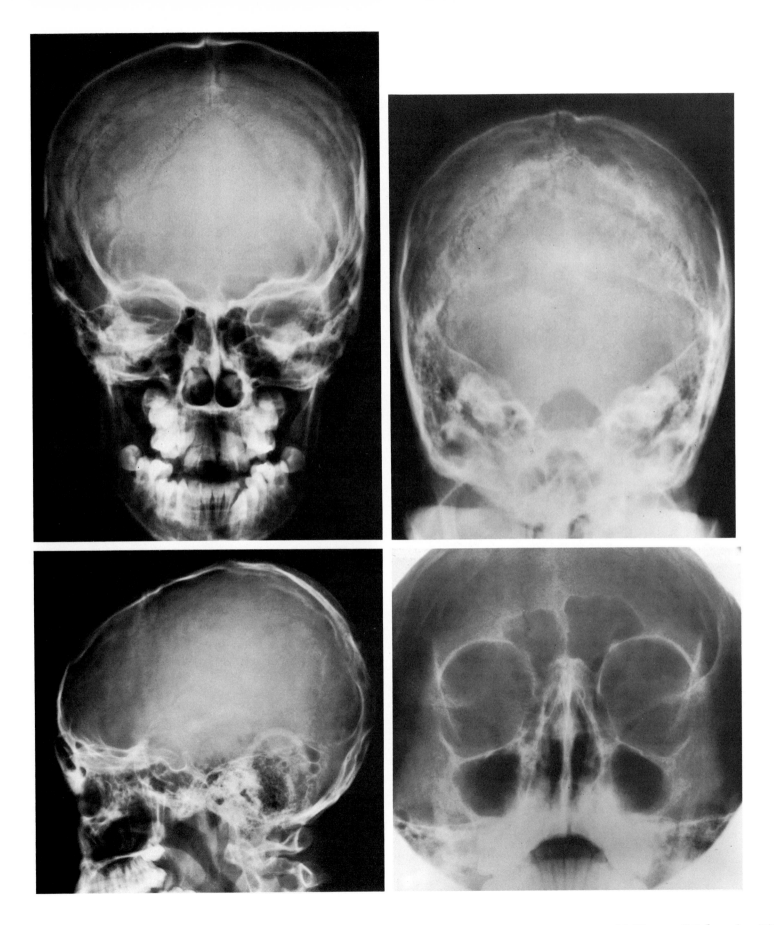

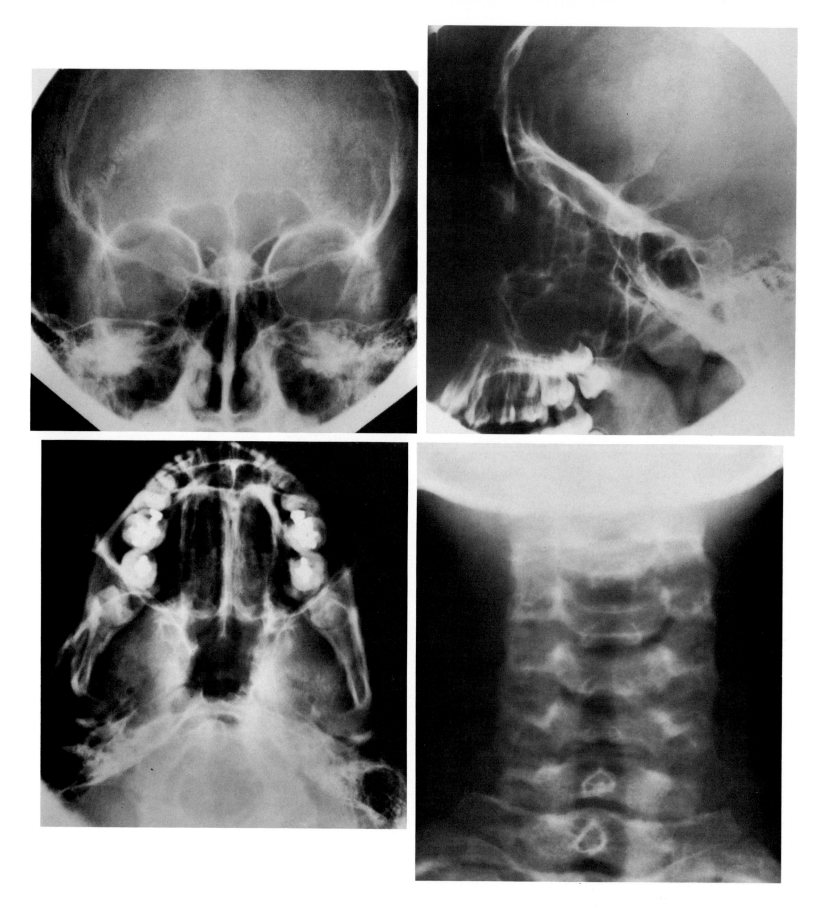

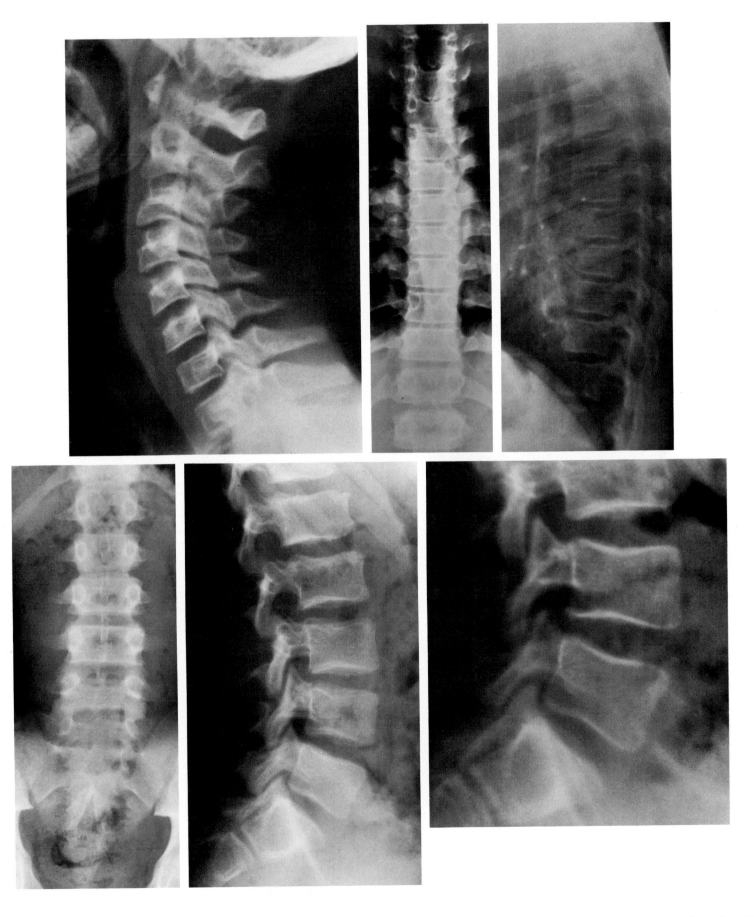

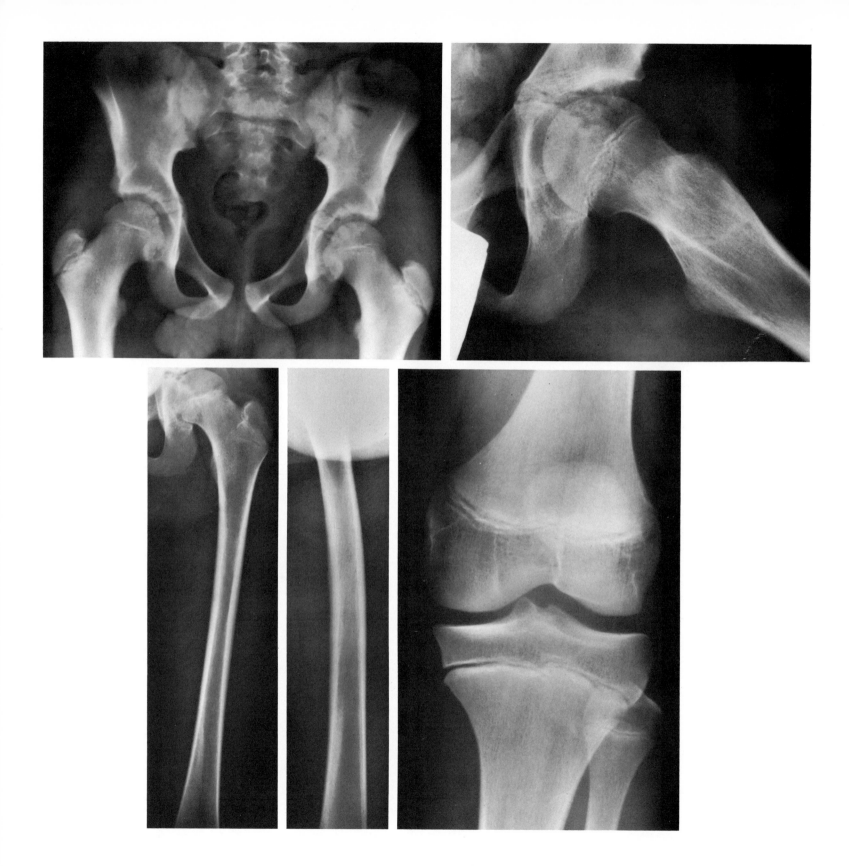

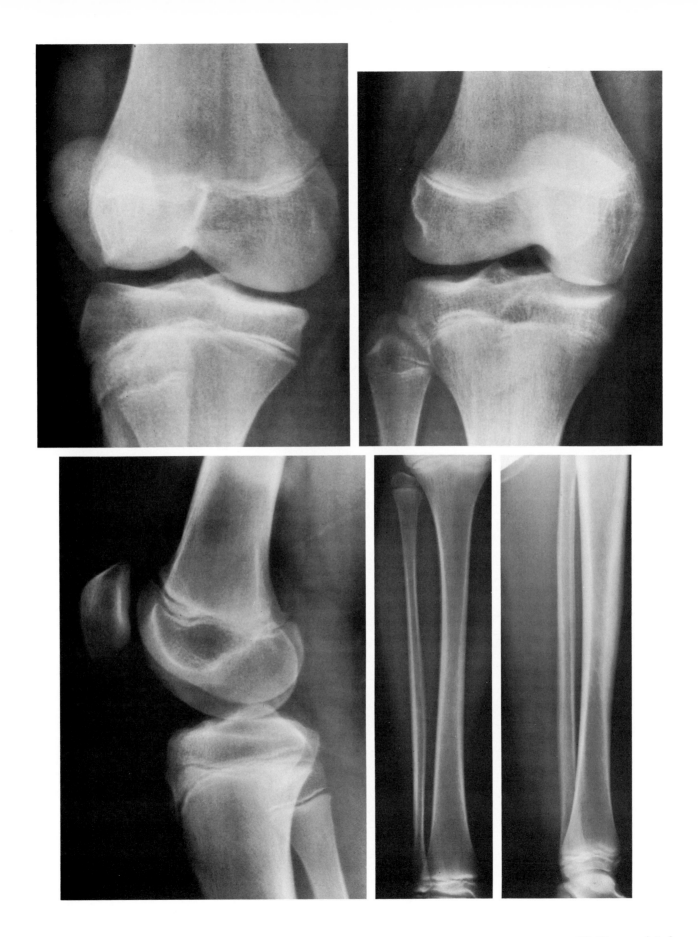

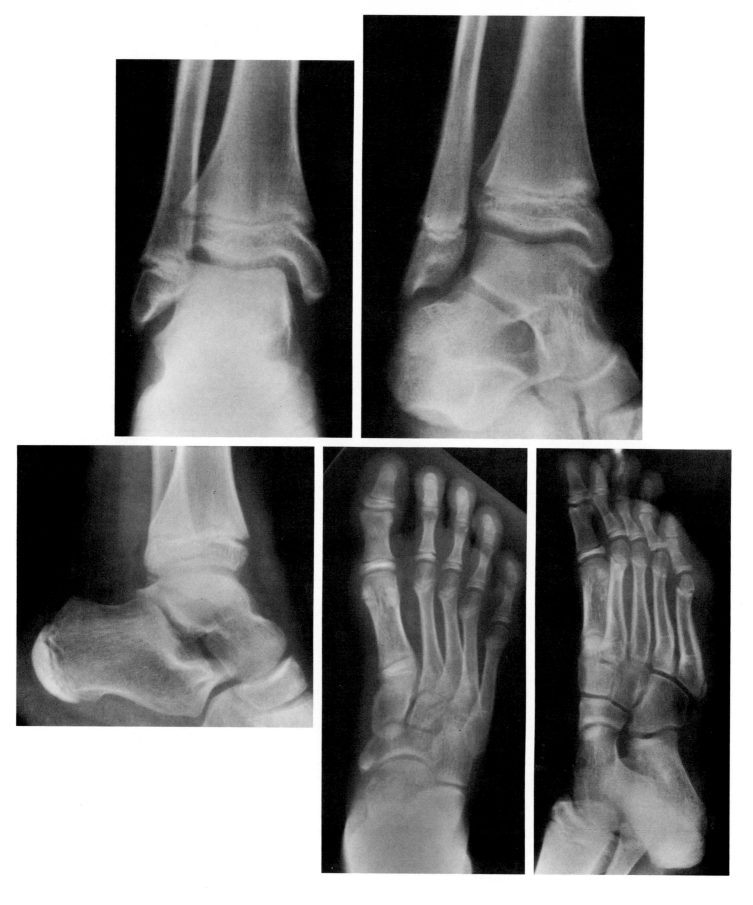

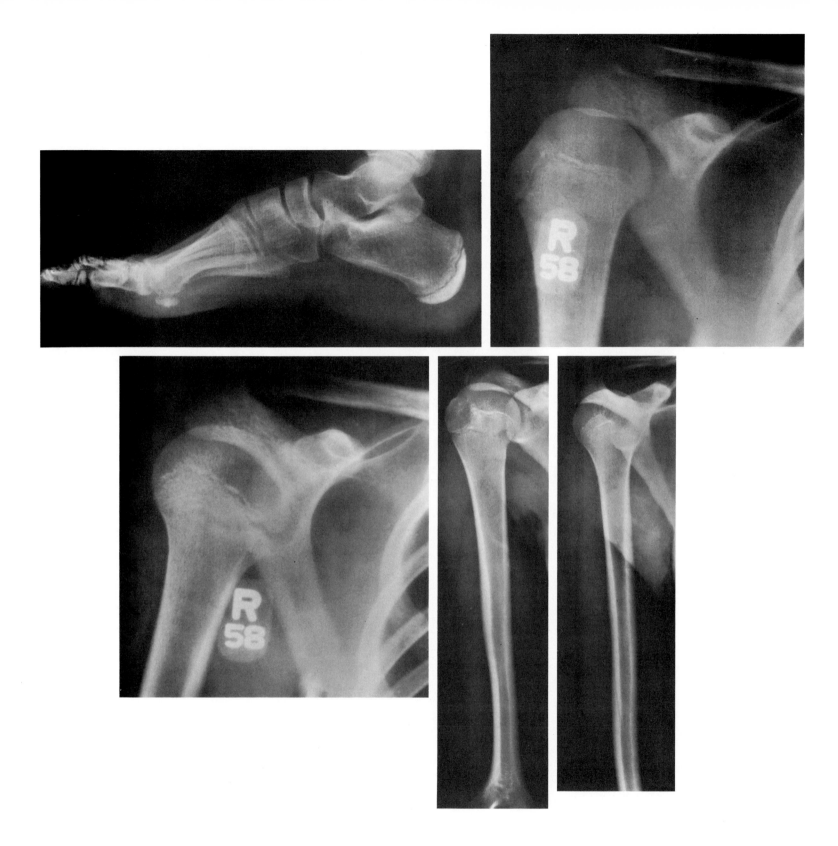

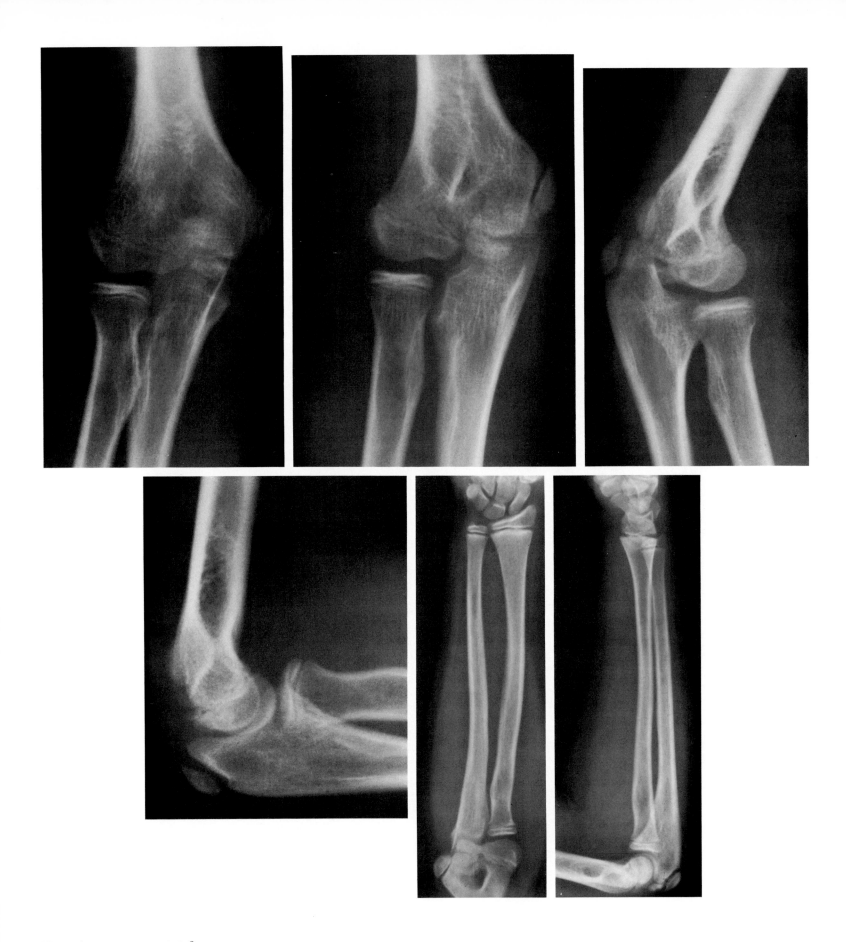

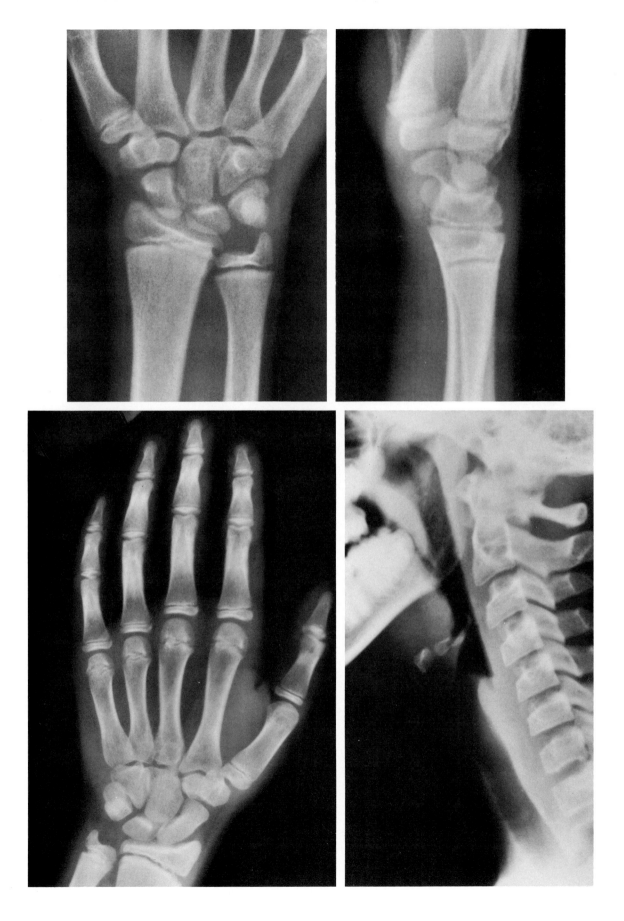

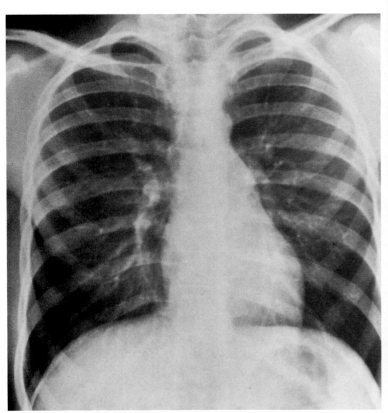
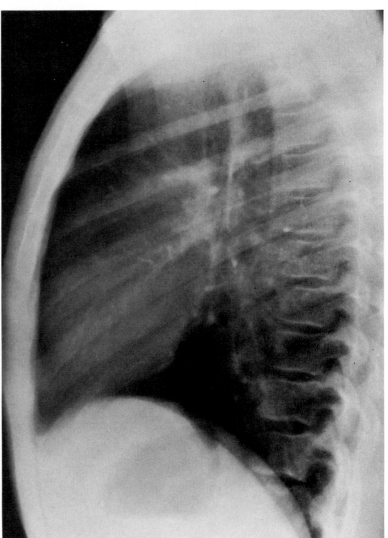

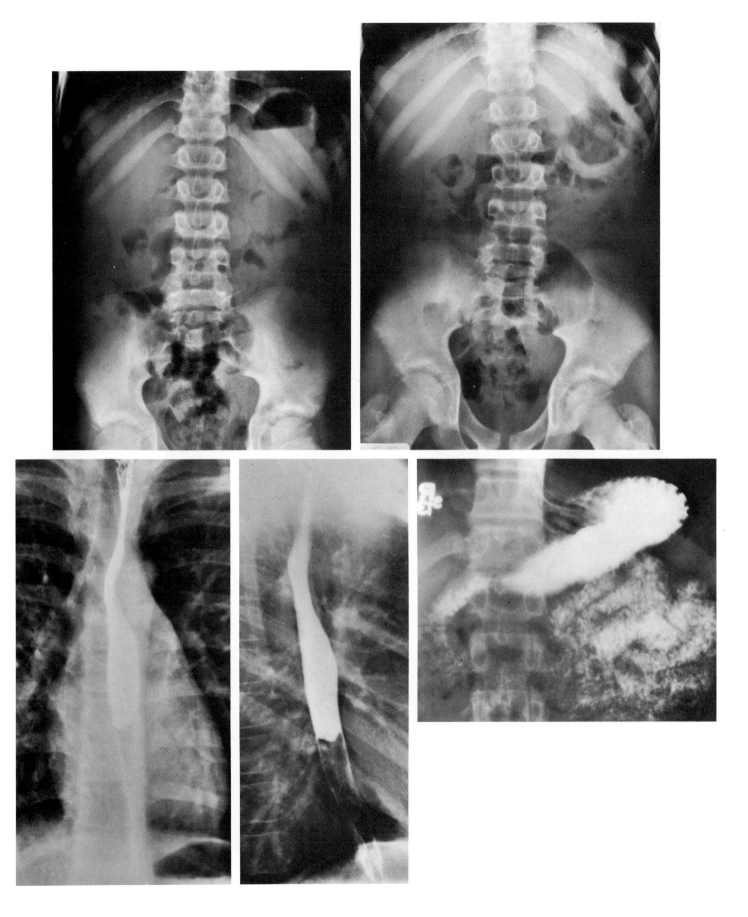

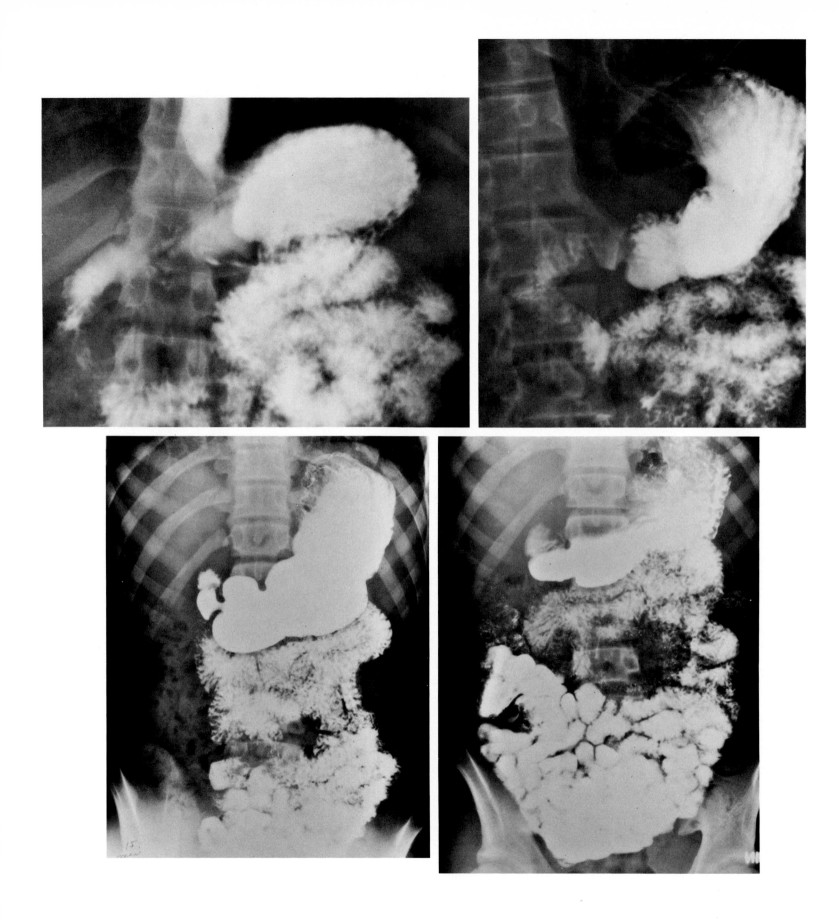

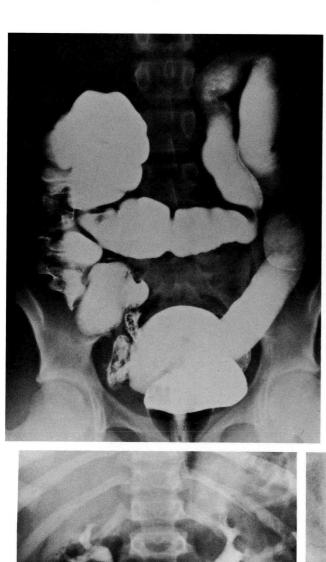

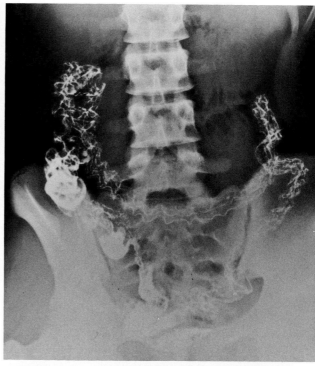

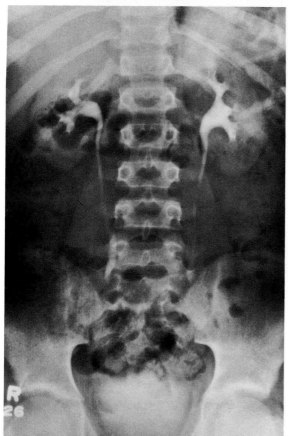

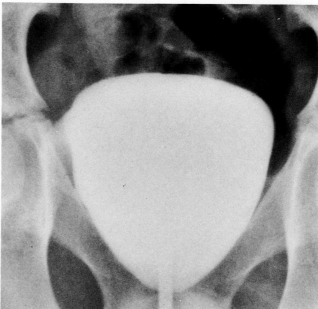

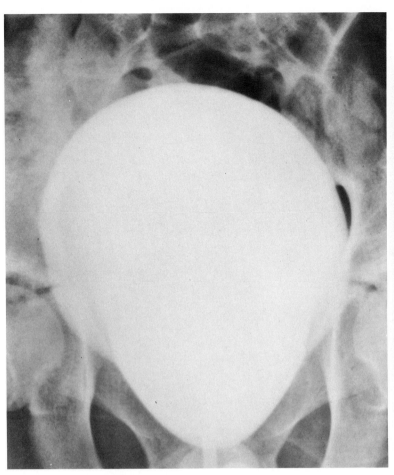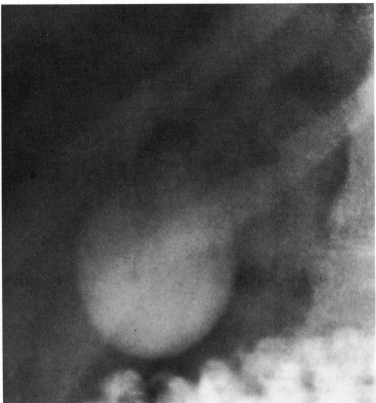

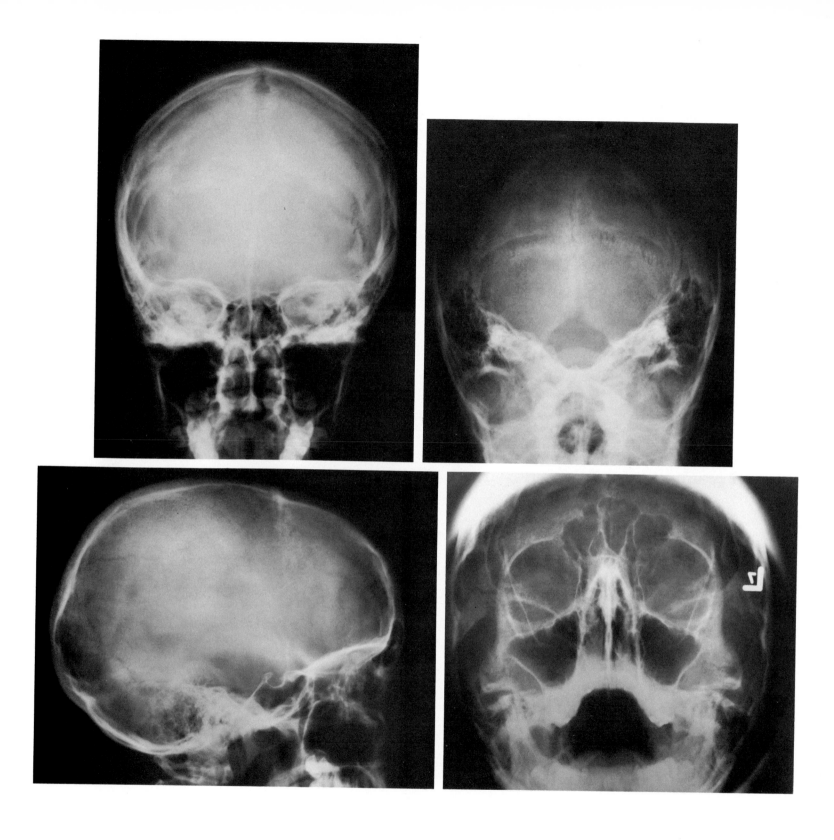

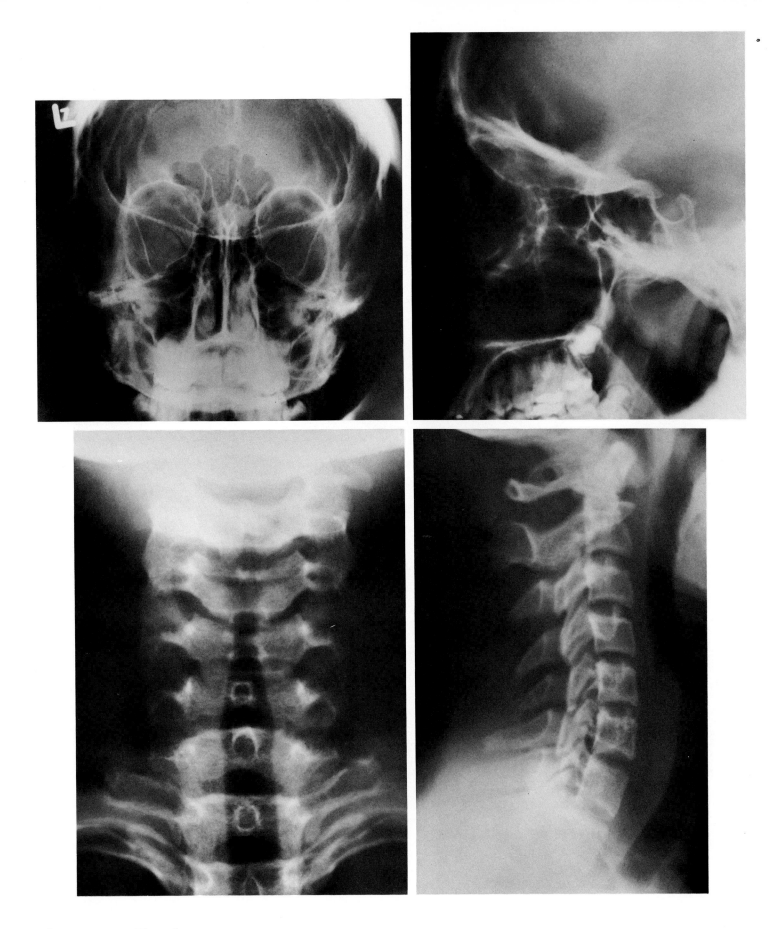

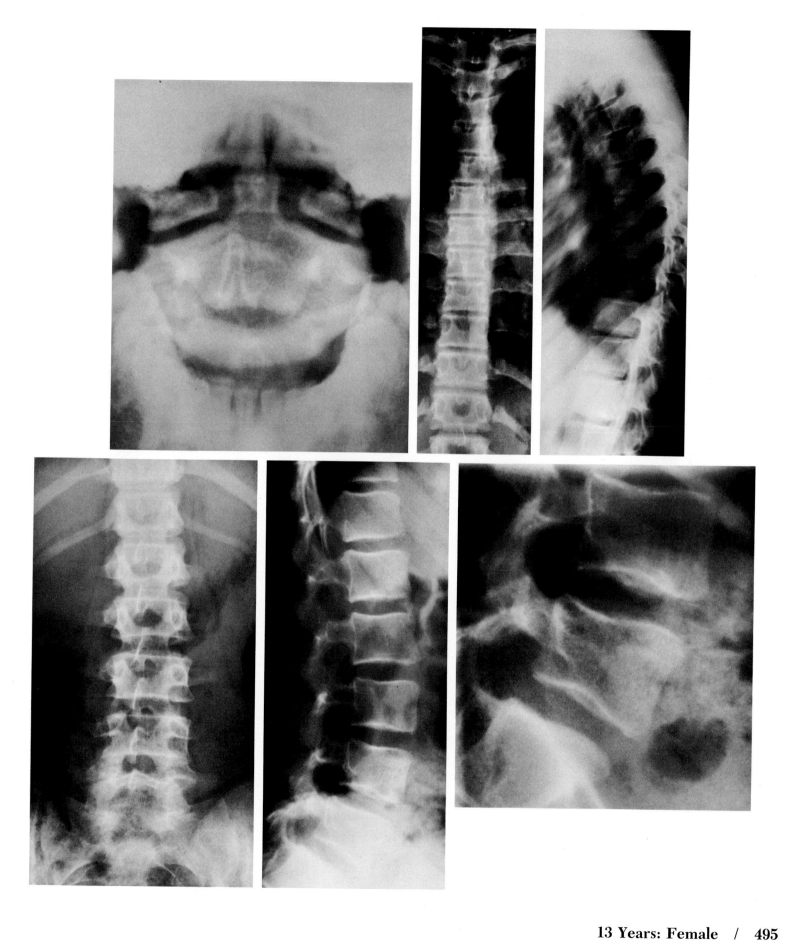

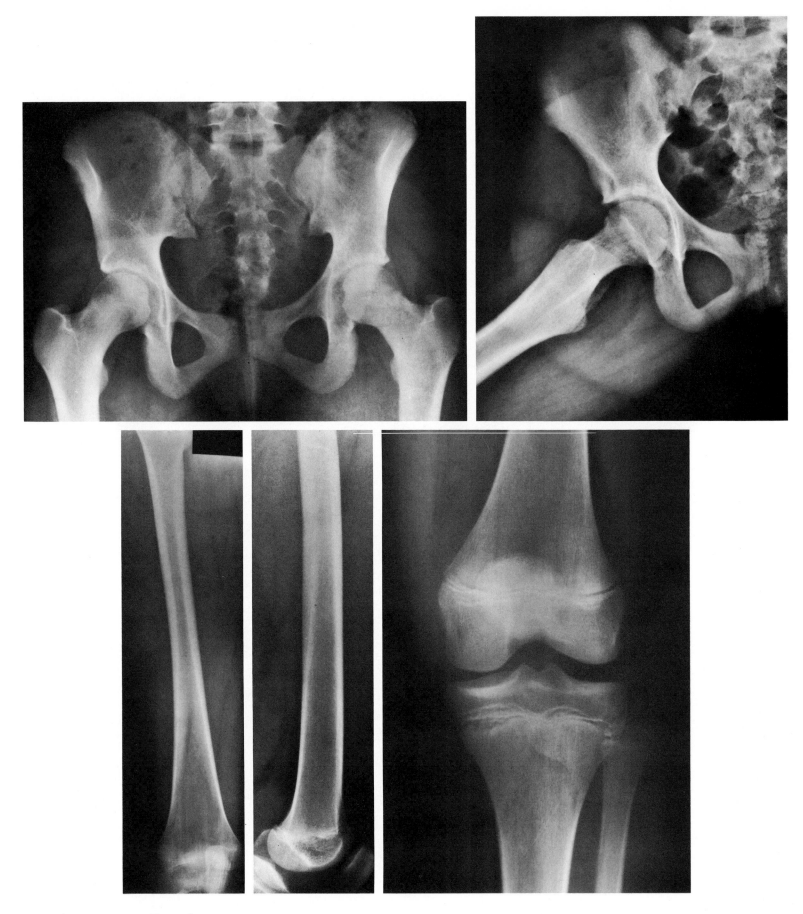

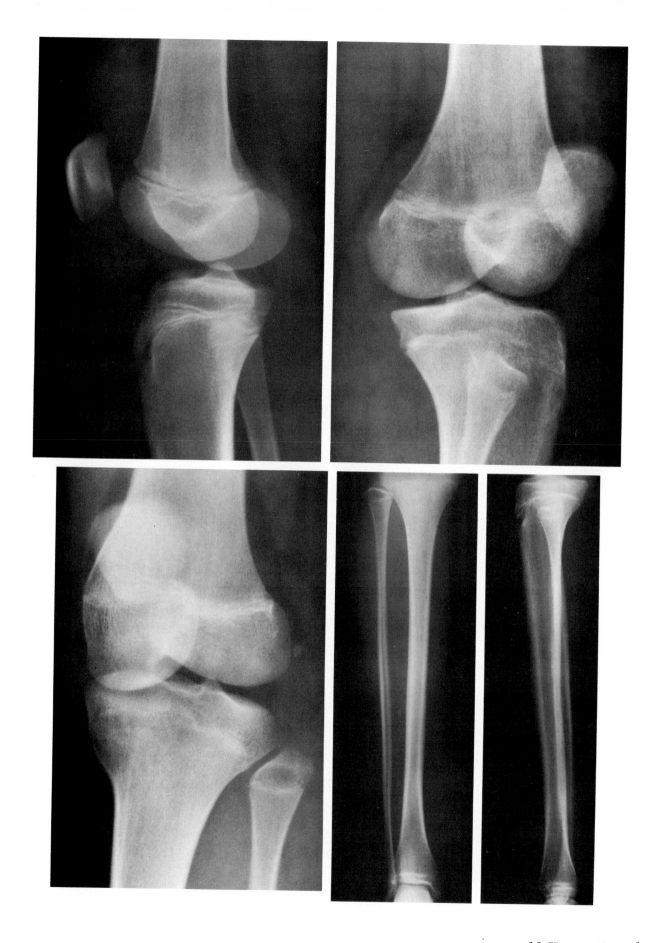

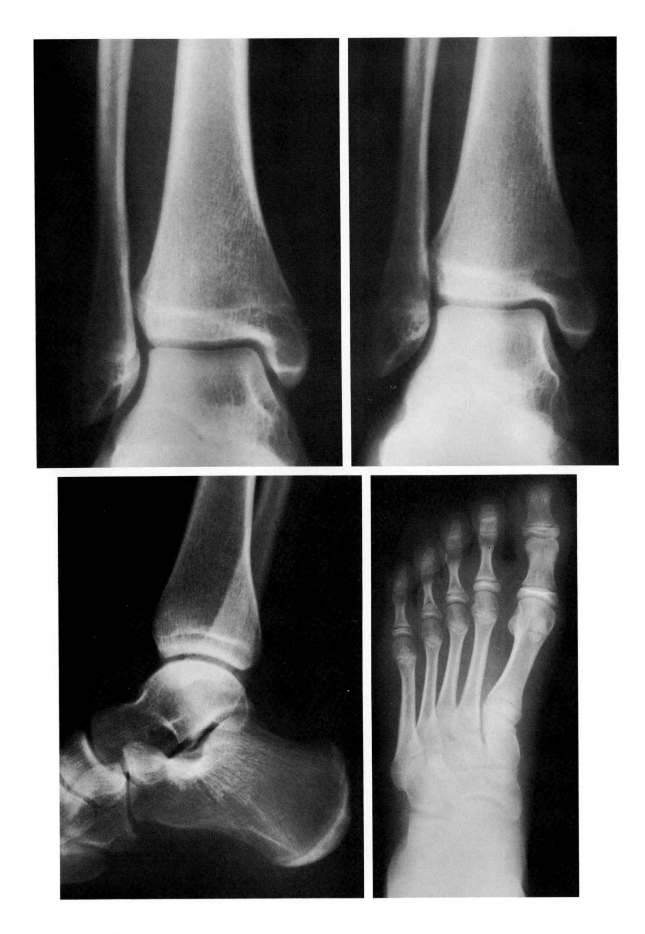

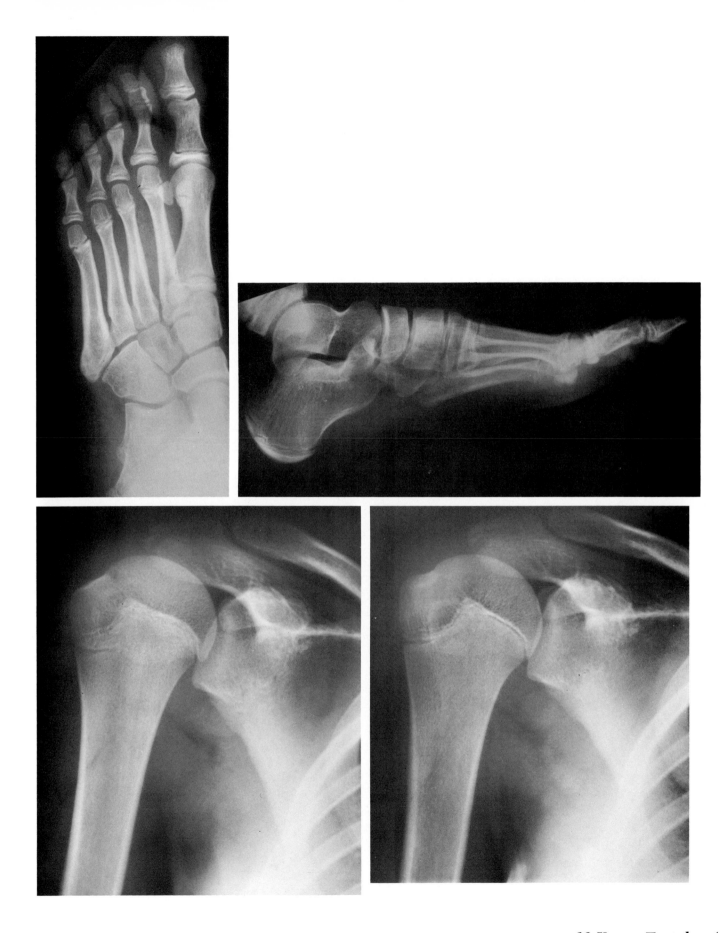

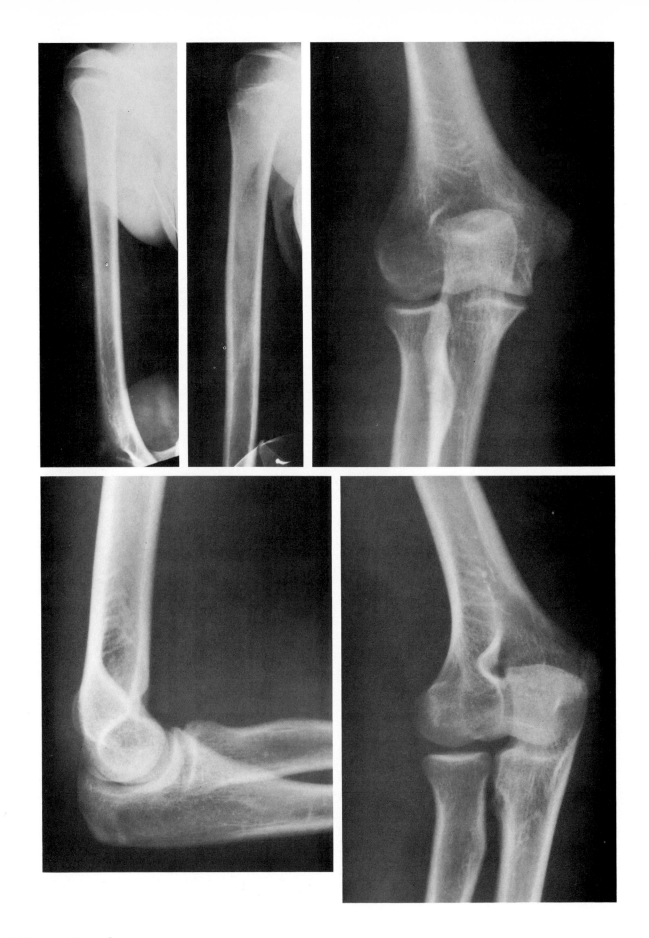

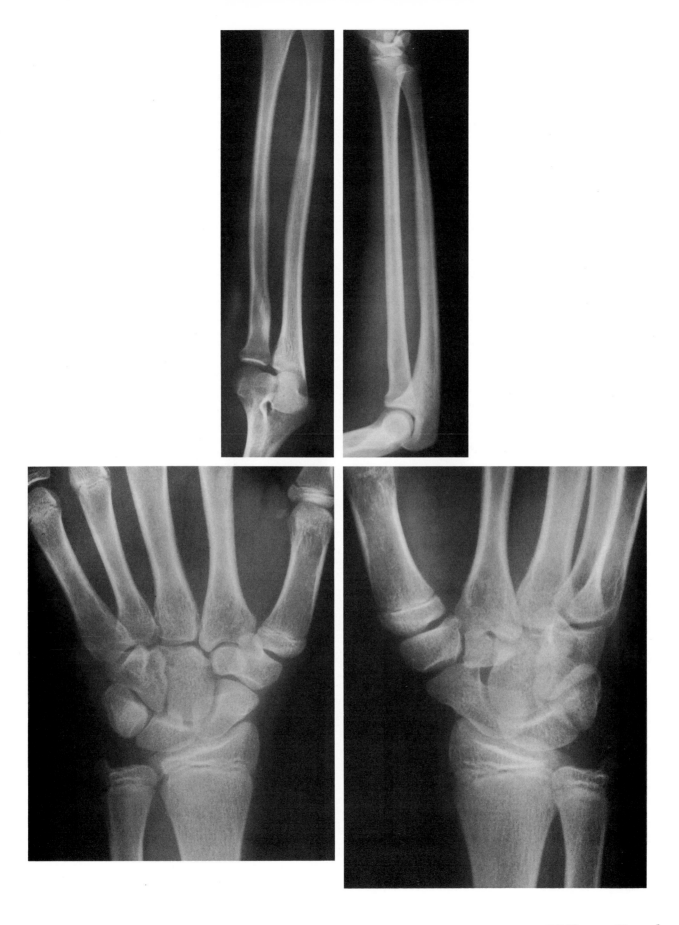

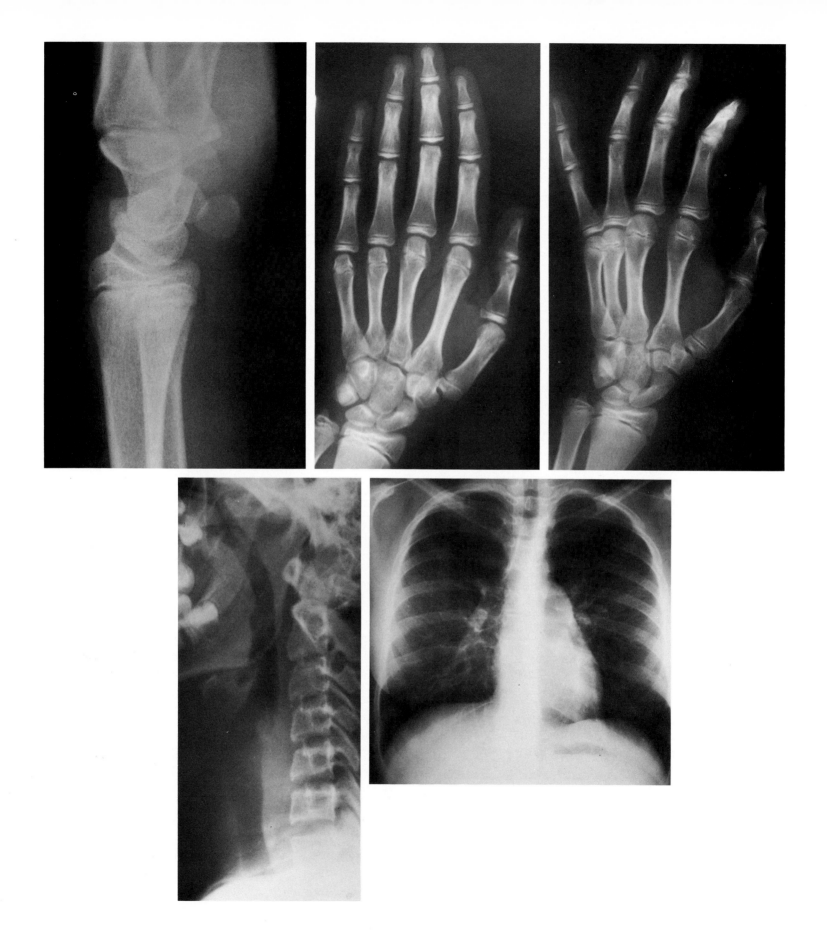

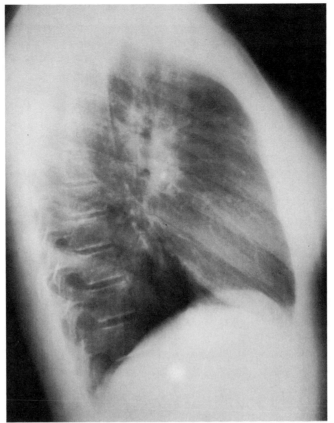

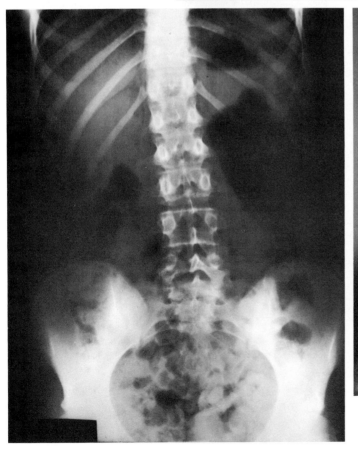

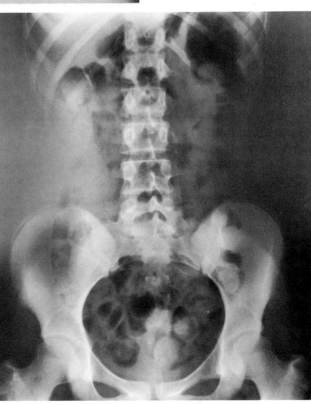

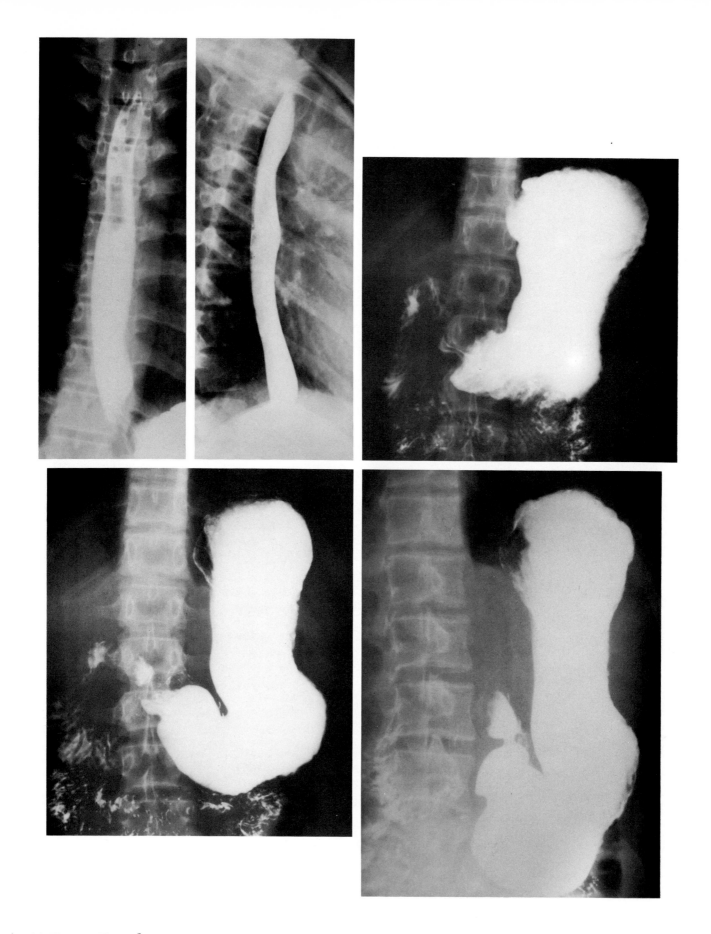

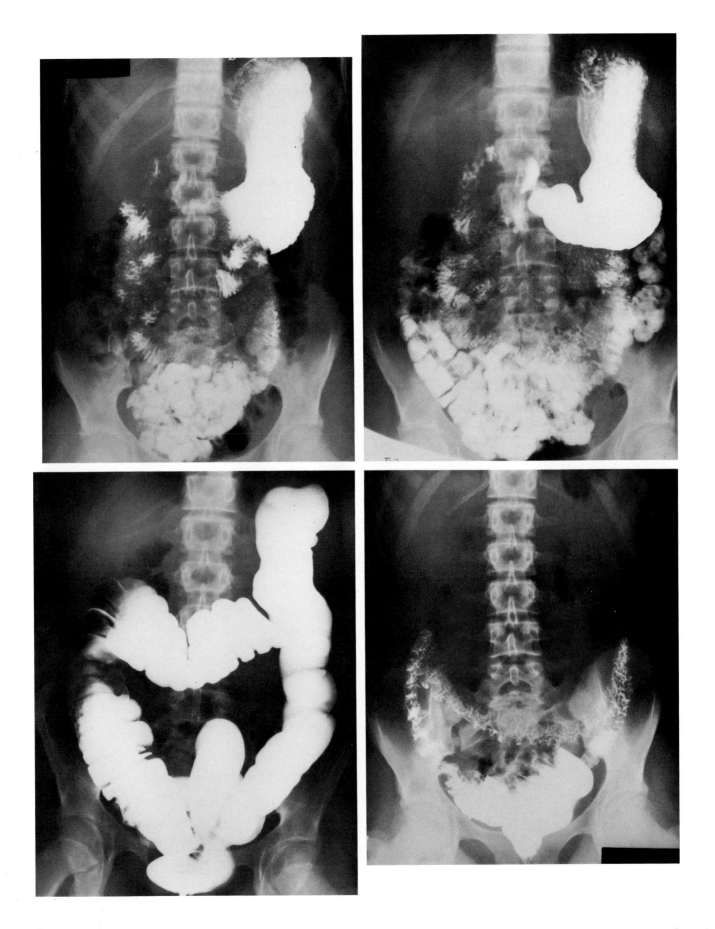

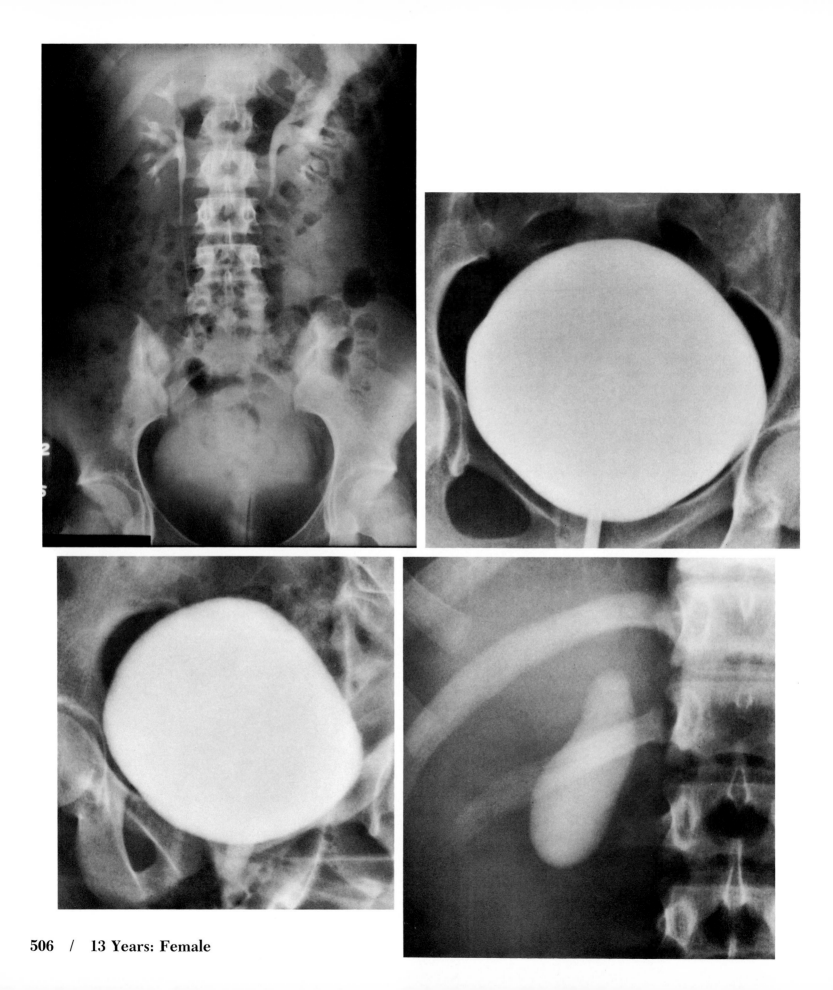

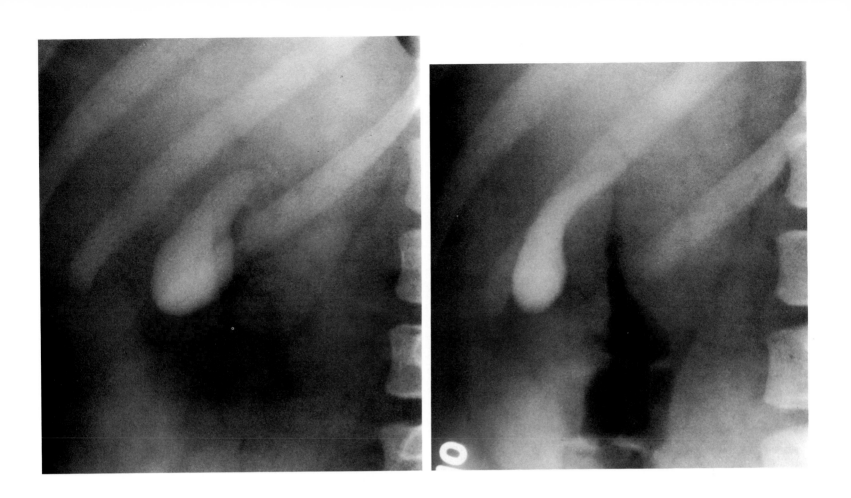

22

14 YEARS

The sphenoid sinus is now completely pneumatized. The cervical vertebrae are still somewhat wedged, particularly in the male. The accelerated development of the female, contrasted to the male, is becoming clearer. The epiphyses at the elbow and the calcaneal apophysis may be open in the male, but closed in the female. These differences are seen in the shoulder, elbow, feet, and hands.

The secondary ossification centers for the acetabula are evident. The iliac apophyses approximate the ilia, but are not yet fixed.

The mobility of the colon is more apparent, particularly in the transverse portion. The urinary bladder is more deeply seated in the pelvis.

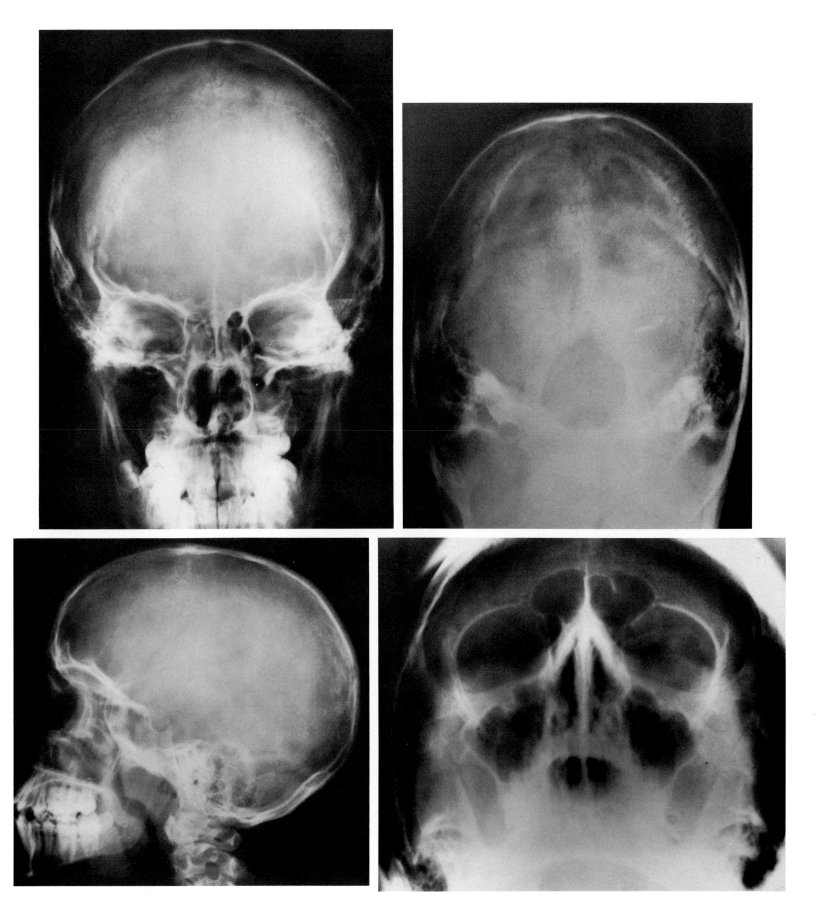

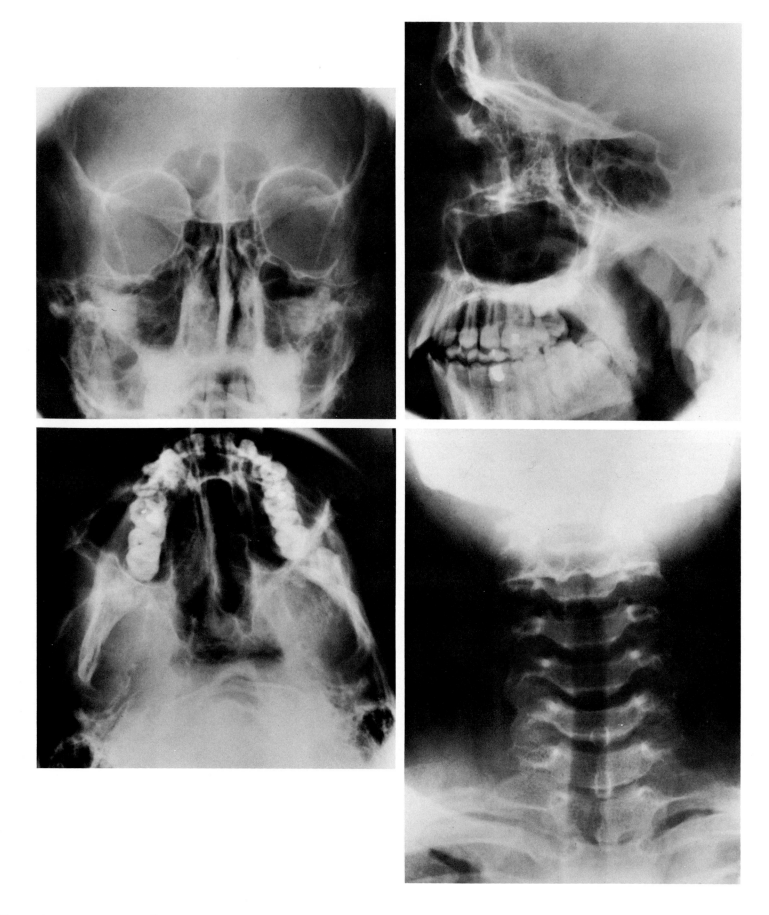

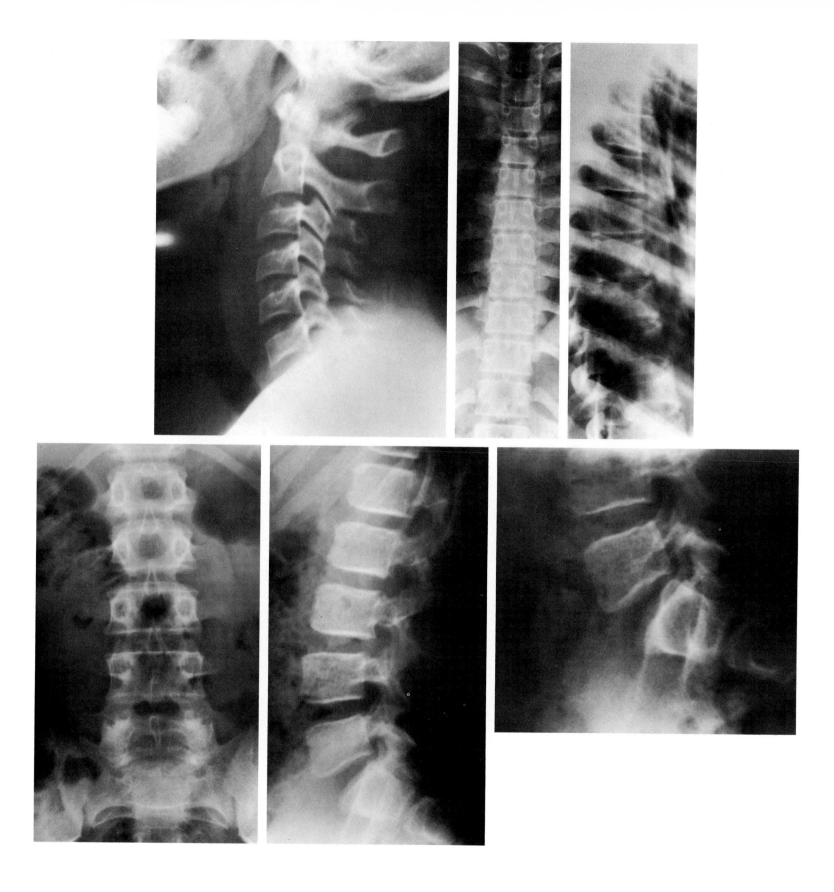

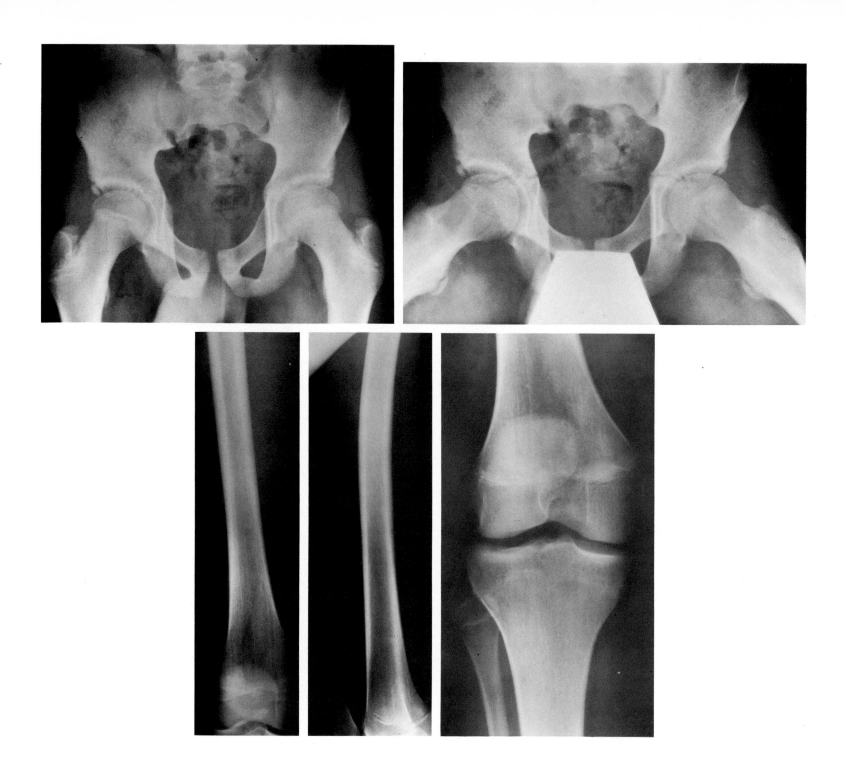

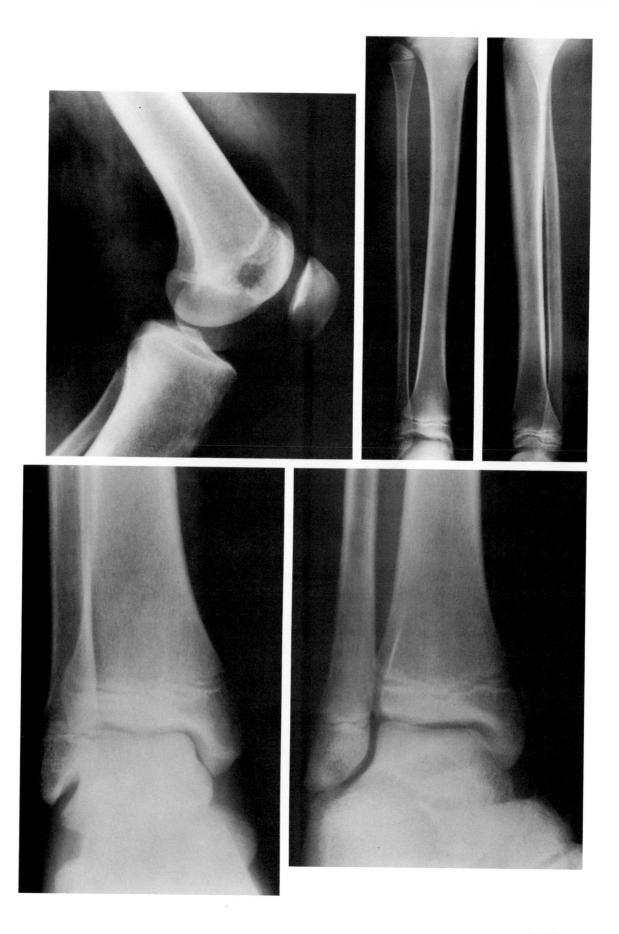

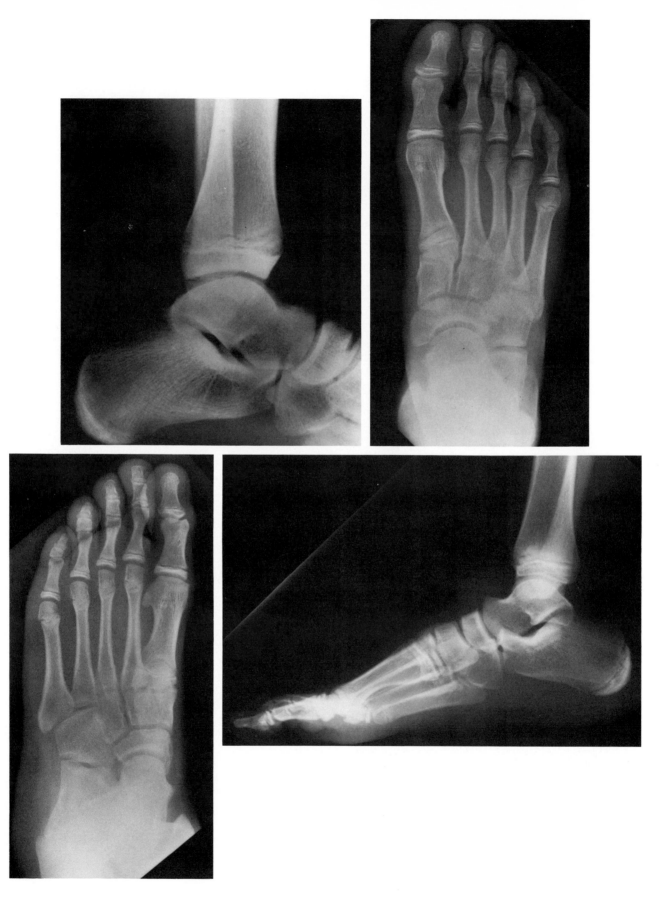

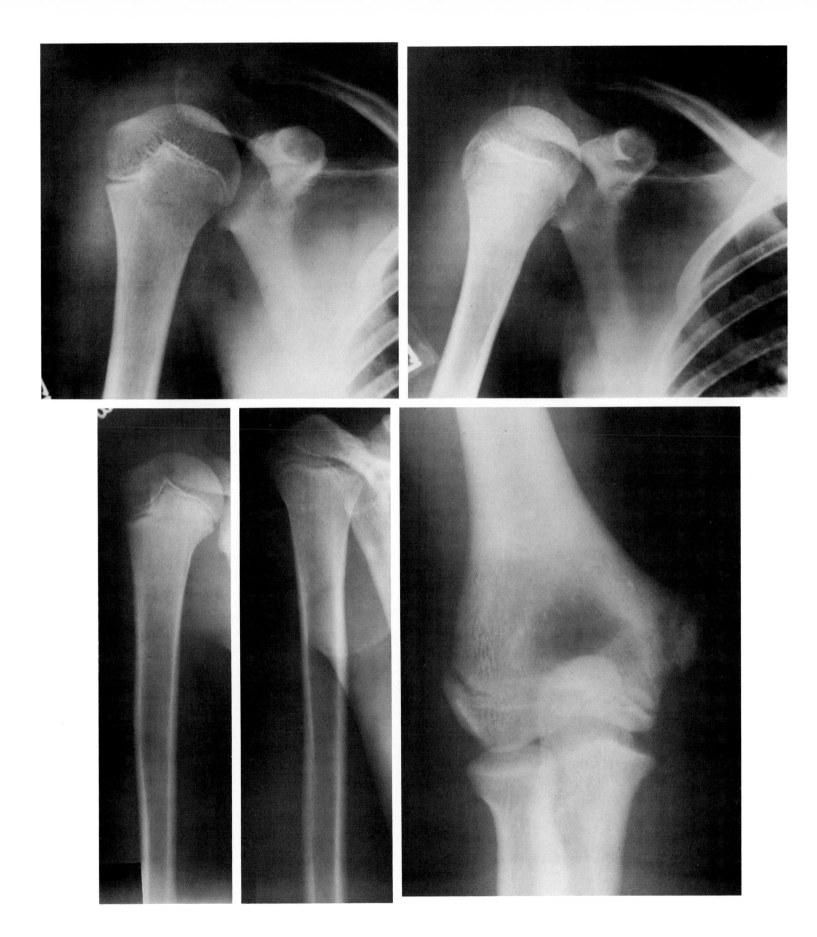

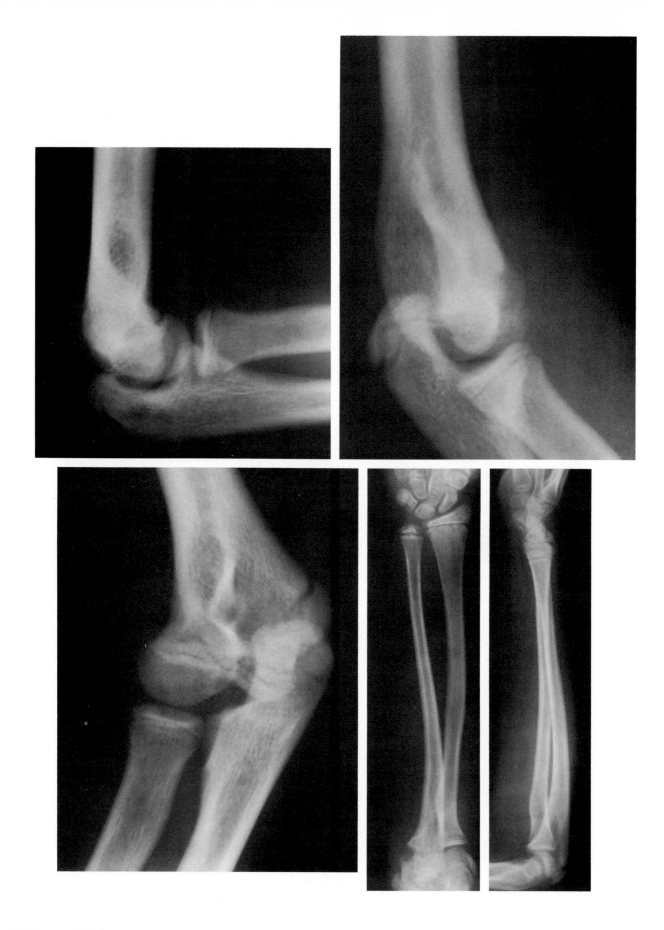

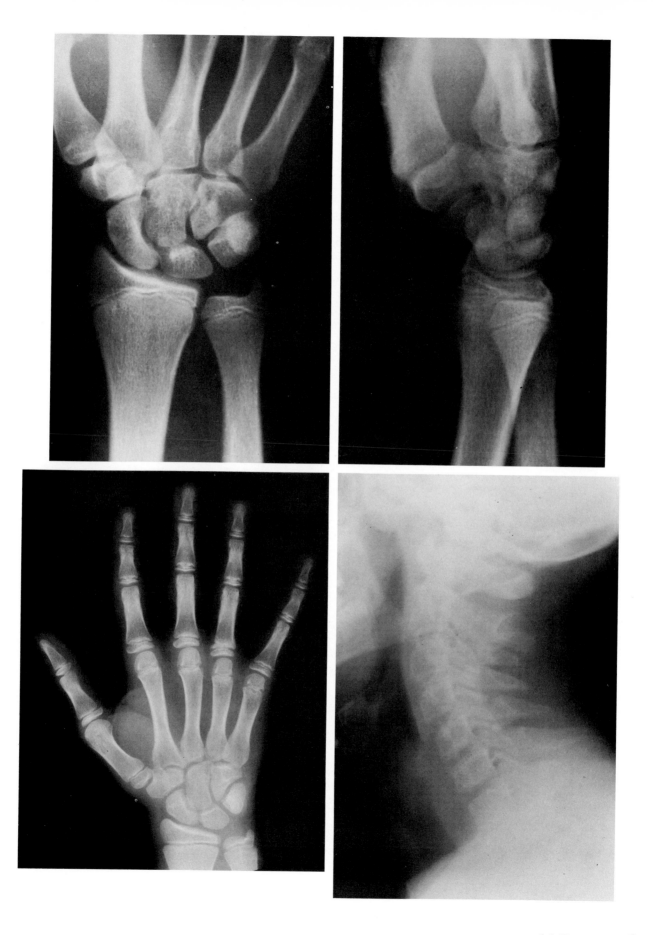

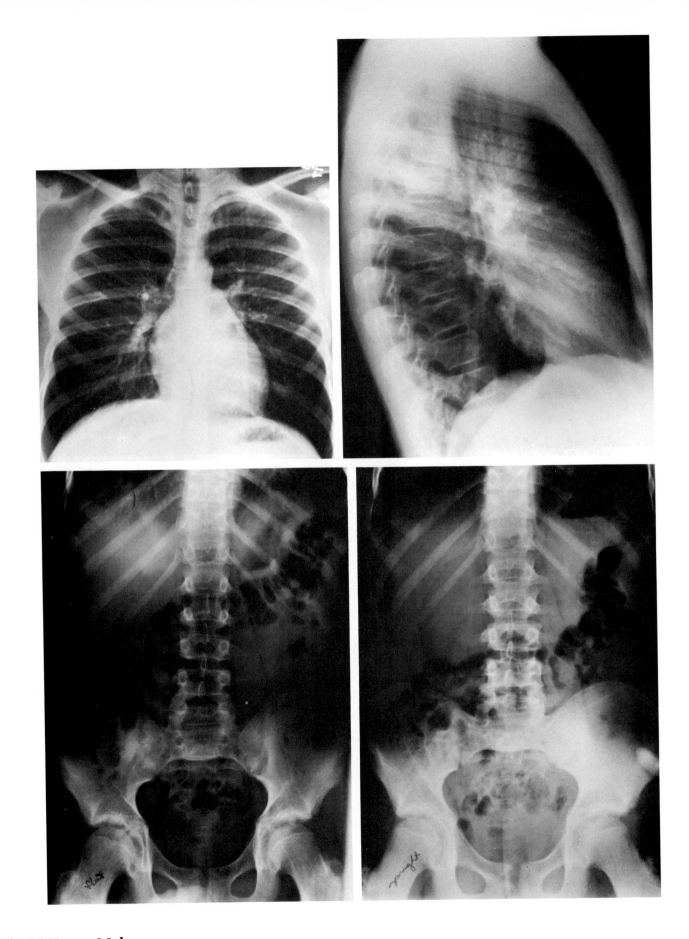

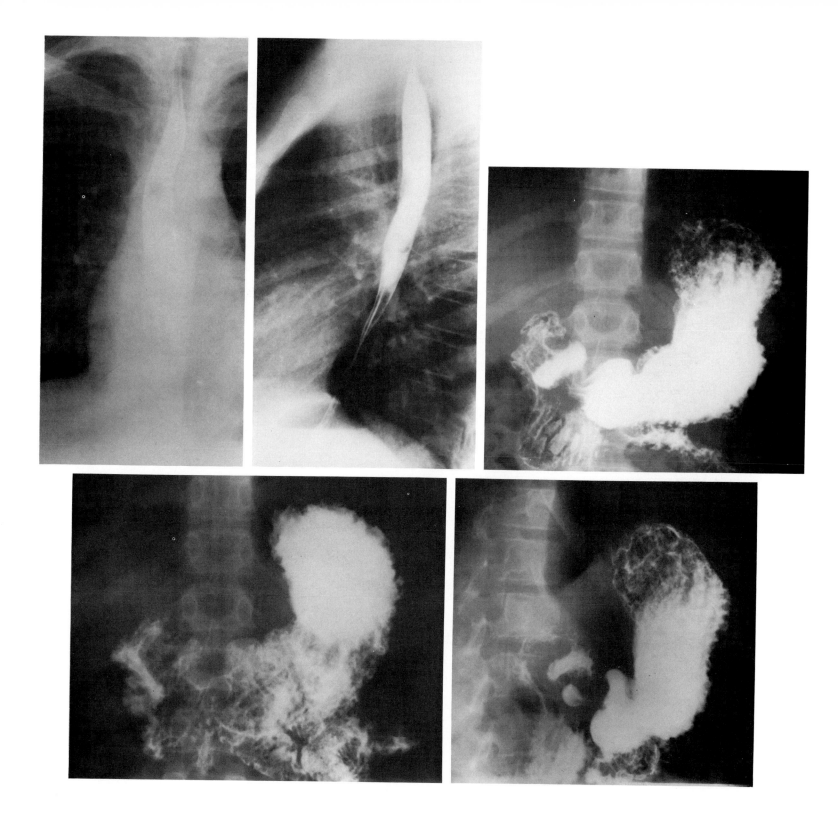

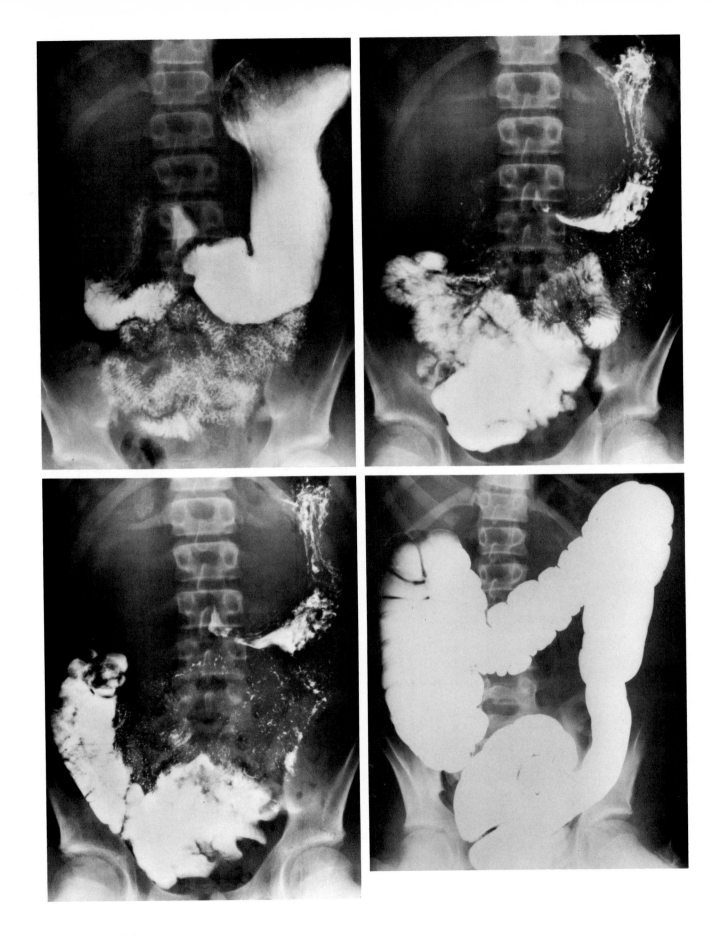

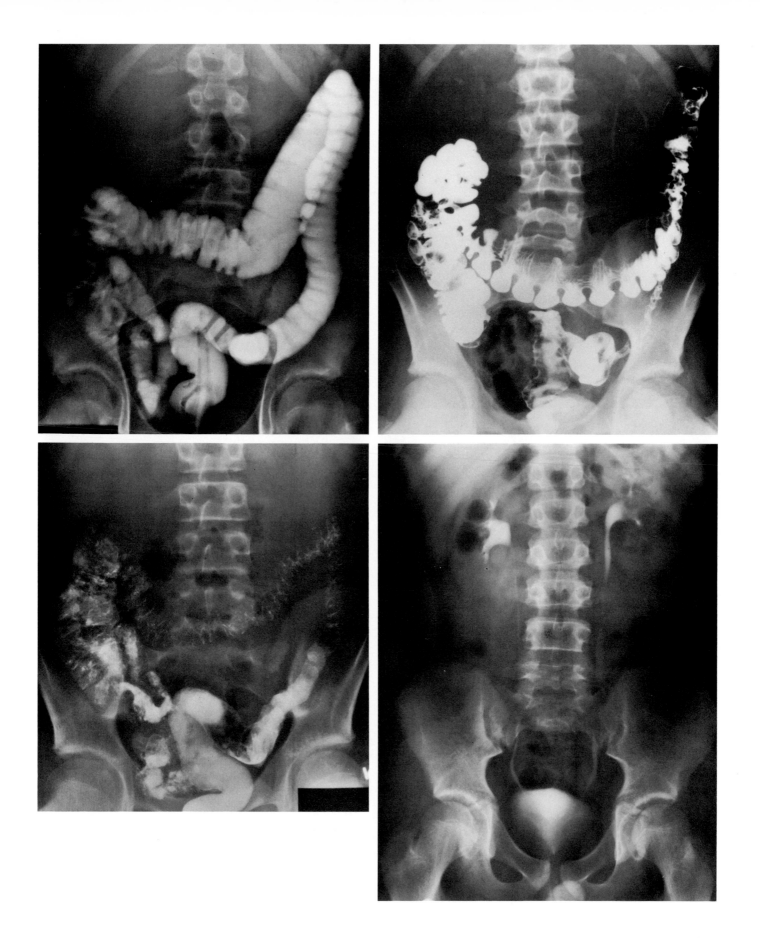

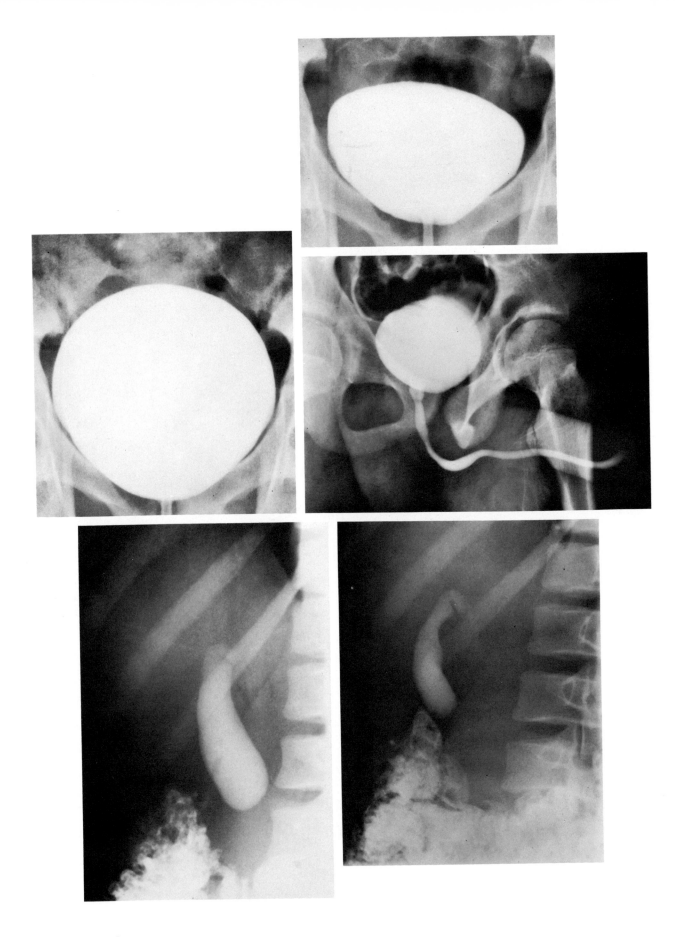

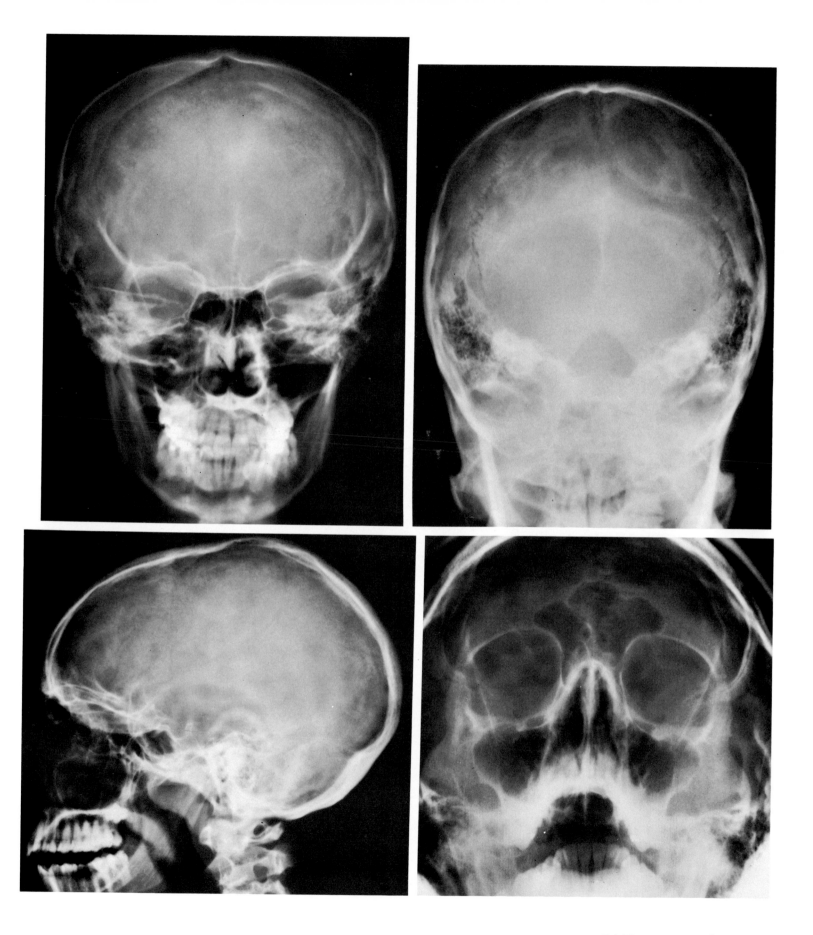

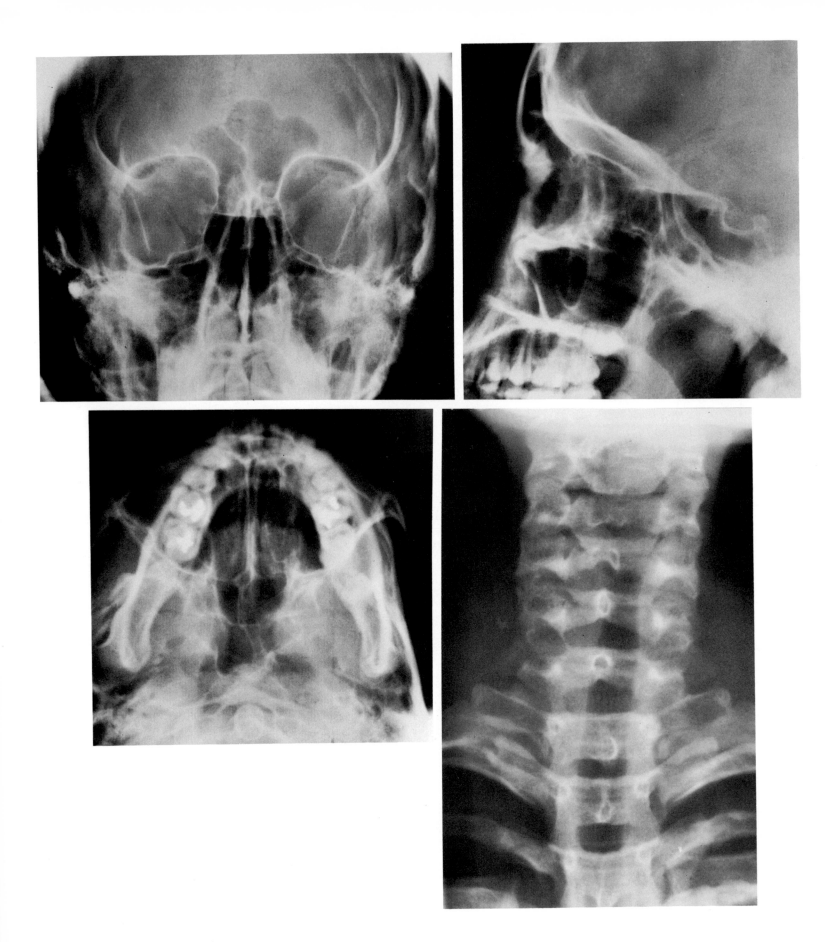

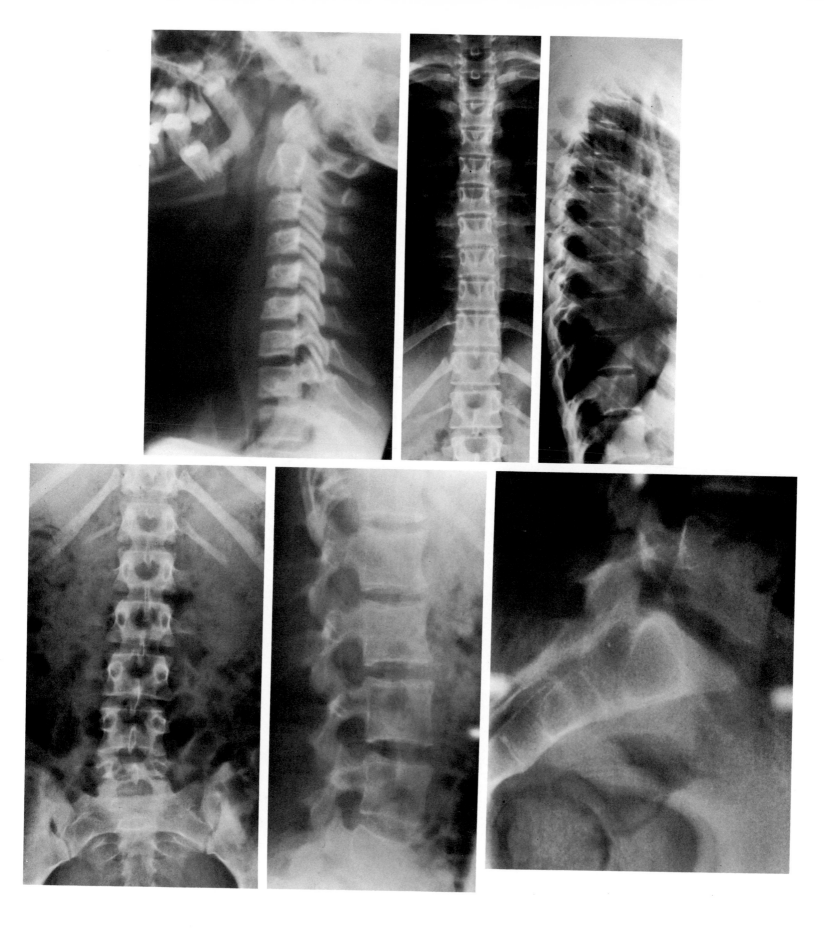

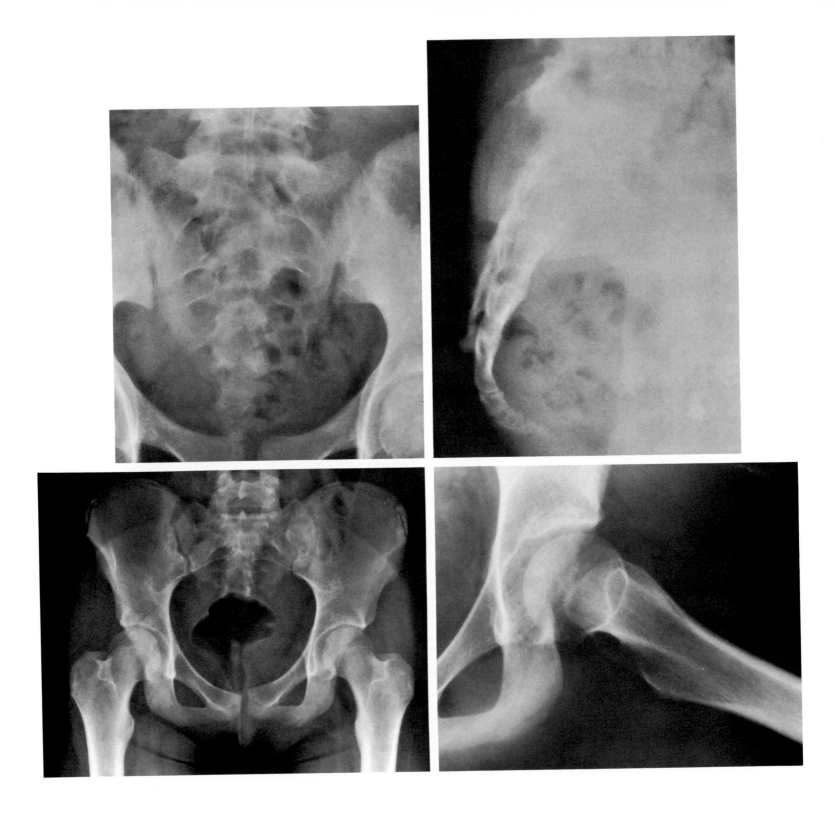

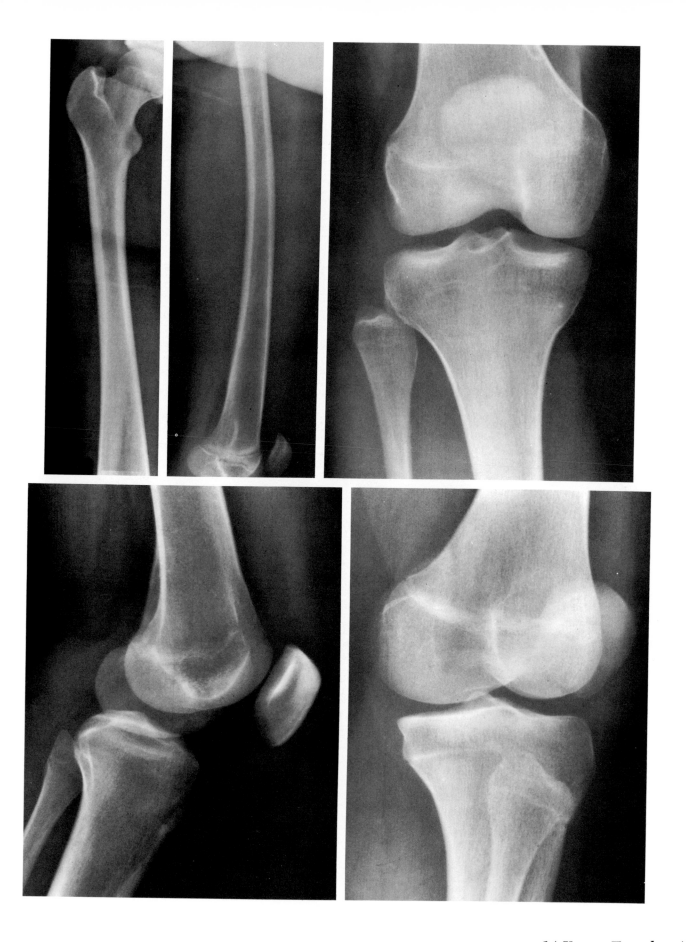

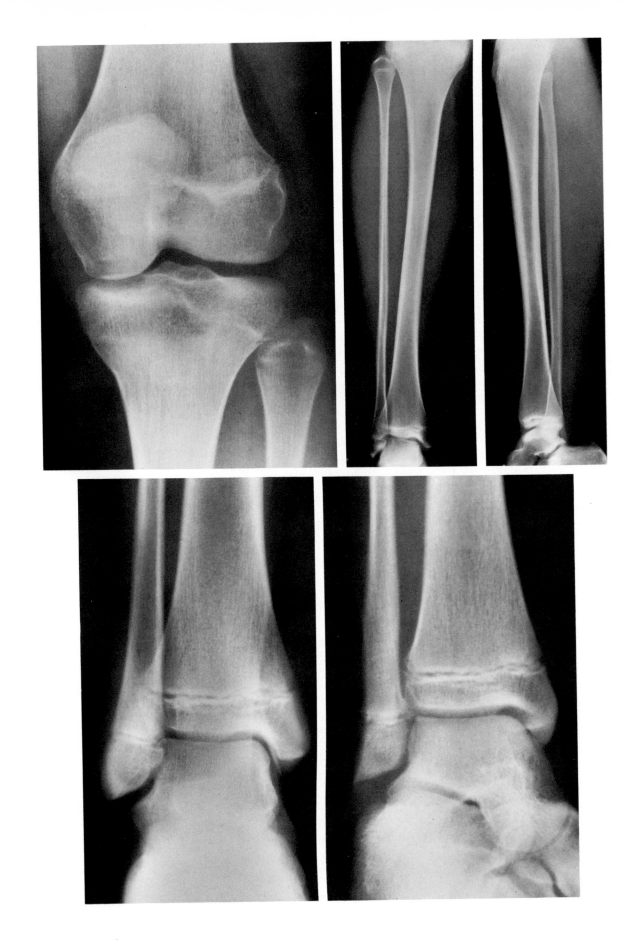

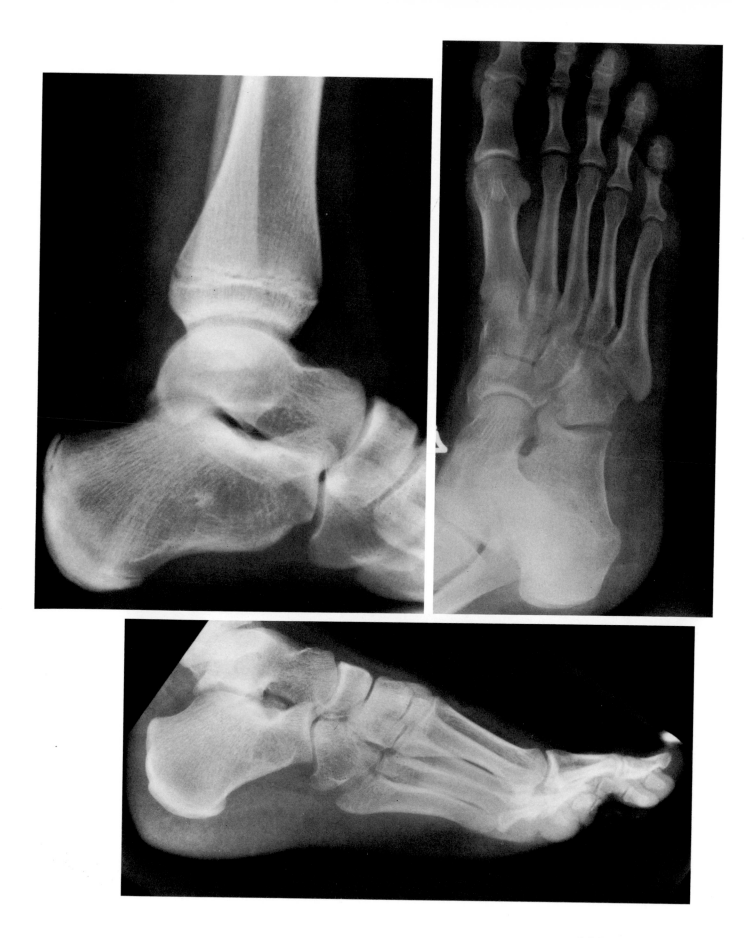

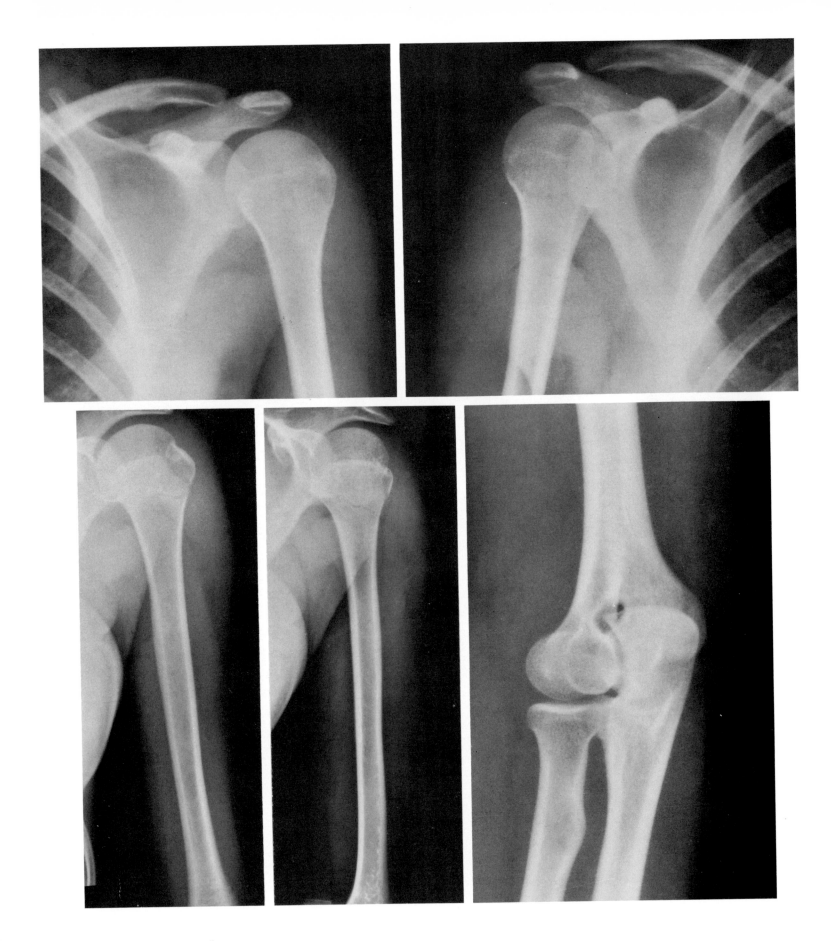

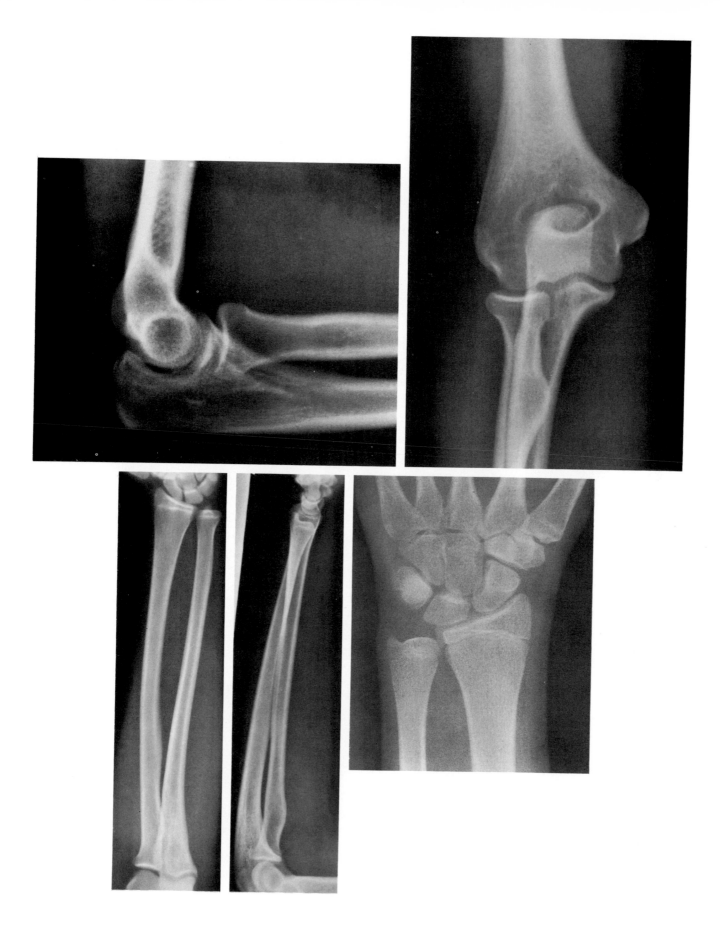

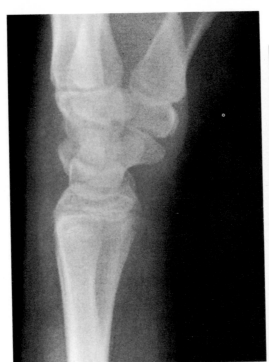
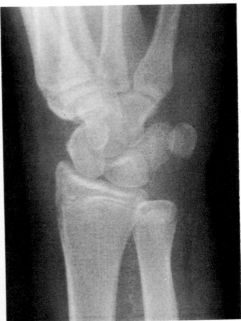
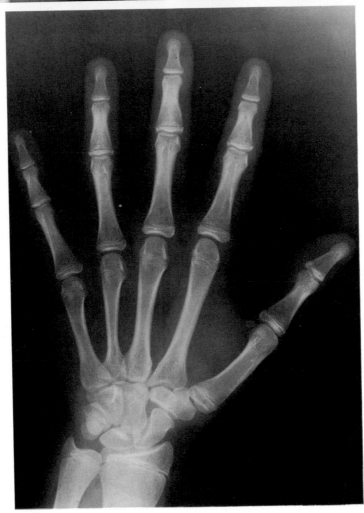

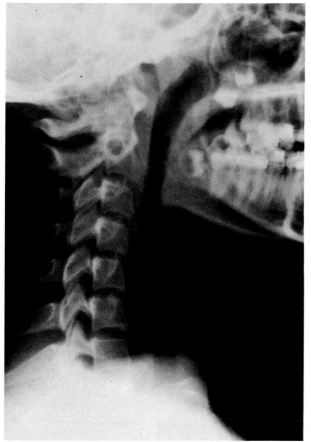

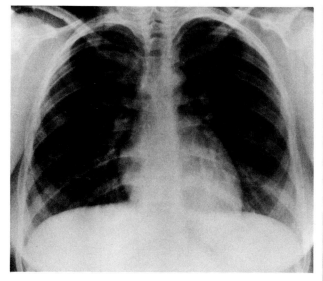

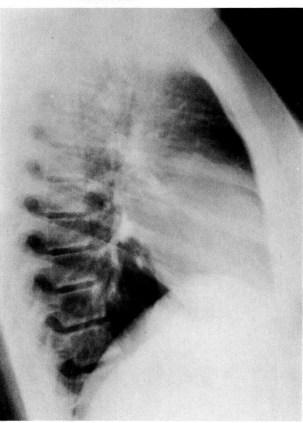

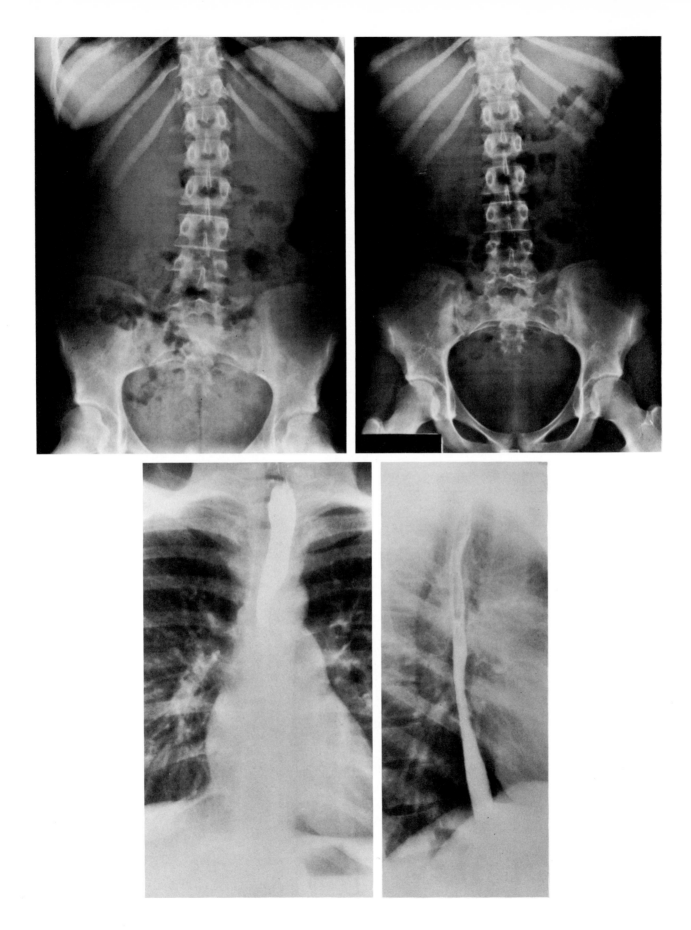

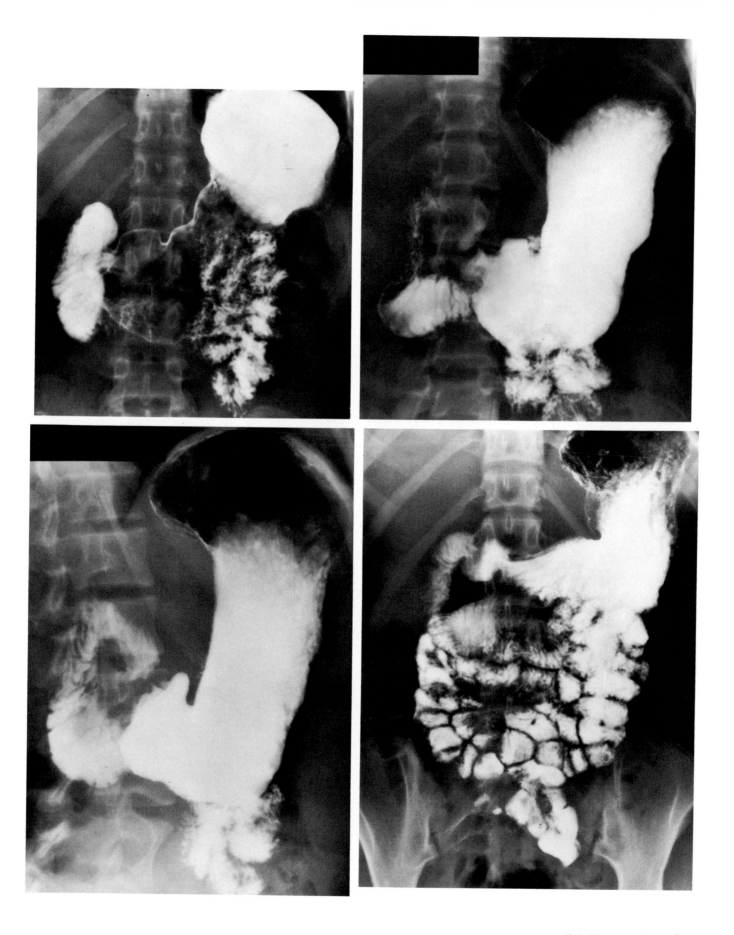

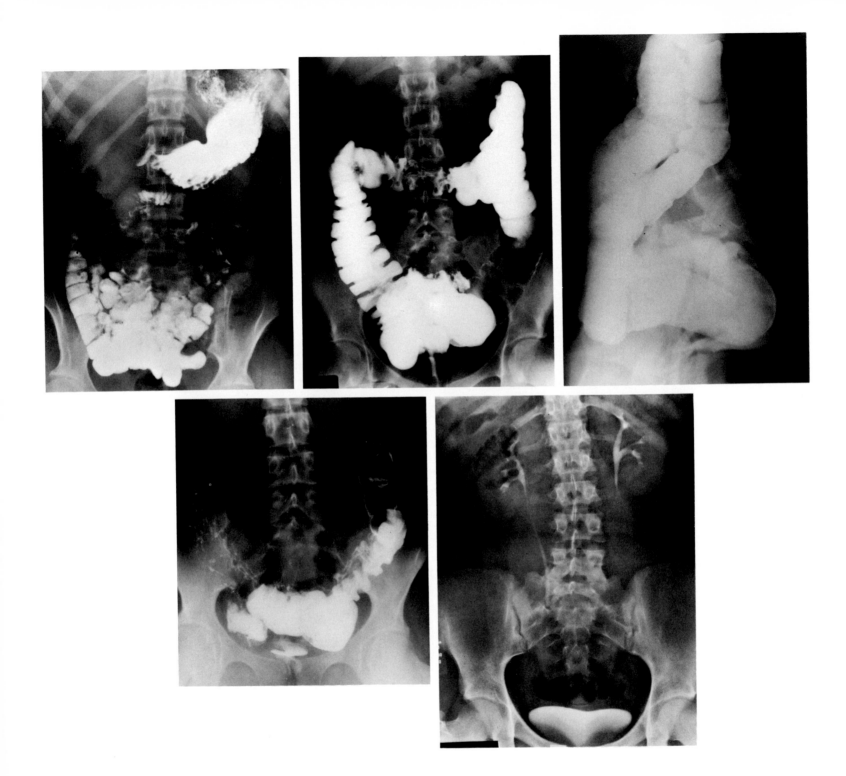

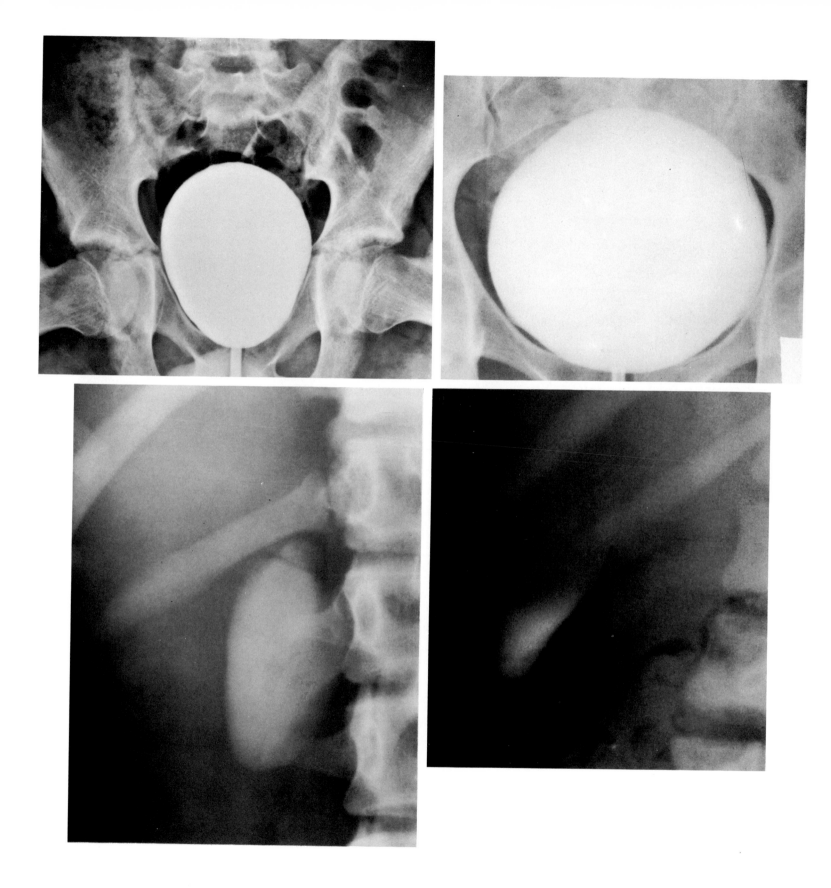

23

15 YEARS

The cervical vertebrae are less wedge-shaped. The ring apophyses of the dorsal vertebrae may be seen. The ilial apophyses are fusing. The physiologic protrusio acetabuli are no longer present. The configuration of the female pelvis is adult-like. The anterior extension of the distal tibial epiphysis is still present and encroaches on the outline of the epiphyseal plate. The calcaneal apophysis may still be open in the male. The maturation of the male begins to approach that of the female.

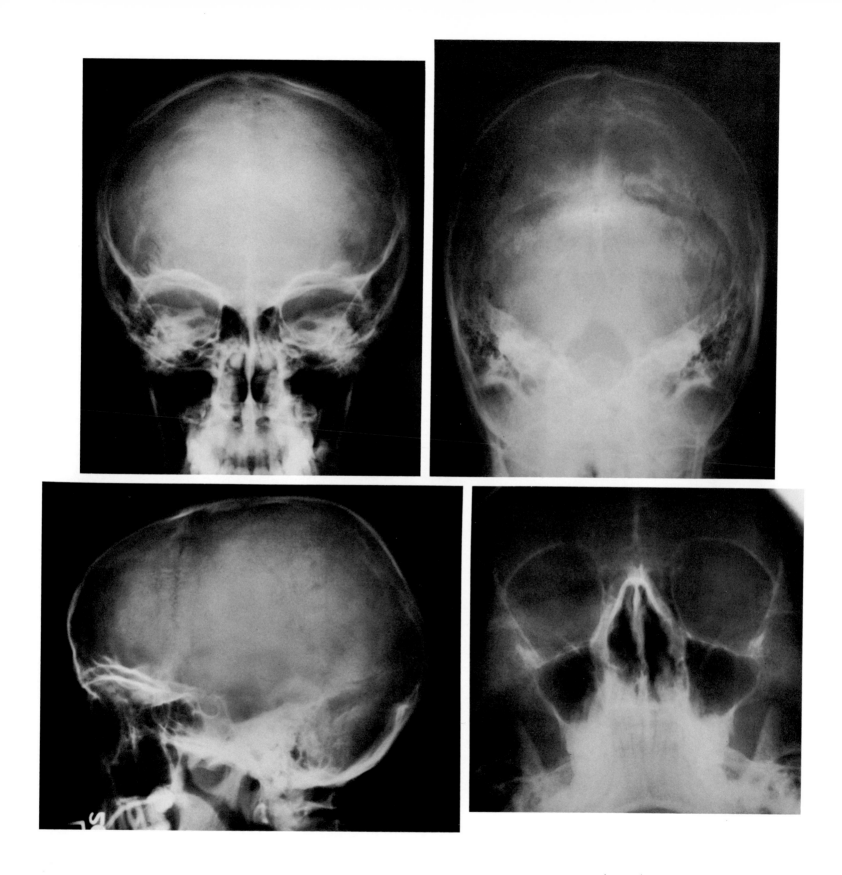

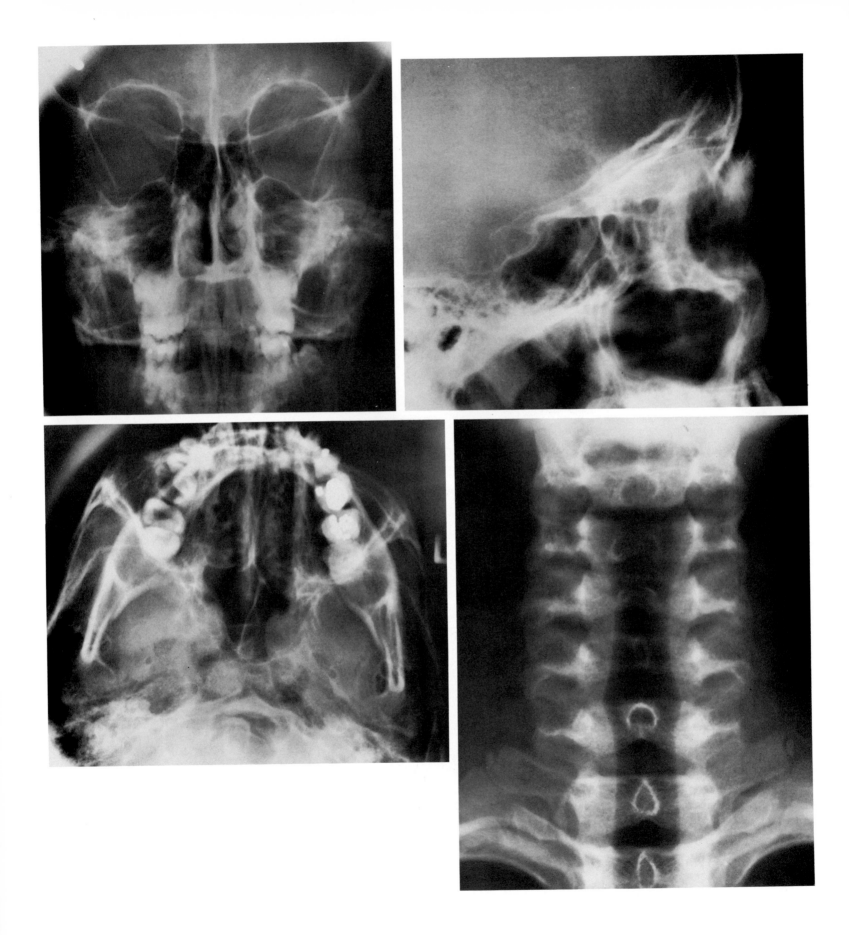

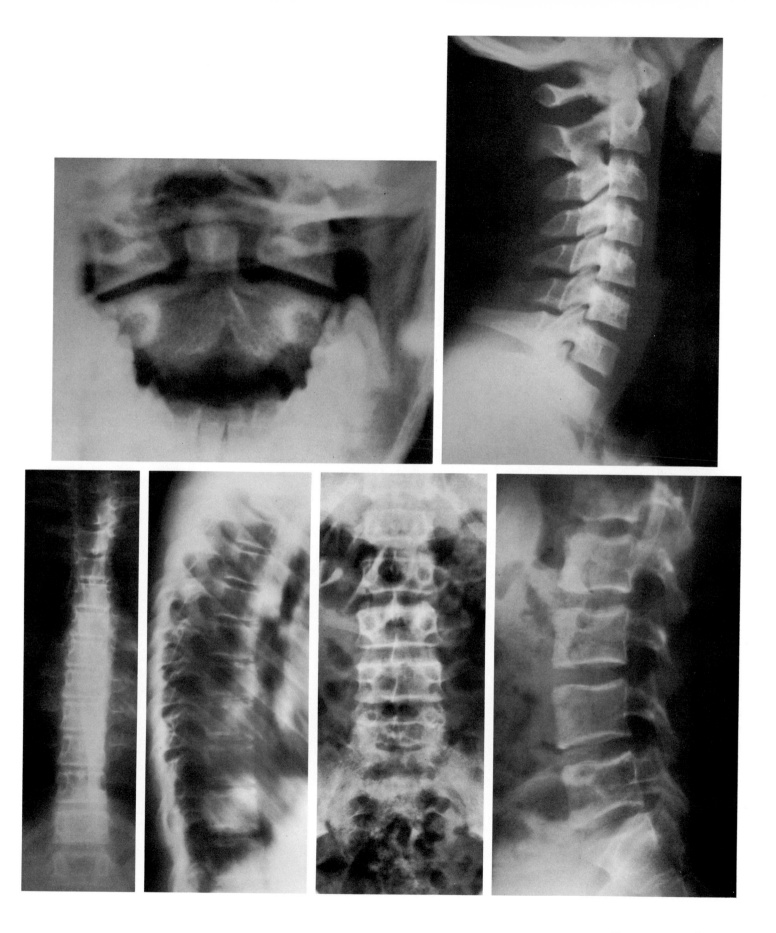

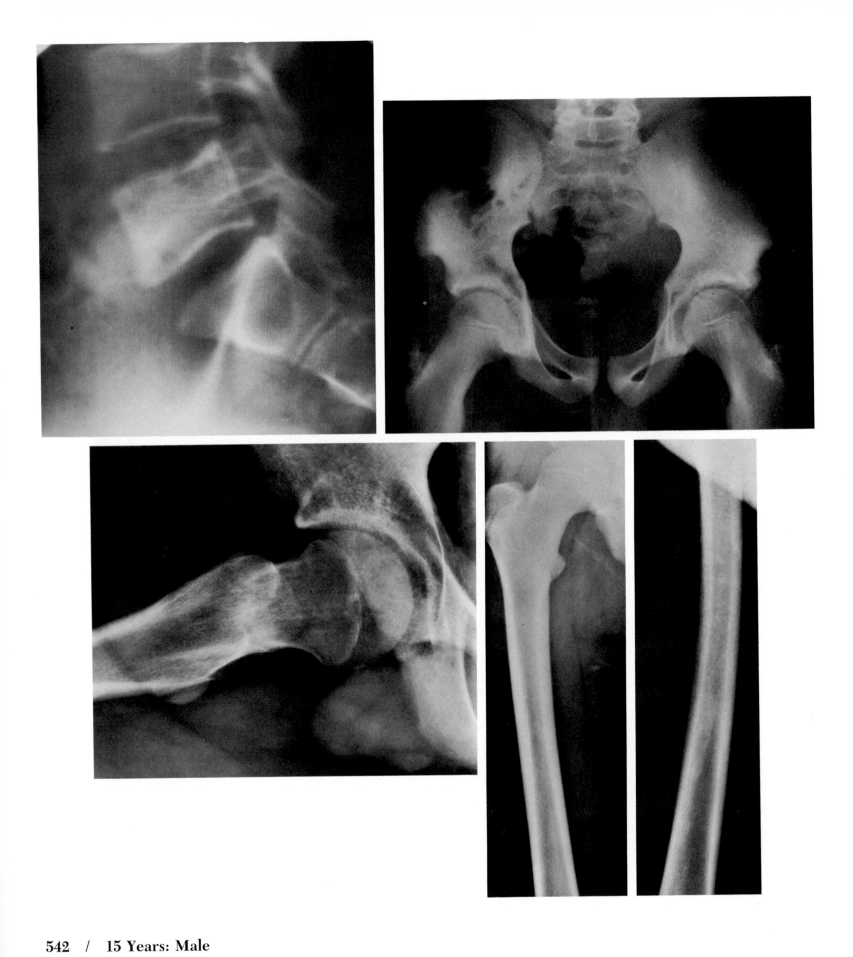

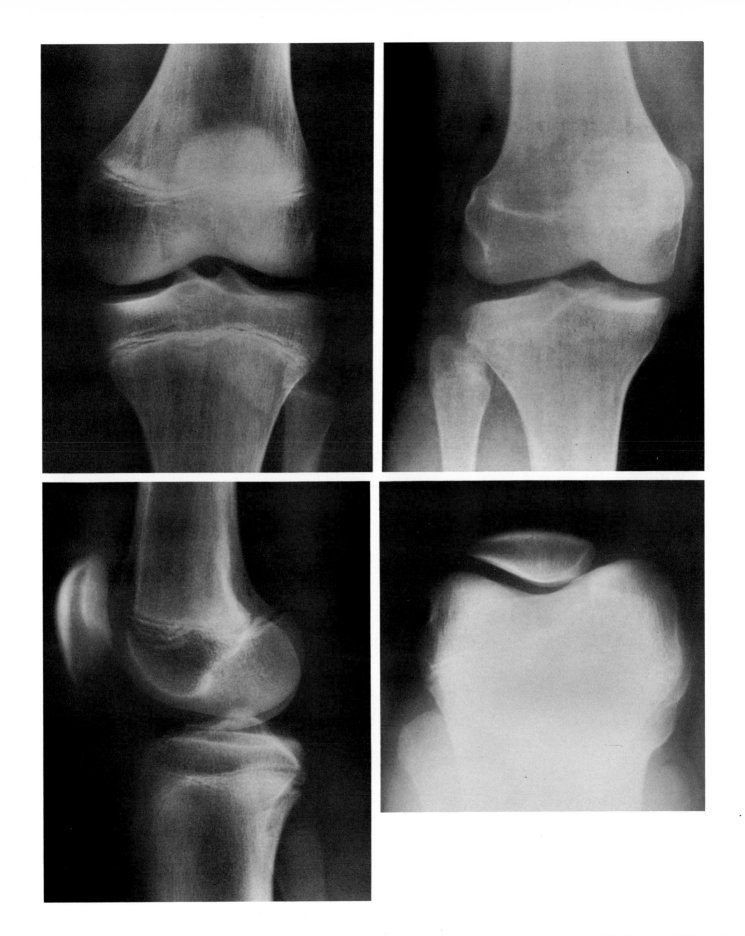

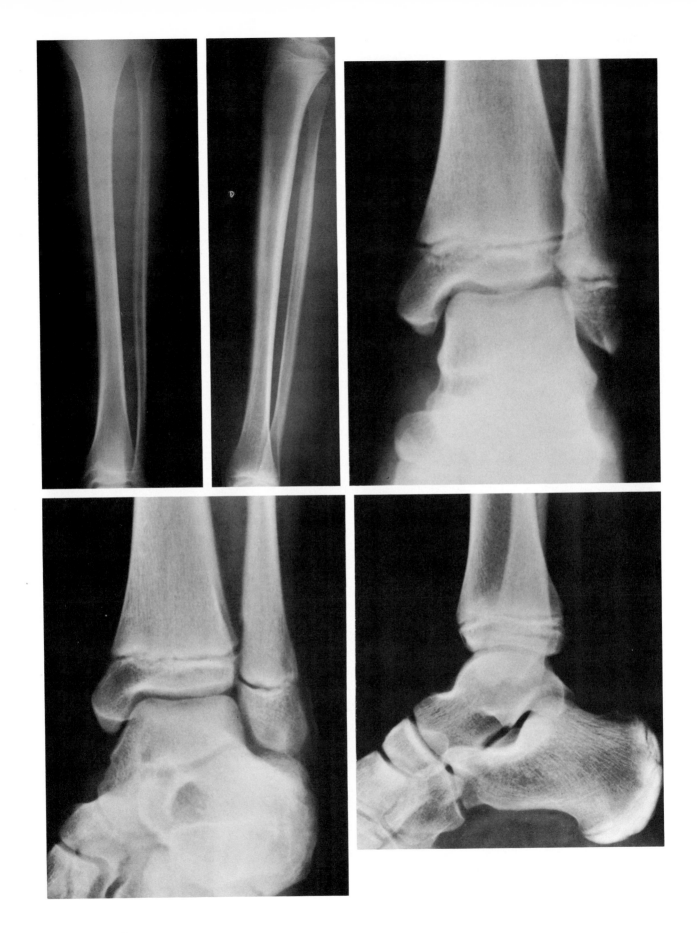

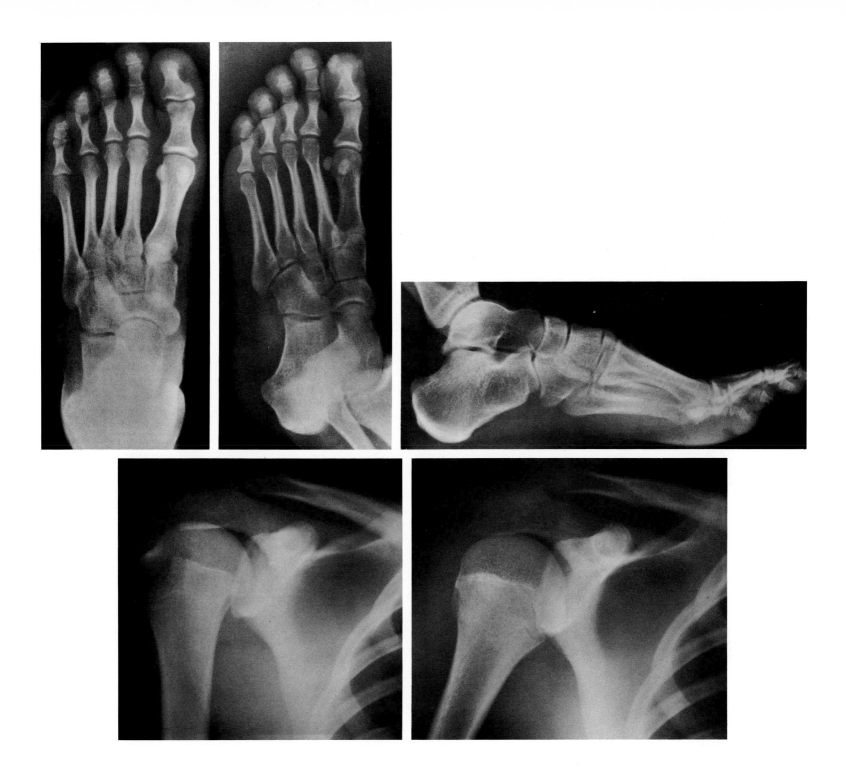

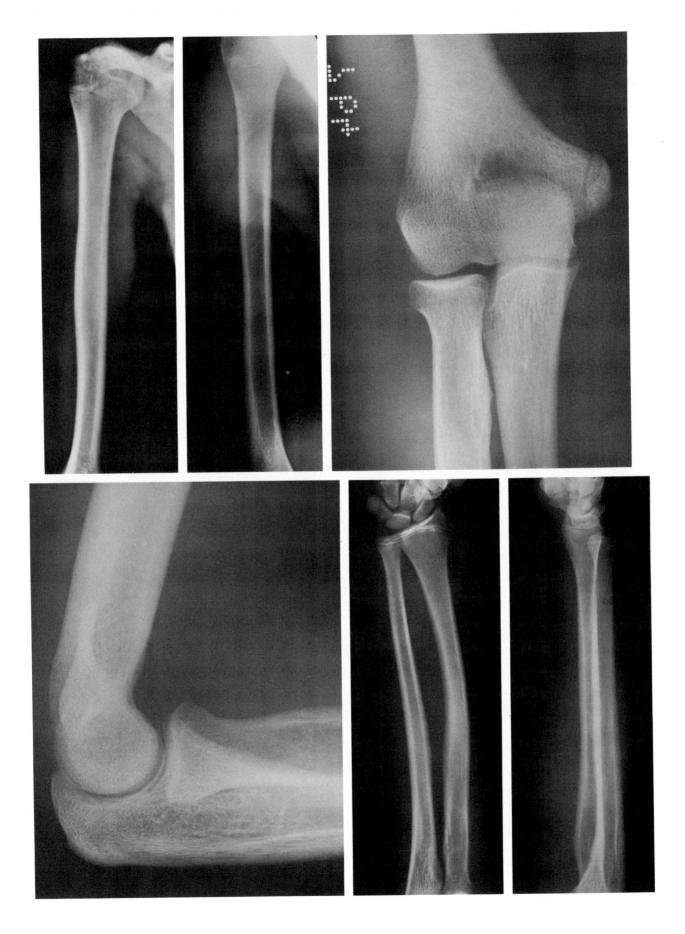

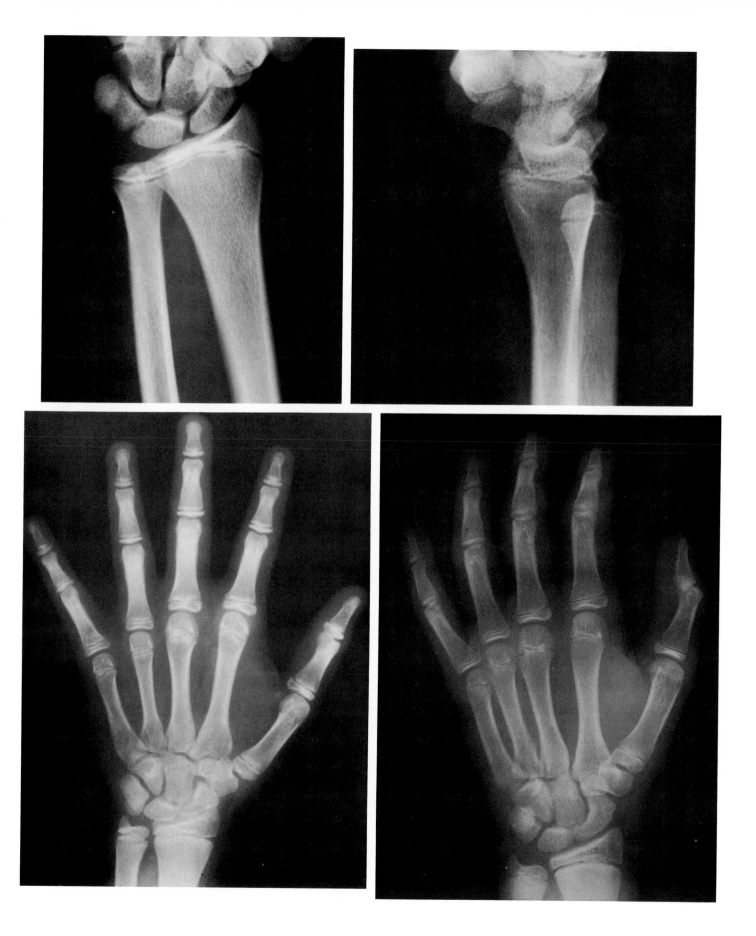

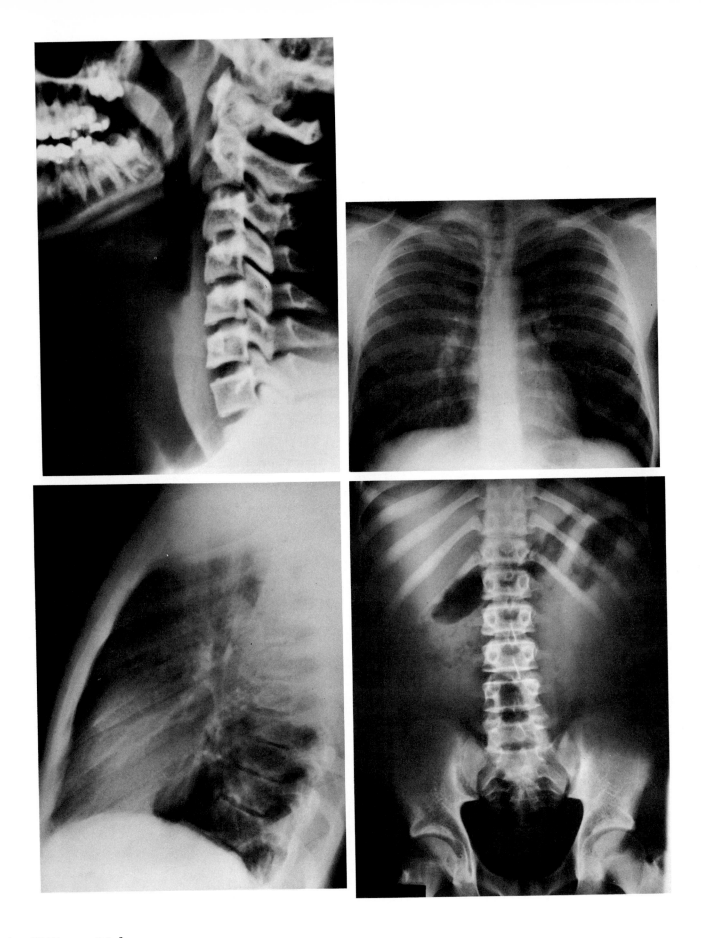

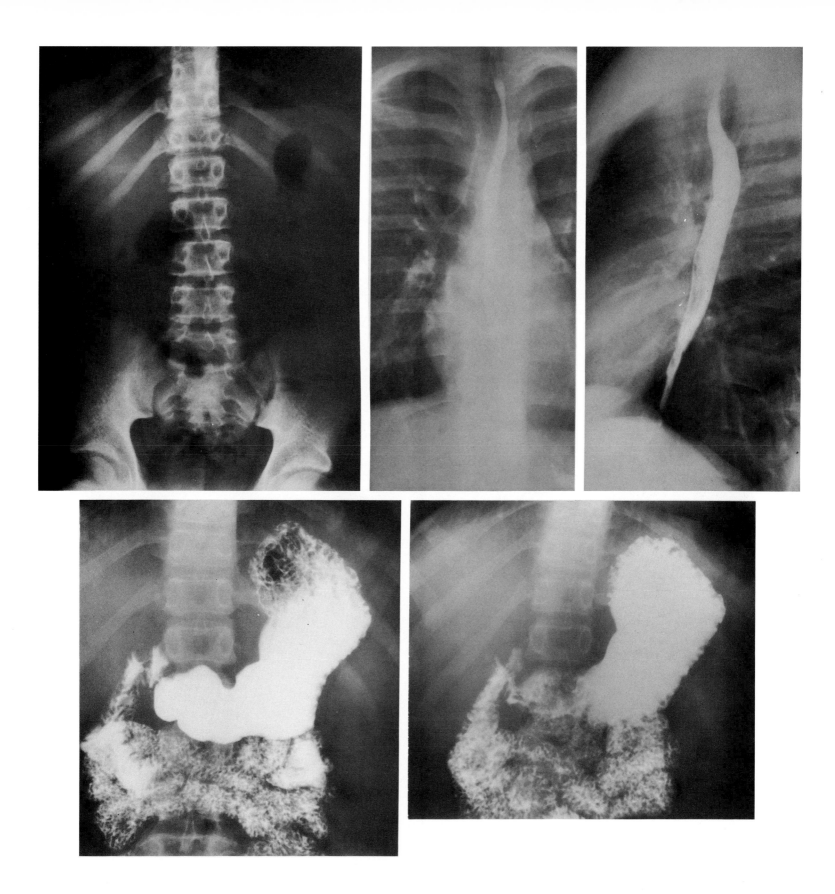

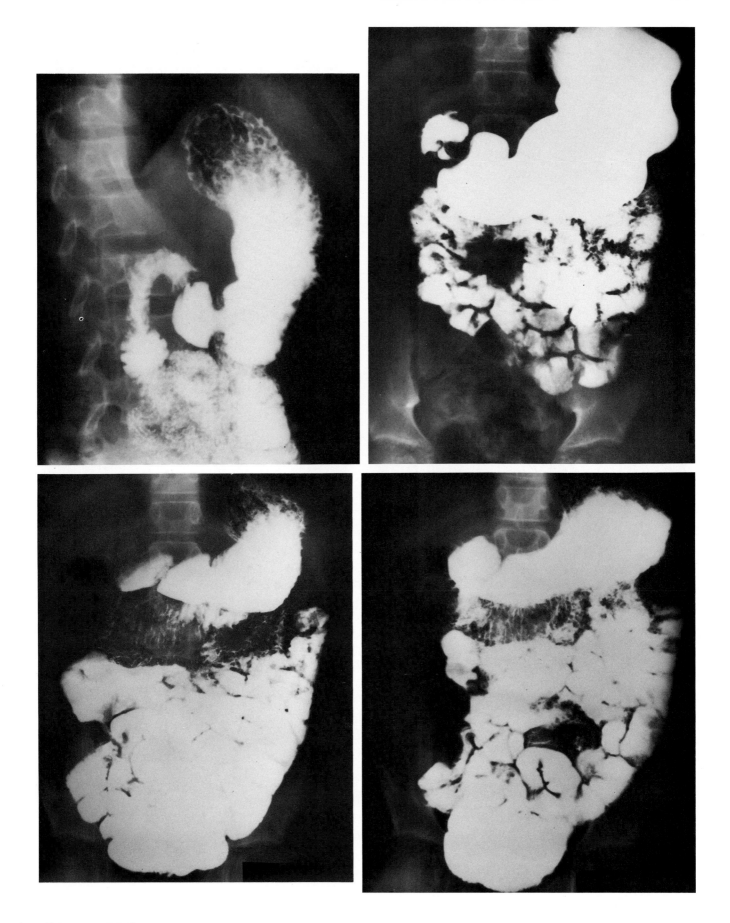

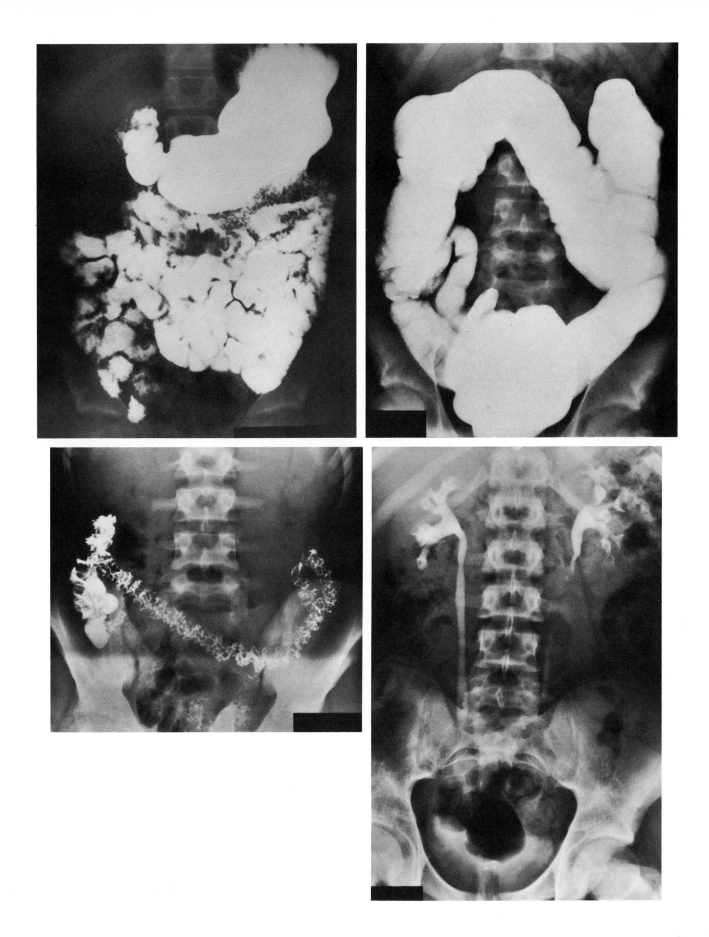

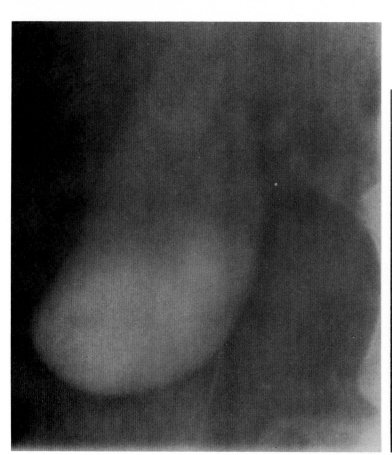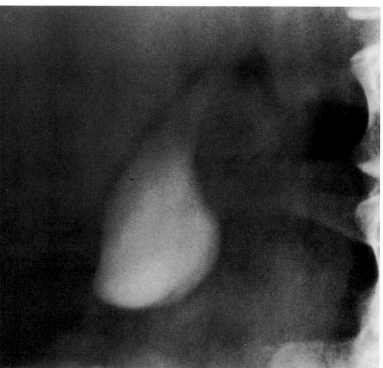

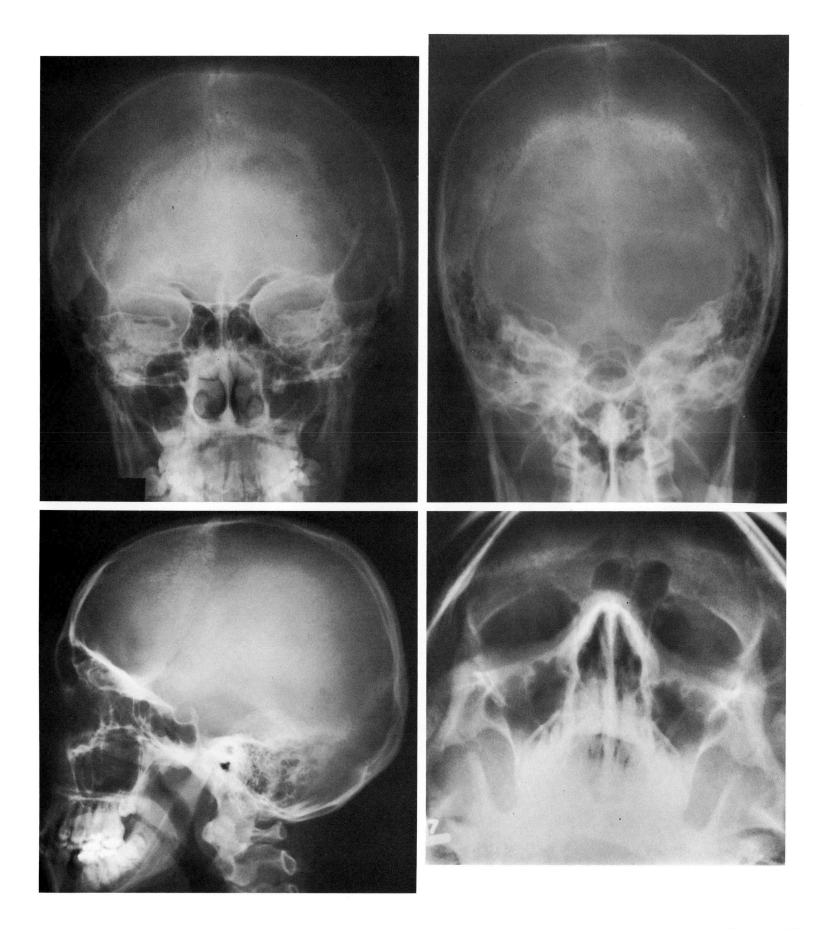

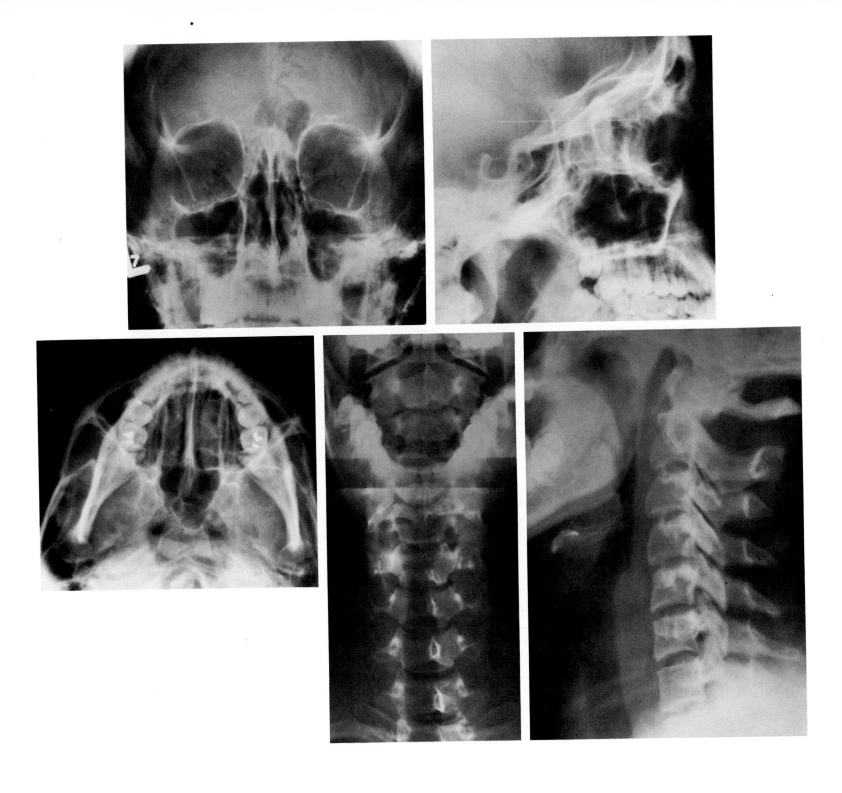

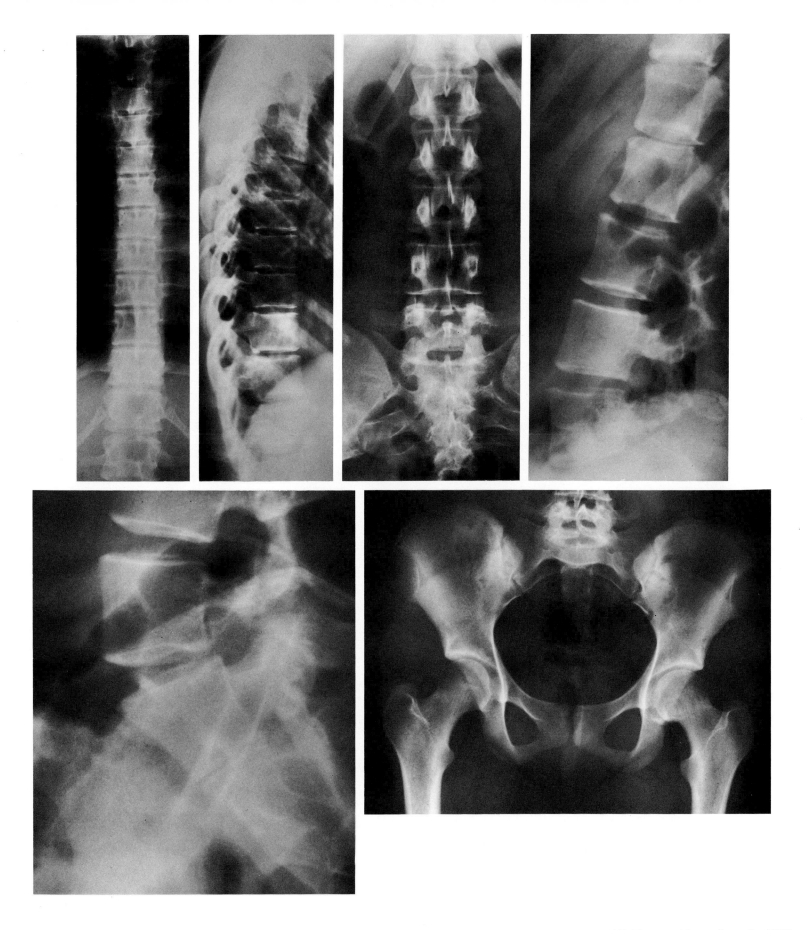

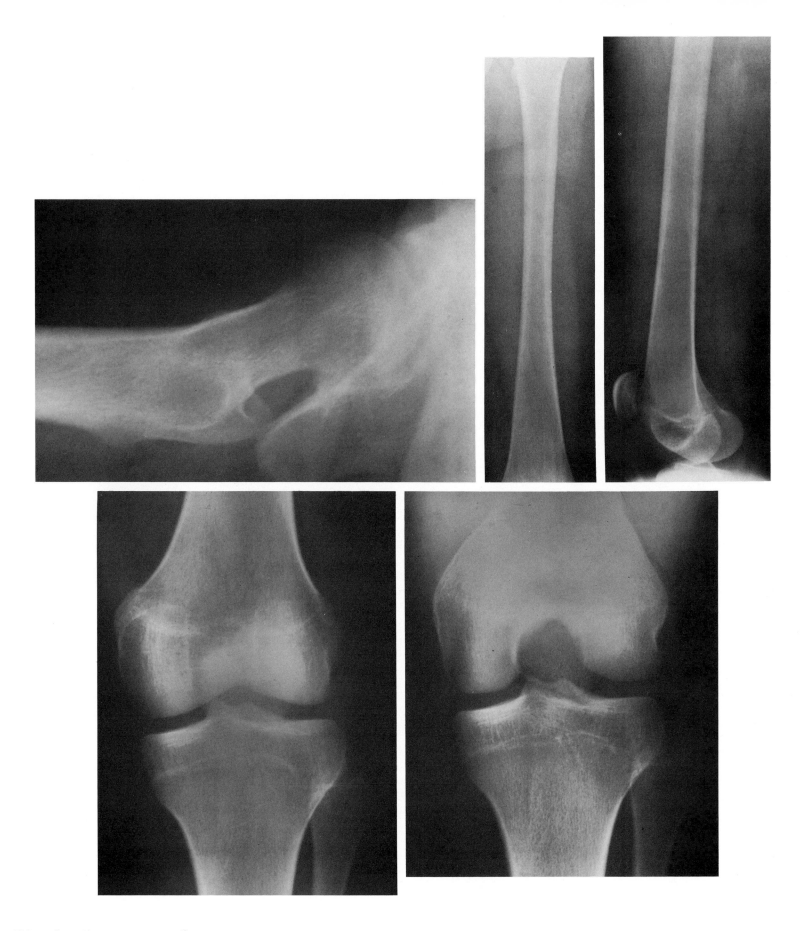

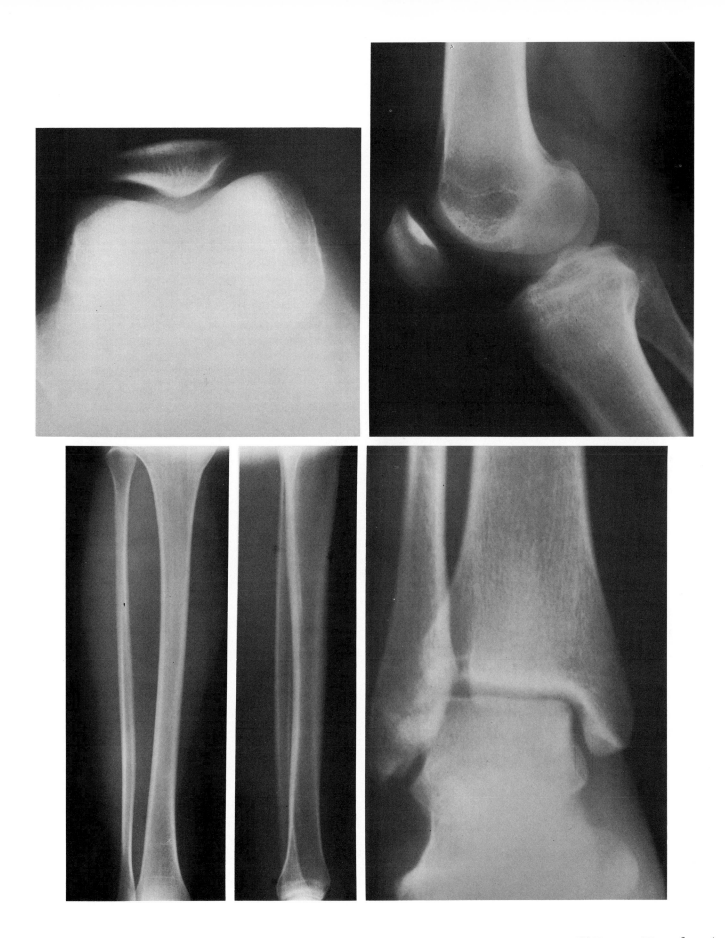

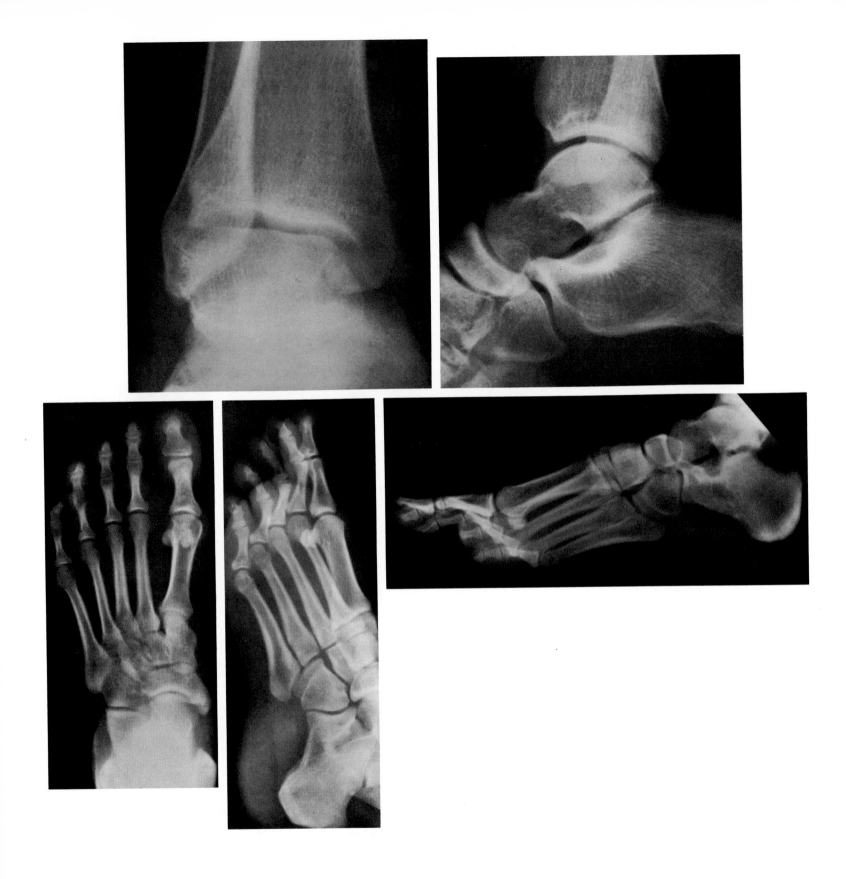

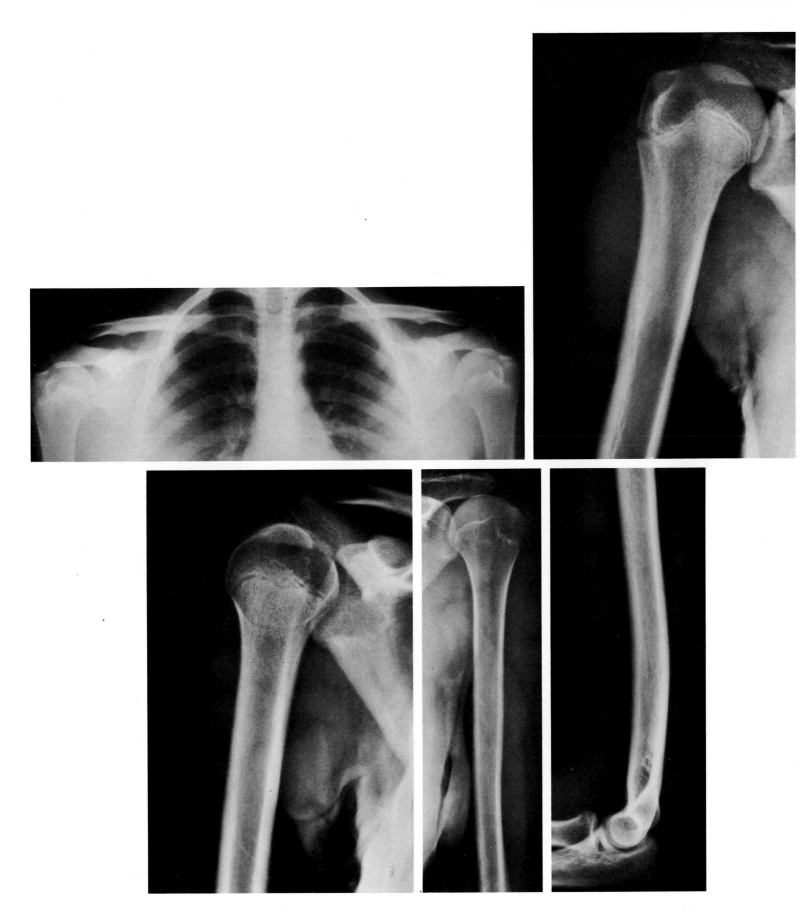

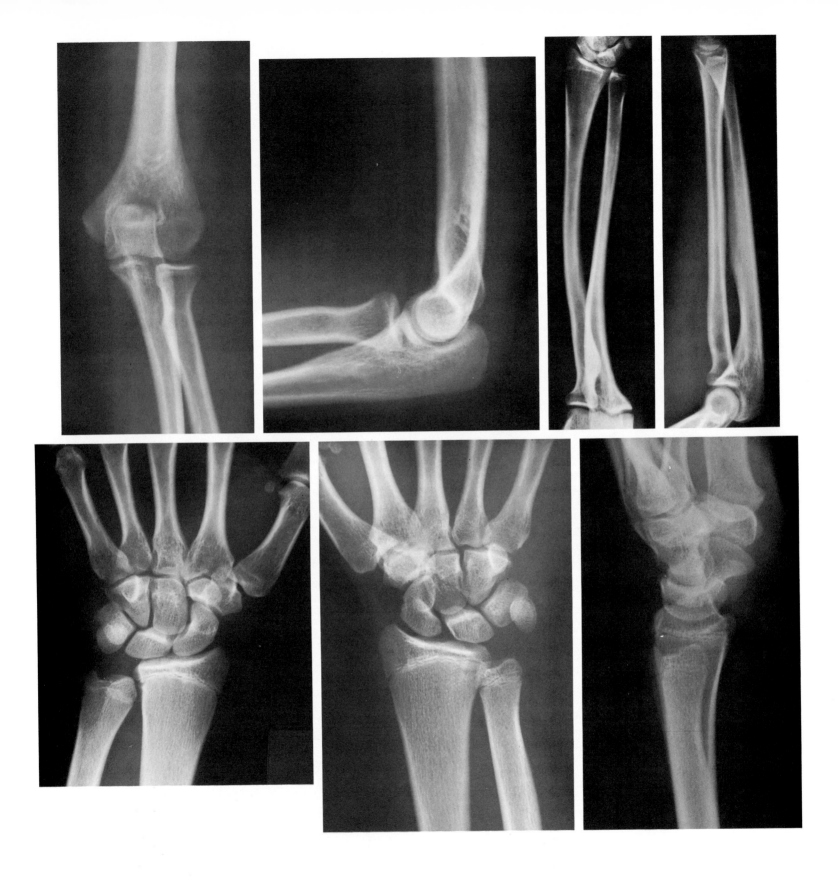

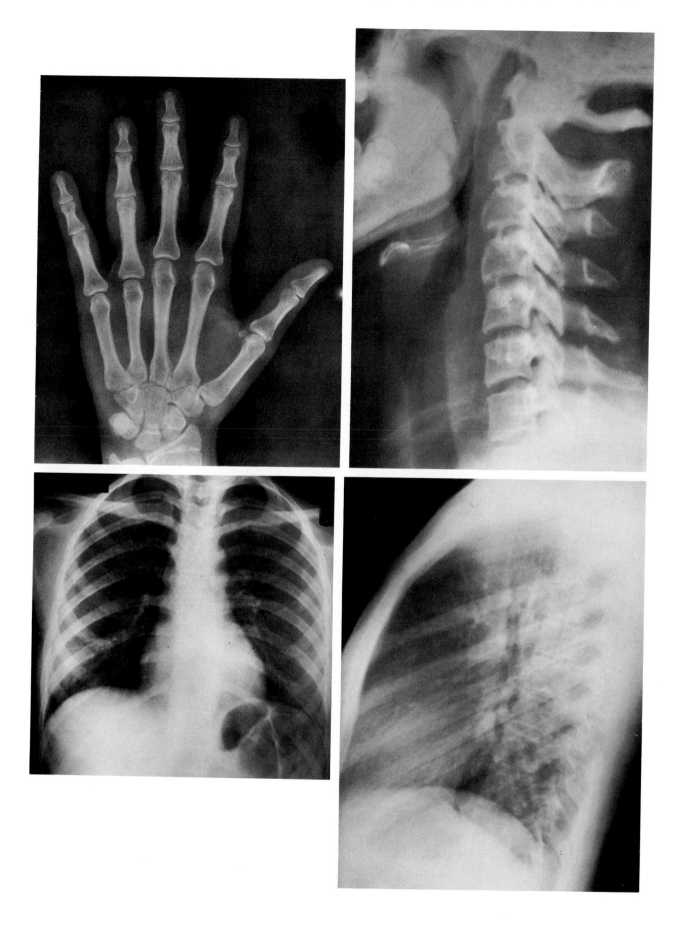

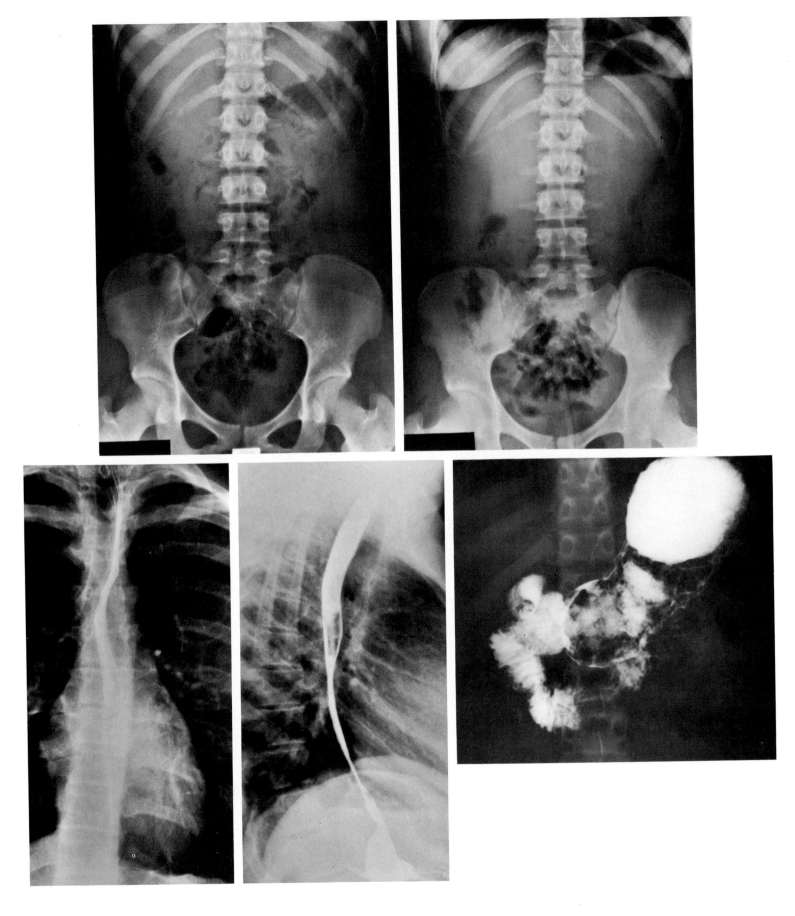

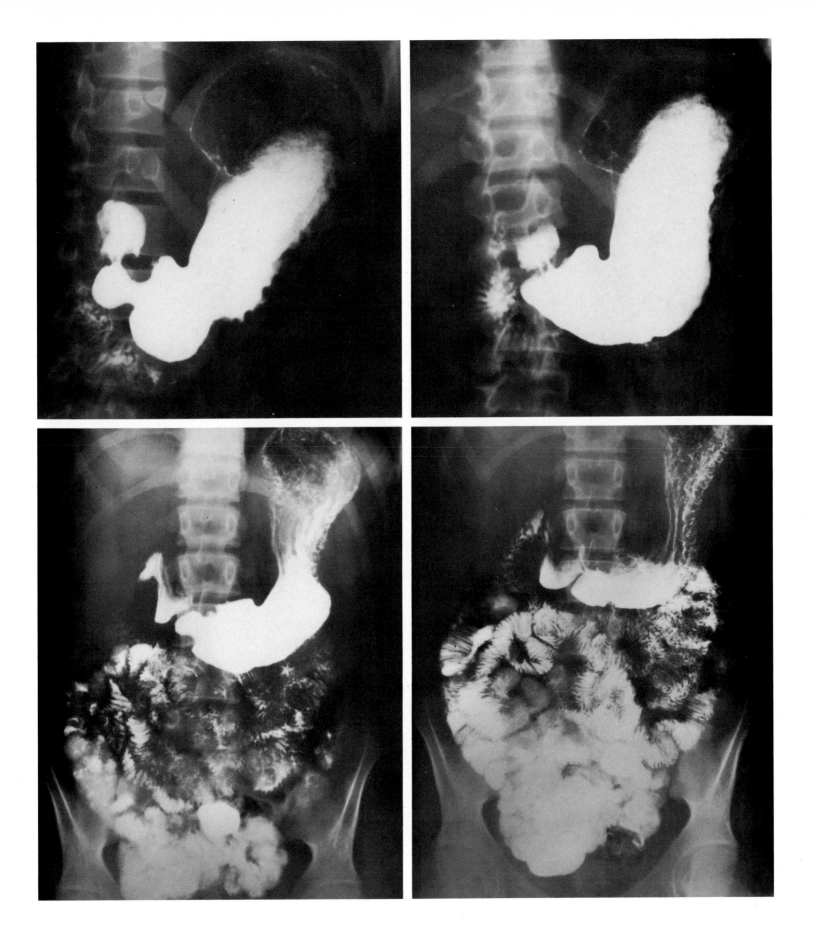

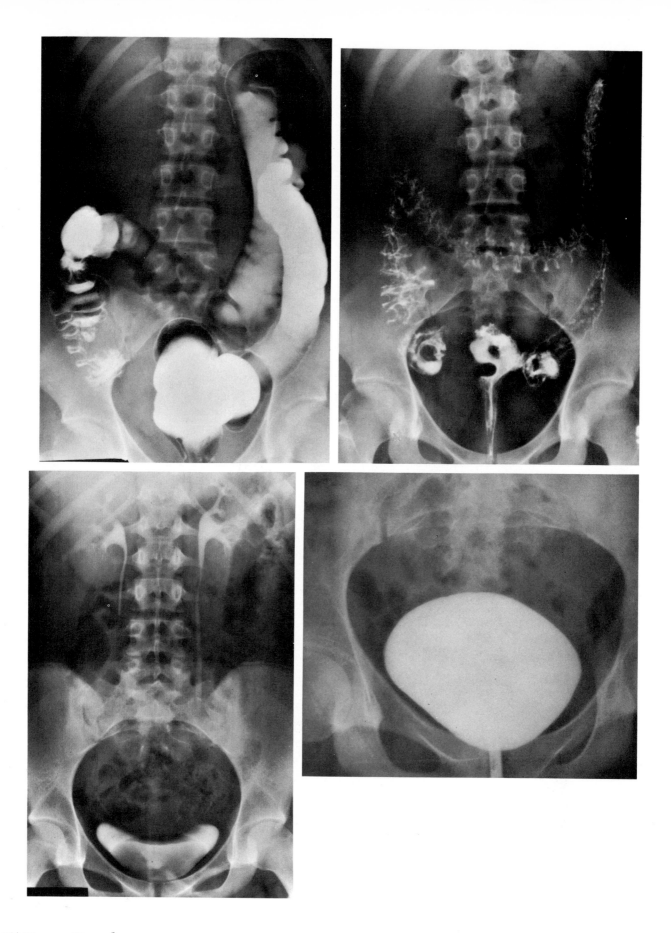

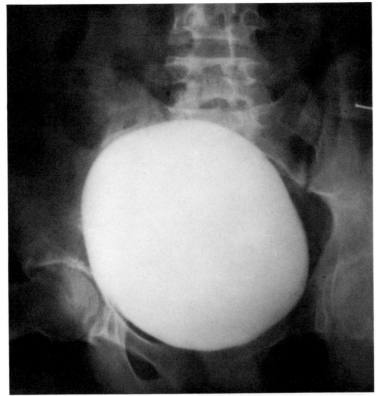

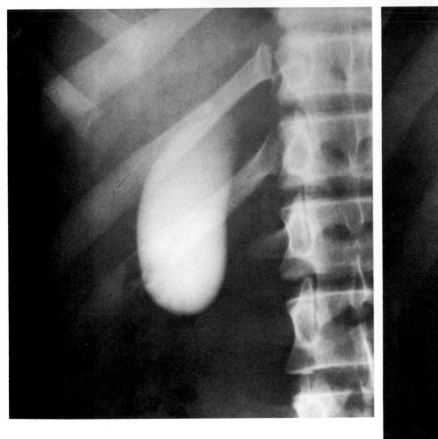

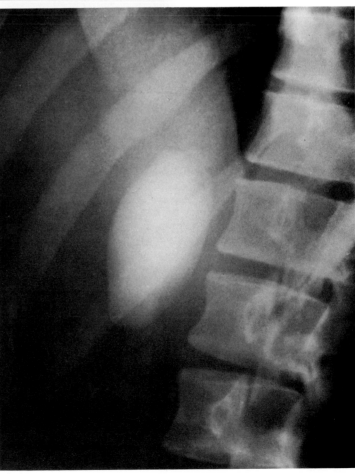

24

16 YEARS

Calvarial vascular channels are evident. Wedging of the cervical vertebrae is now largely confined to C-3. The ring apophyses of the vertebrae are closing. The cervical and lumbar lordoses are accentuated. The pelves of both sexes are adult-like. The epiphyses of the ilium may still be seen in the male. The distal tibial epiphysis is closing in the male and closed in the female. The proximal humeral epiphysis is closed. Growth at the elbow is complete. The distal radial epiphysis is closing. The calcaneal apophysis may be closed, particularly in the female. Physiologic prominence of the pulmonary artery may still be present, particularly in the female.

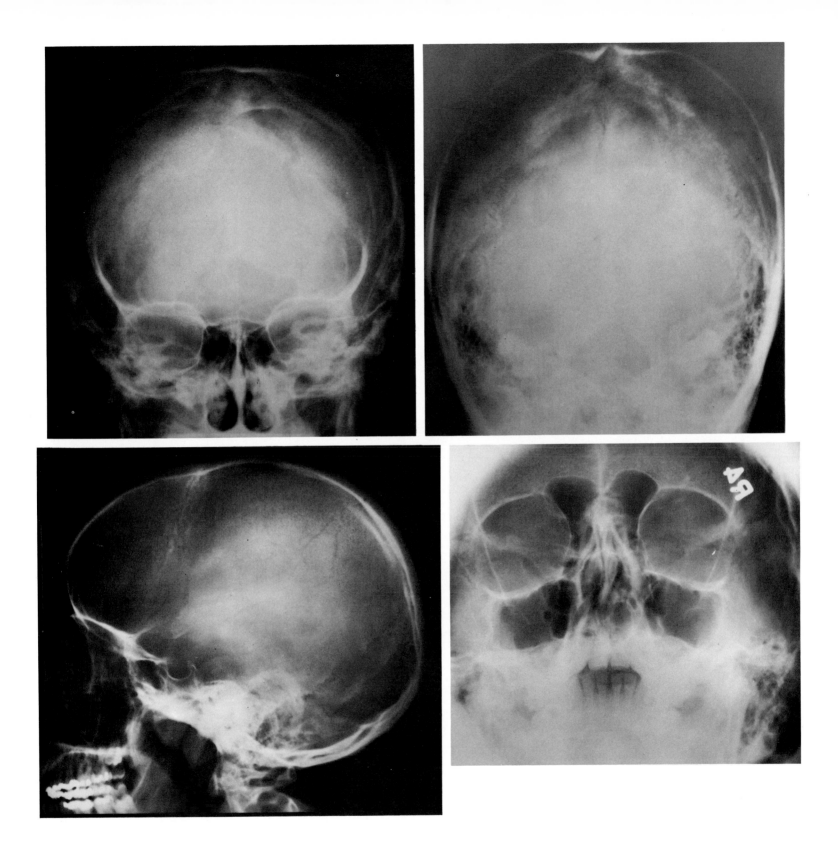

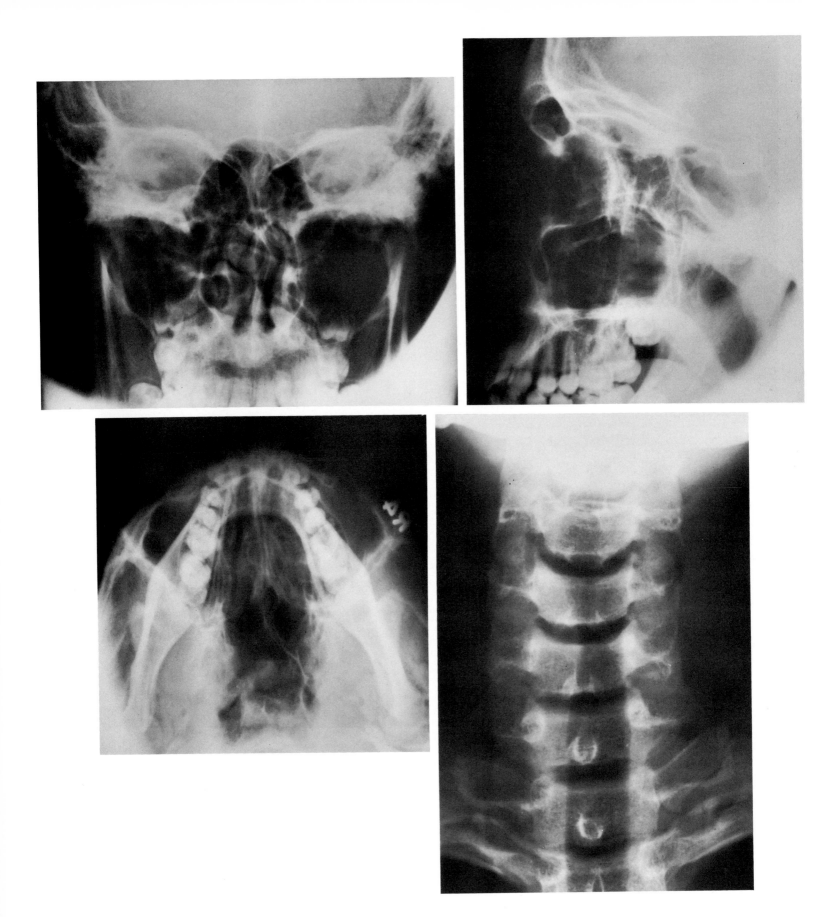

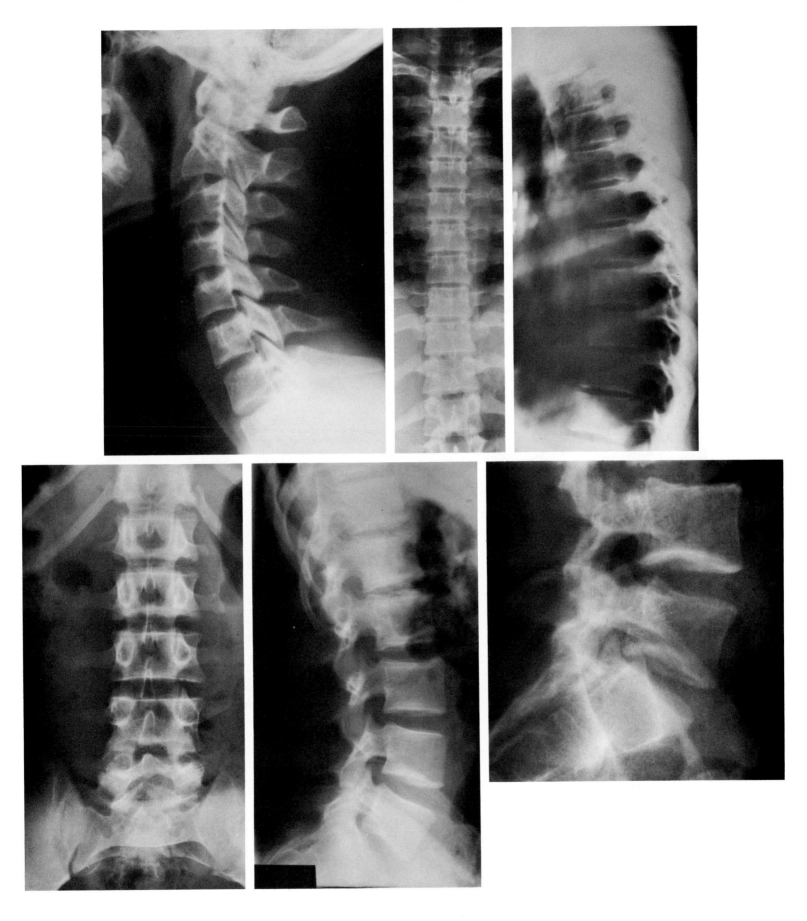

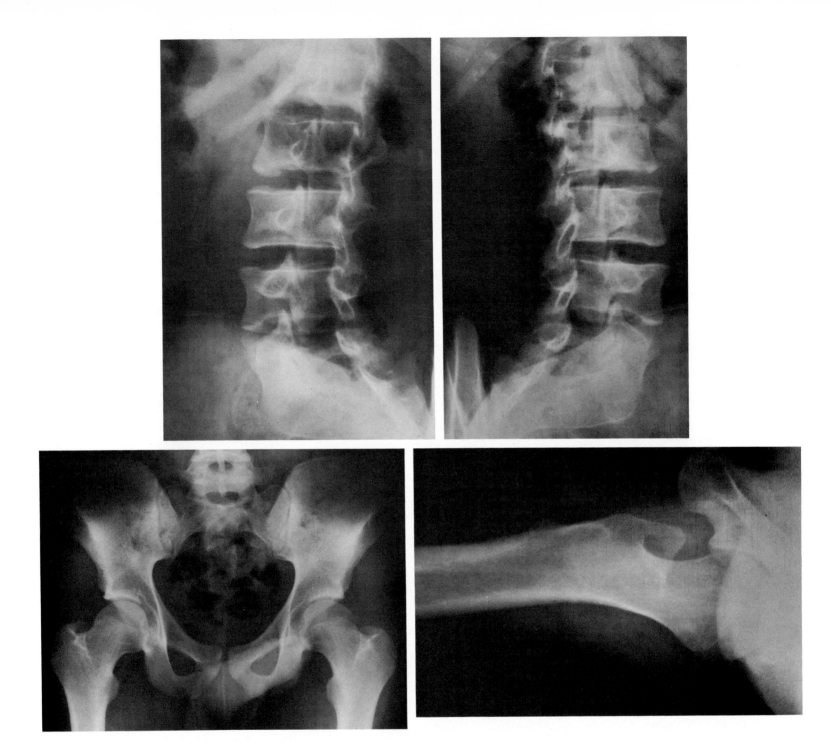

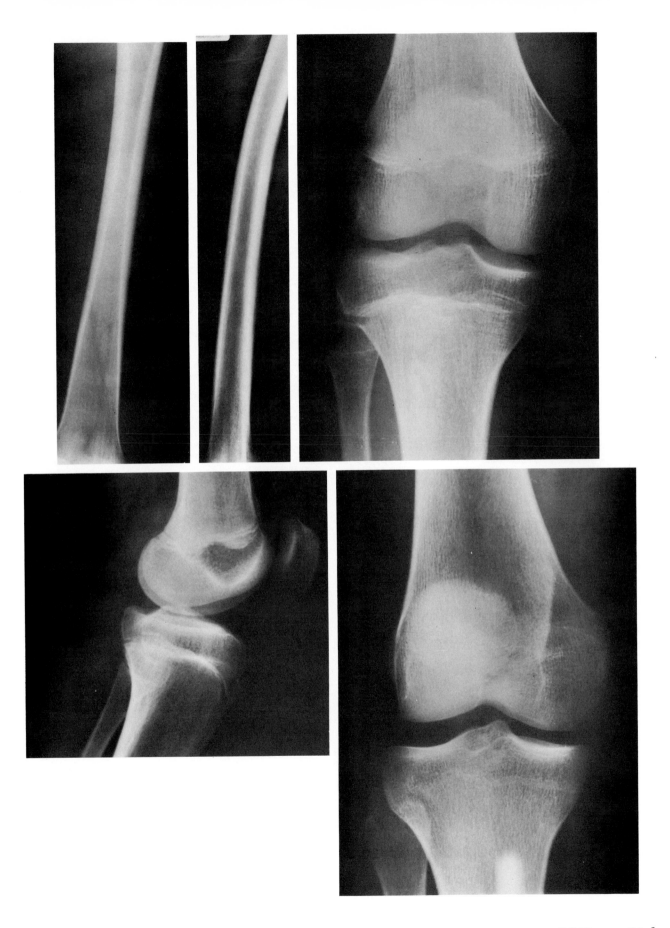

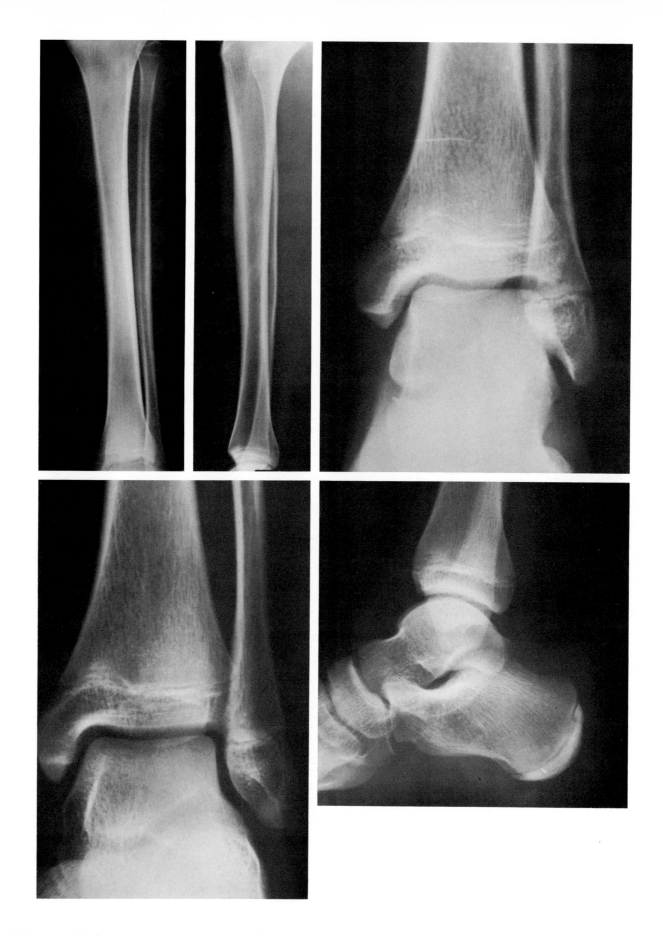

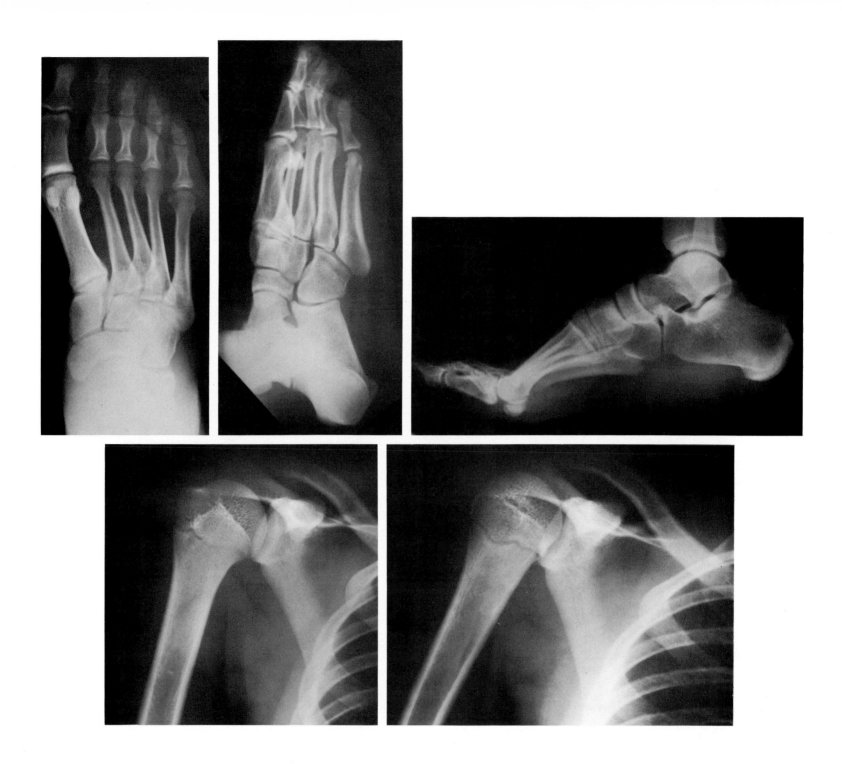

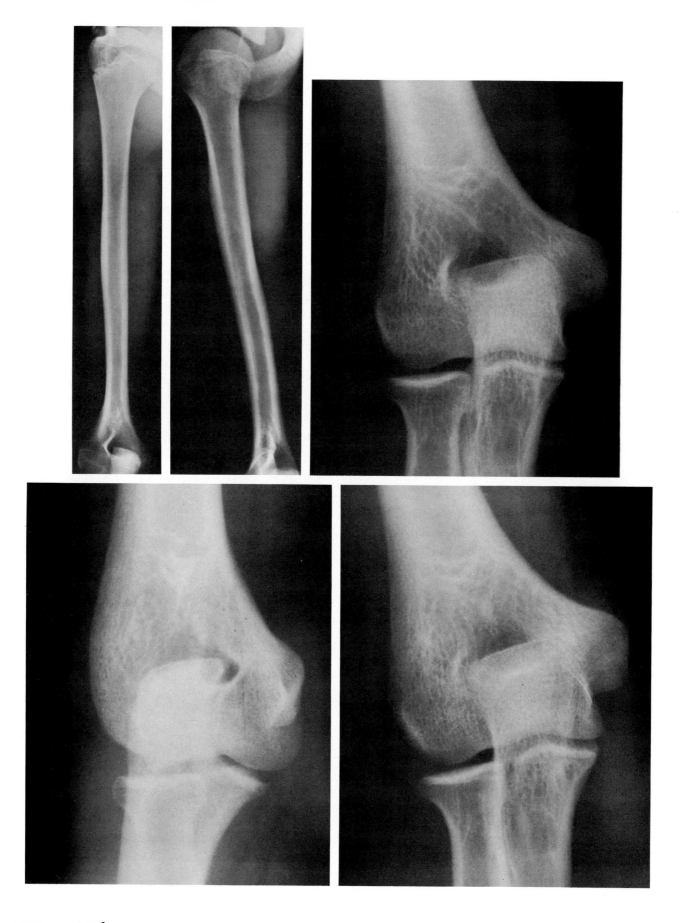

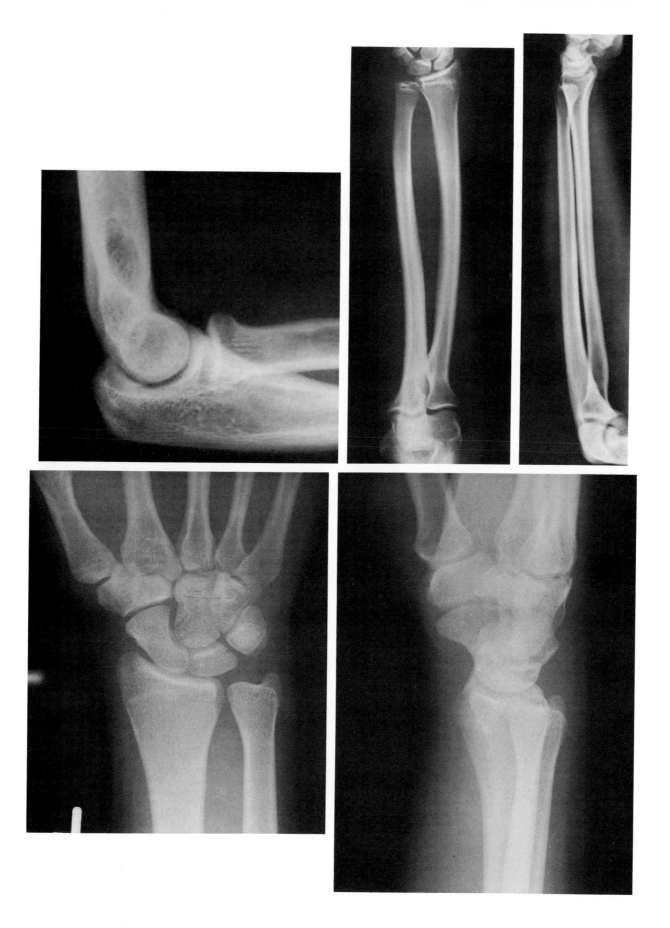

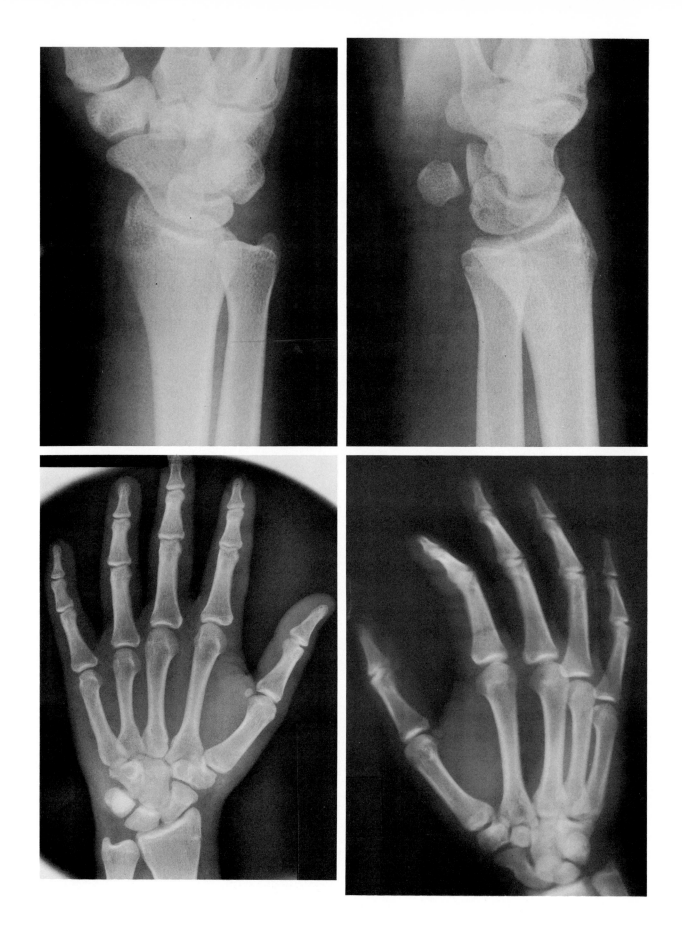

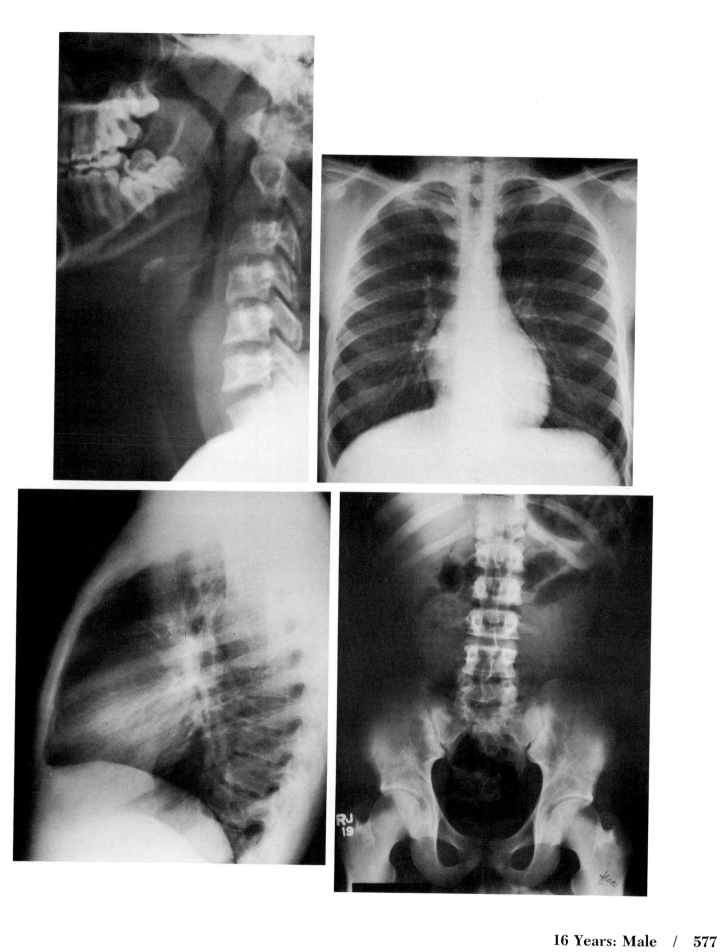

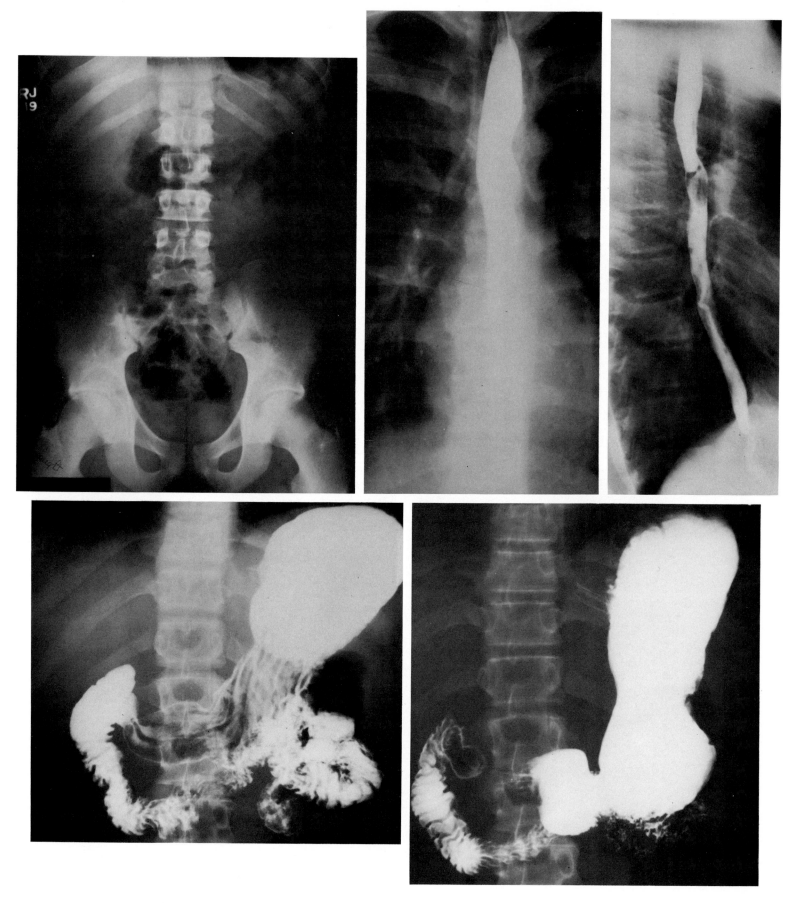

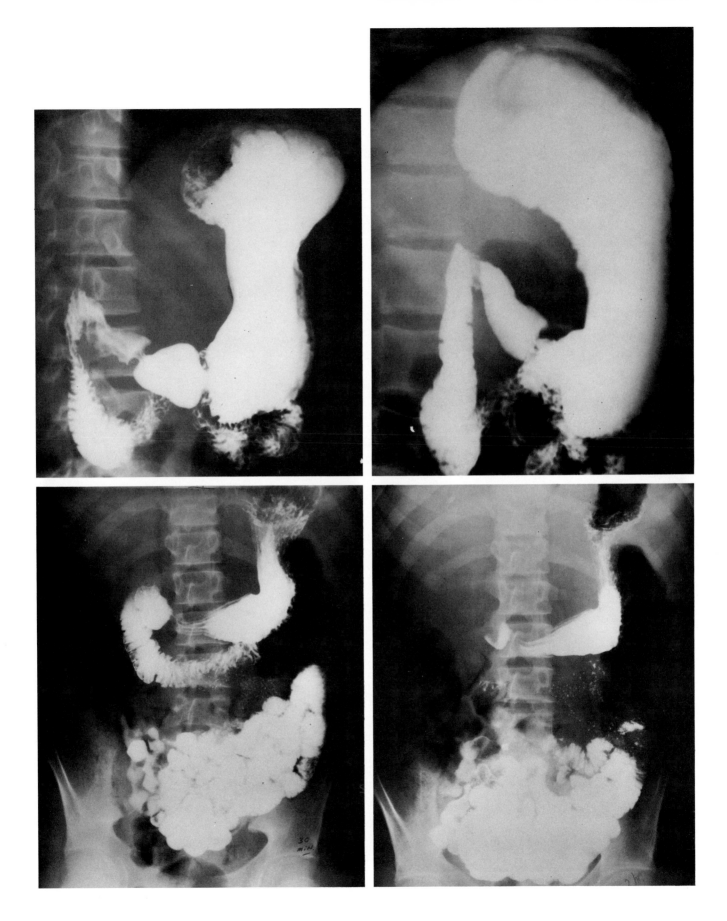

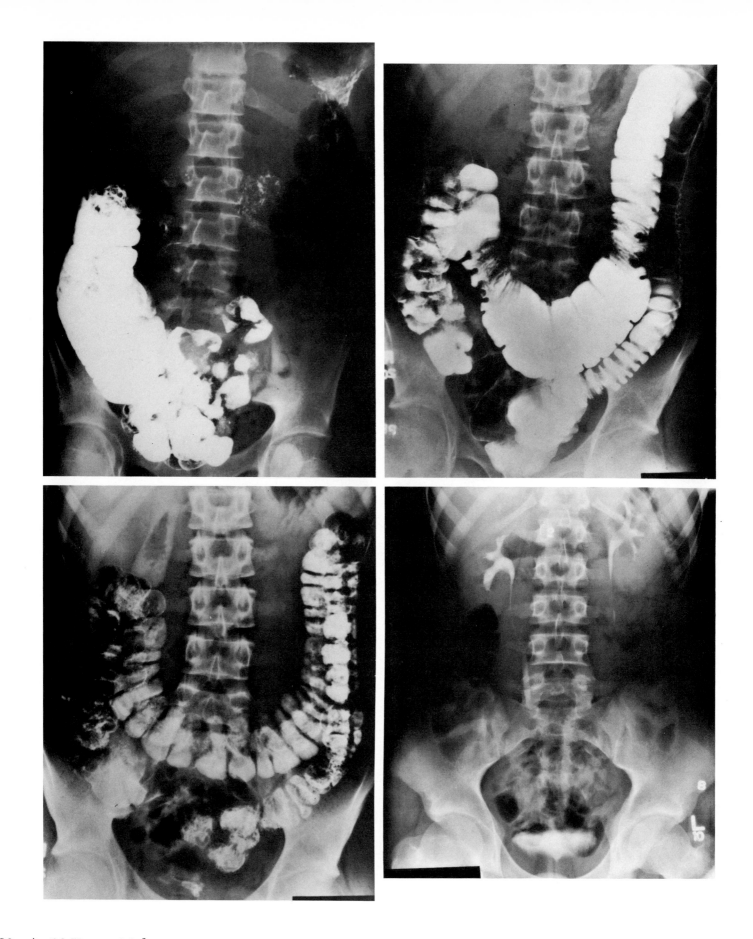

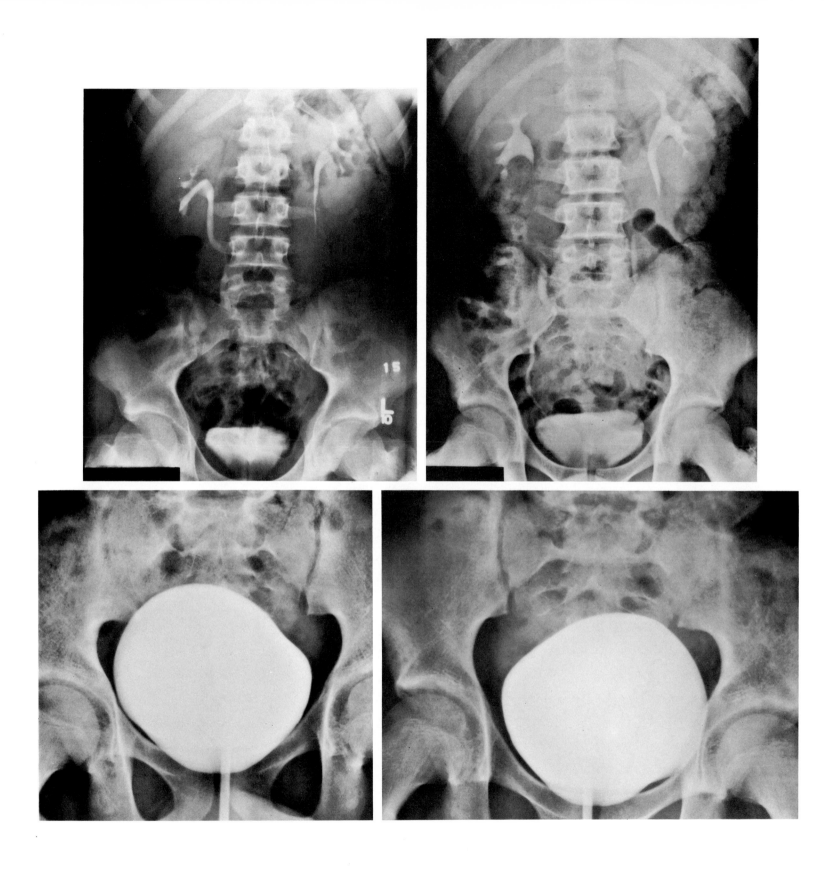

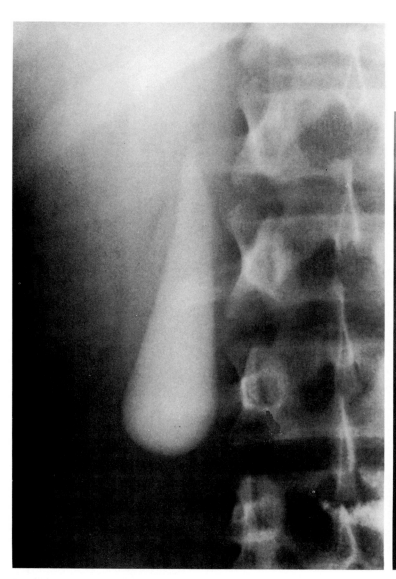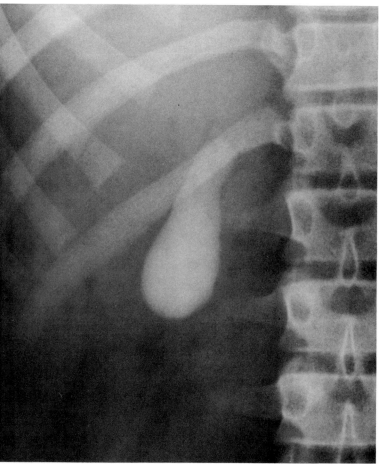

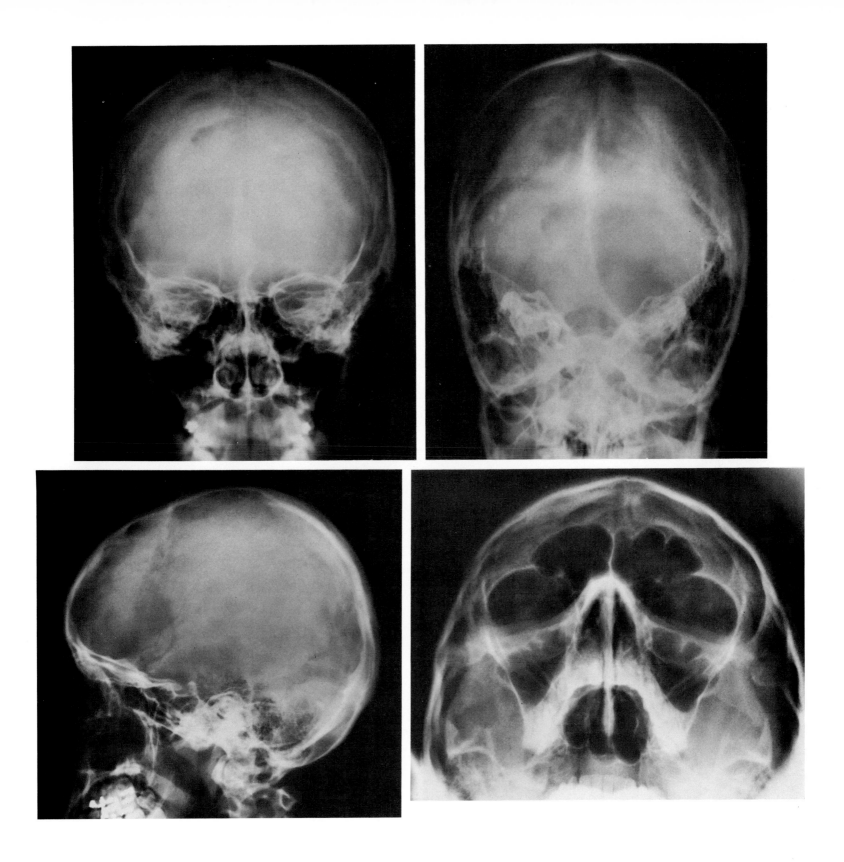

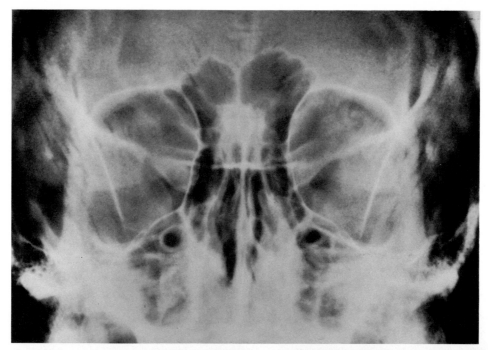

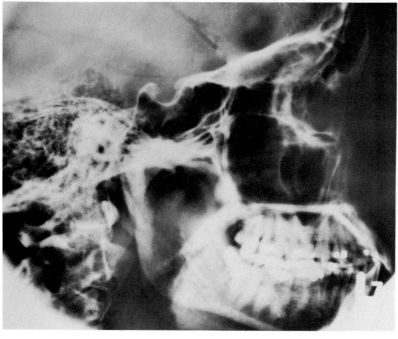

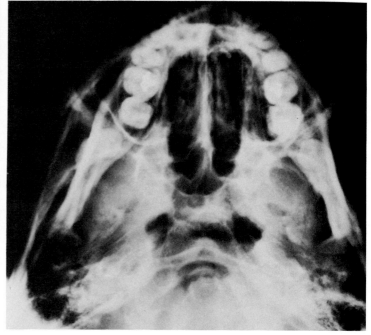

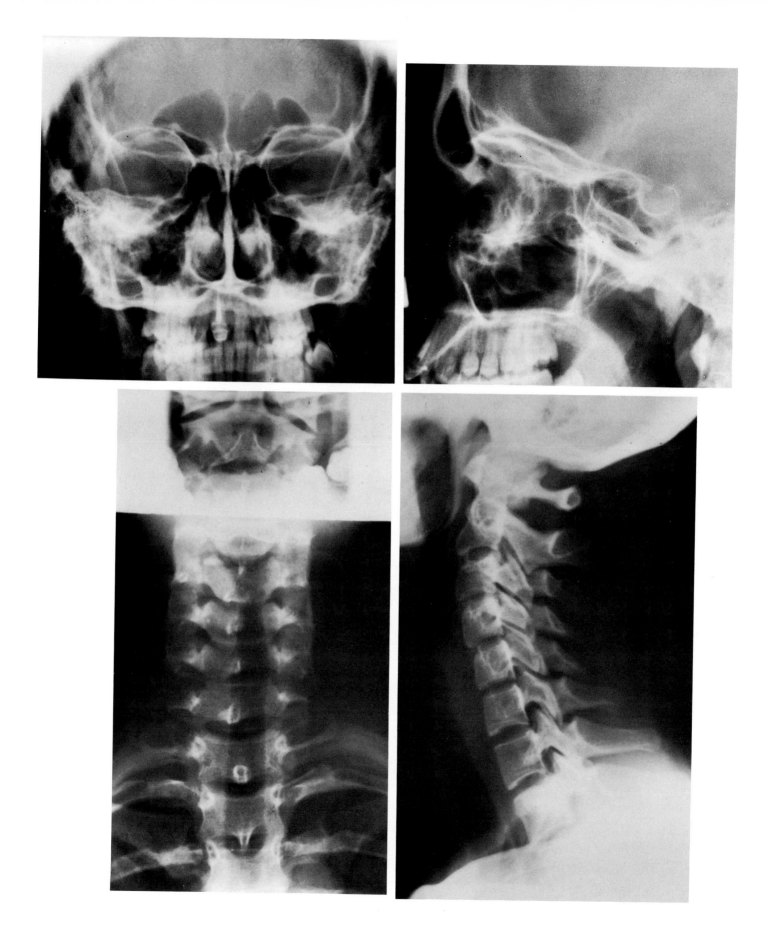

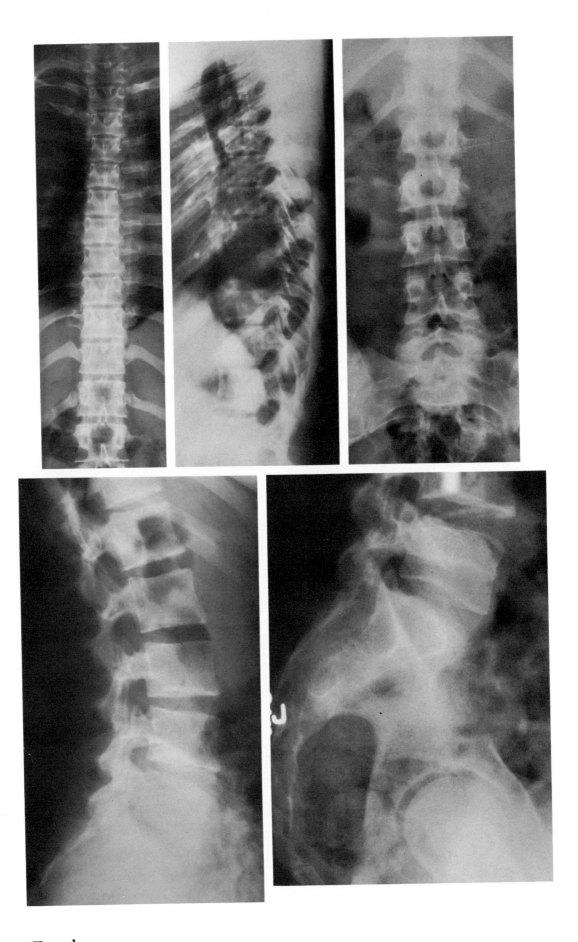

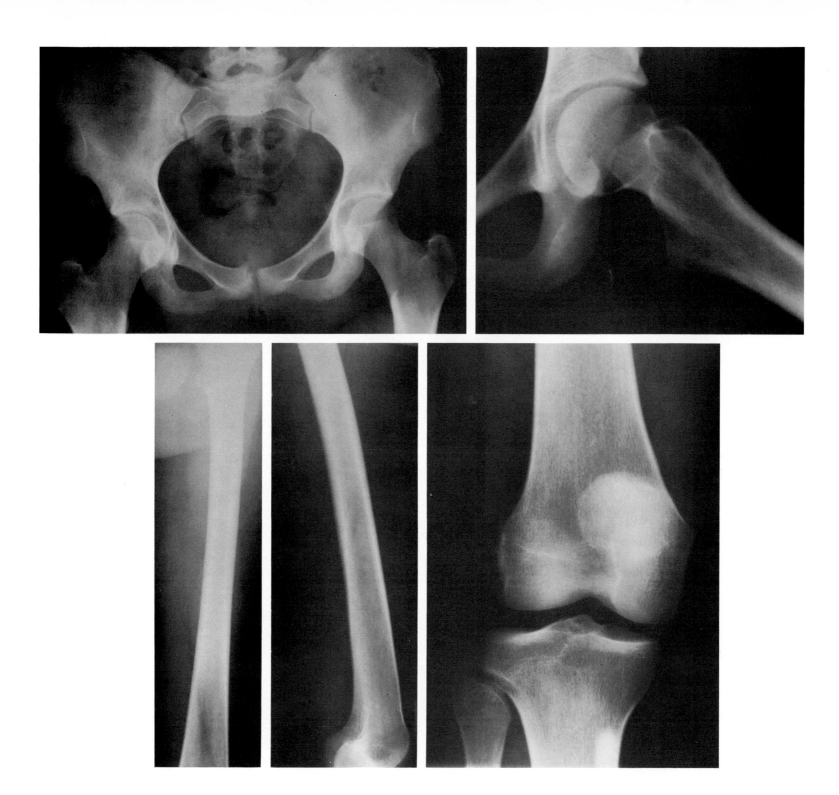

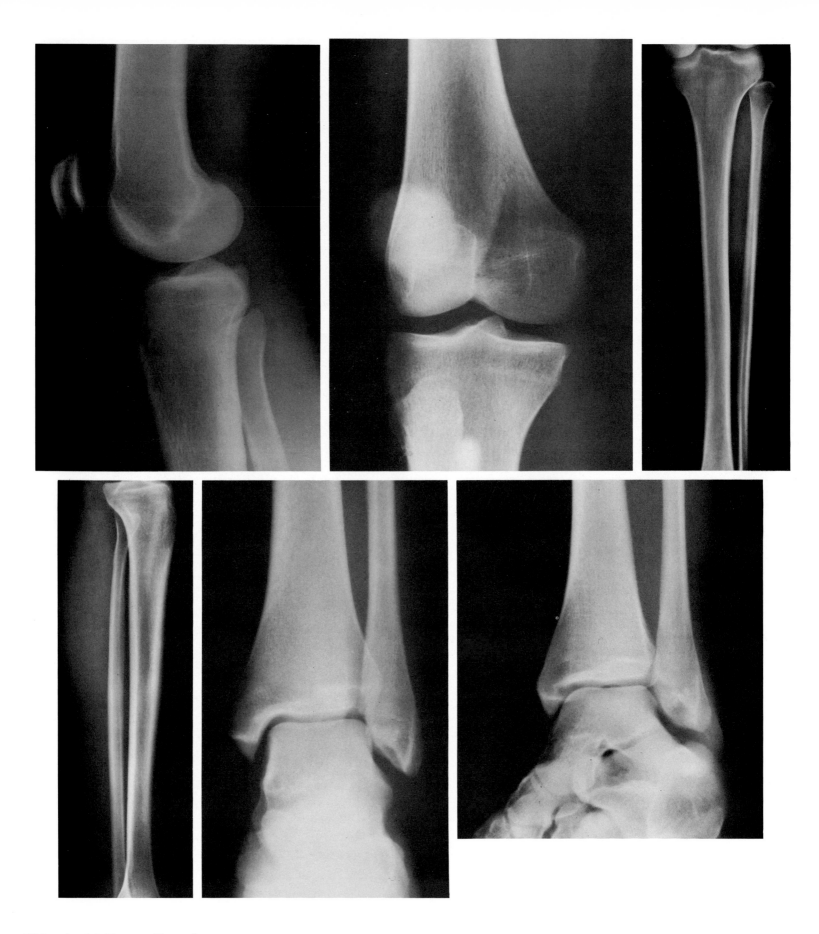

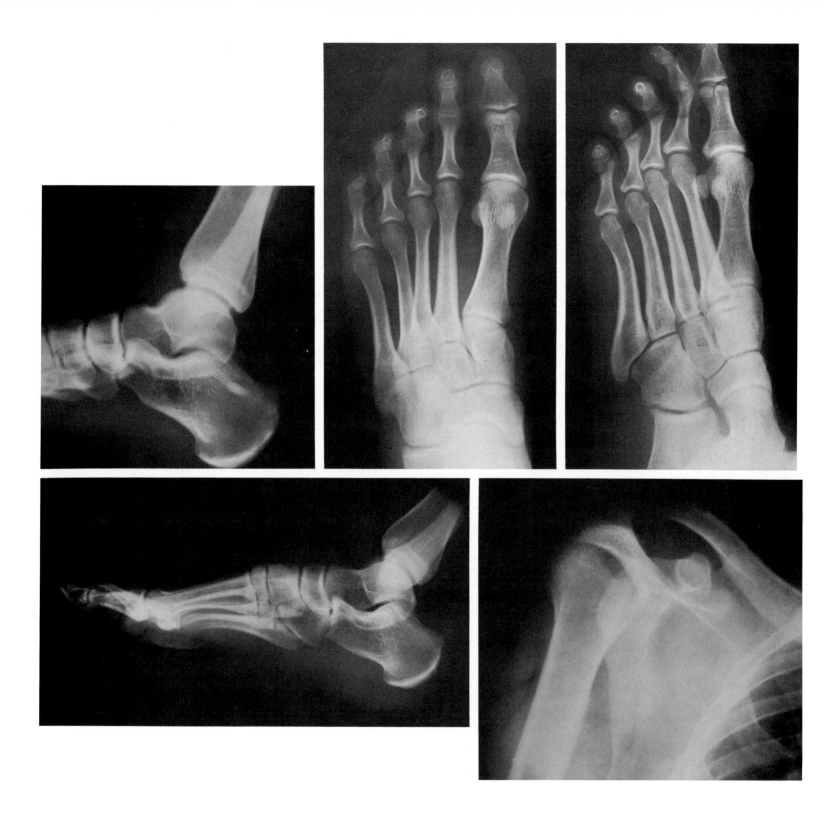

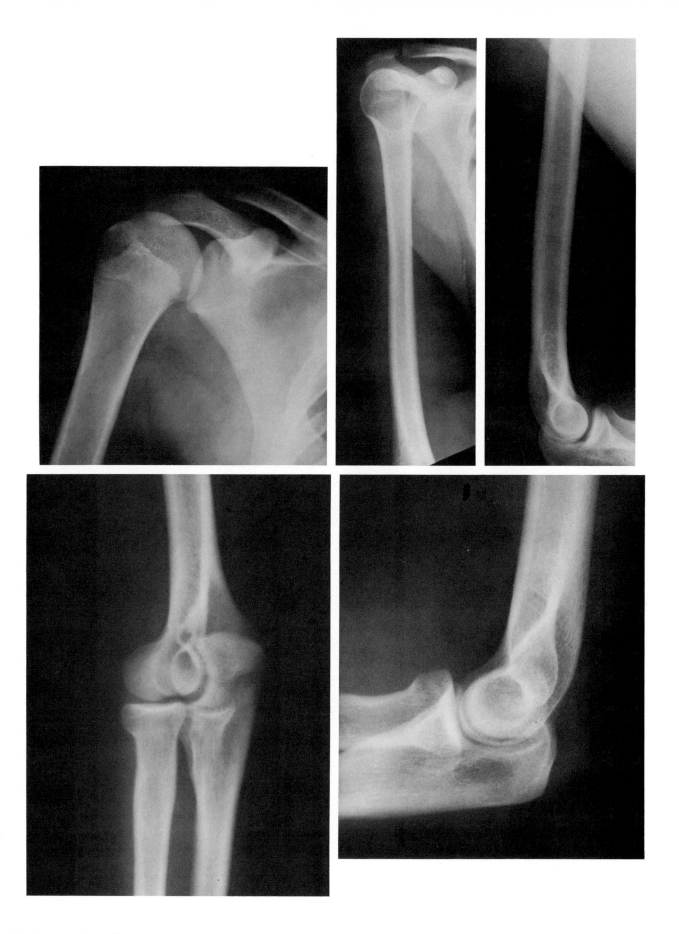

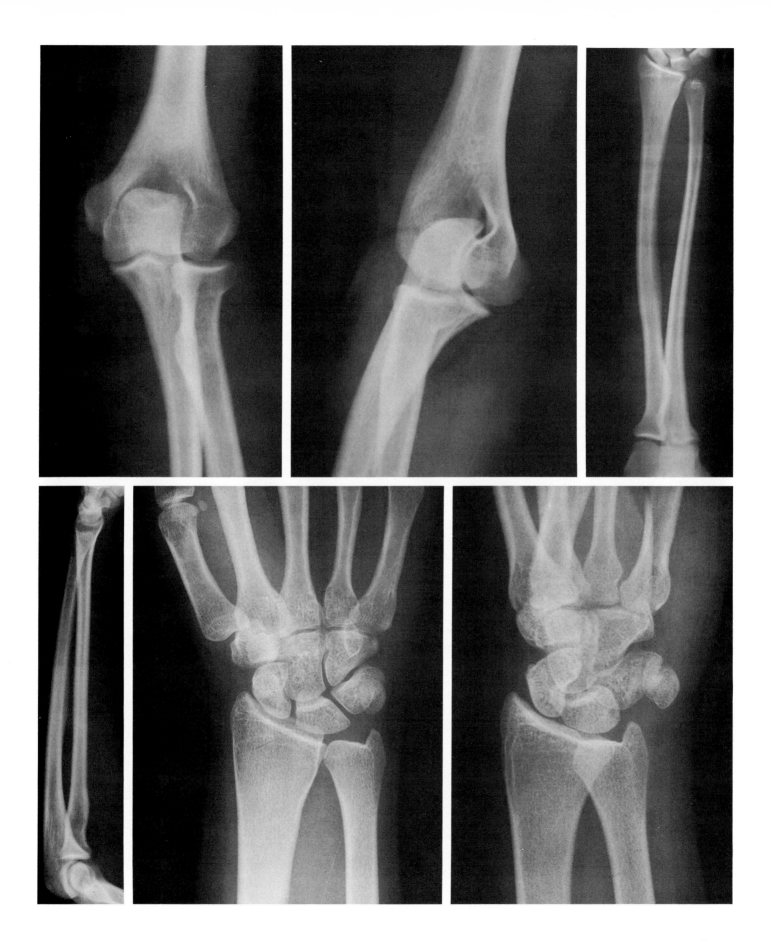

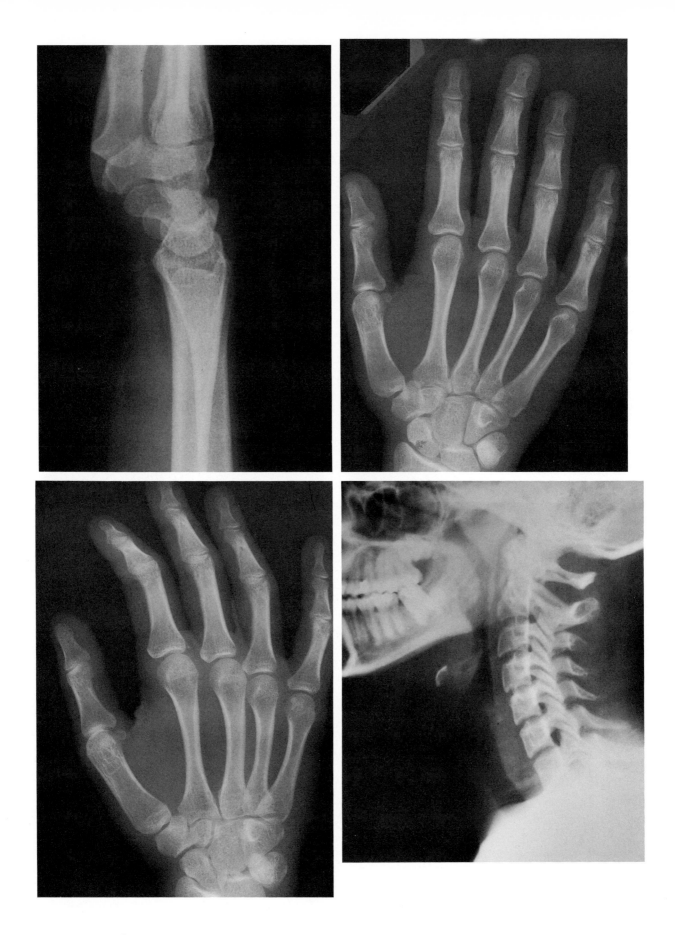

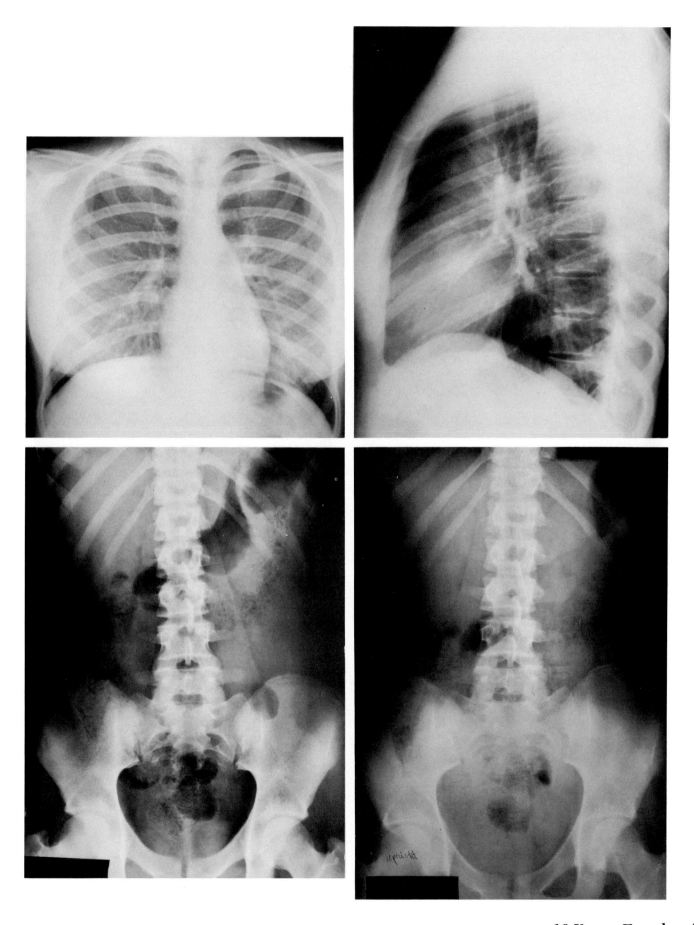

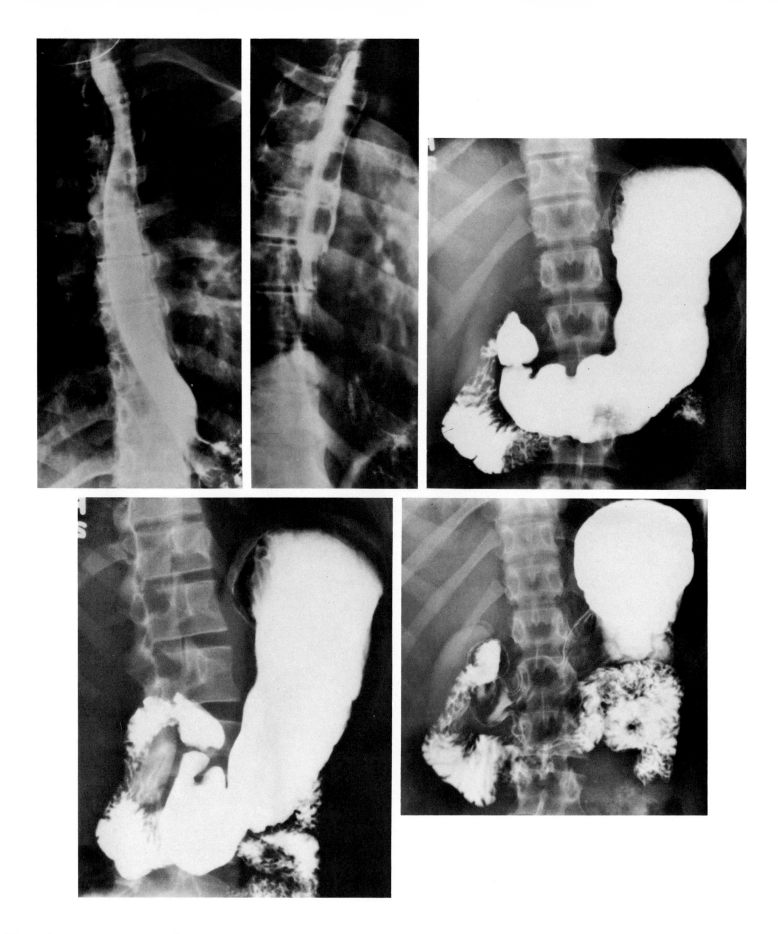

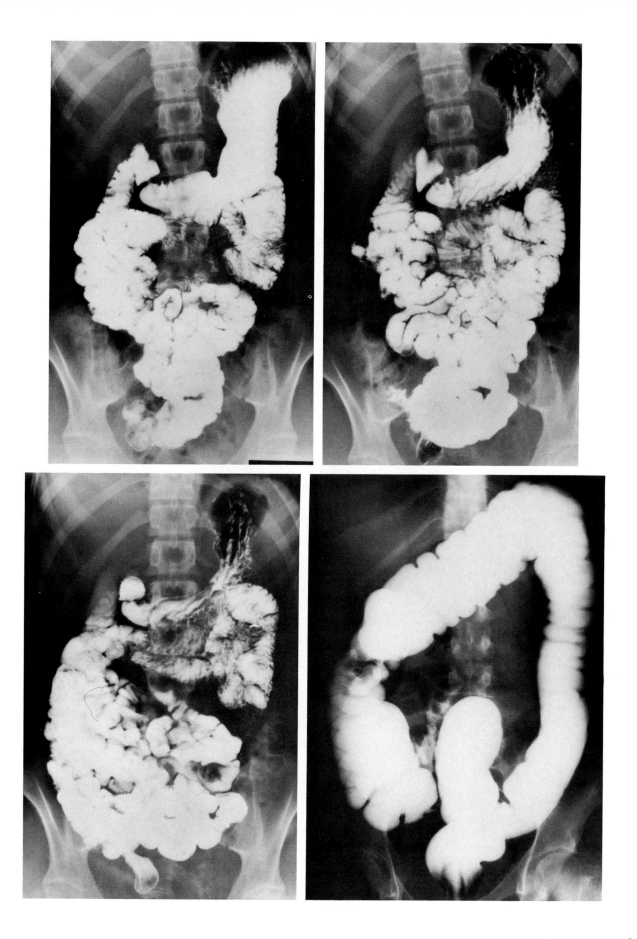

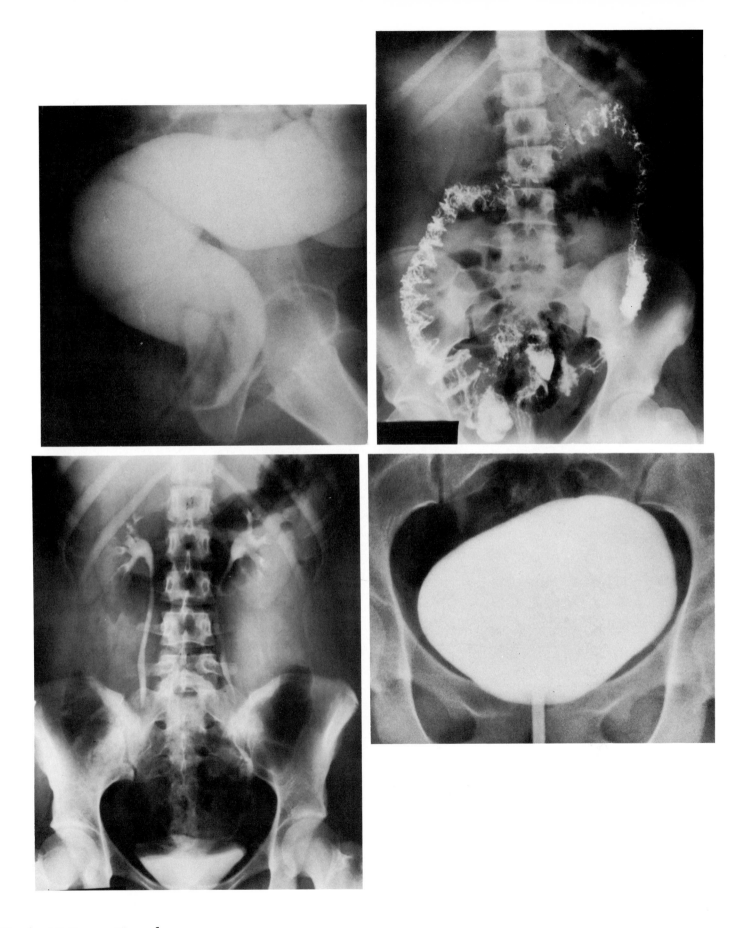

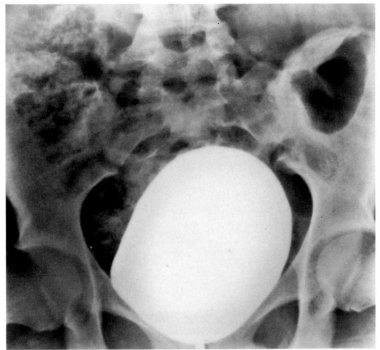

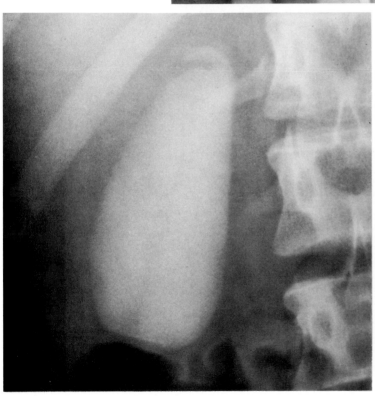

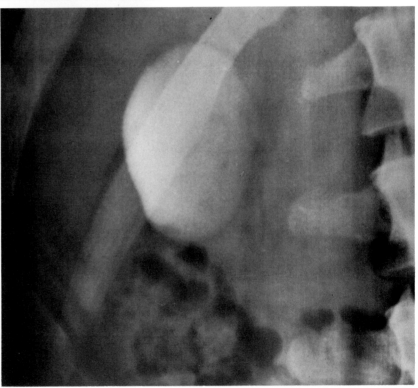

25

17 YEARS

The vertebrae have adult configuration. Physiologic prominence of the pulmonary artery may still be seen. The nasopharyngeal soft tissues are of adult proportions.

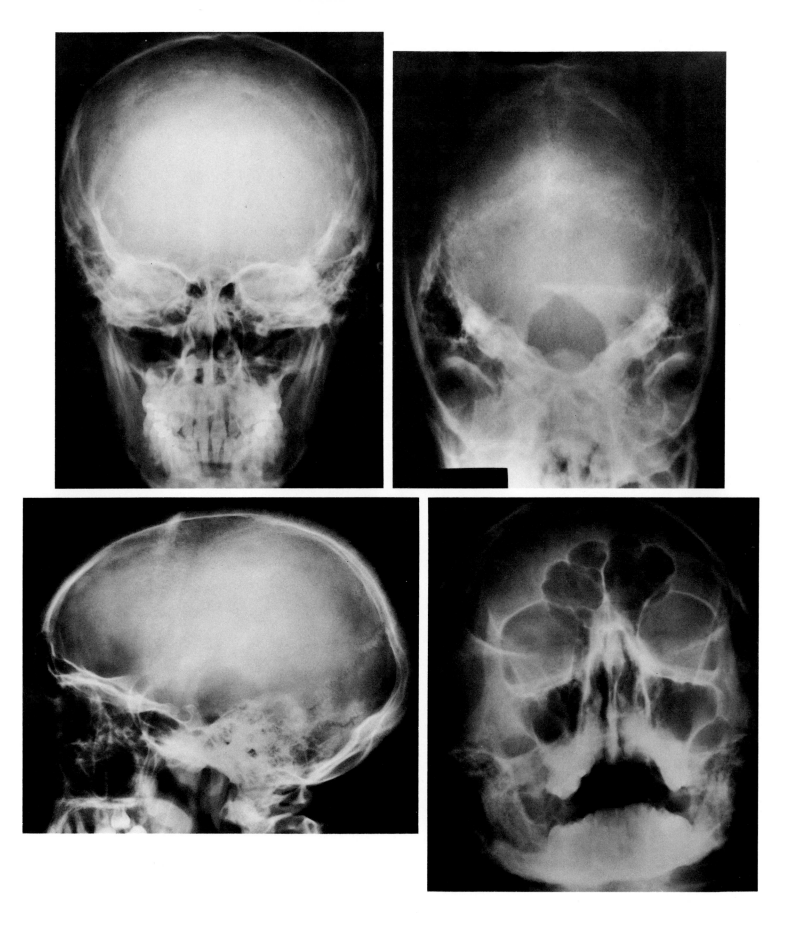

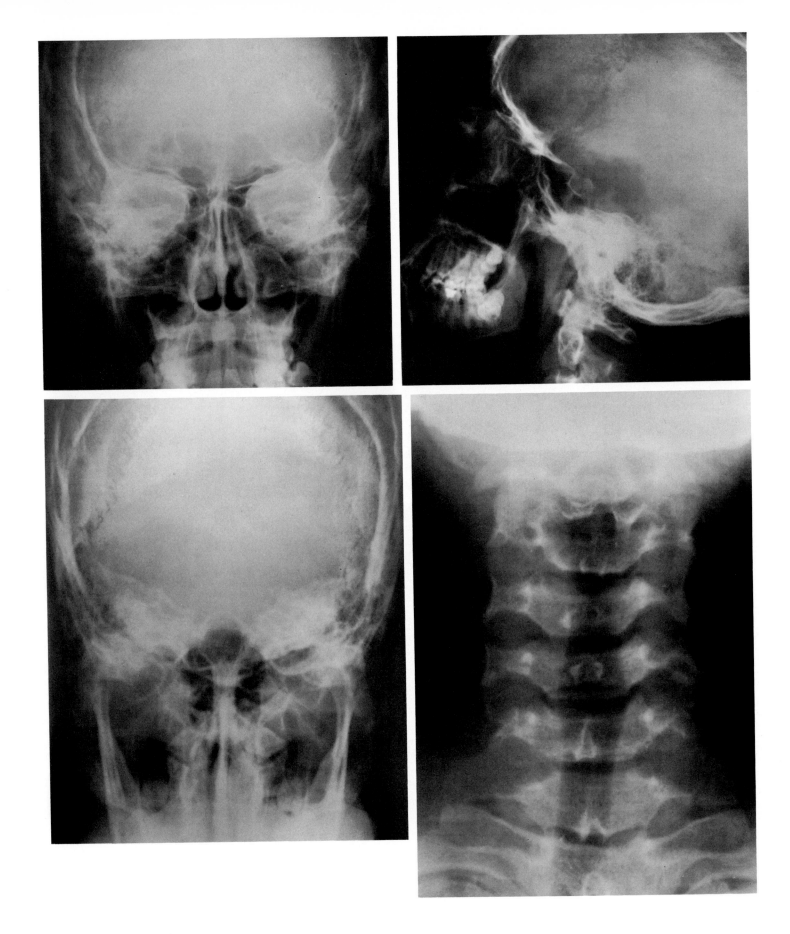

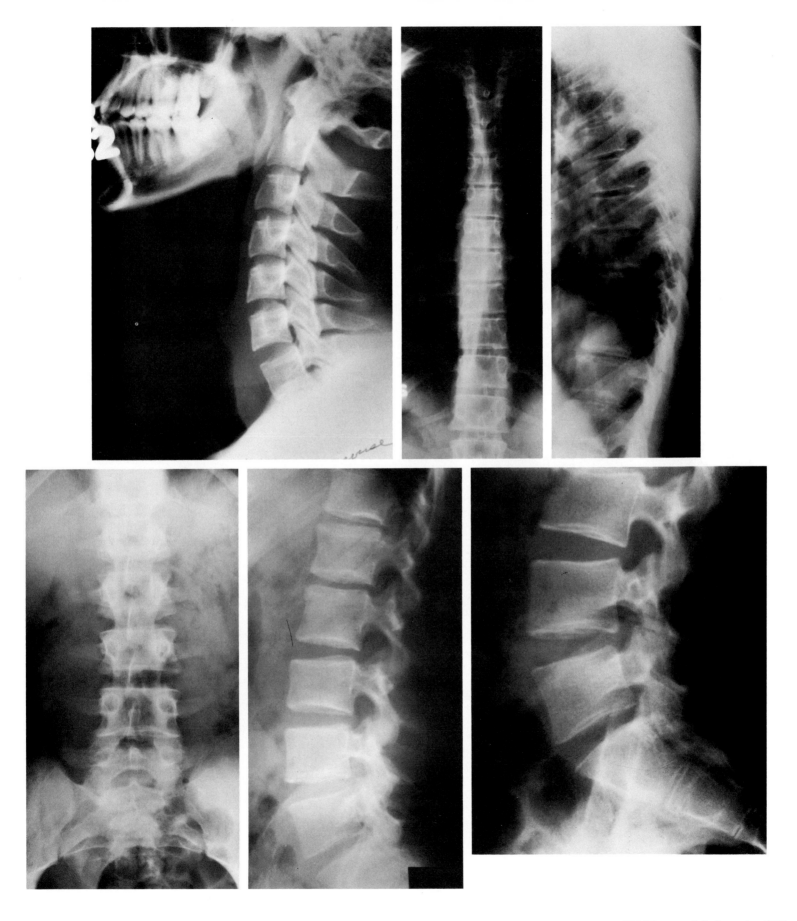

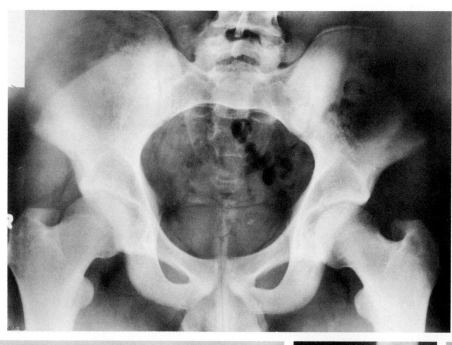

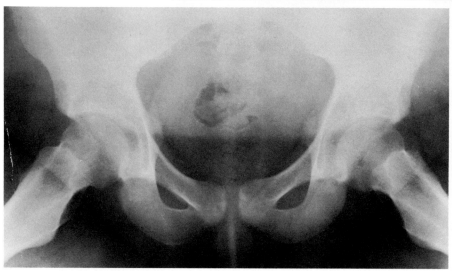

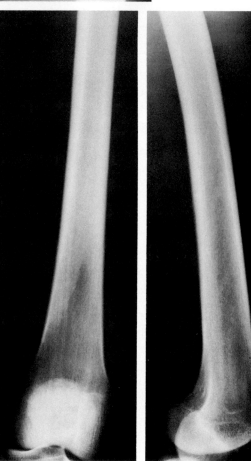

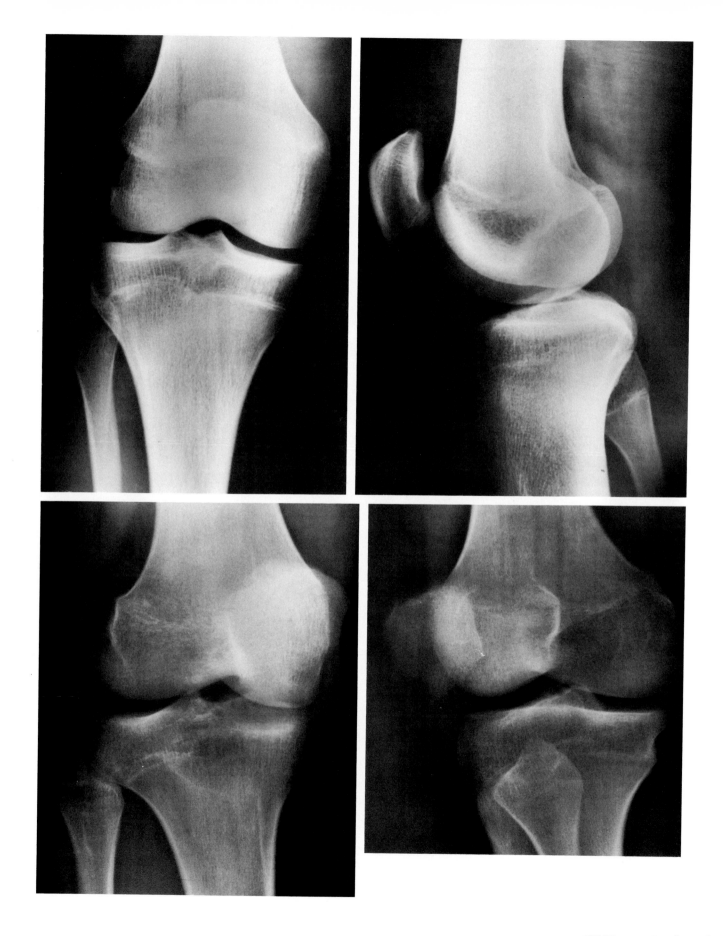

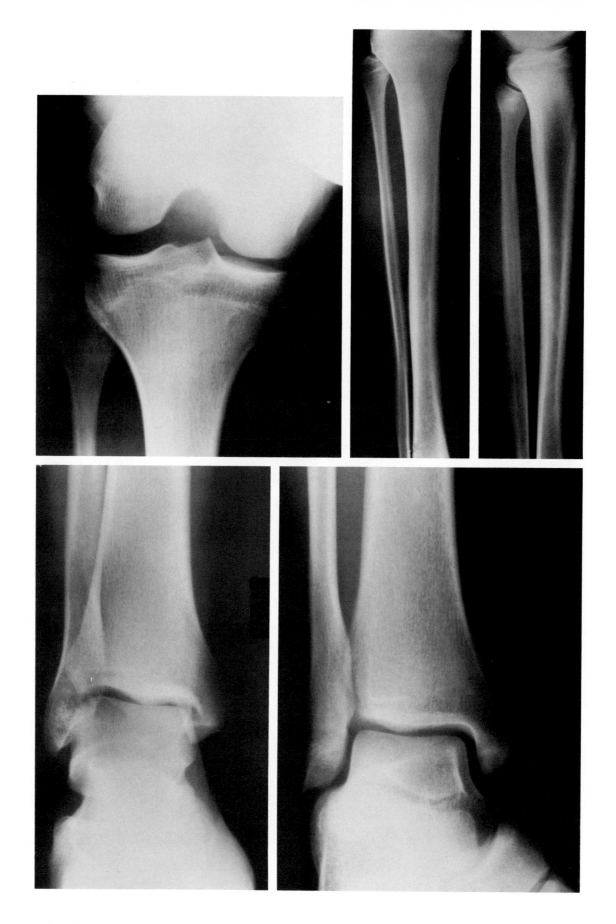

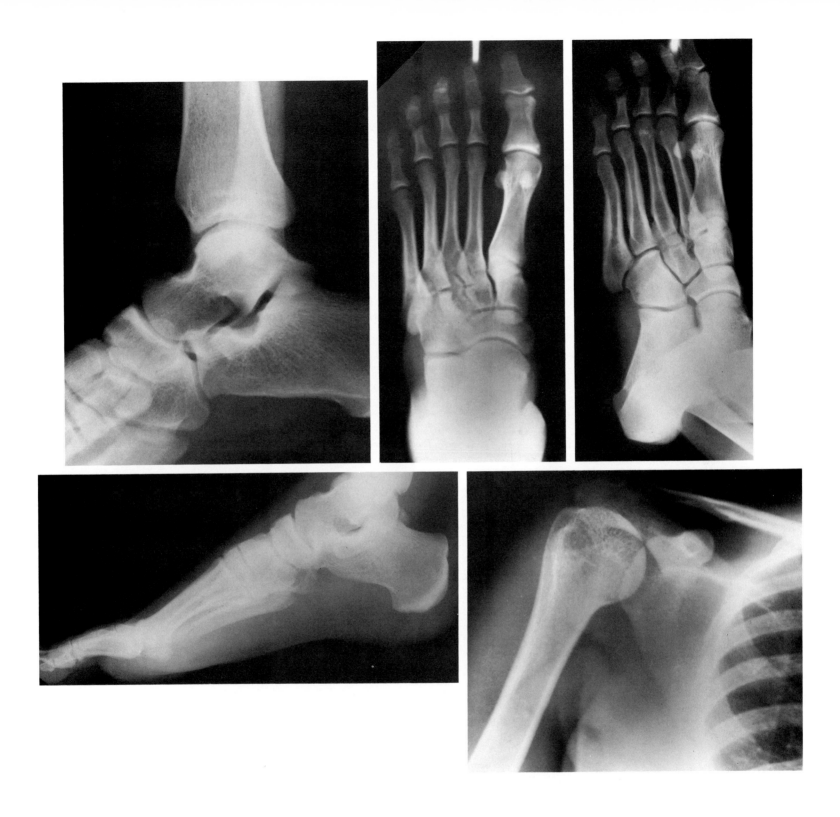

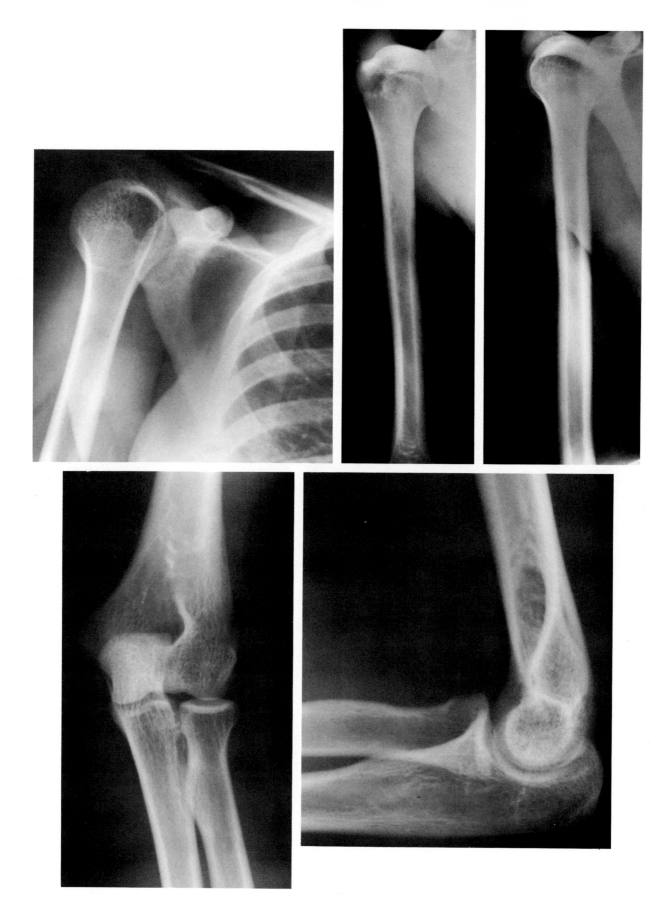

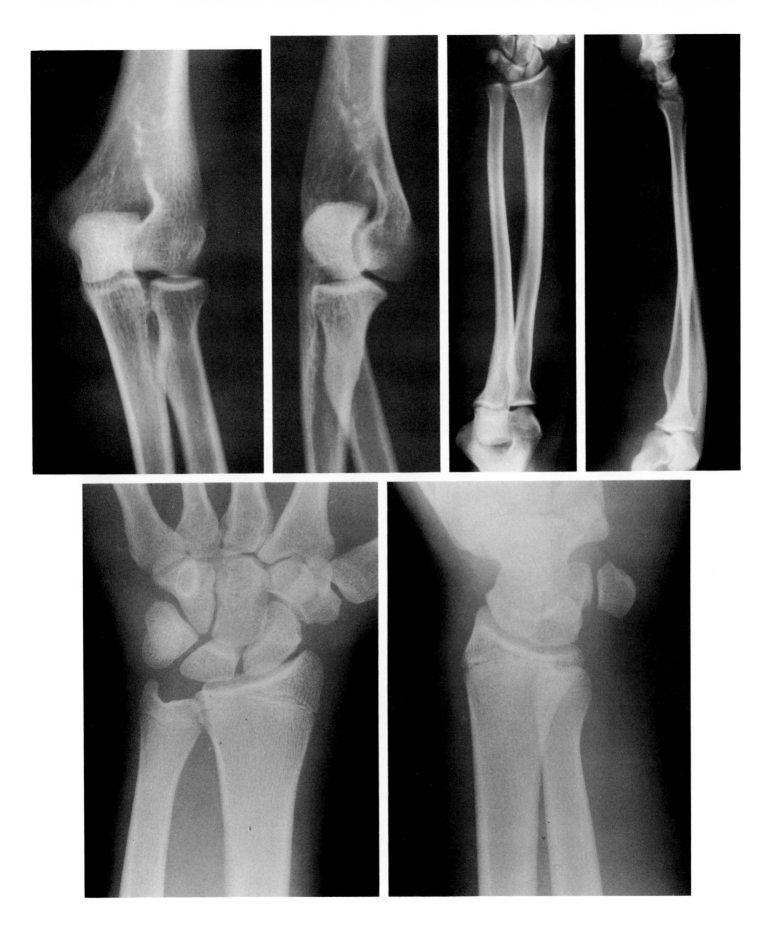

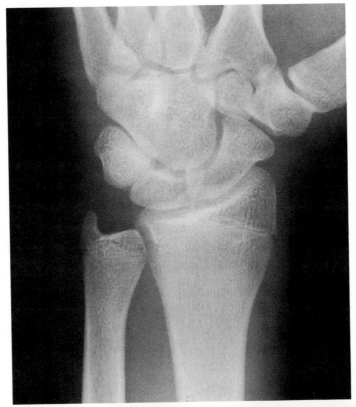

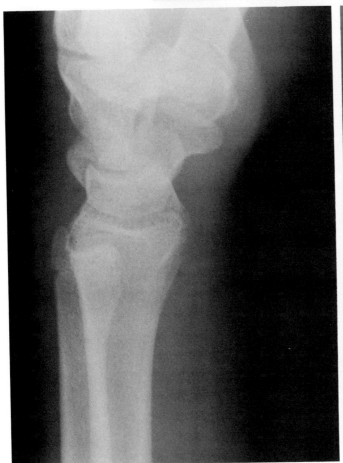

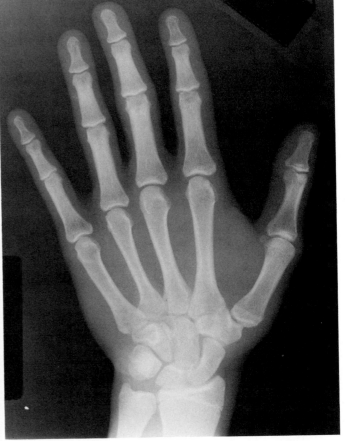

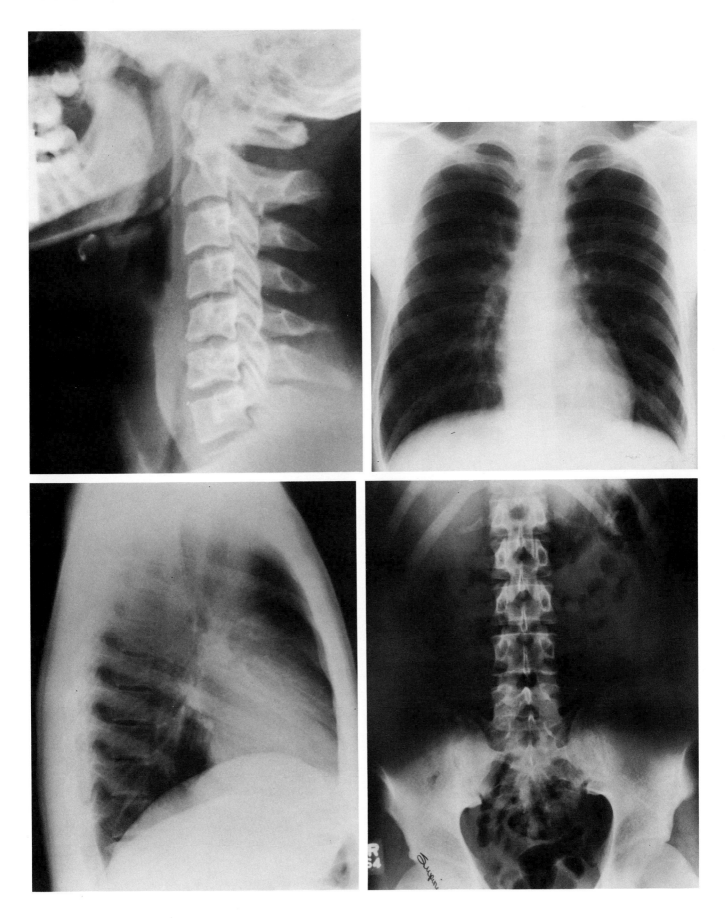

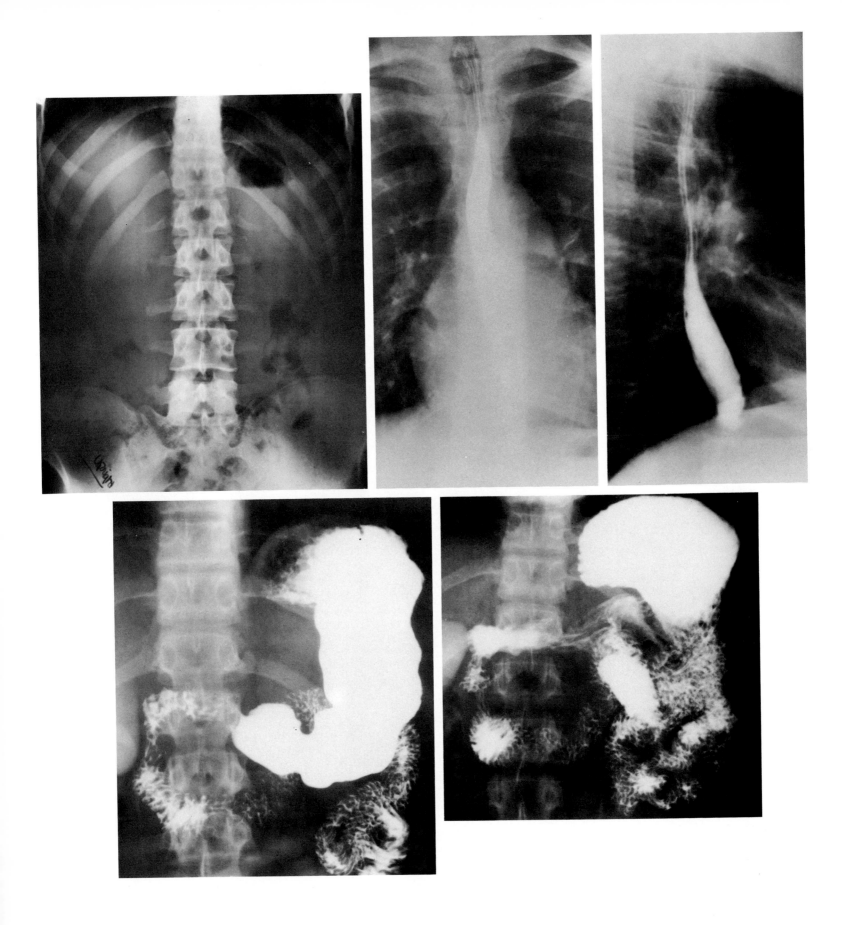

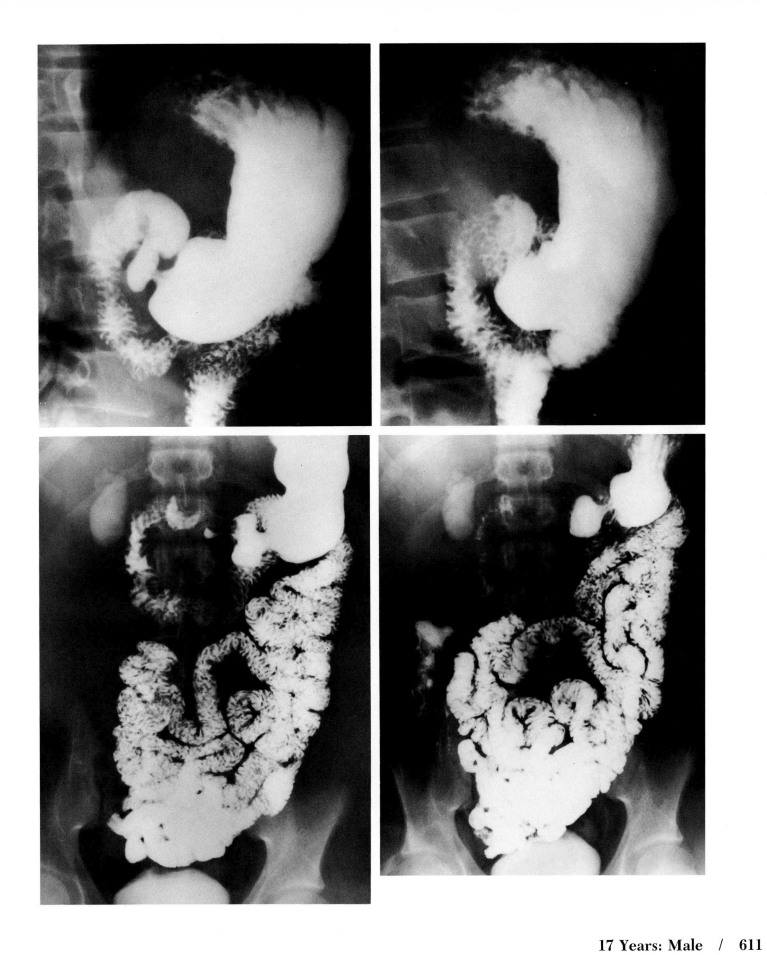

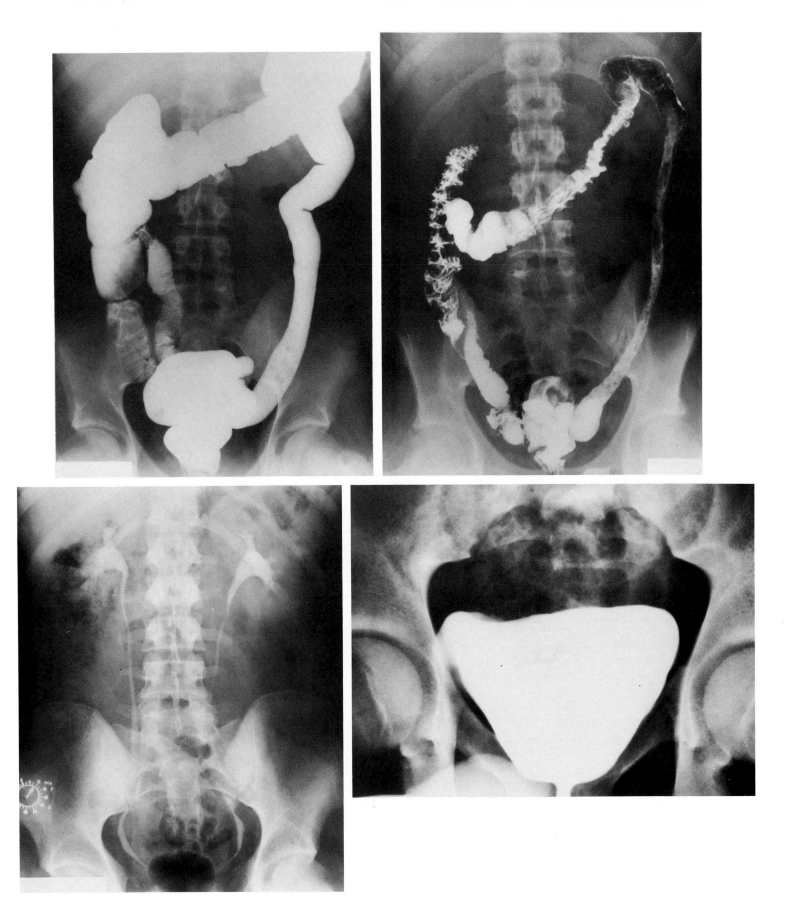

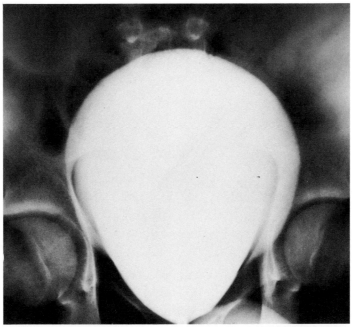

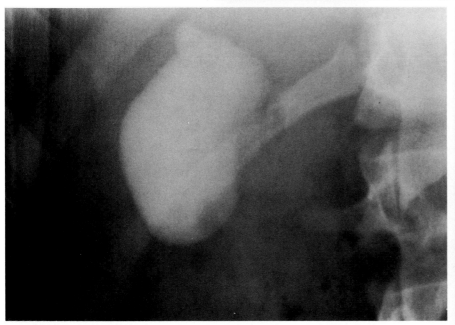

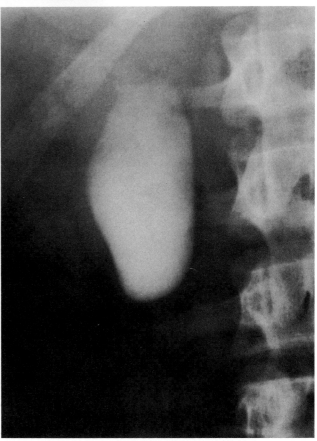

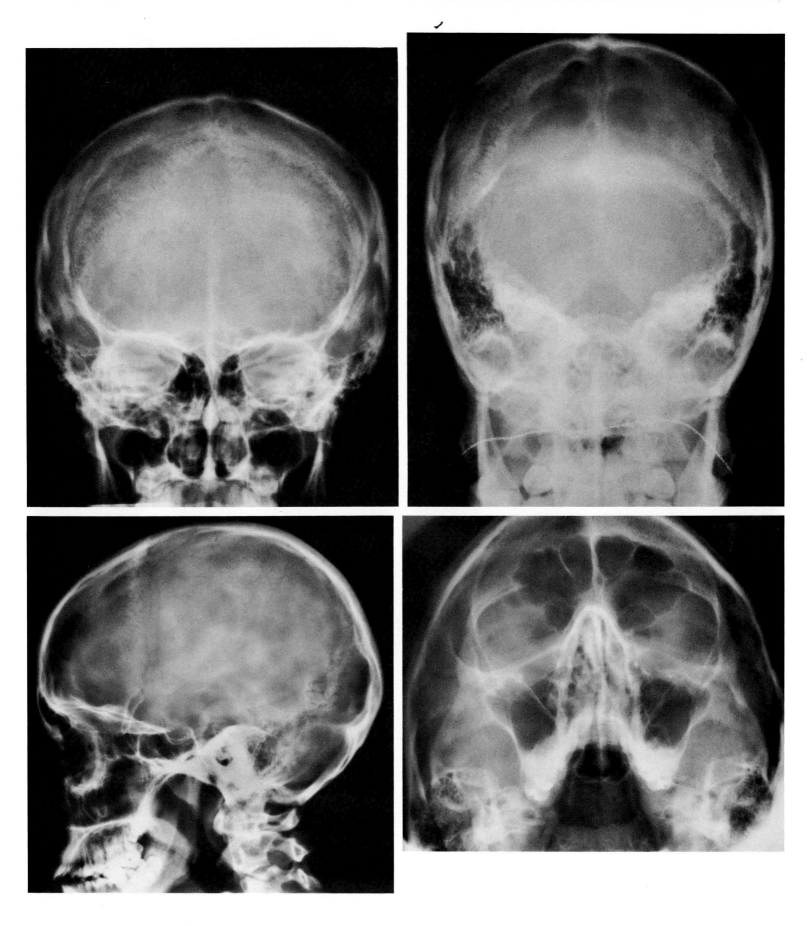

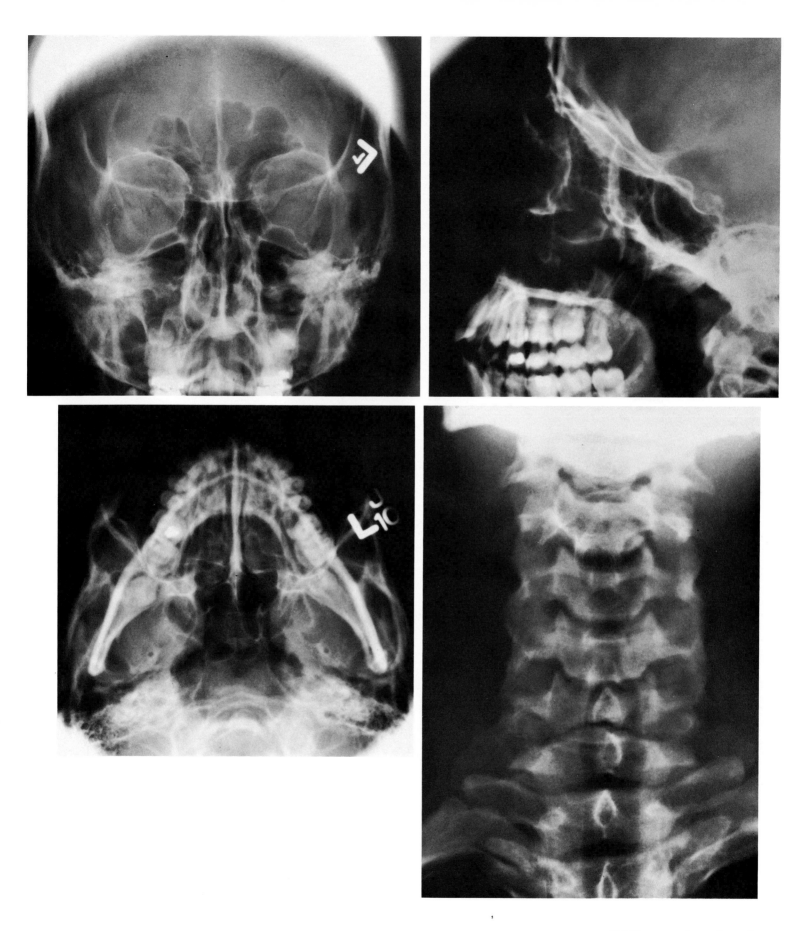

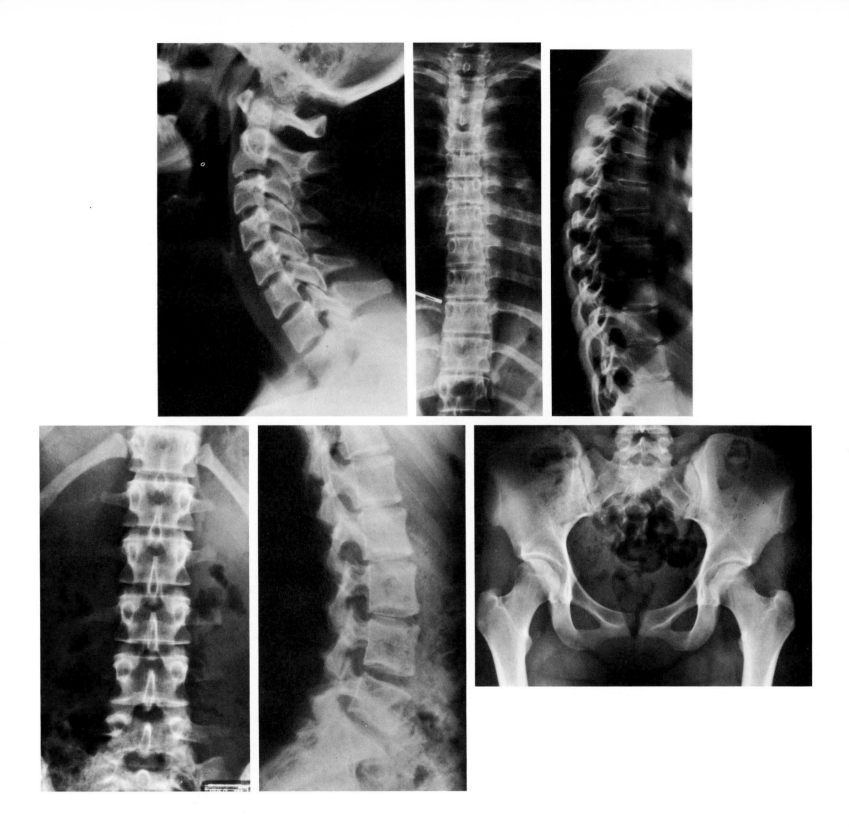

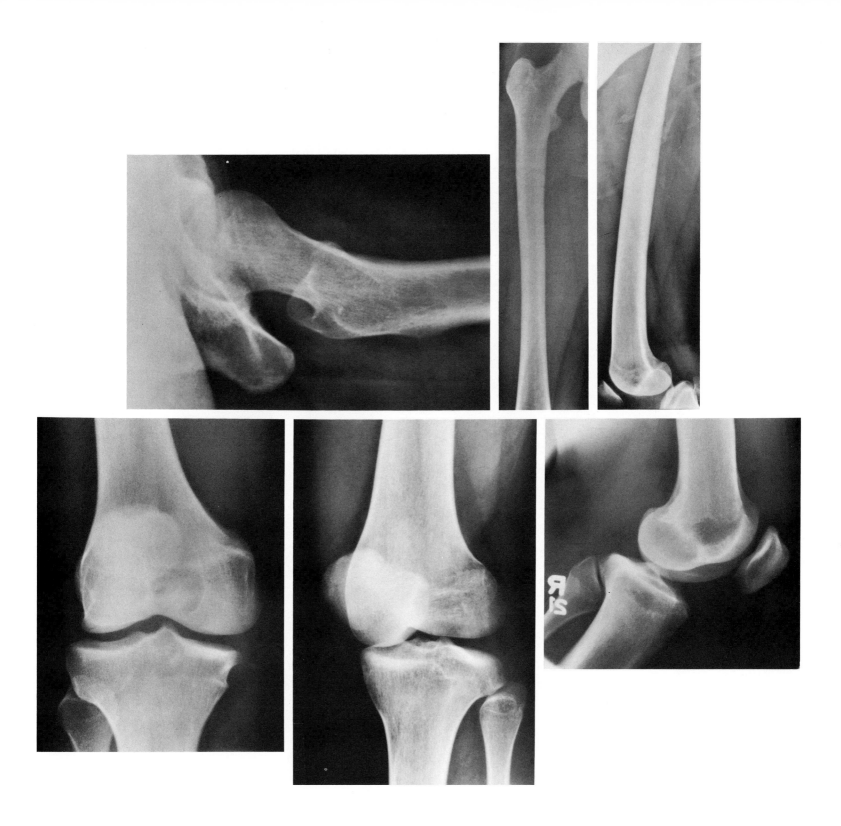

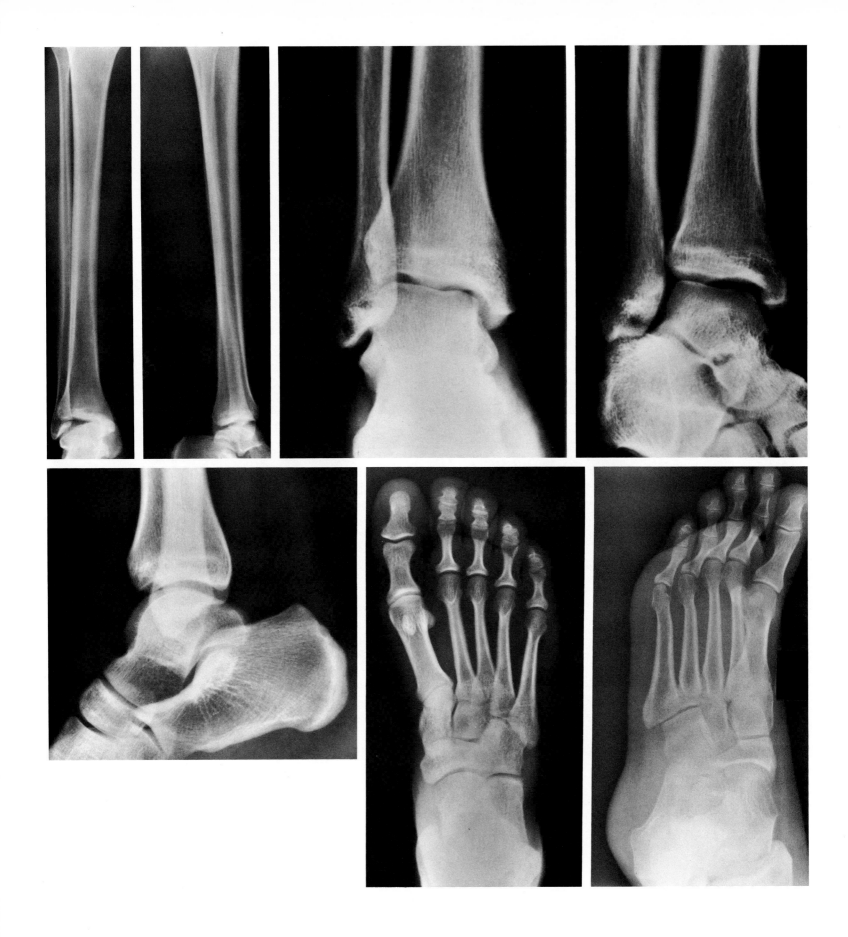

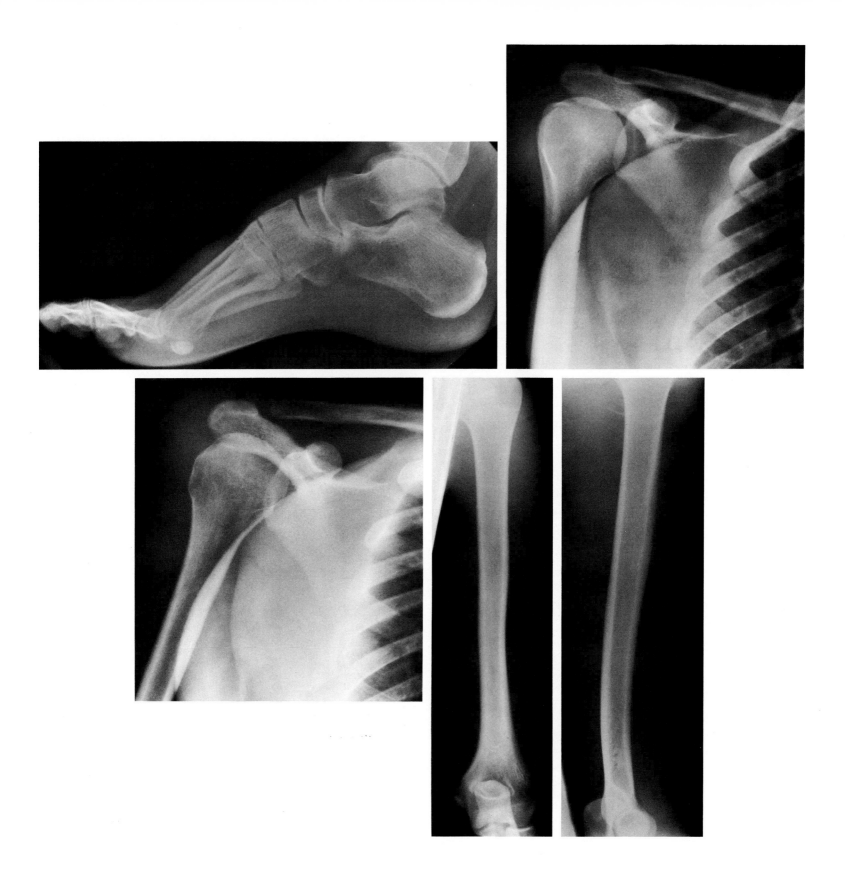

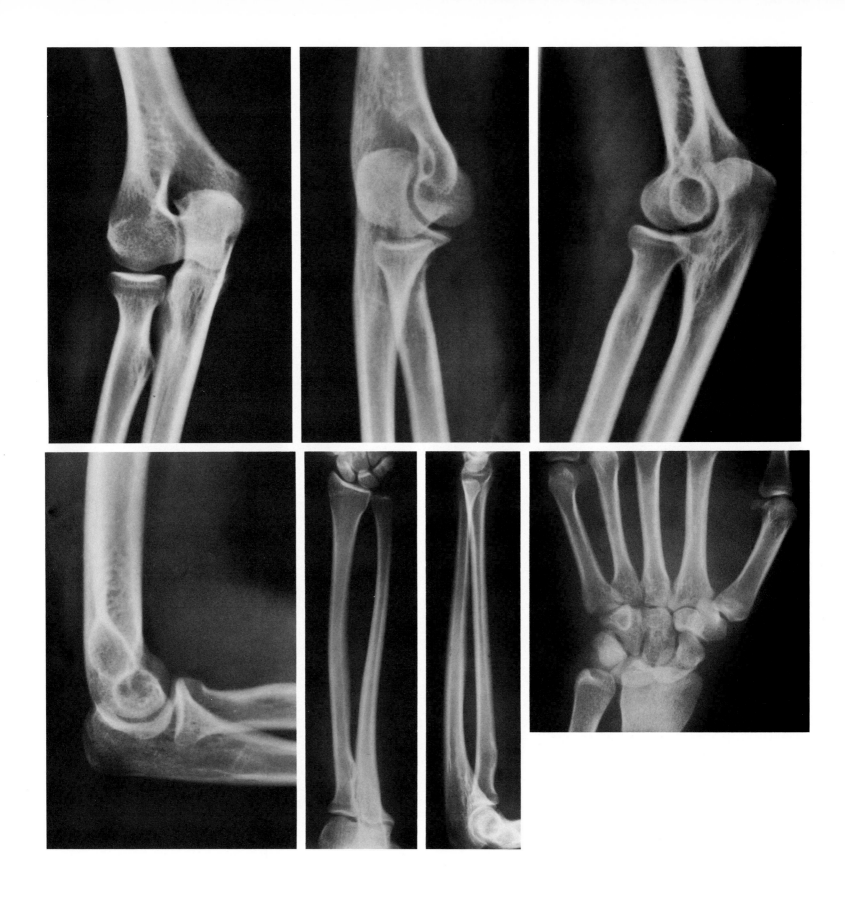

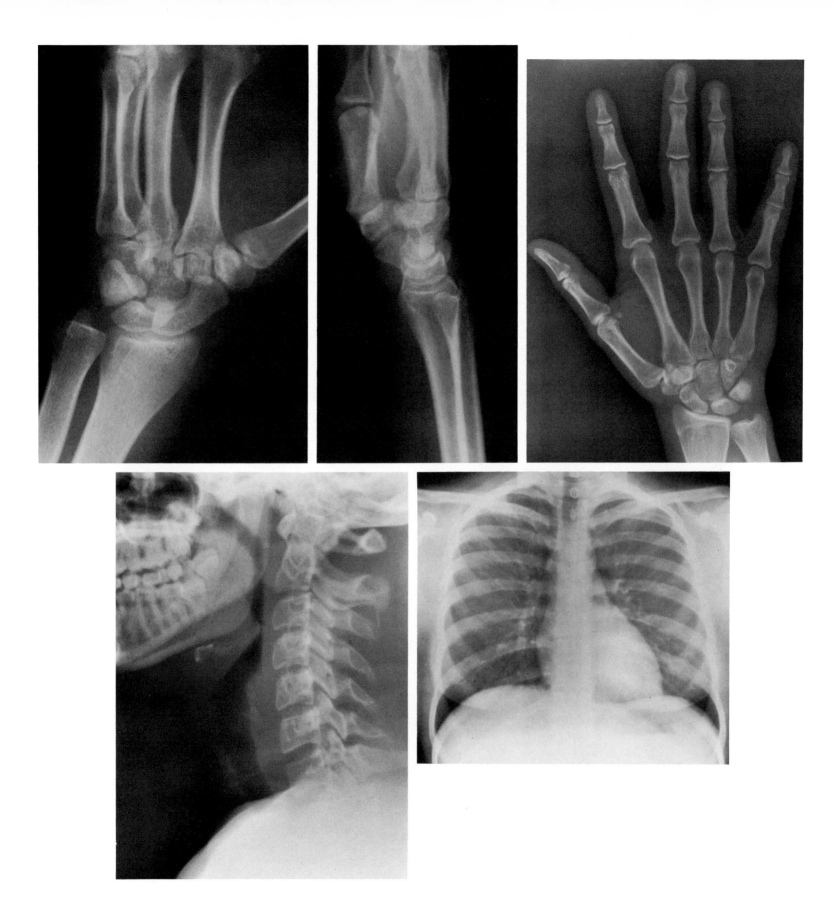

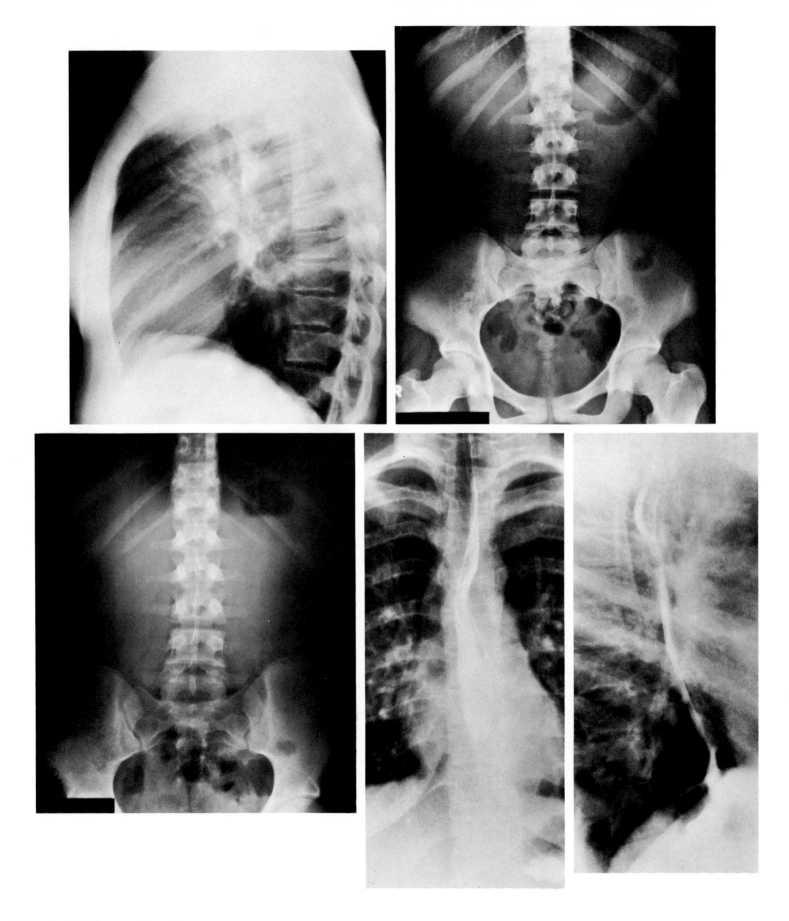

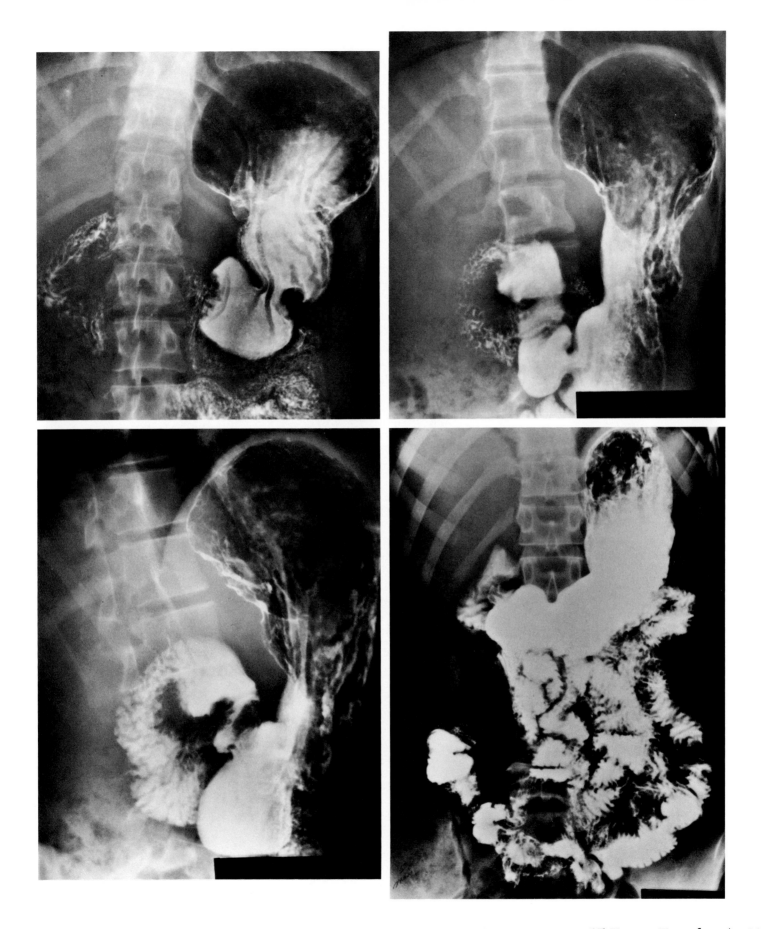

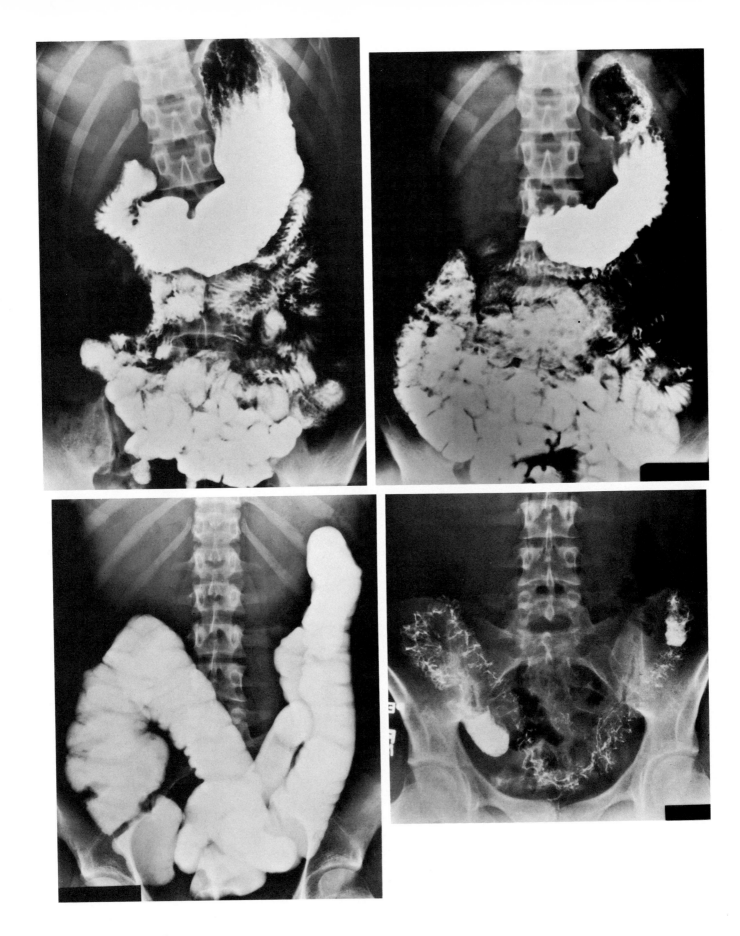

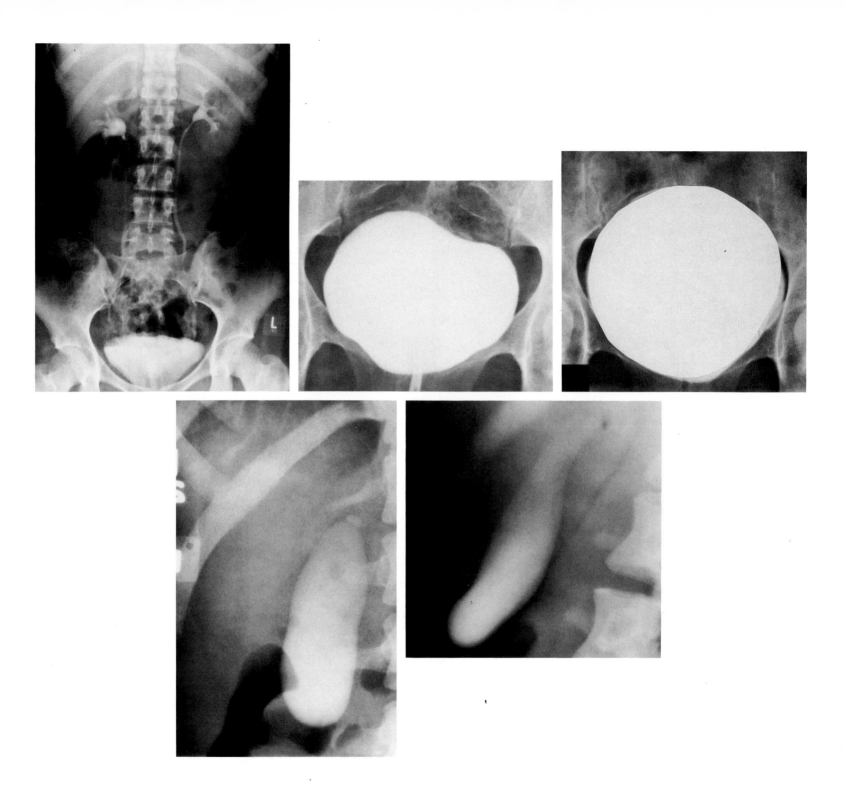

26

18 YEARS

The last remnants of the major epiphyseal plates can still be seen. The skeleton is otherwise adult. The pelvic apophyses are closed.

The heart has assumed adult configuration. The prominence of the pulmonary artery is not as apparent.

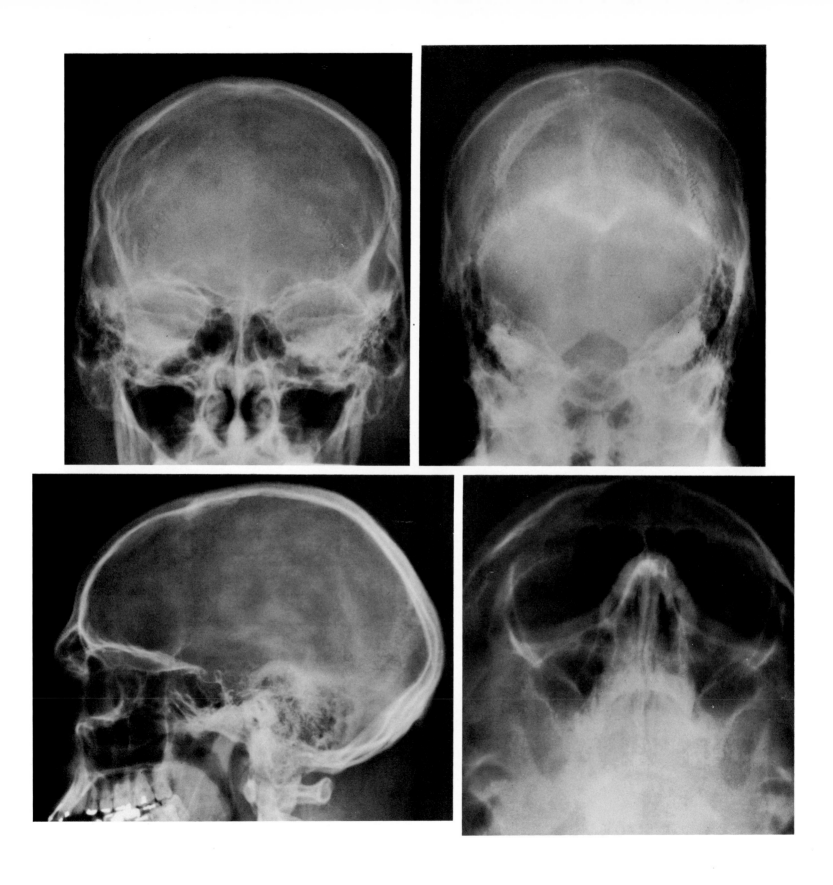

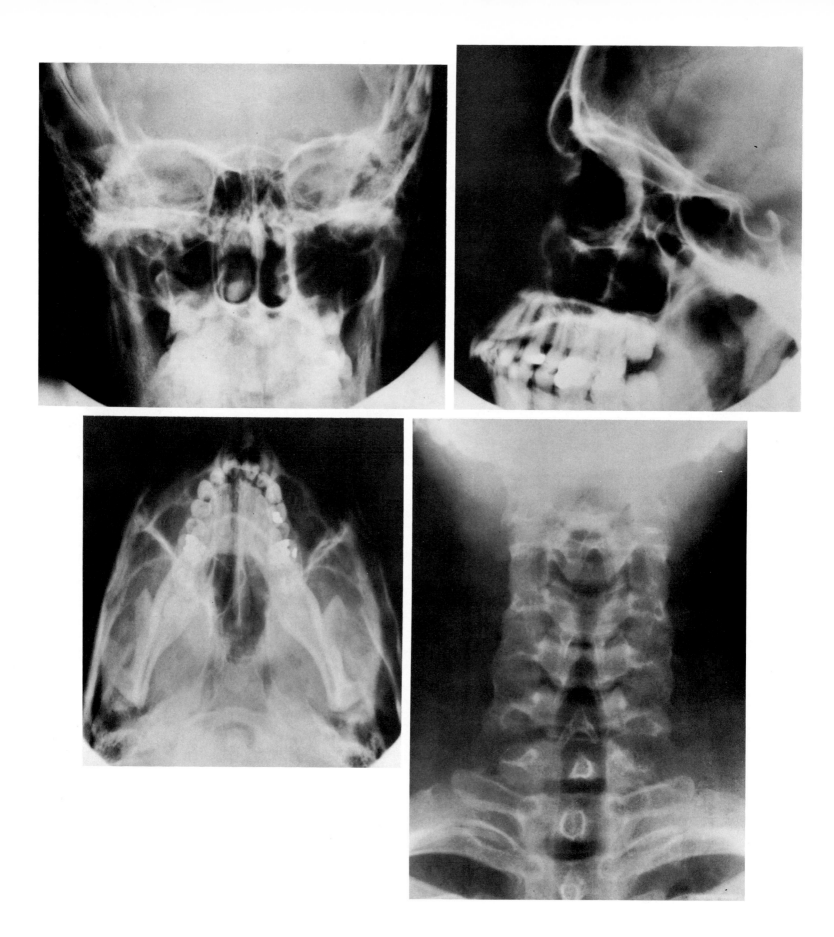

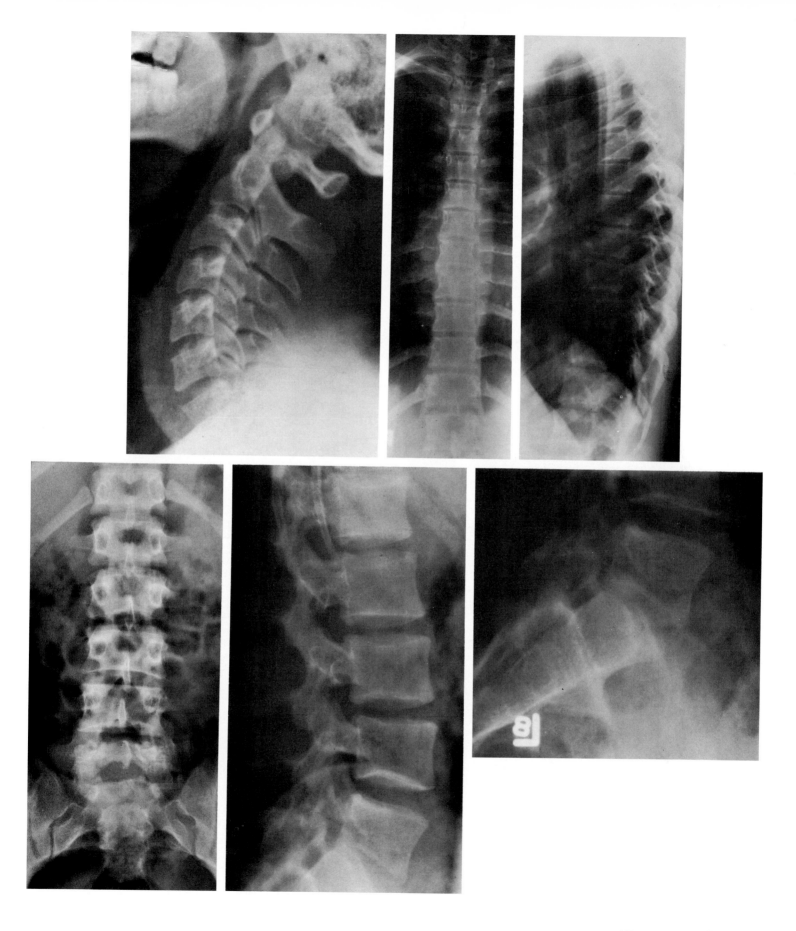

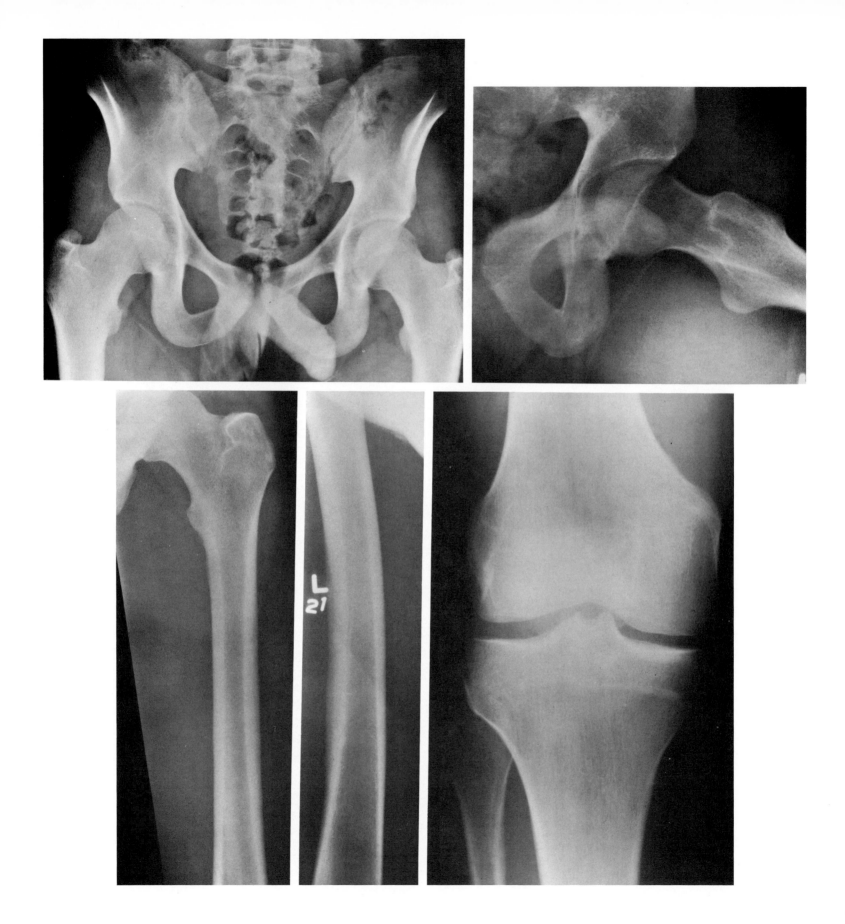

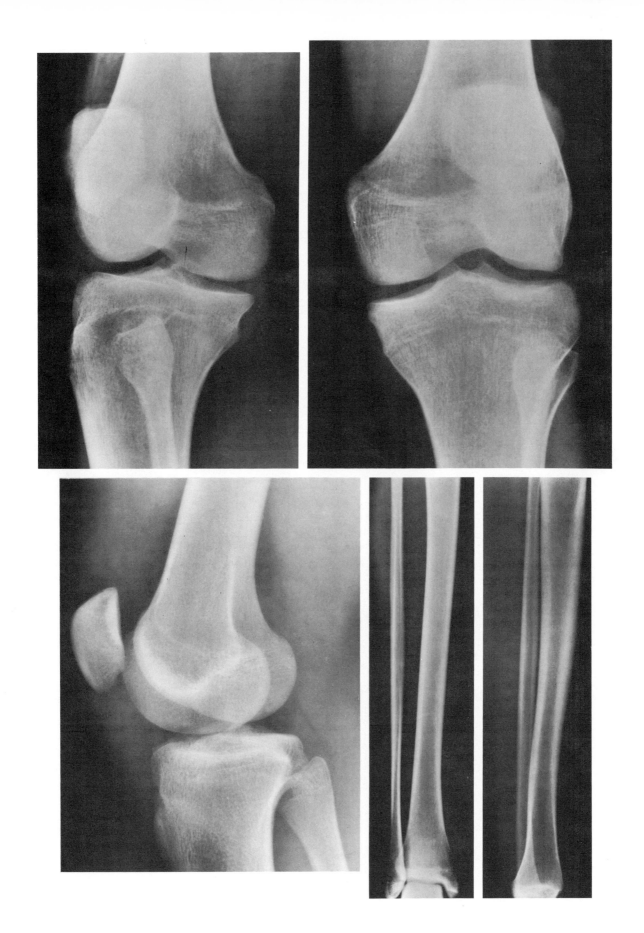

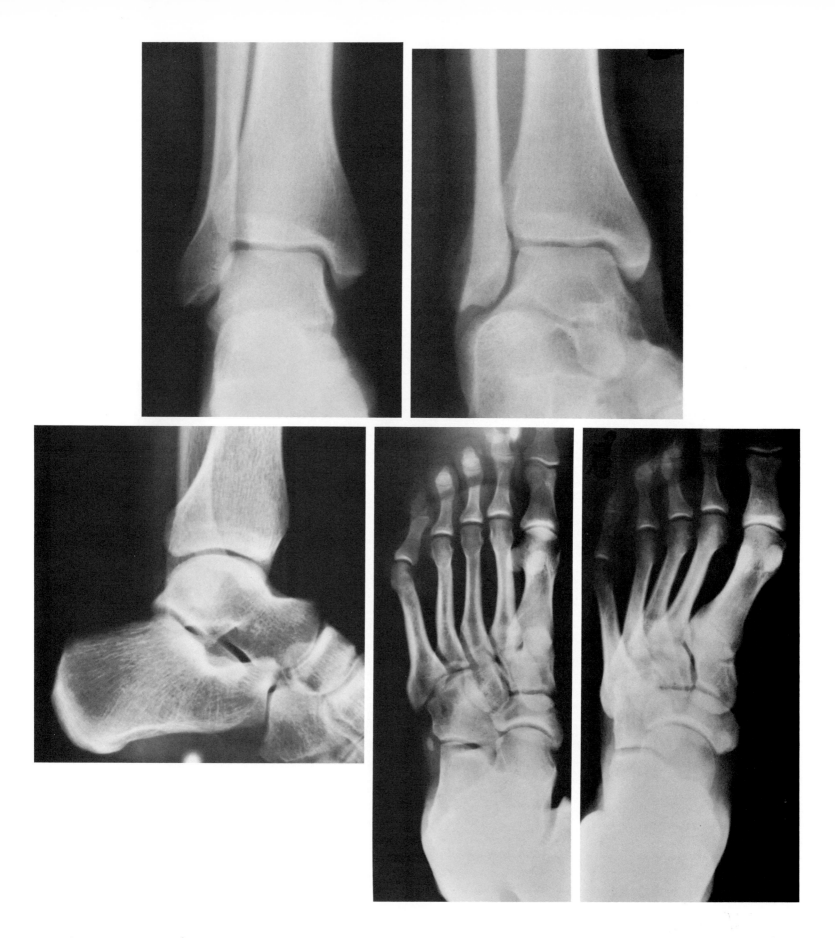

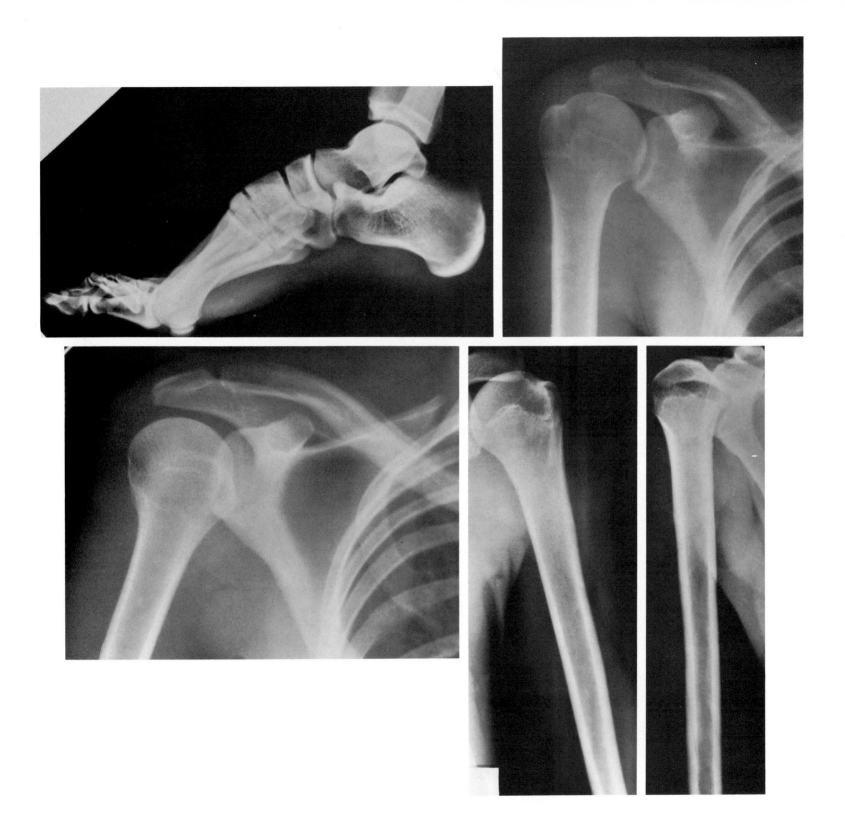

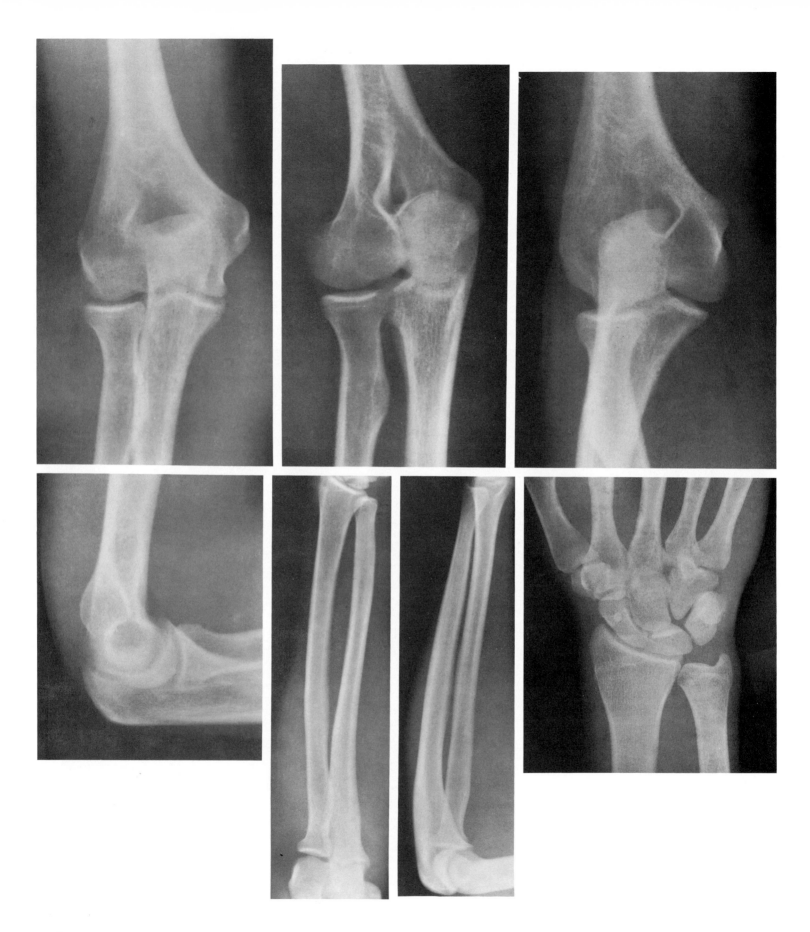

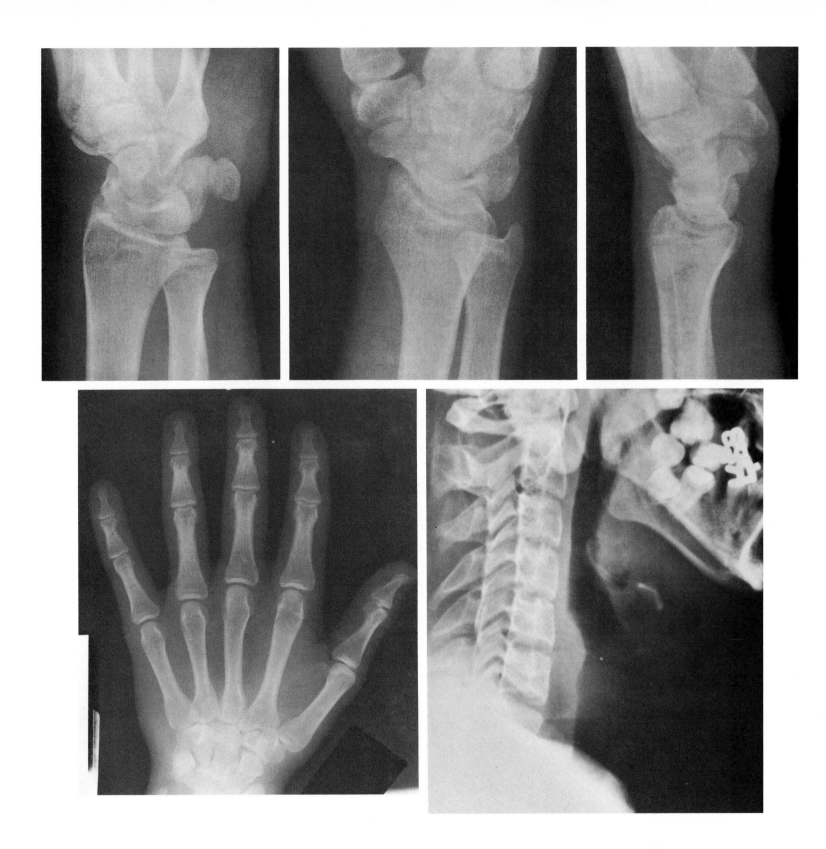

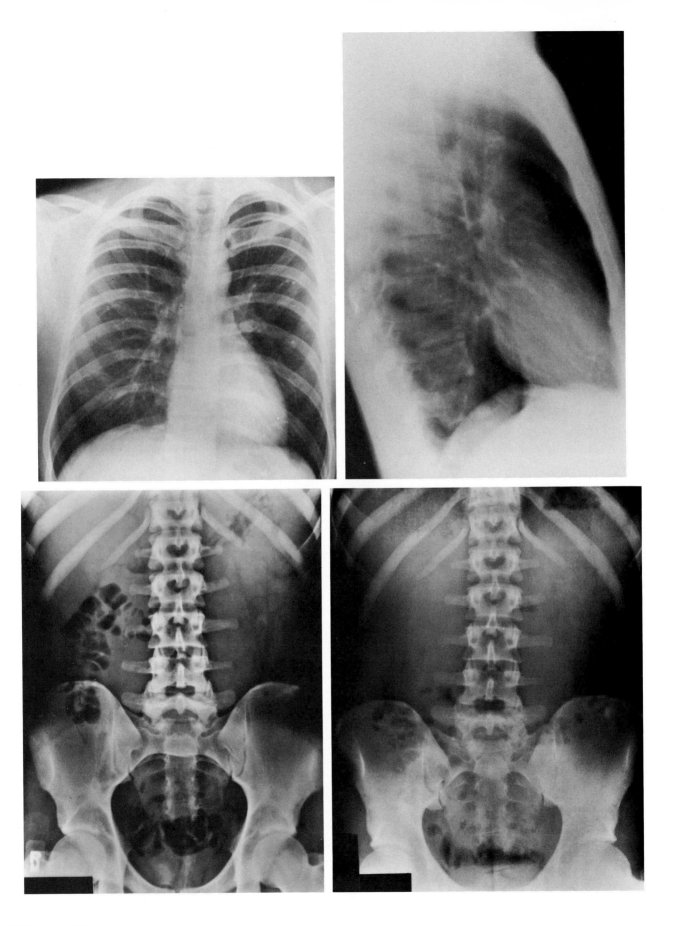

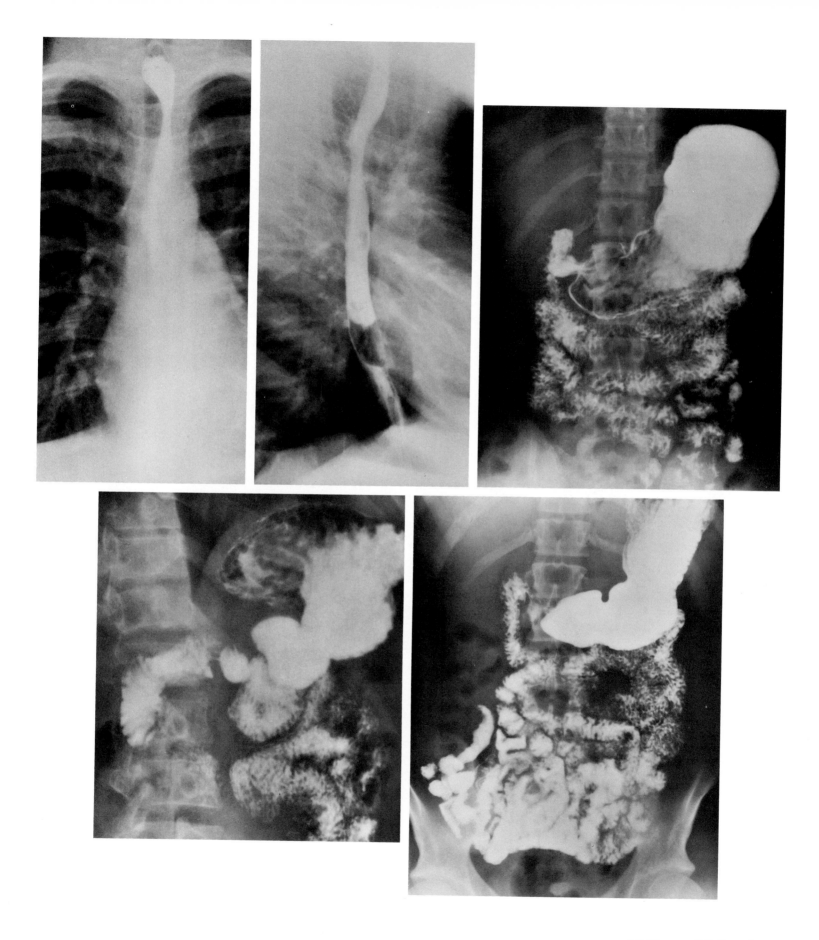

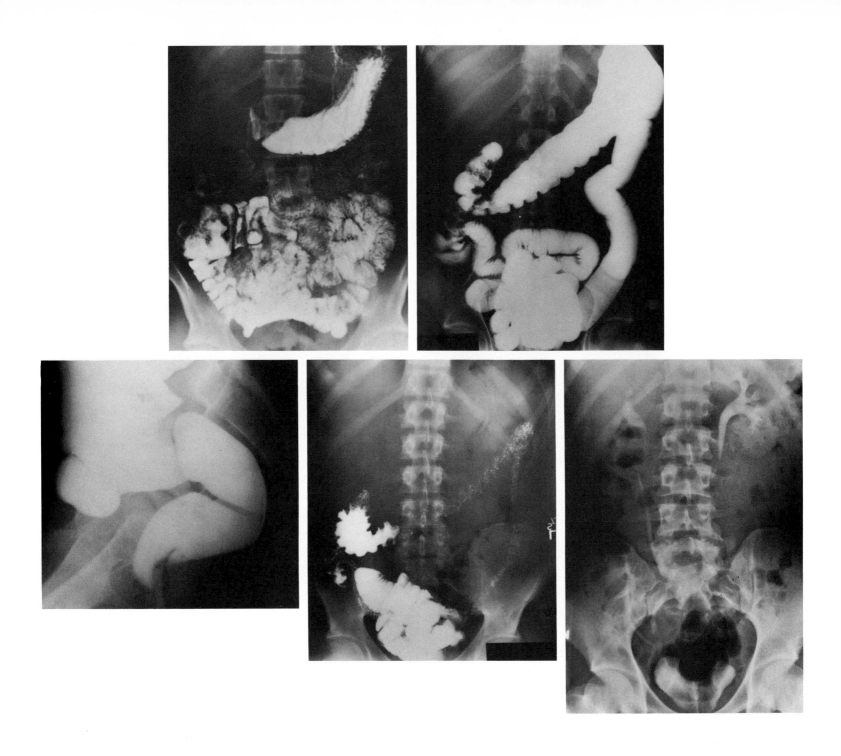

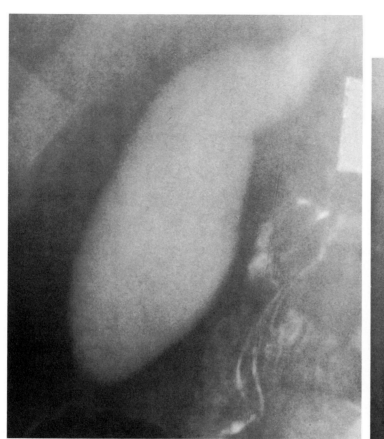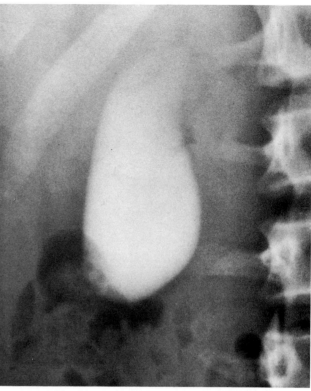

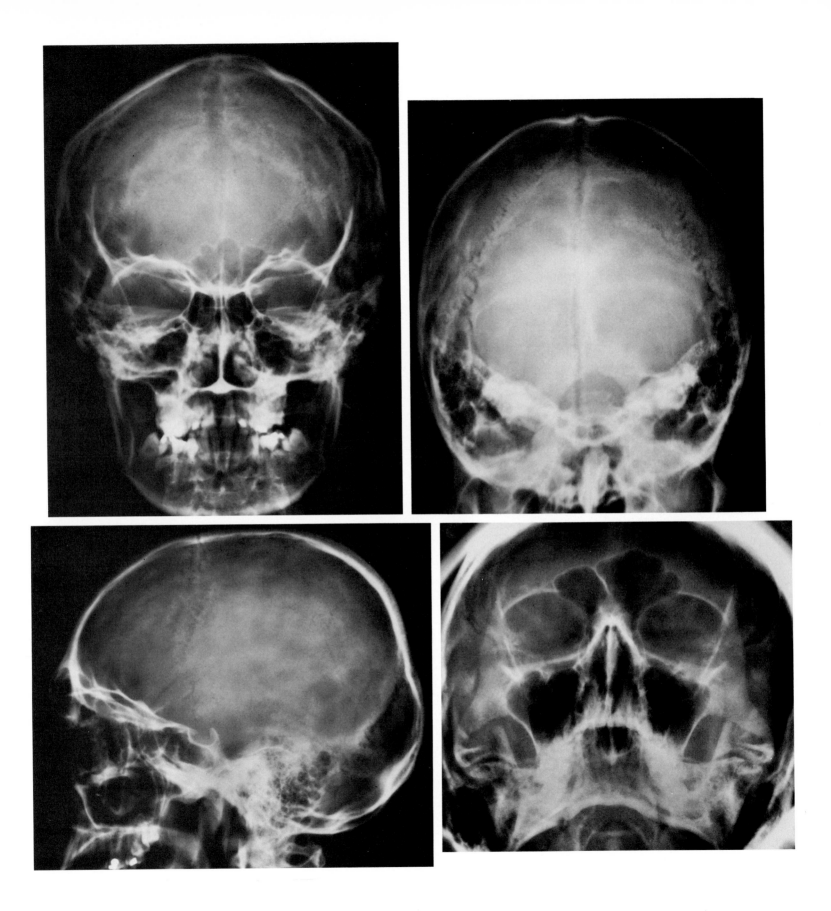

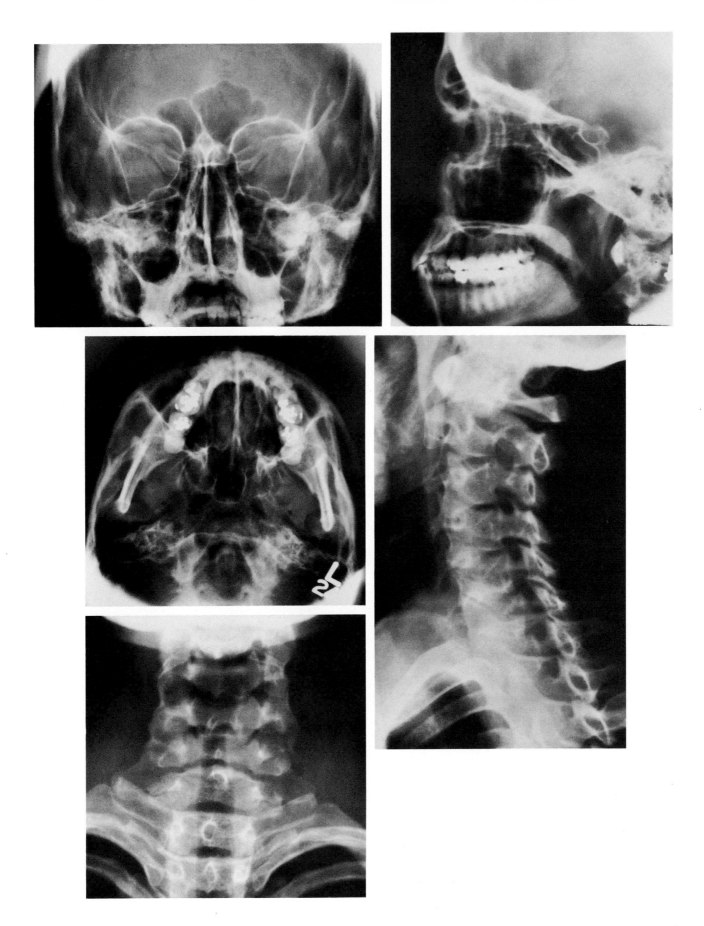

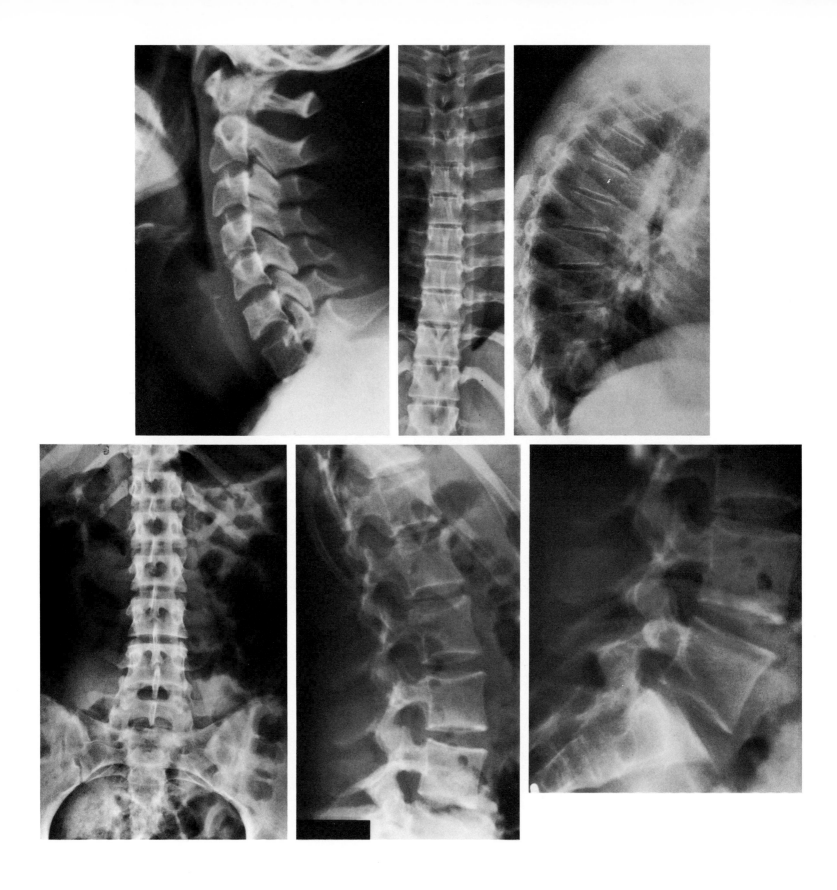

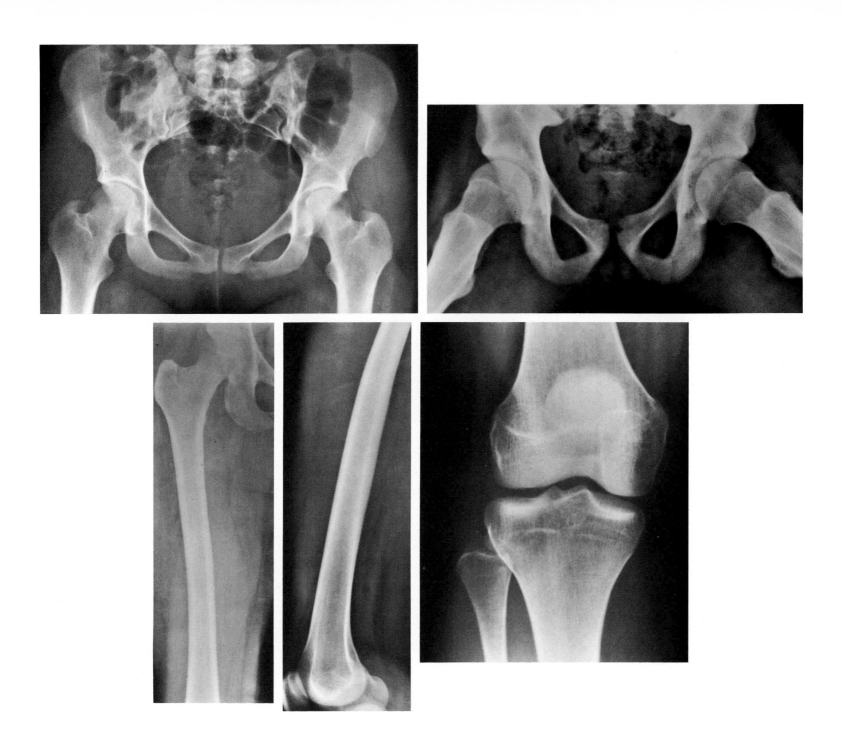

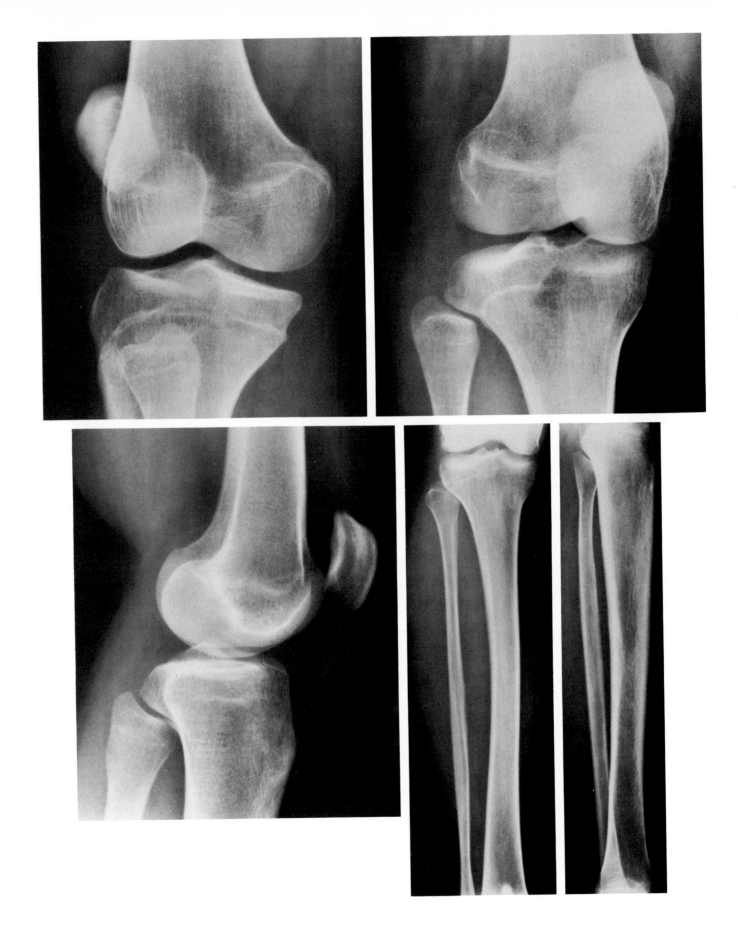

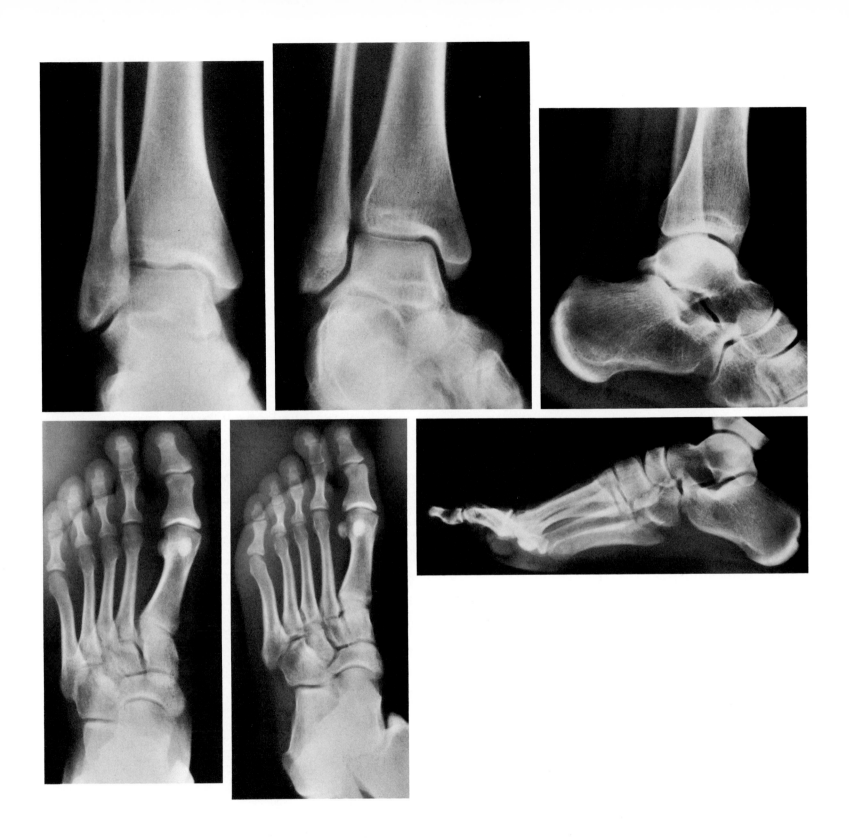

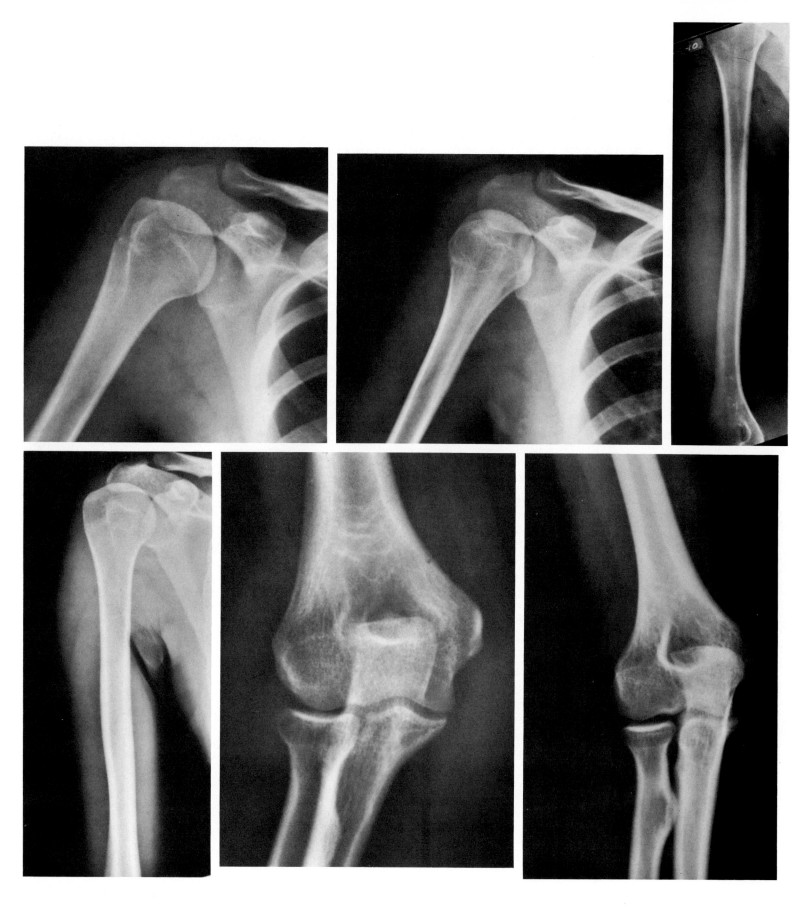

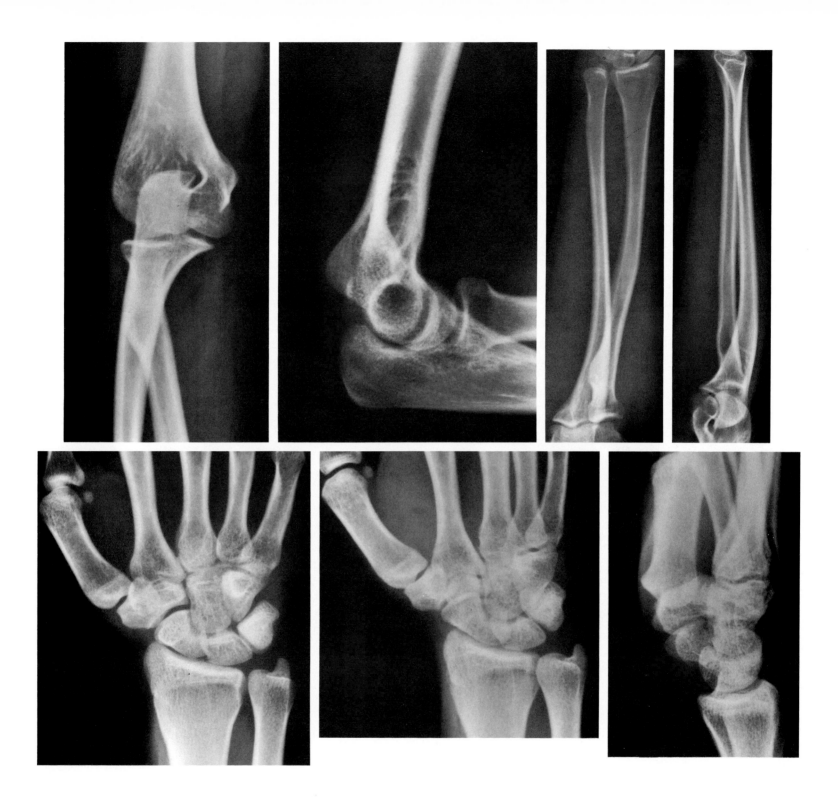

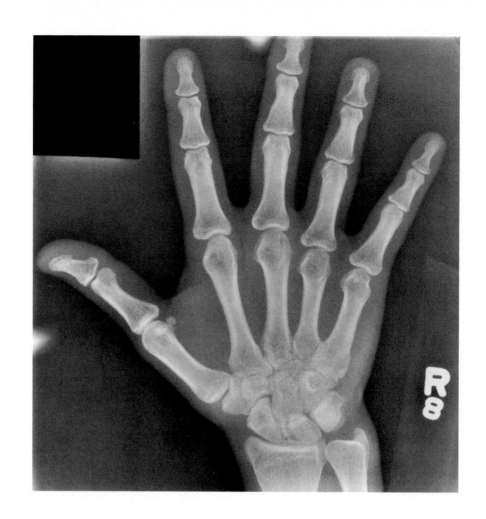

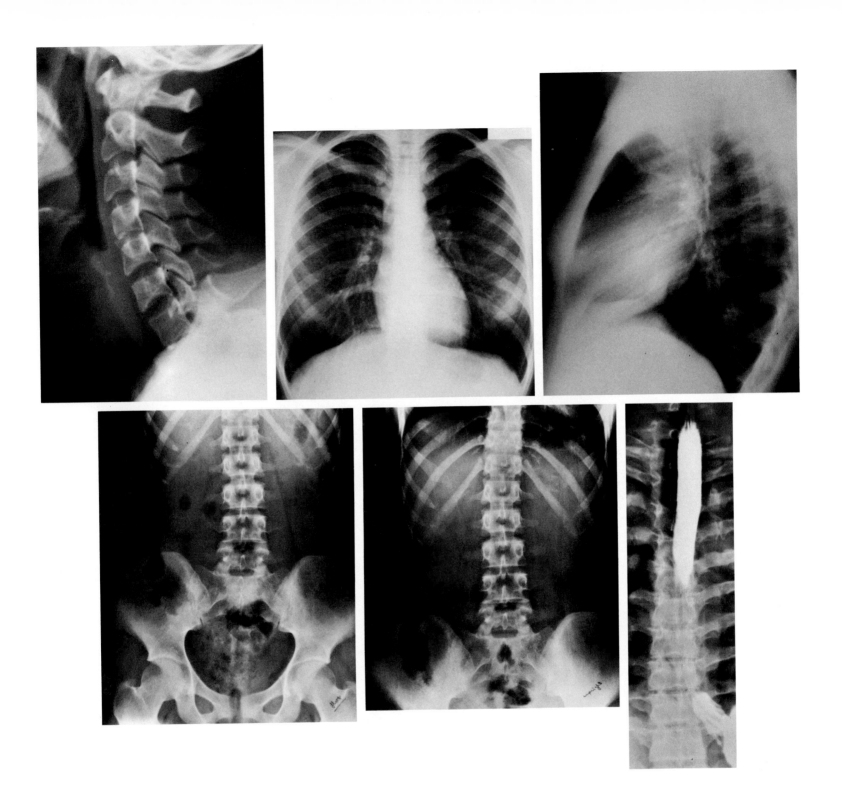

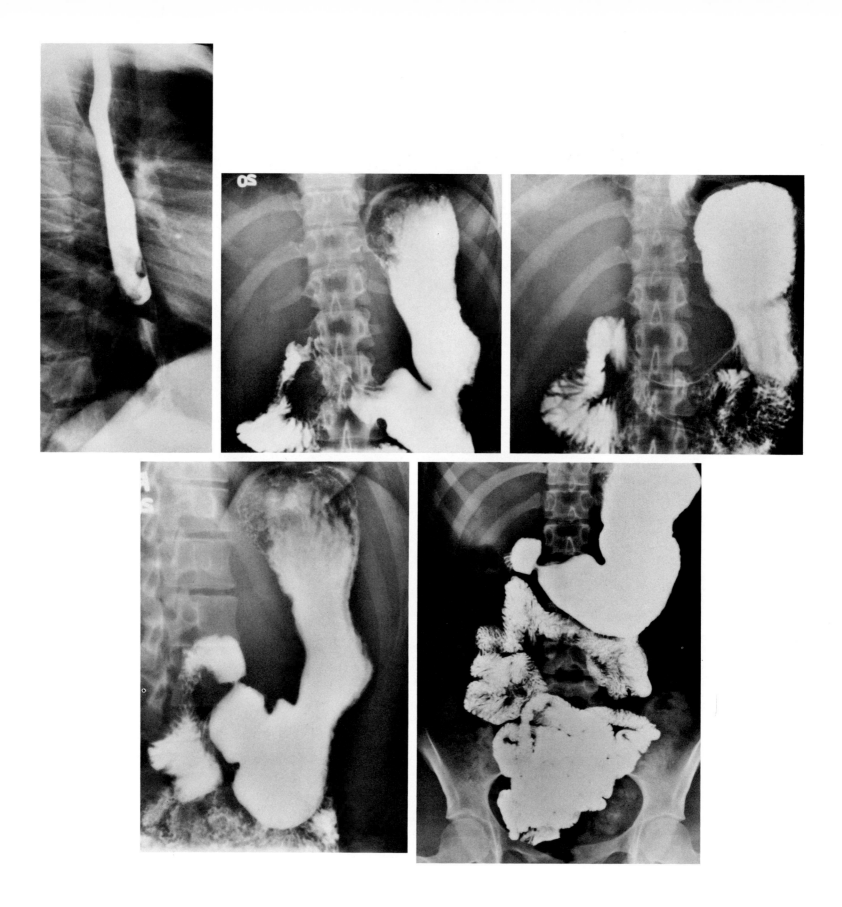

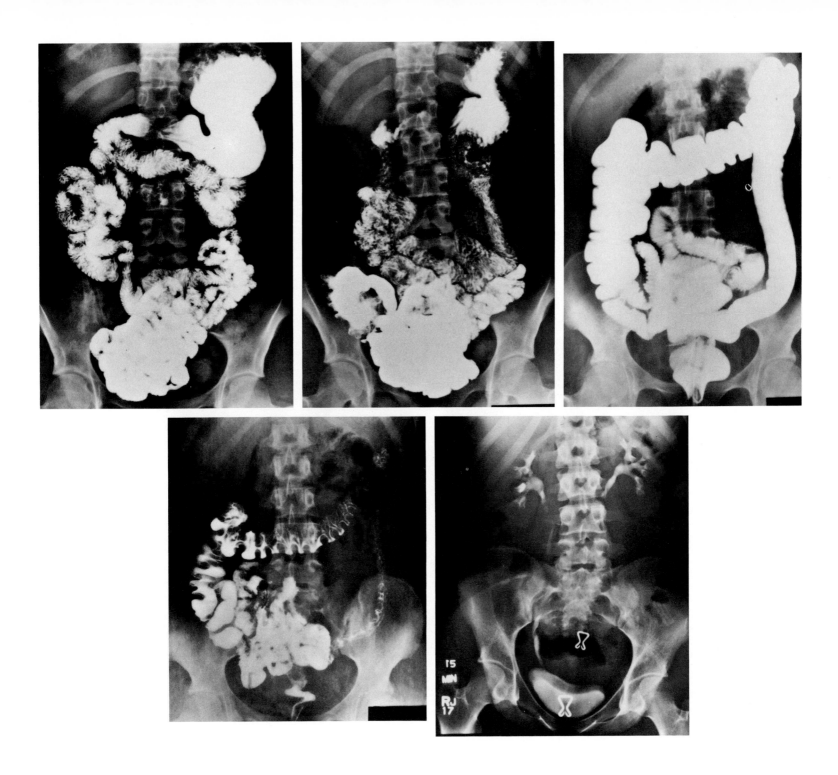

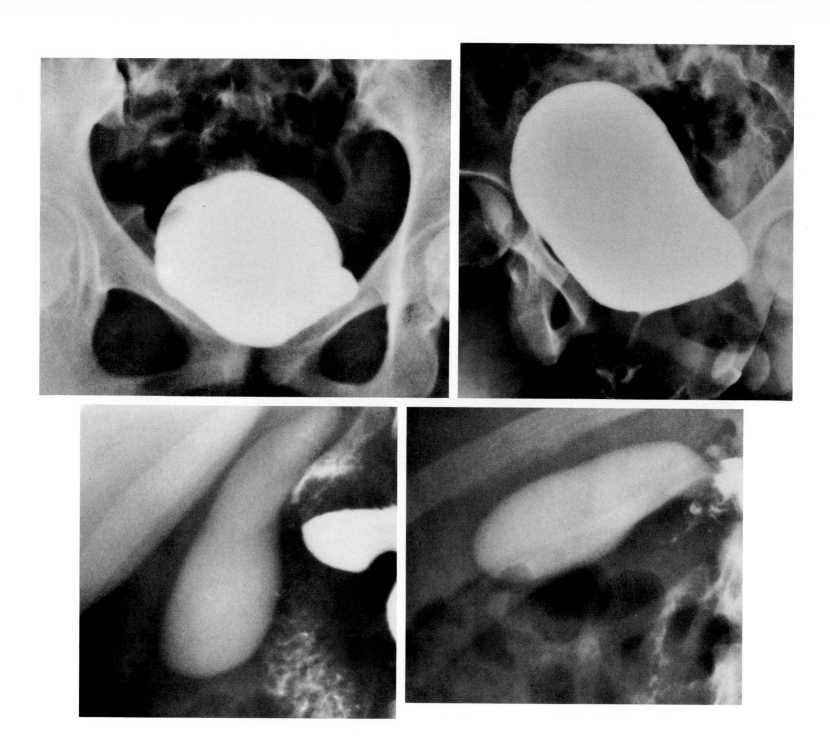

27

19 YEARS

Epiphyses are closed, but the lines of the closed plates are still evident.

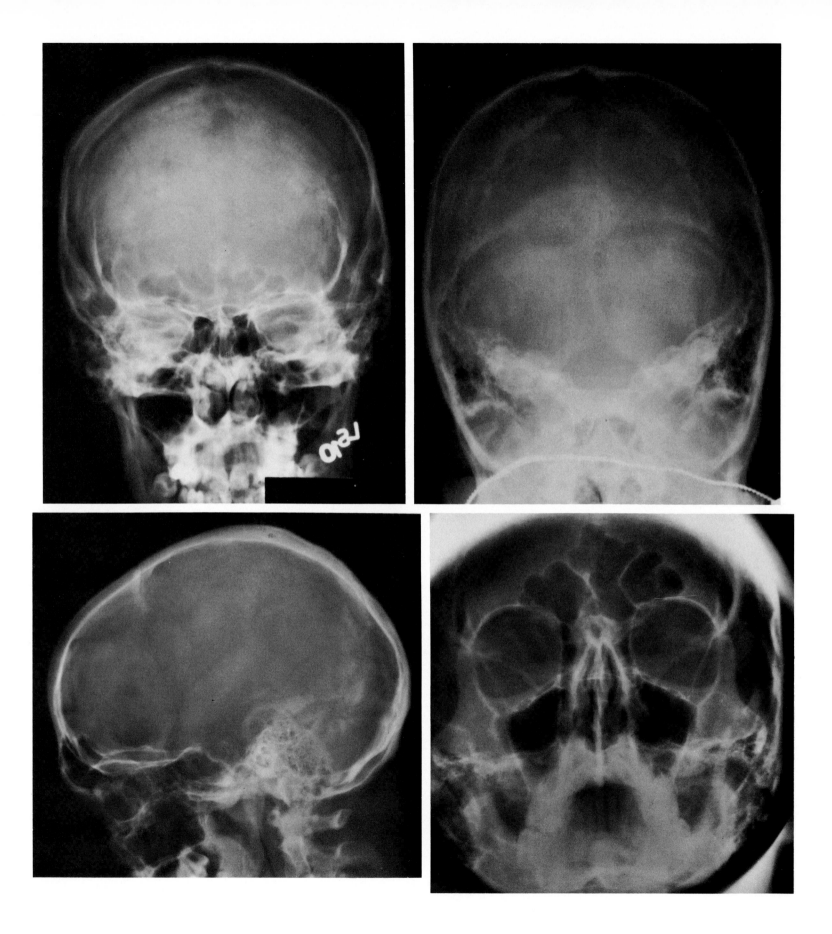

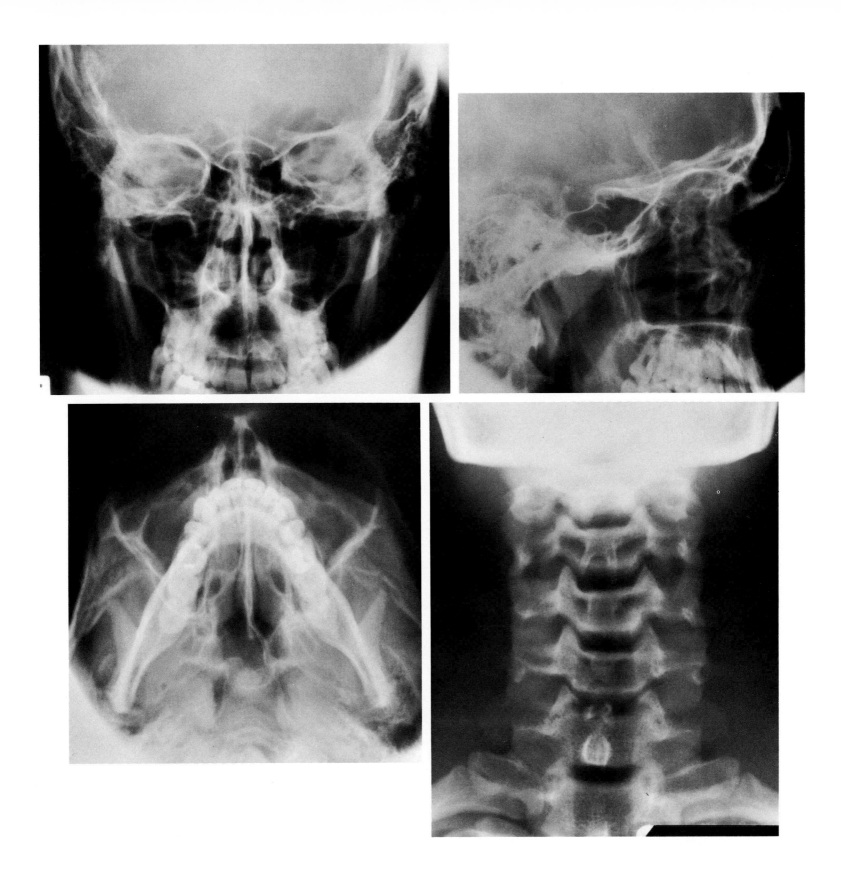

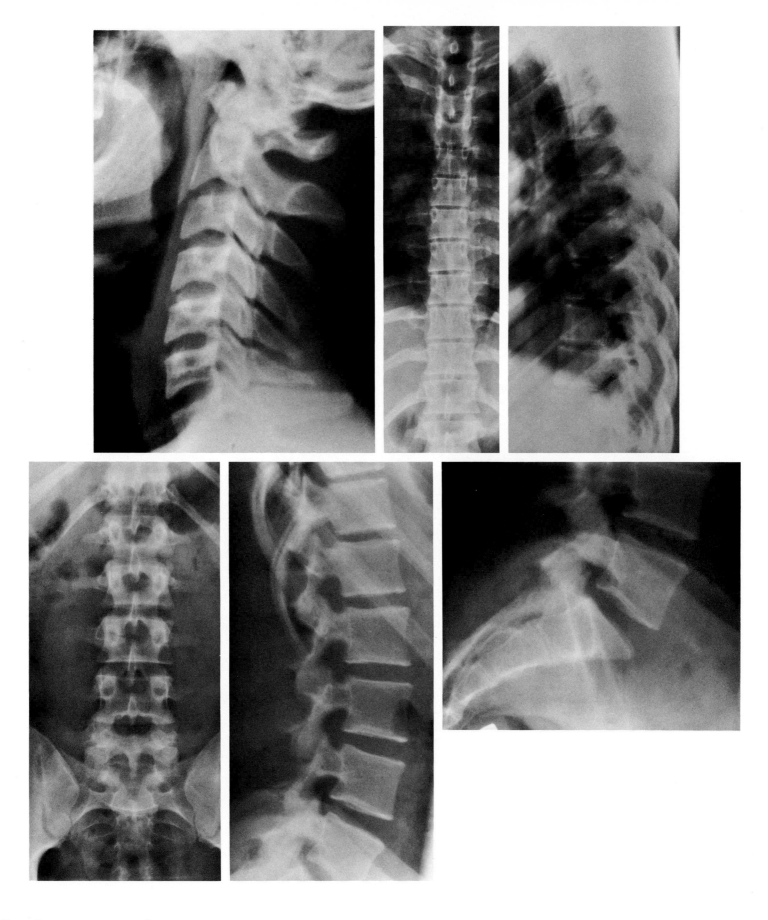

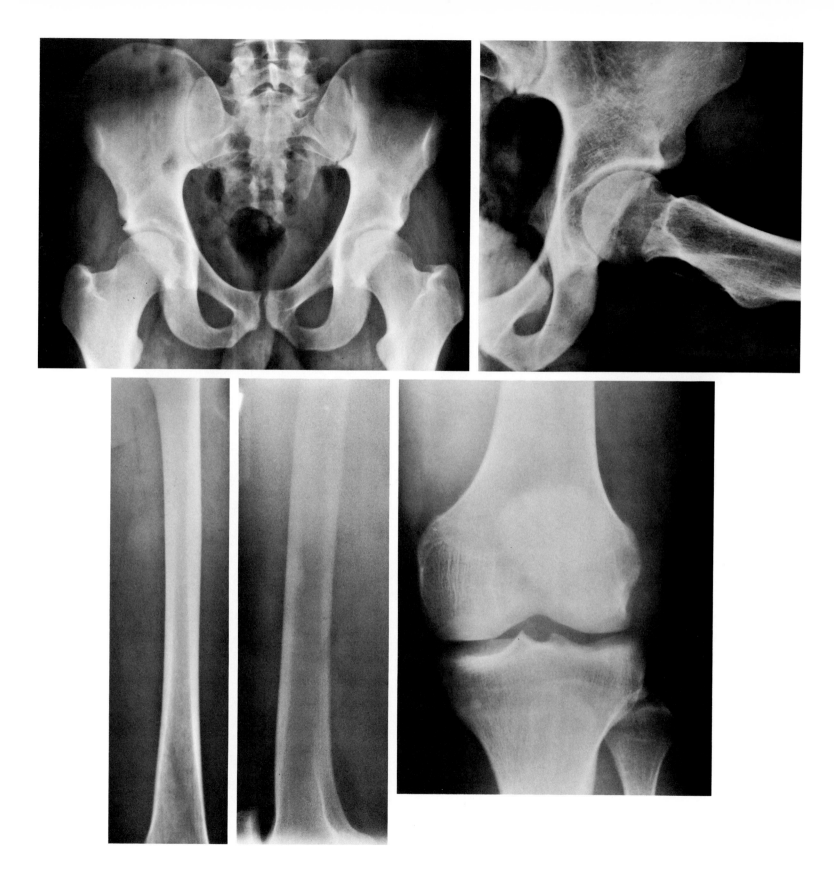

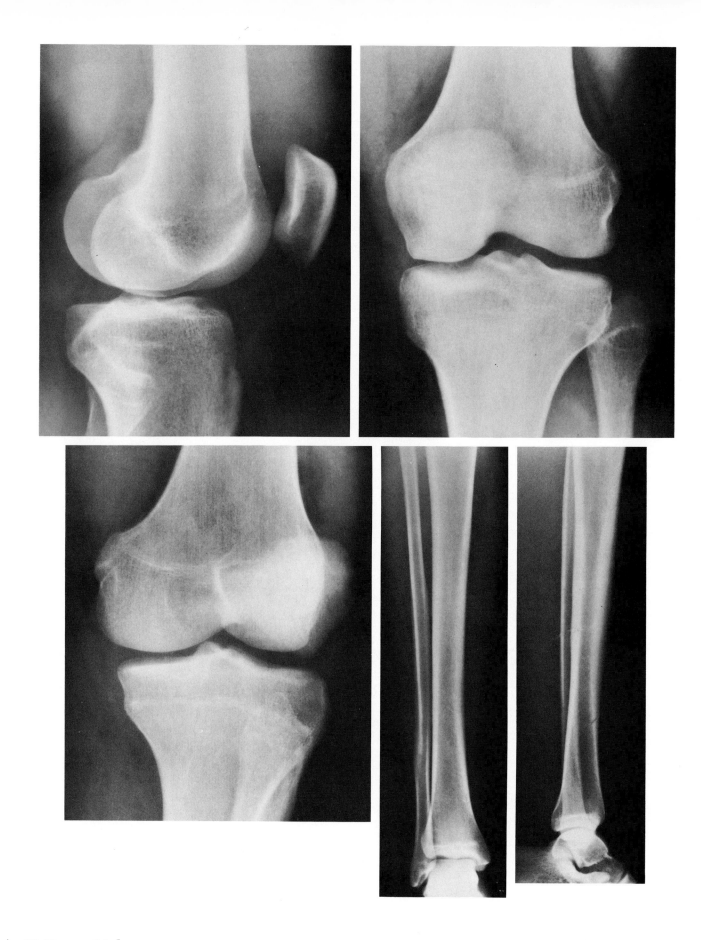

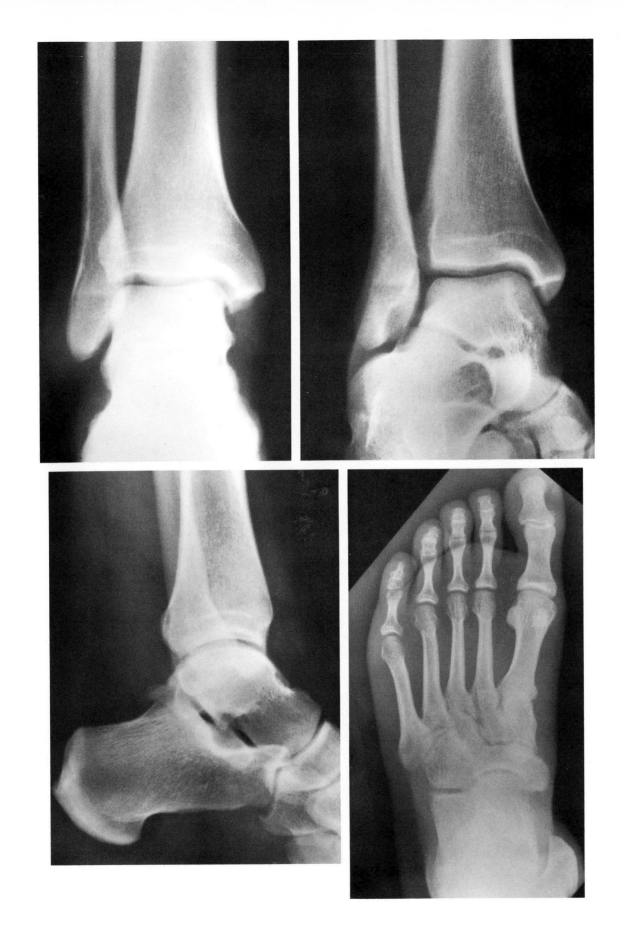

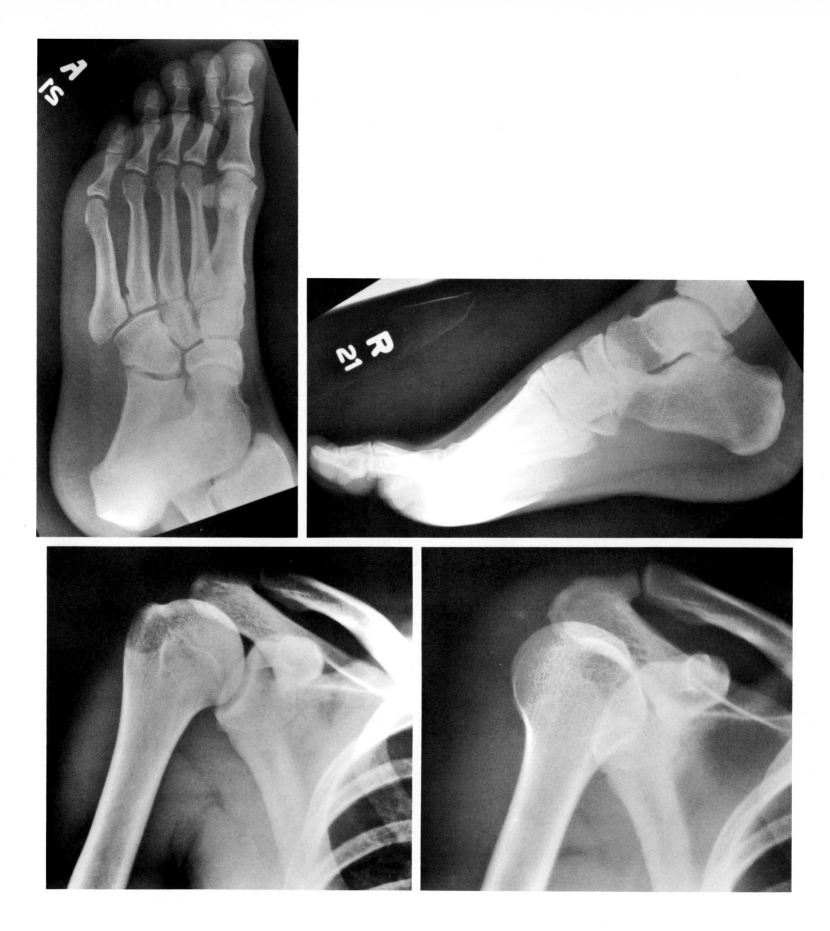

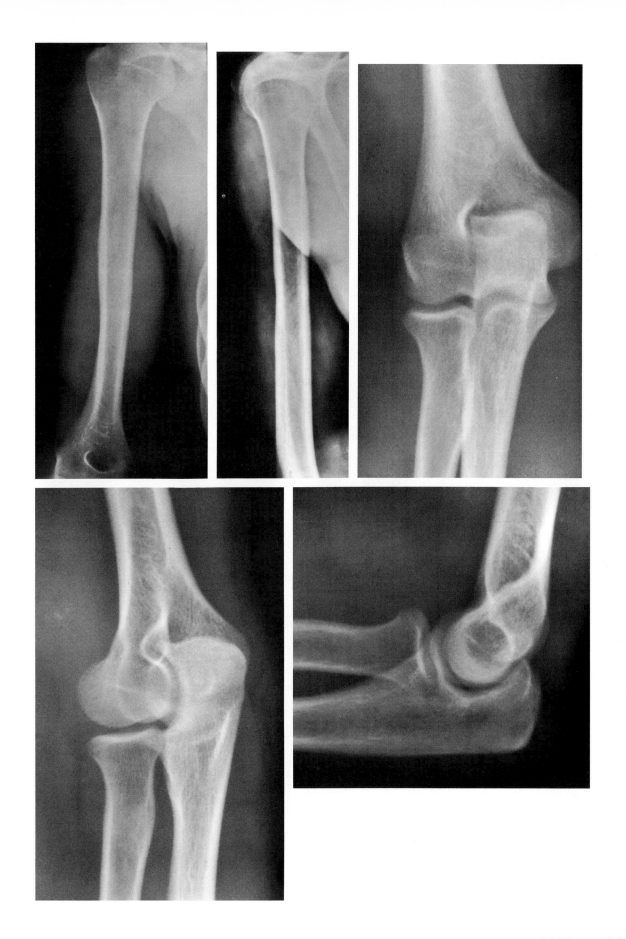

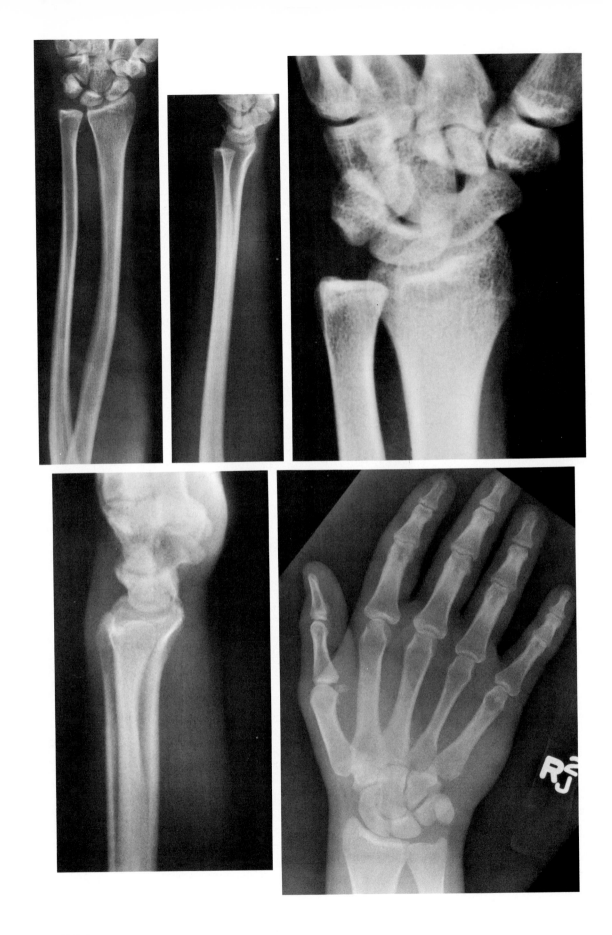

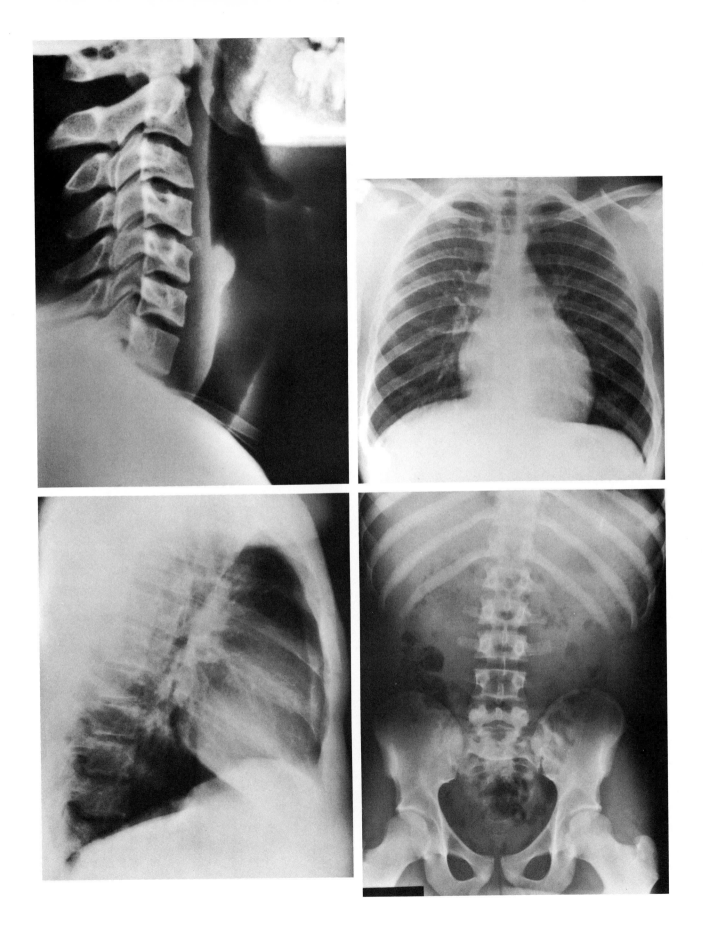

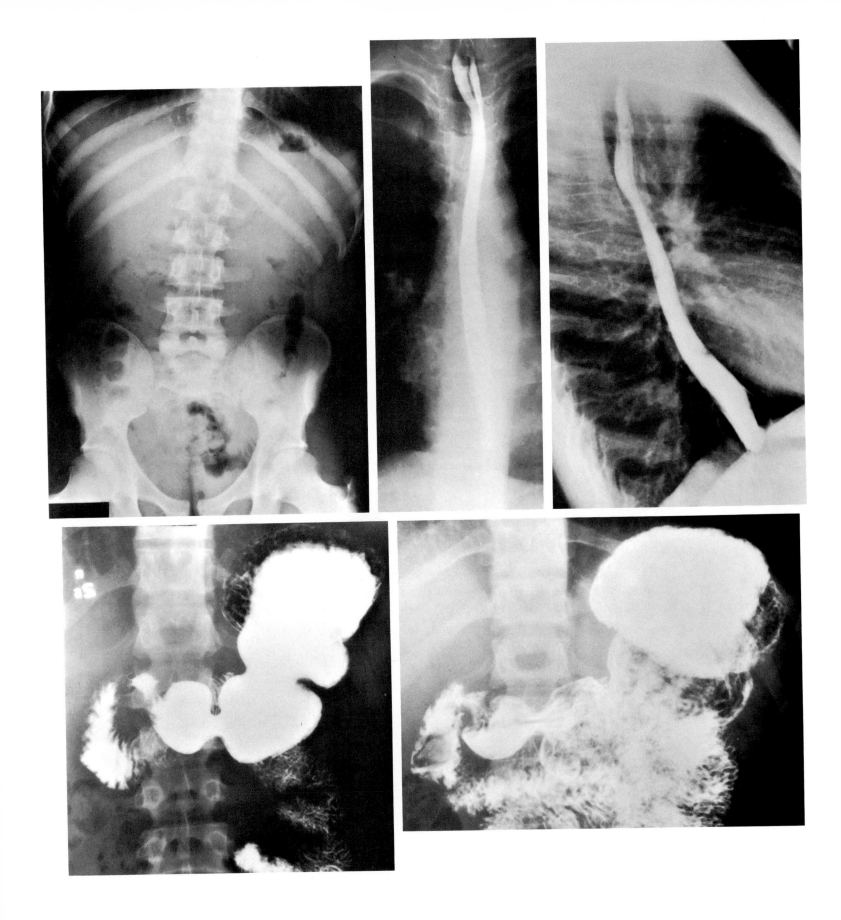

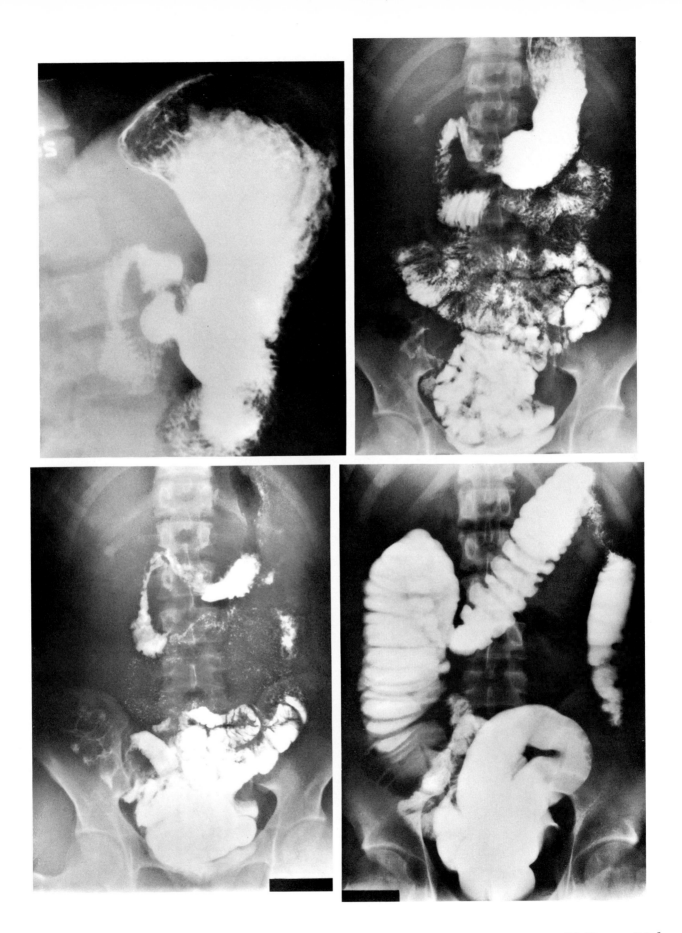

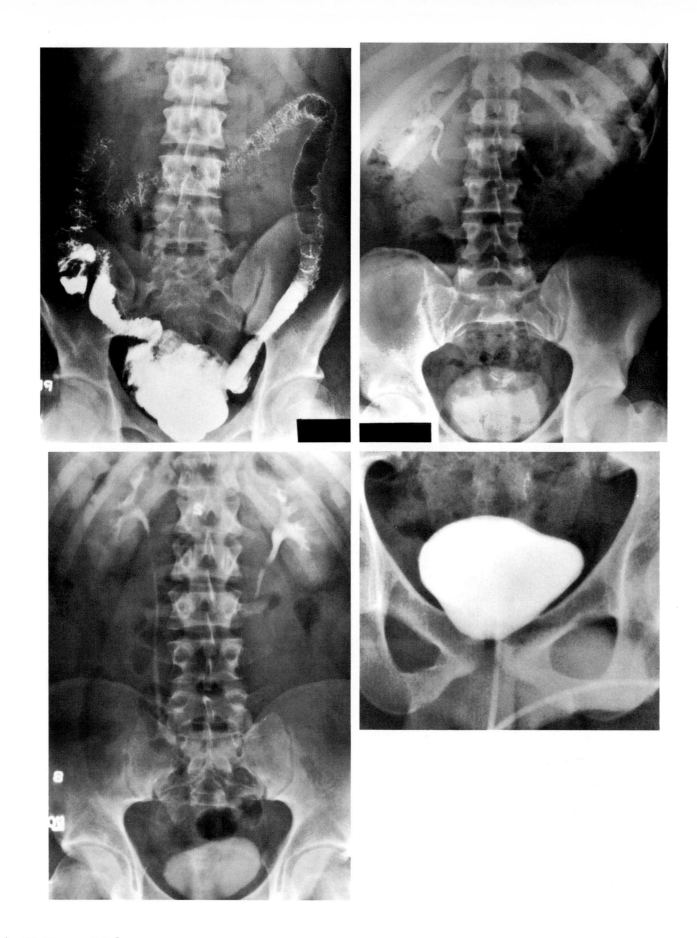

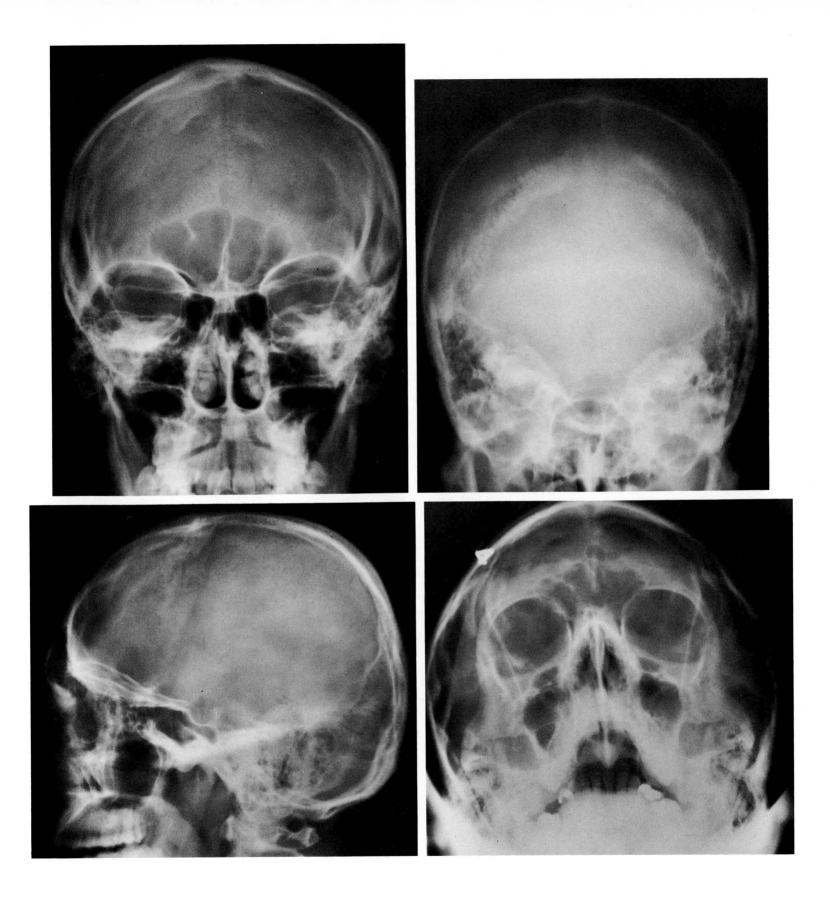

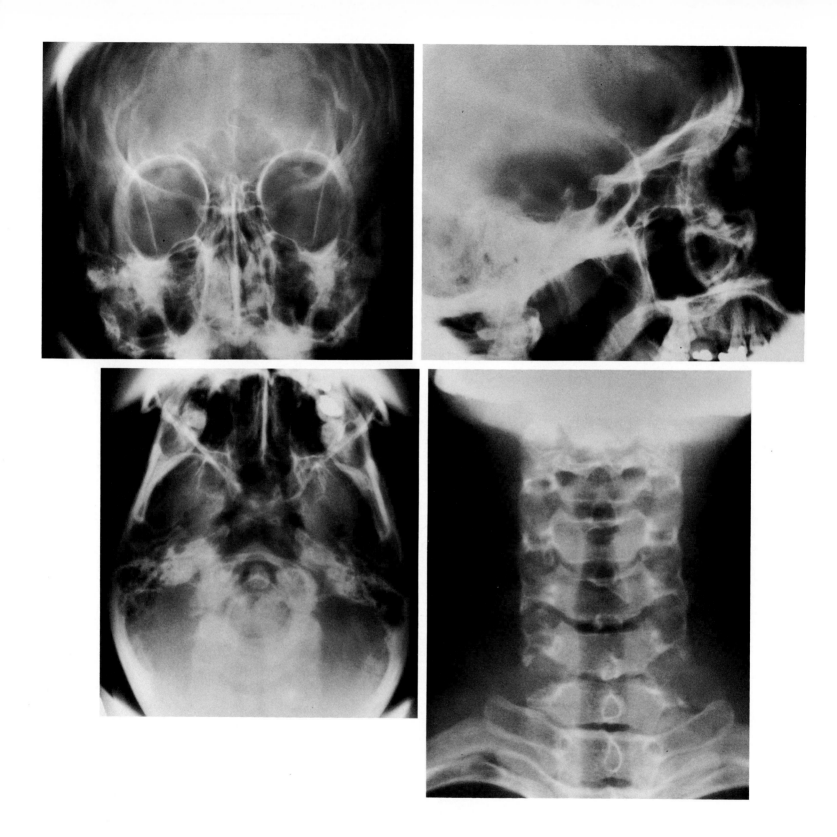

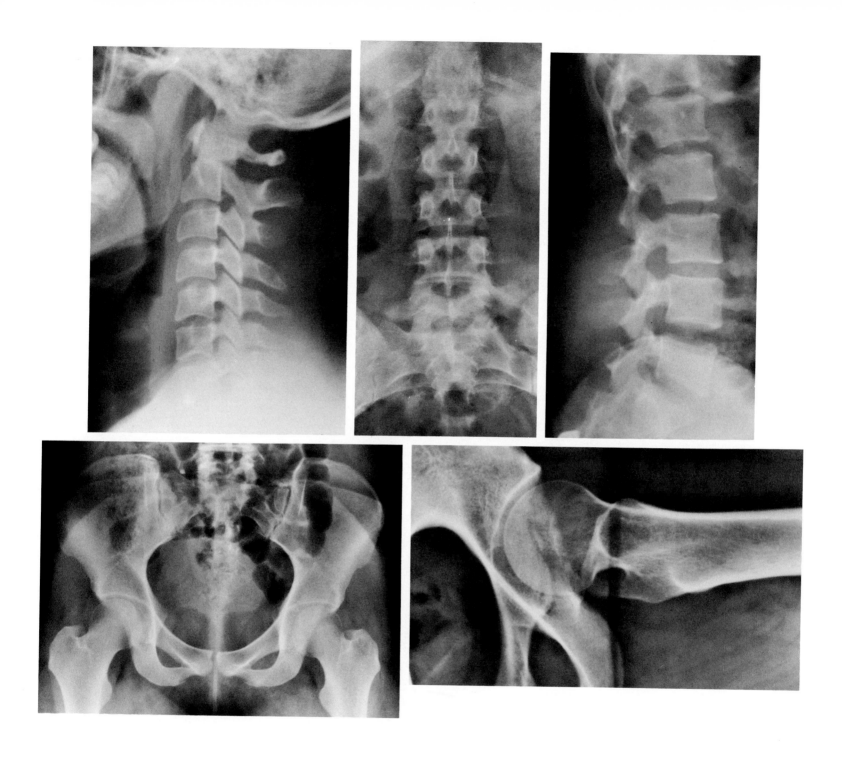

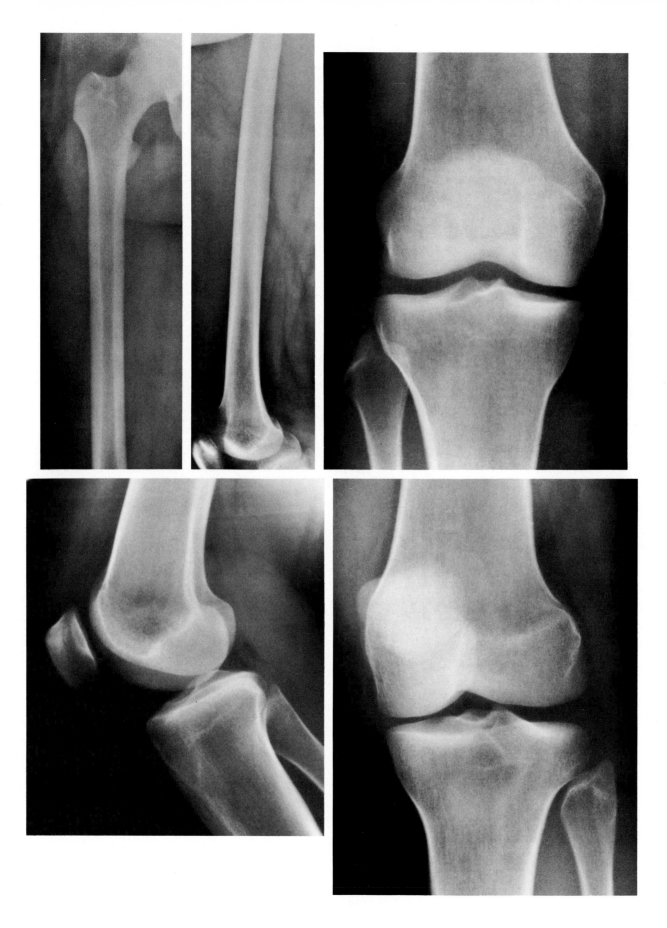

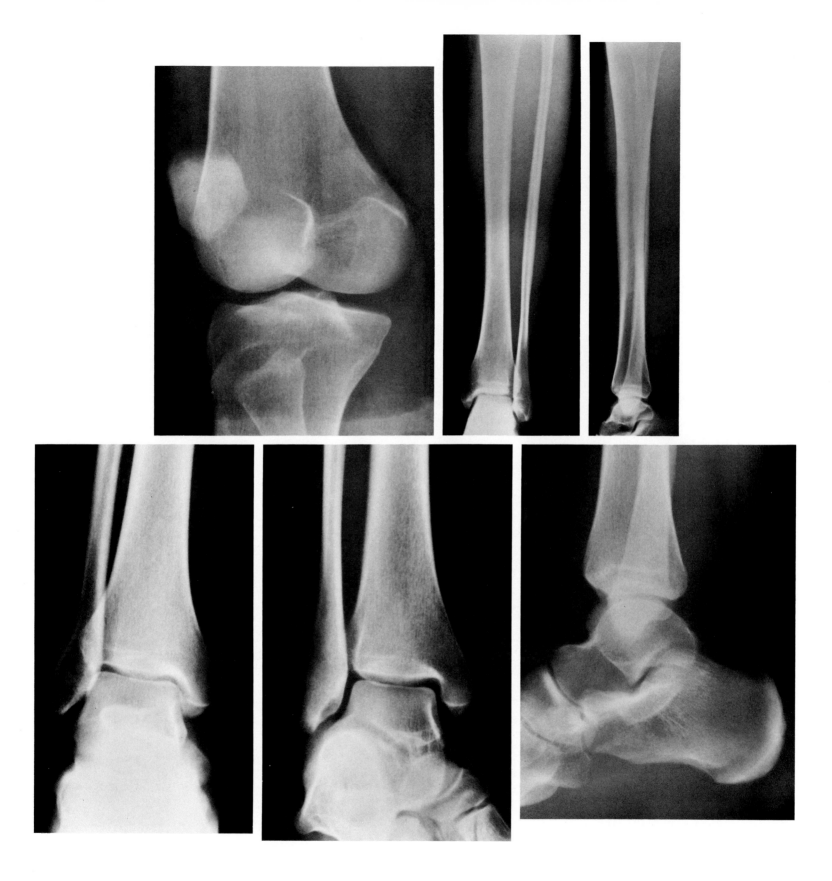

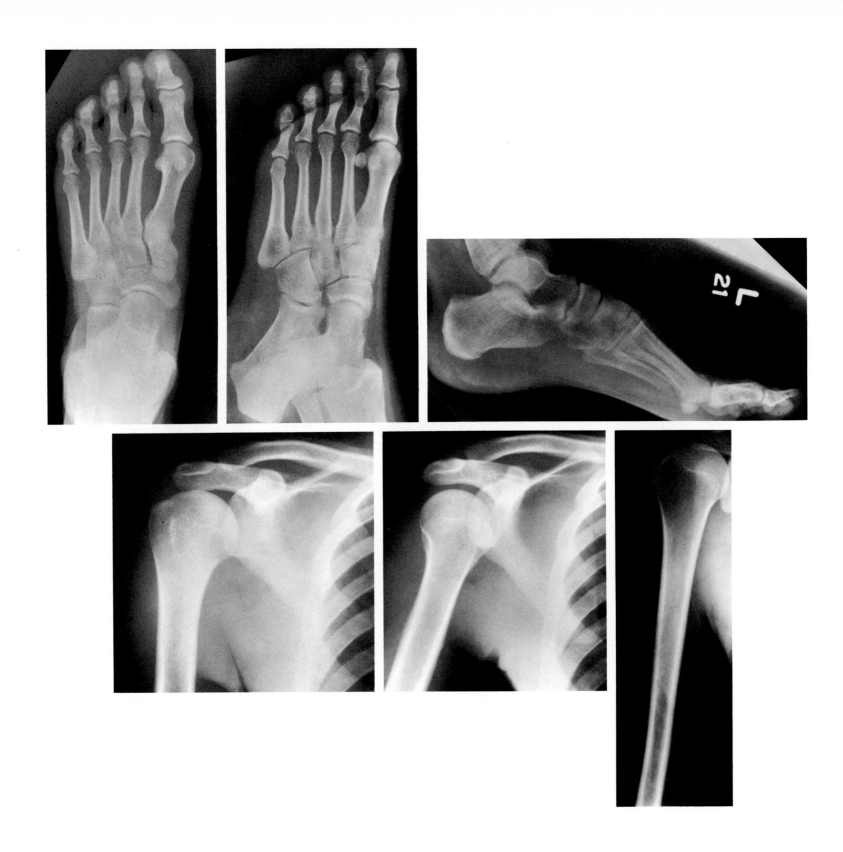

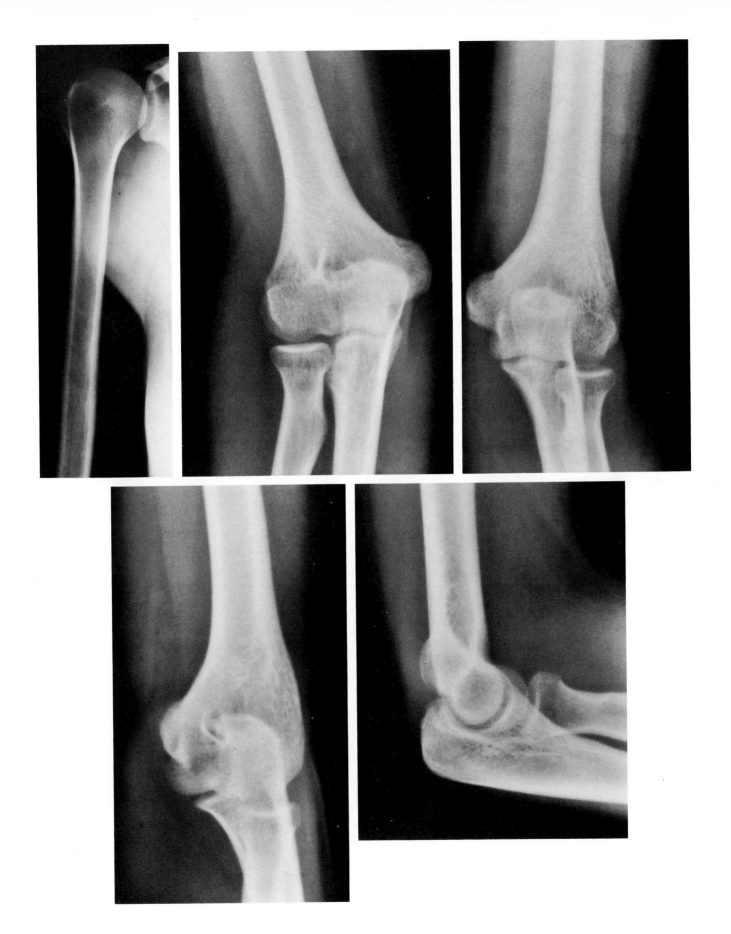

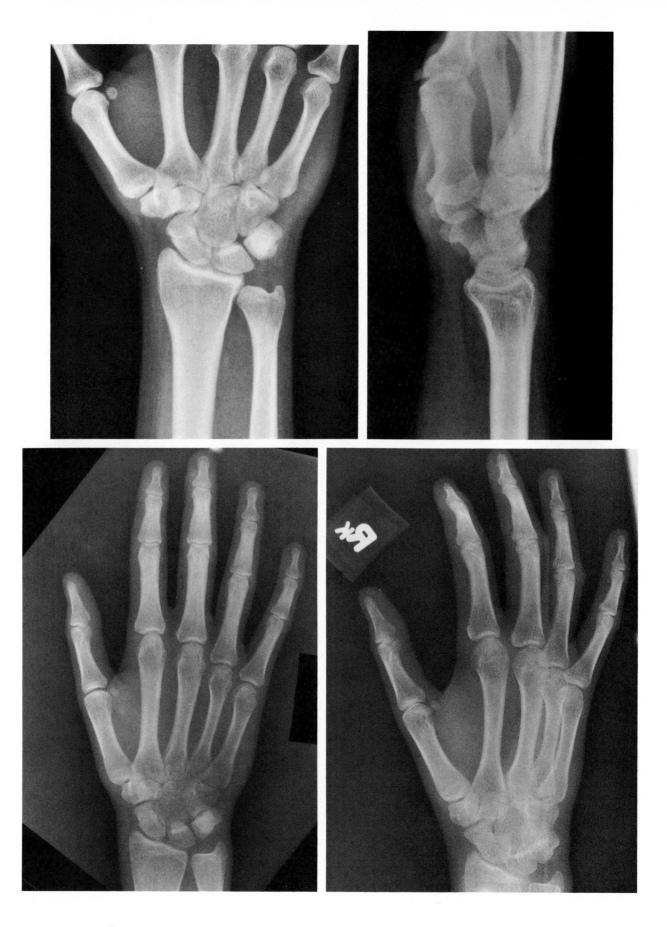

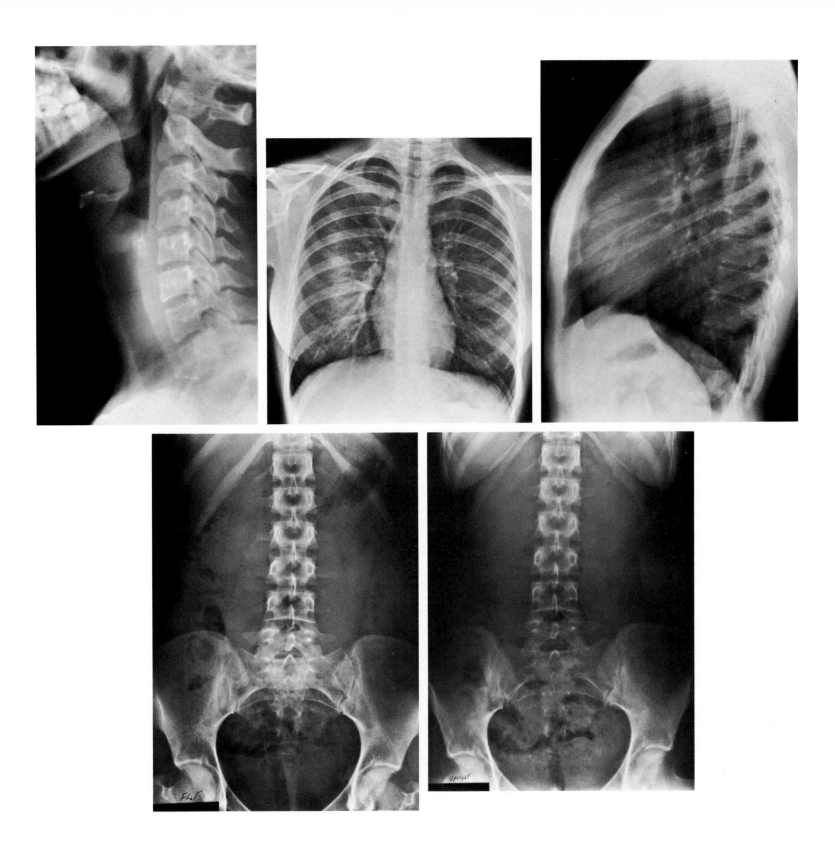

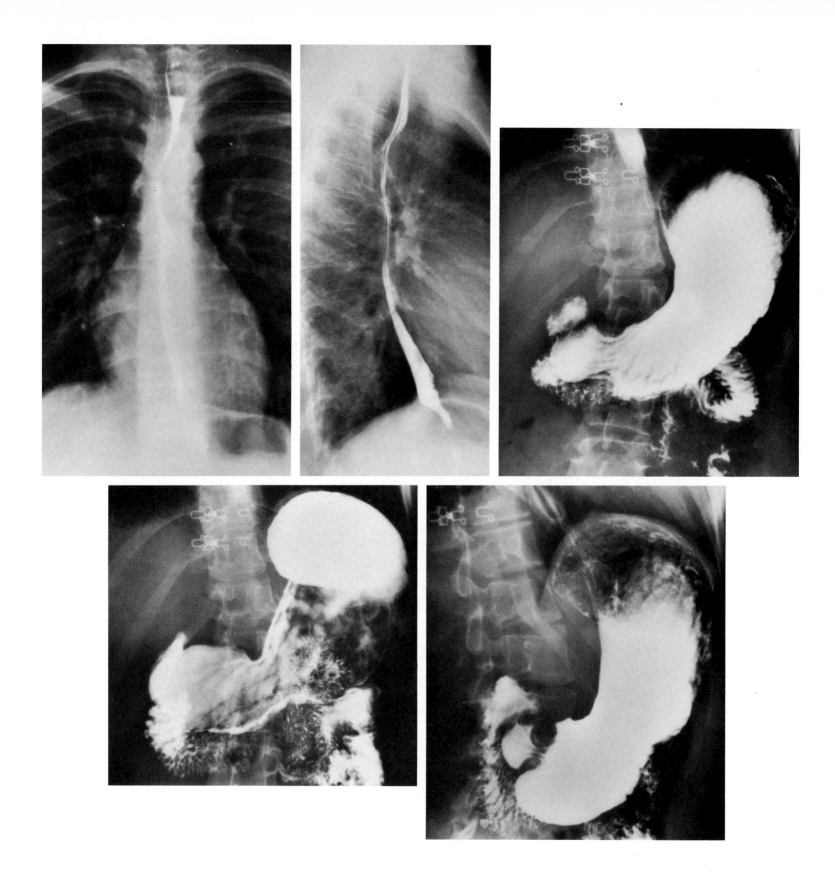

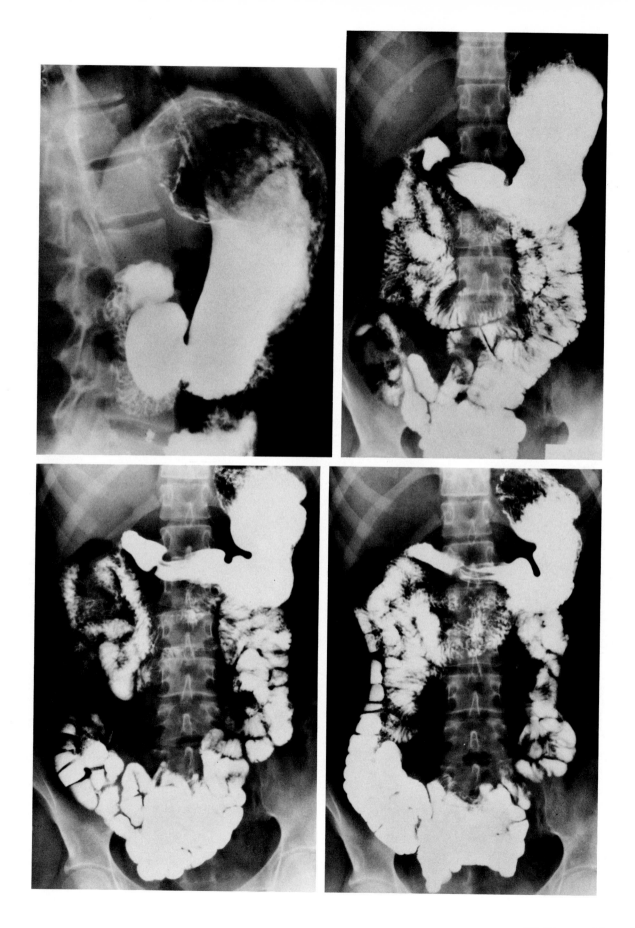

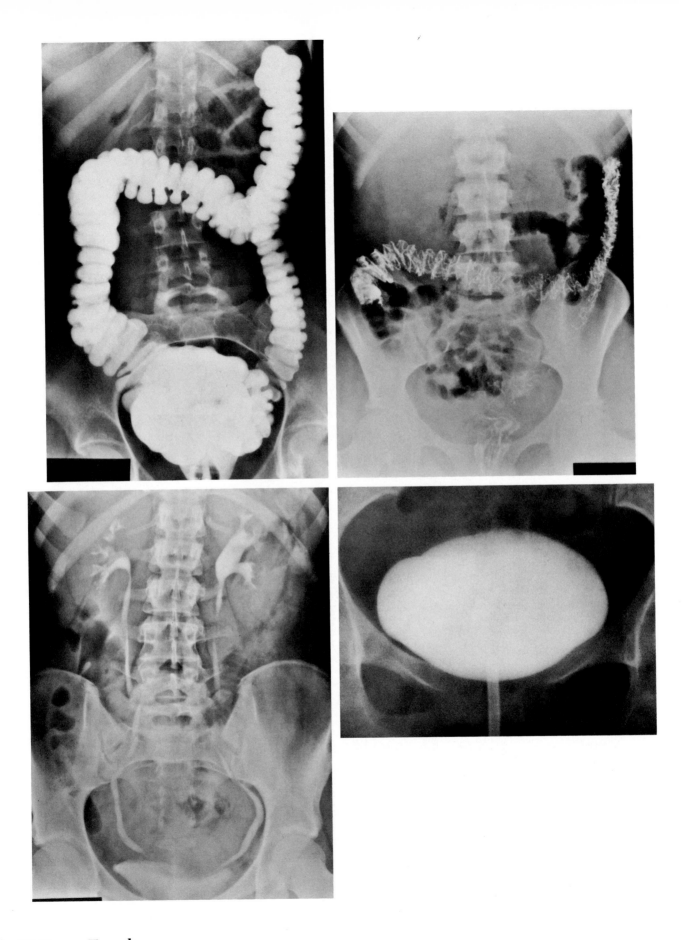

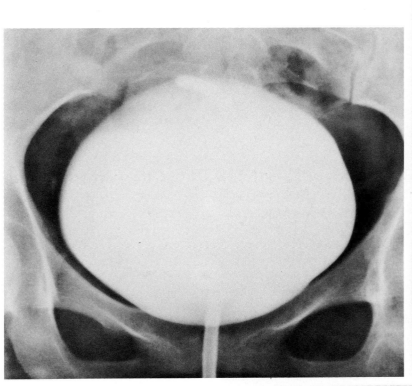

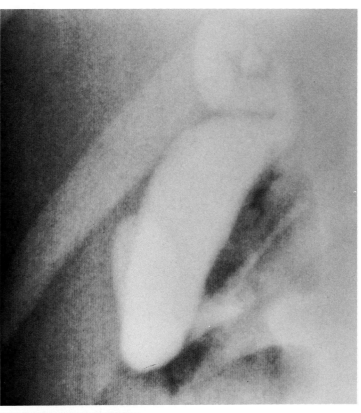

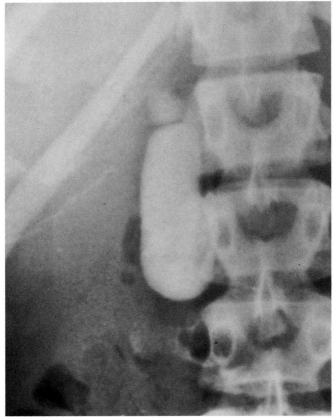

28

20 YEARS

The remnants of the epiphyseal plates are still evident. Otherwise adult criteria apply.

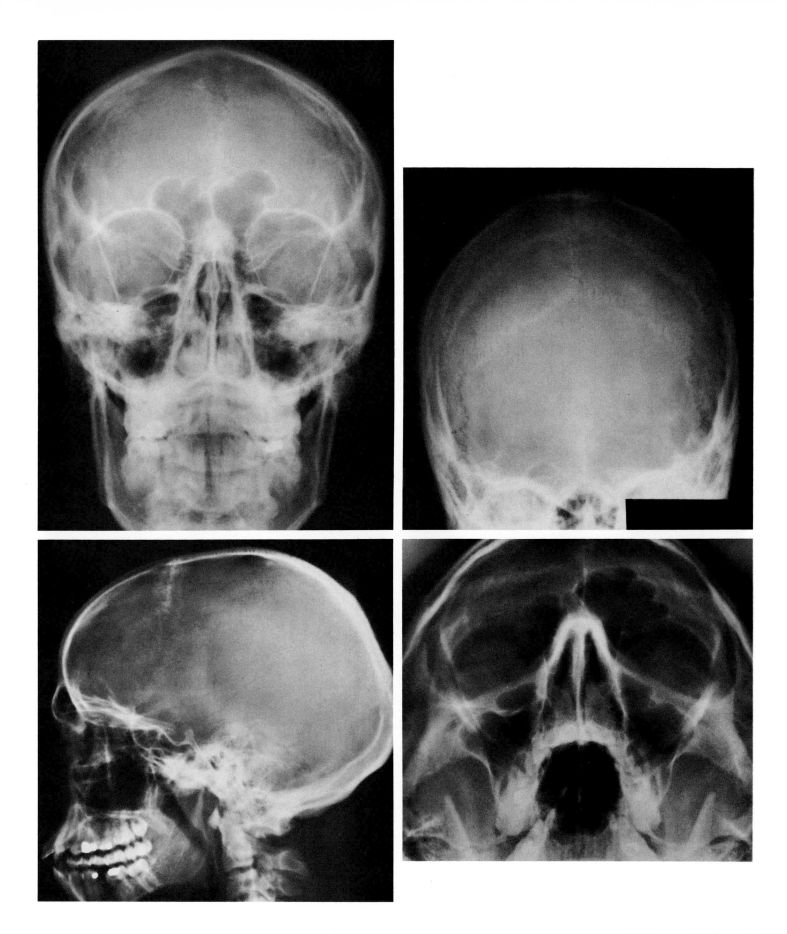

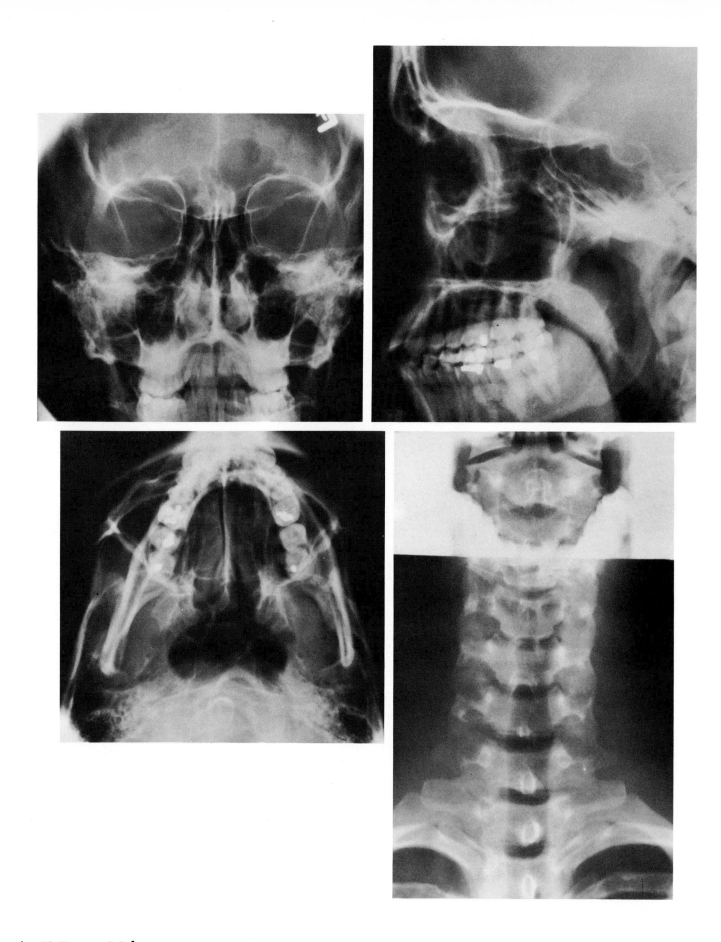

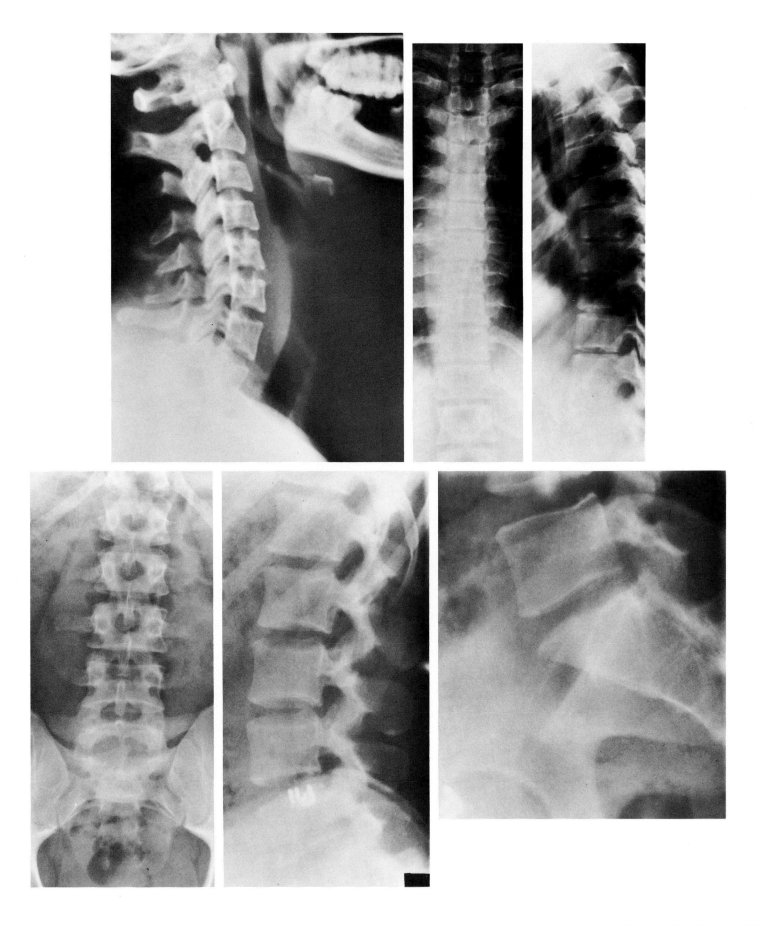

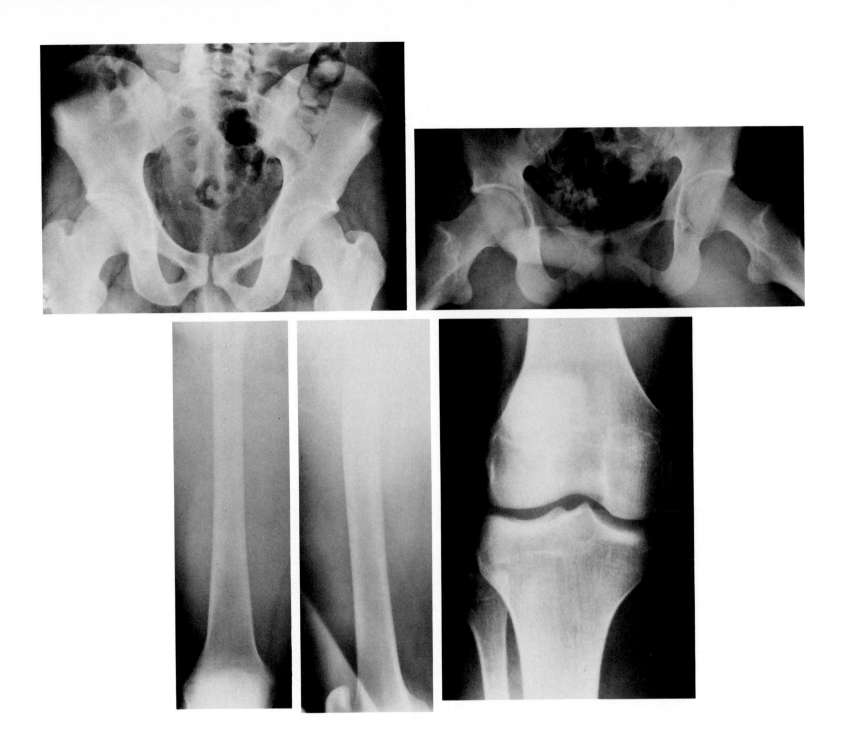

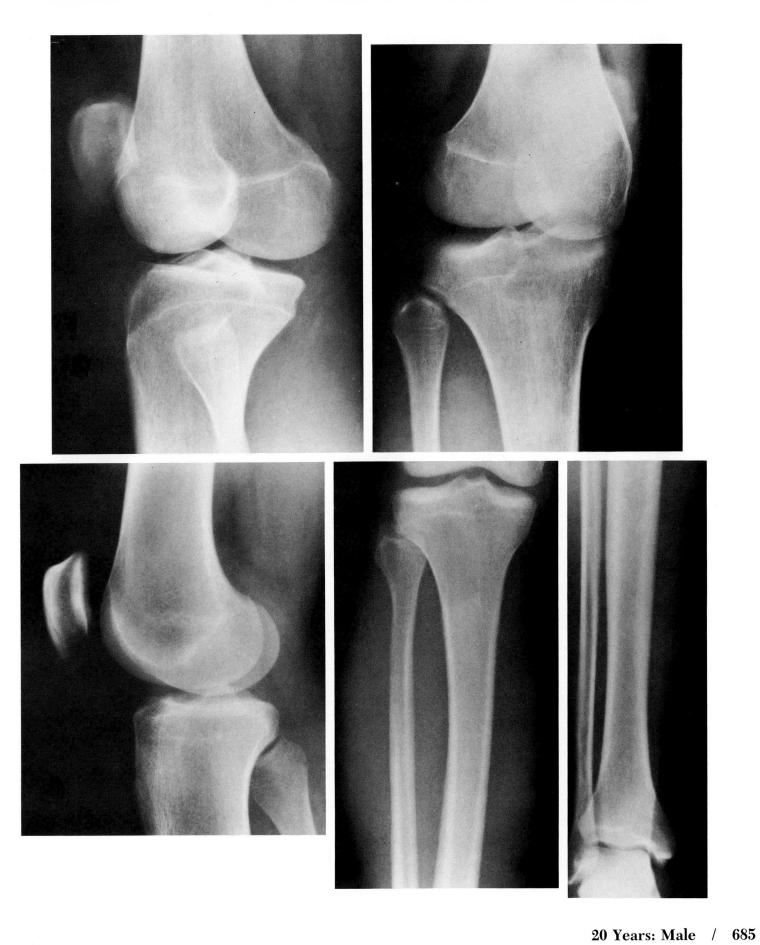

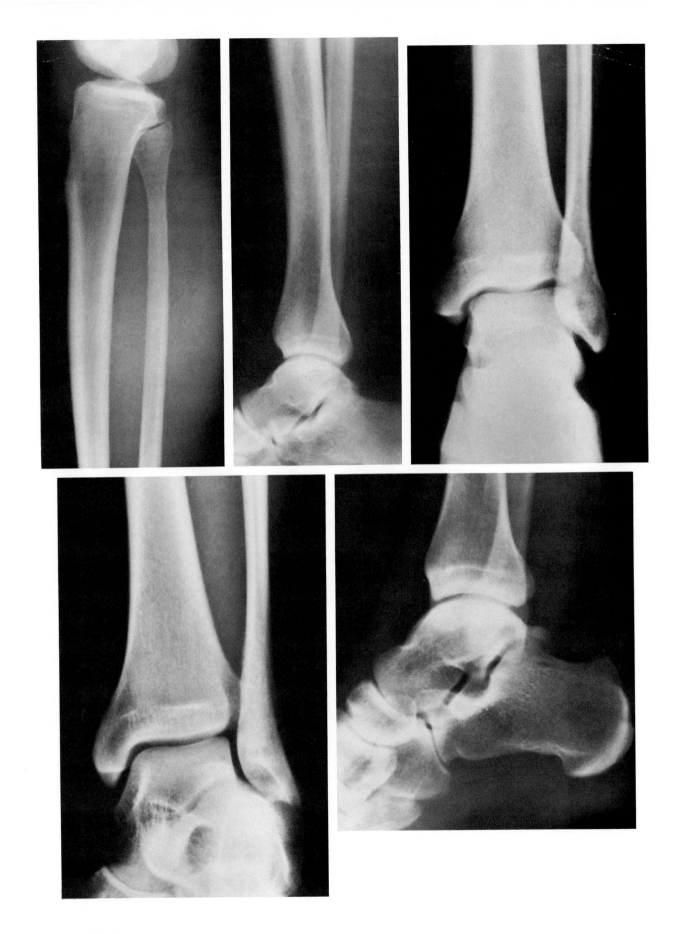

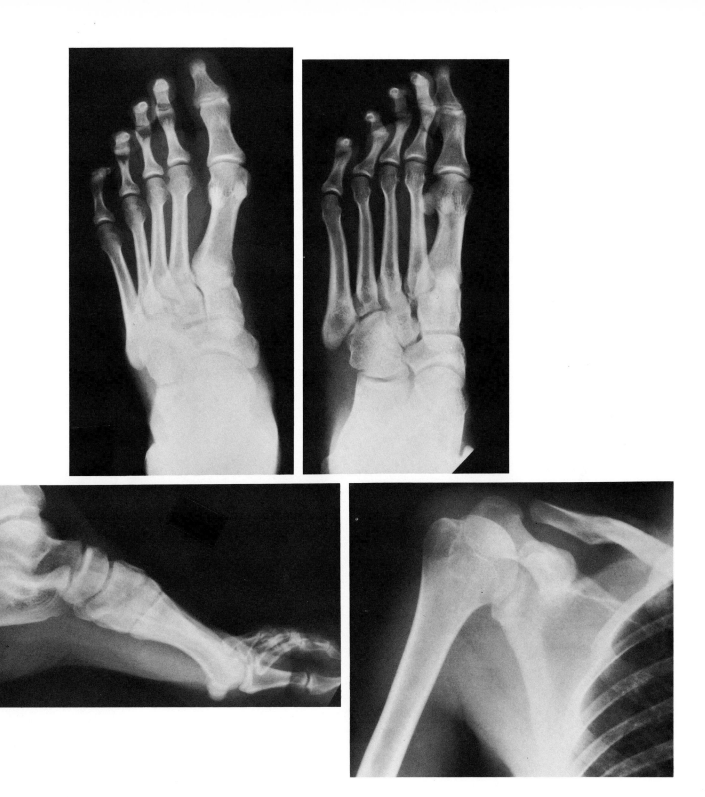

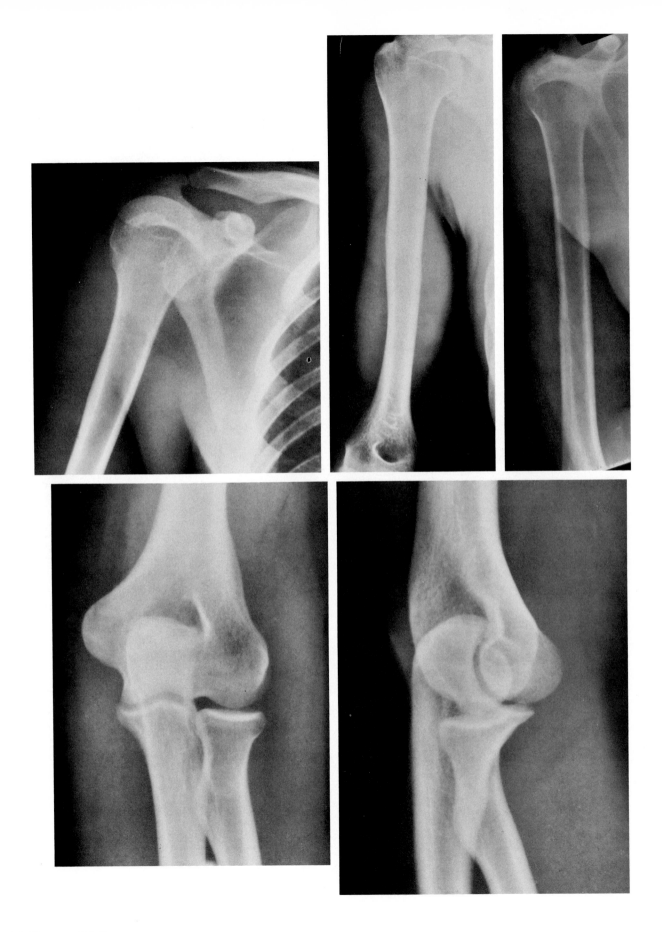

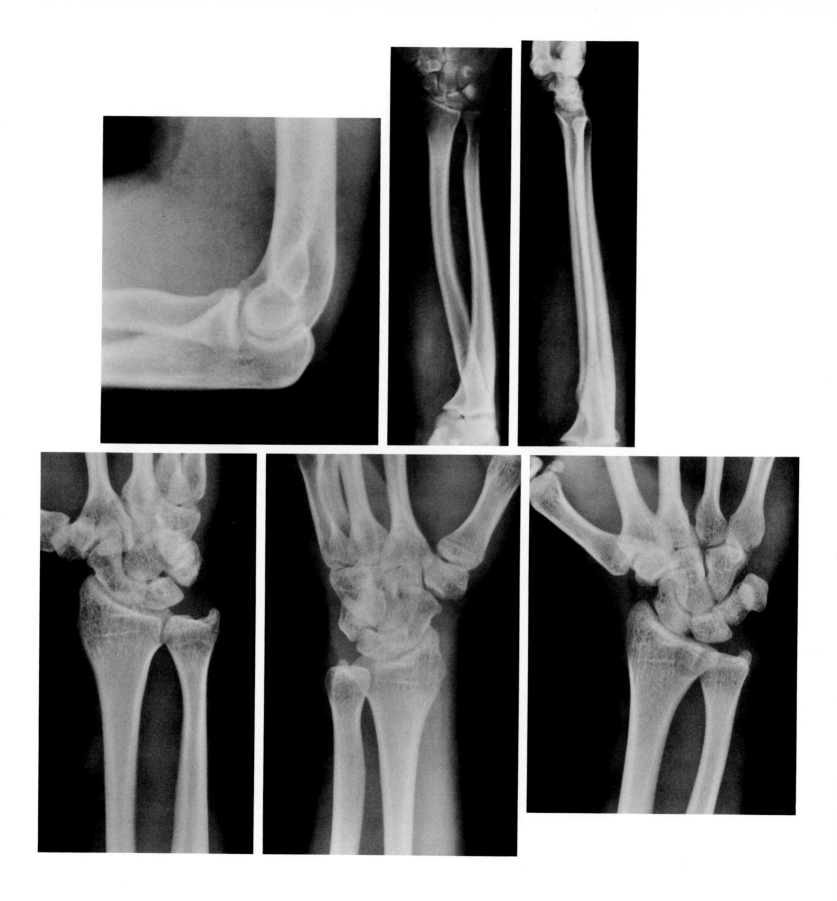

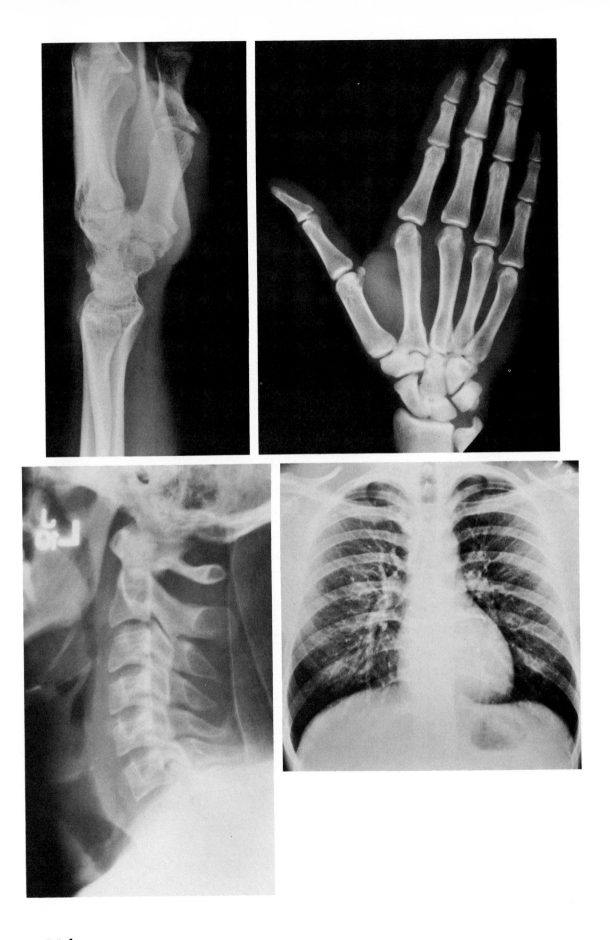

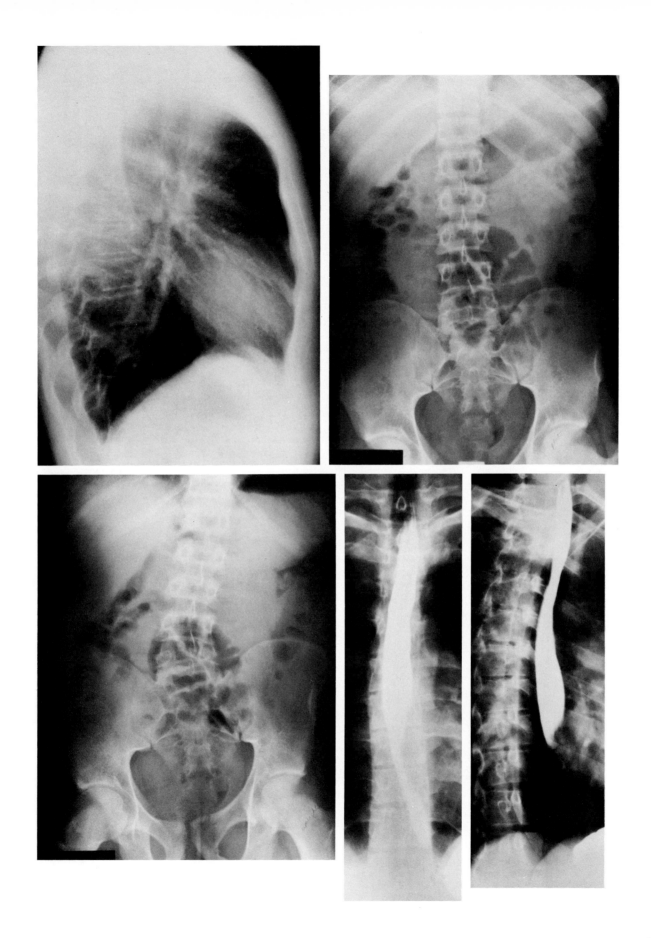

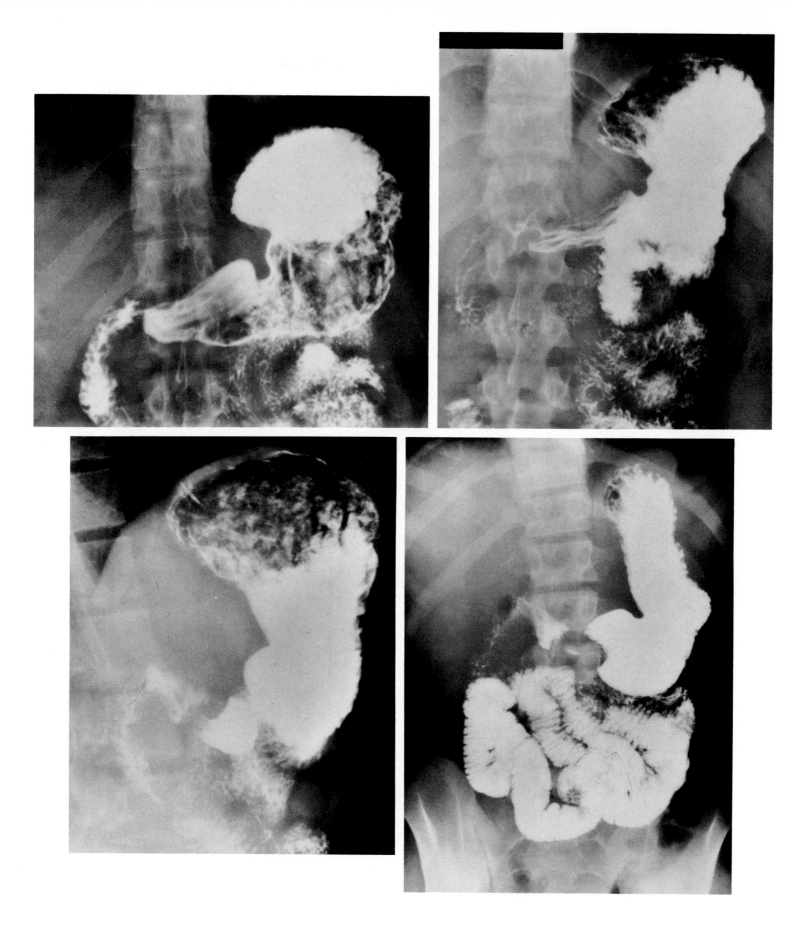

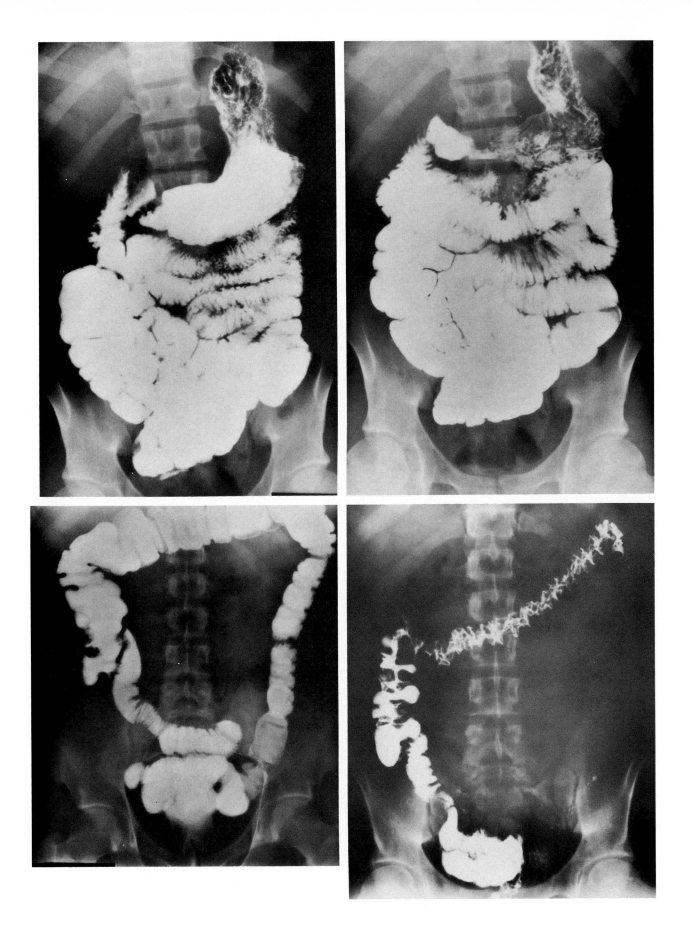

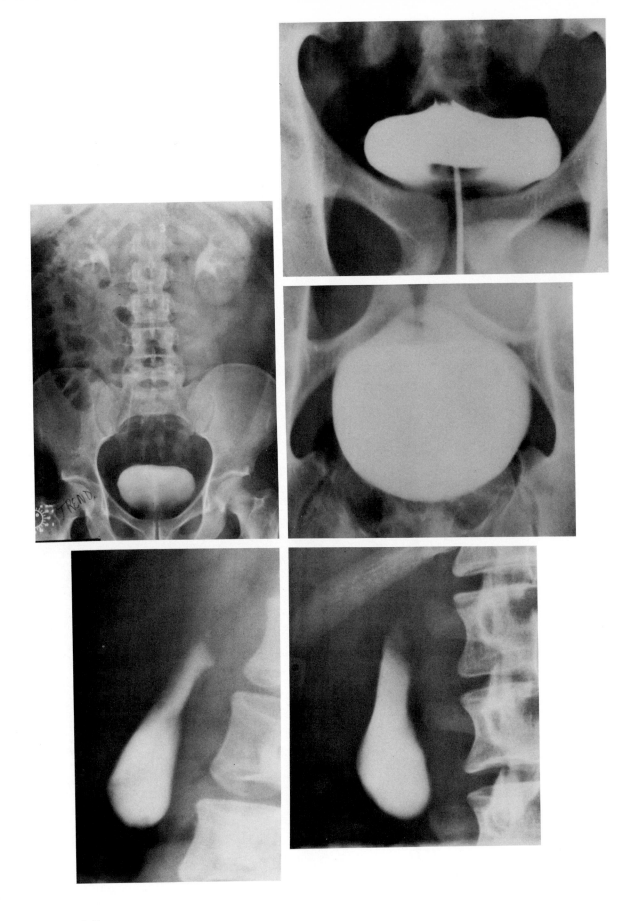

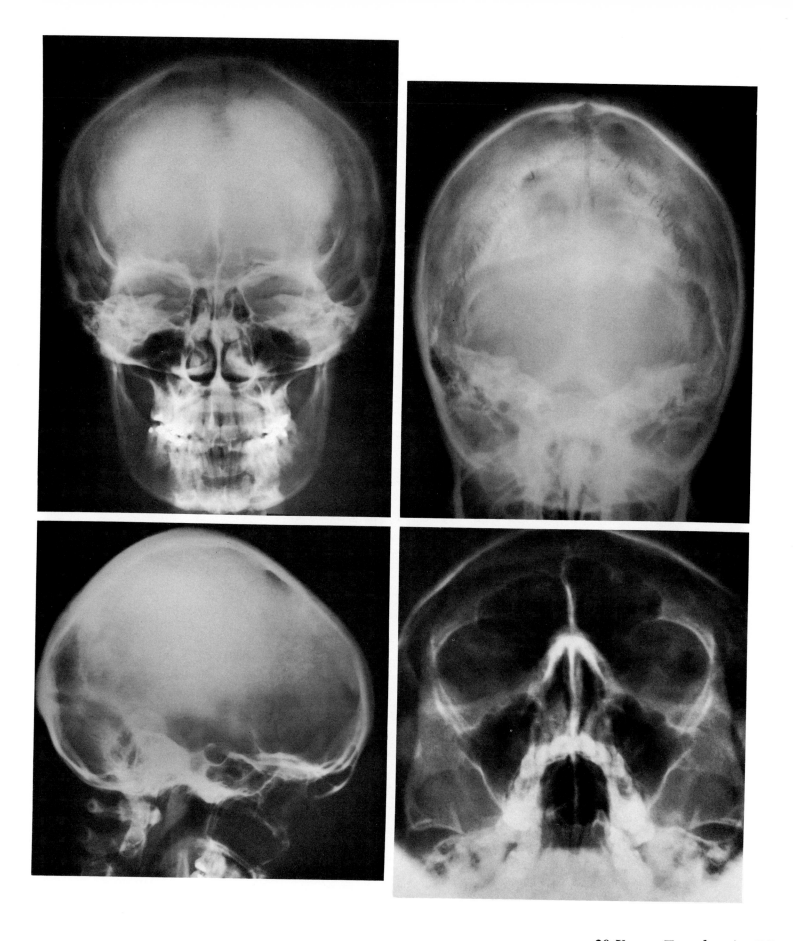

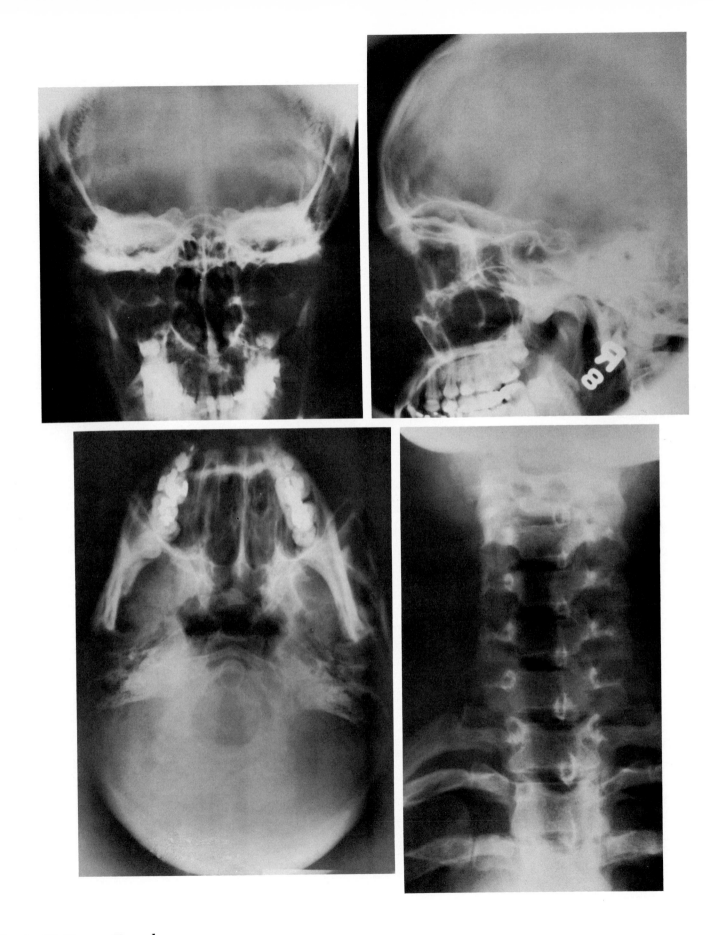

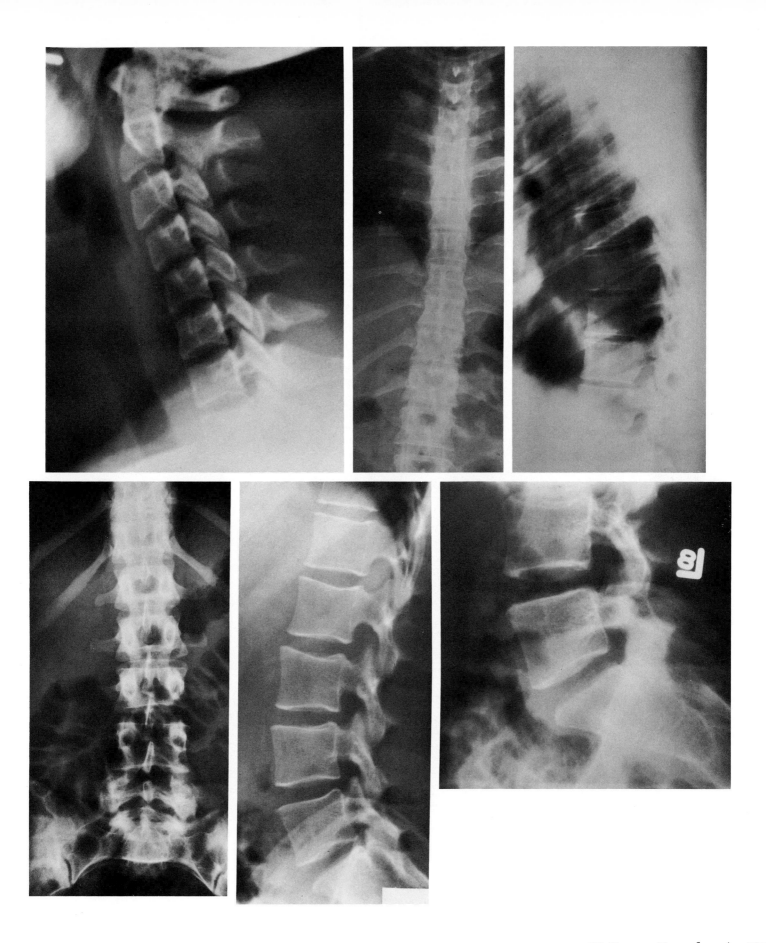

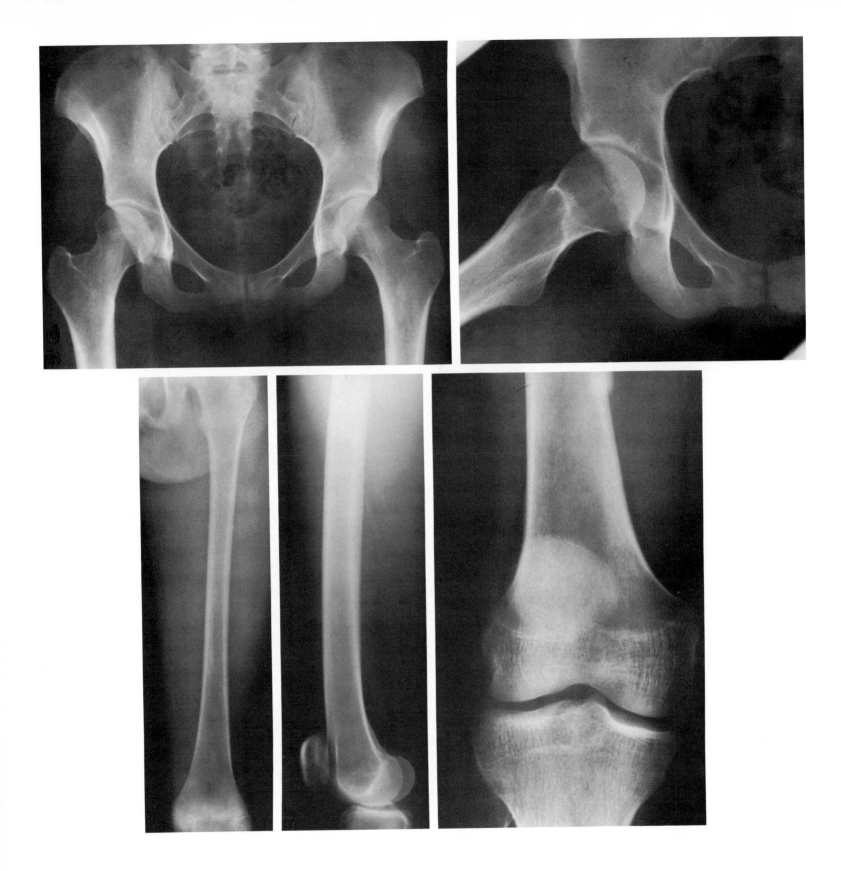

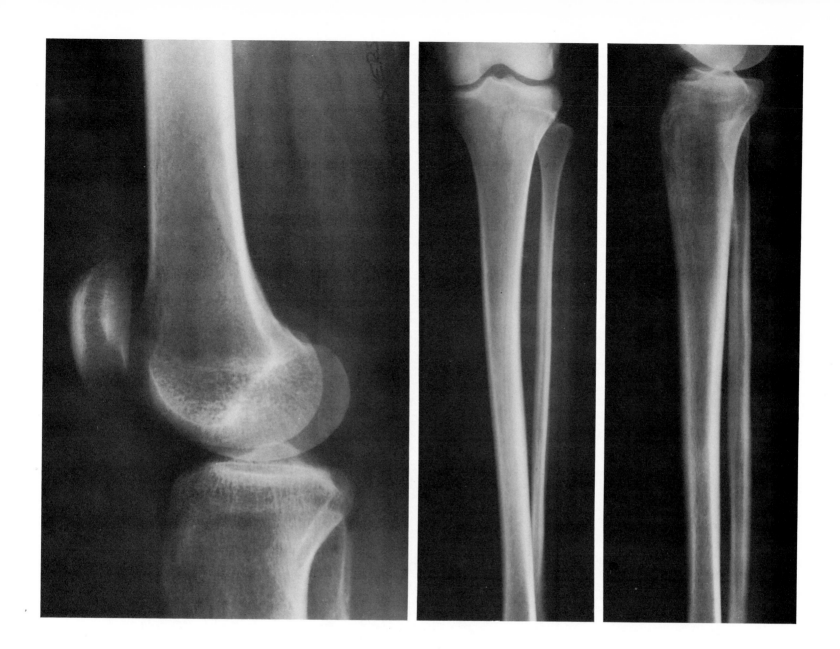

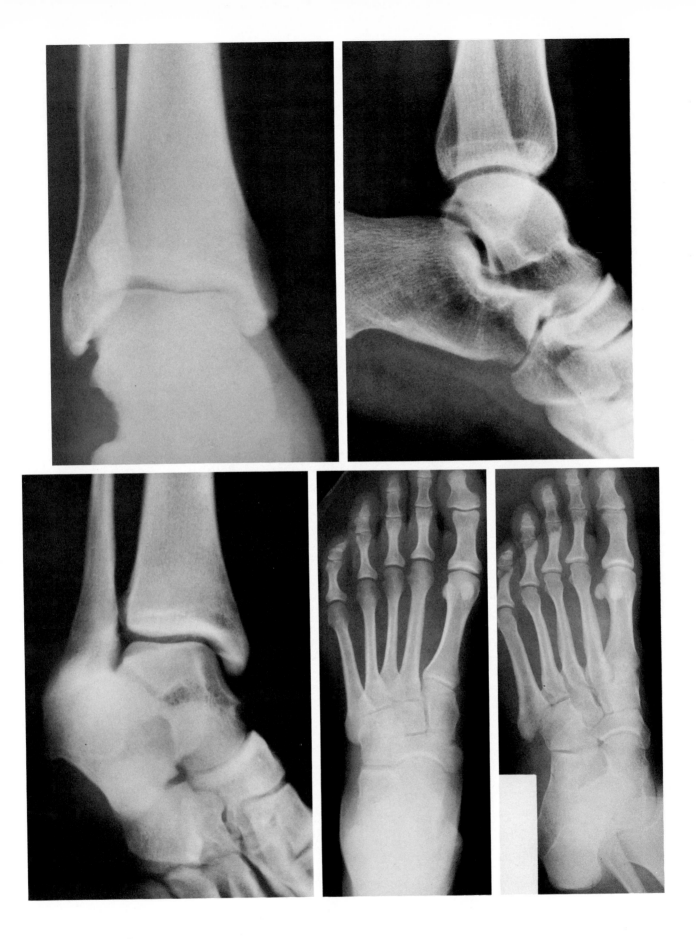

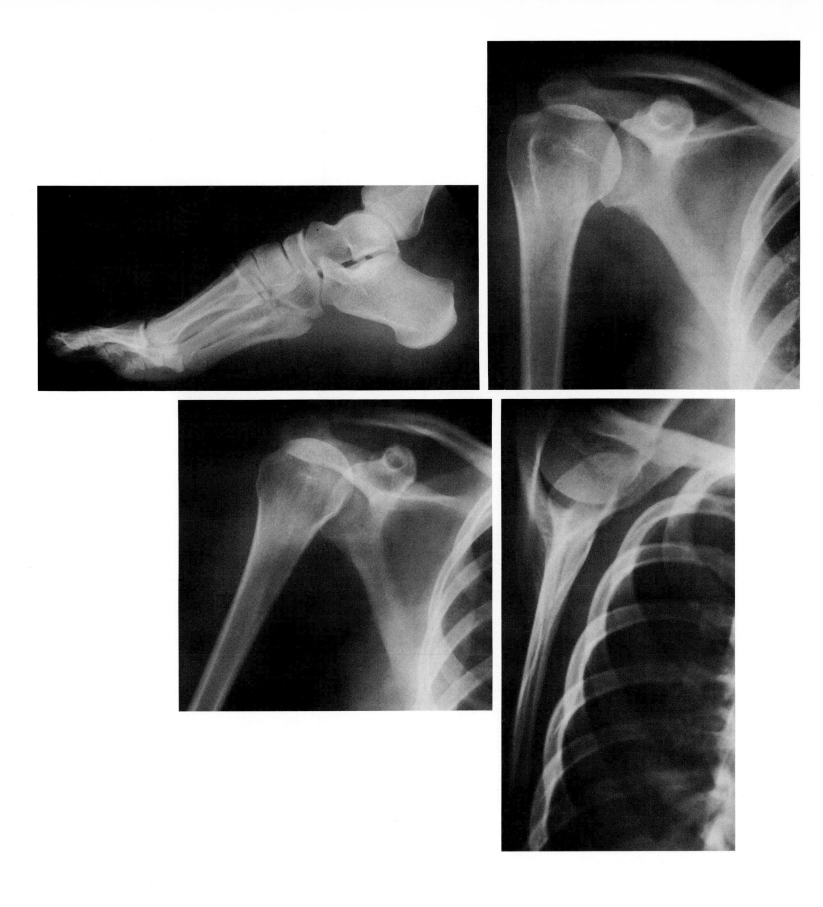

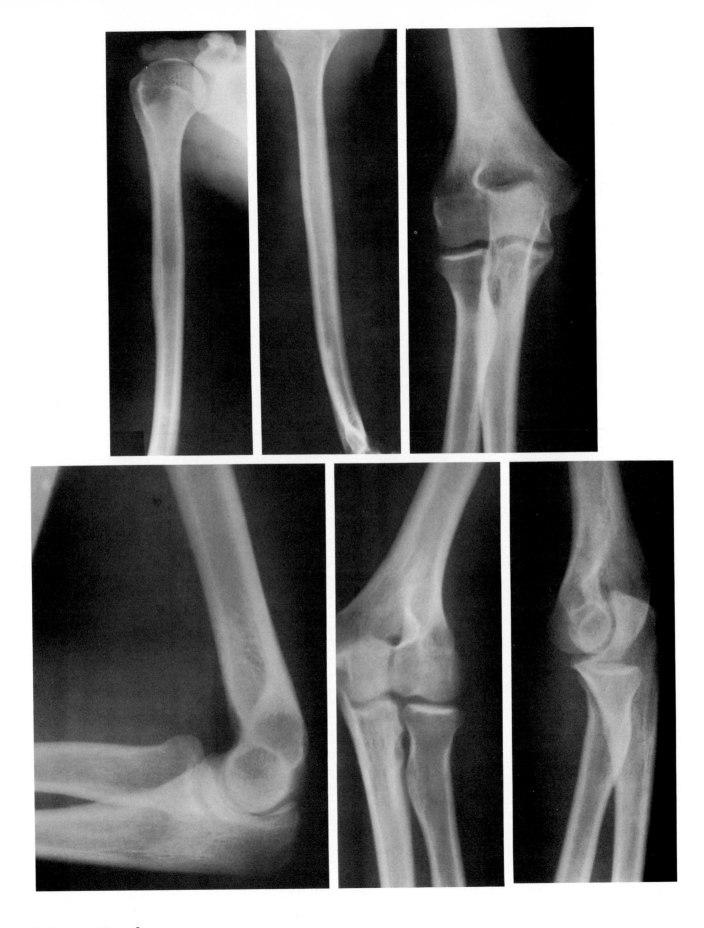

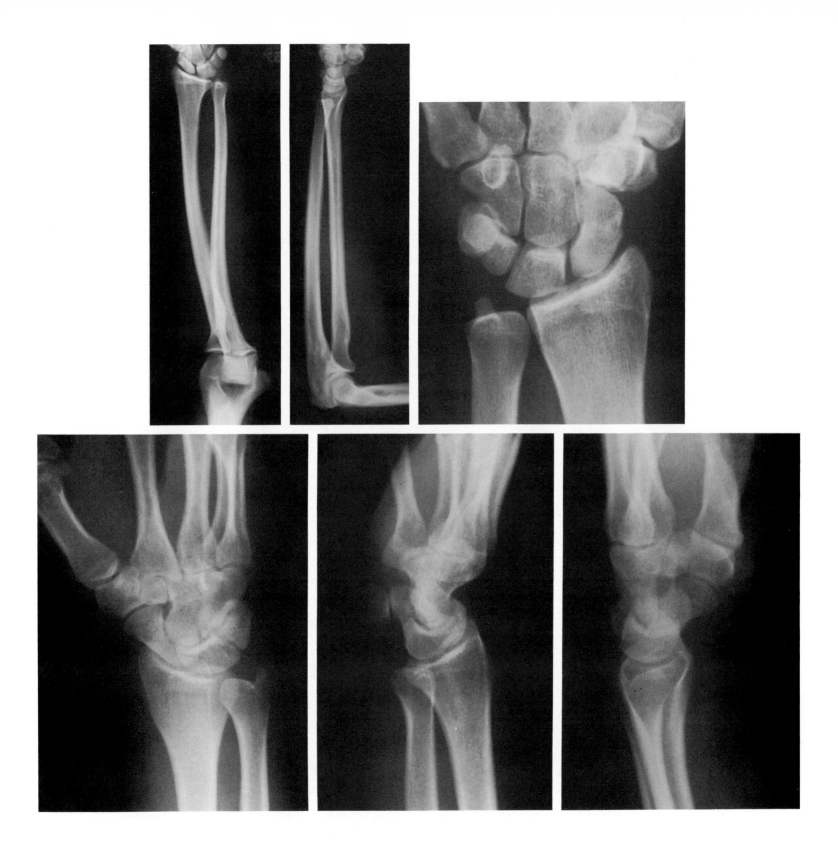

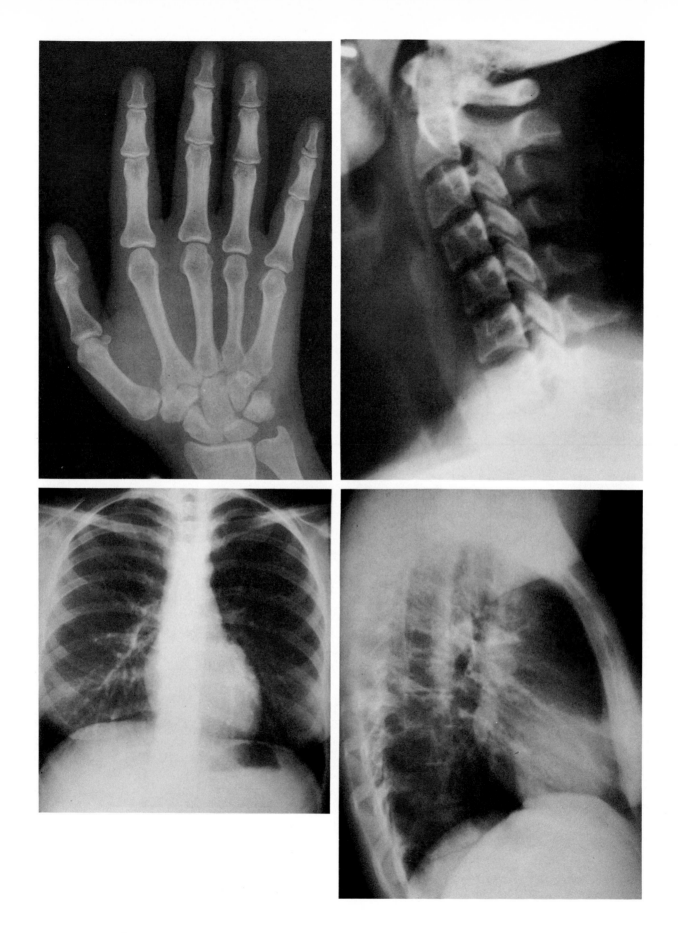

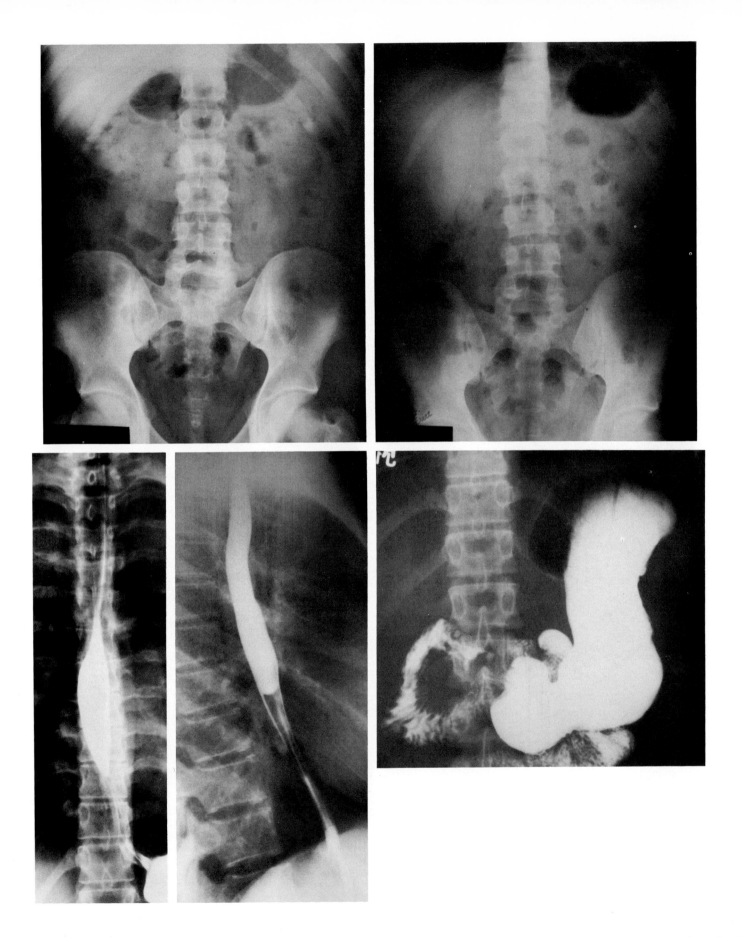

20 Years: Female / 705

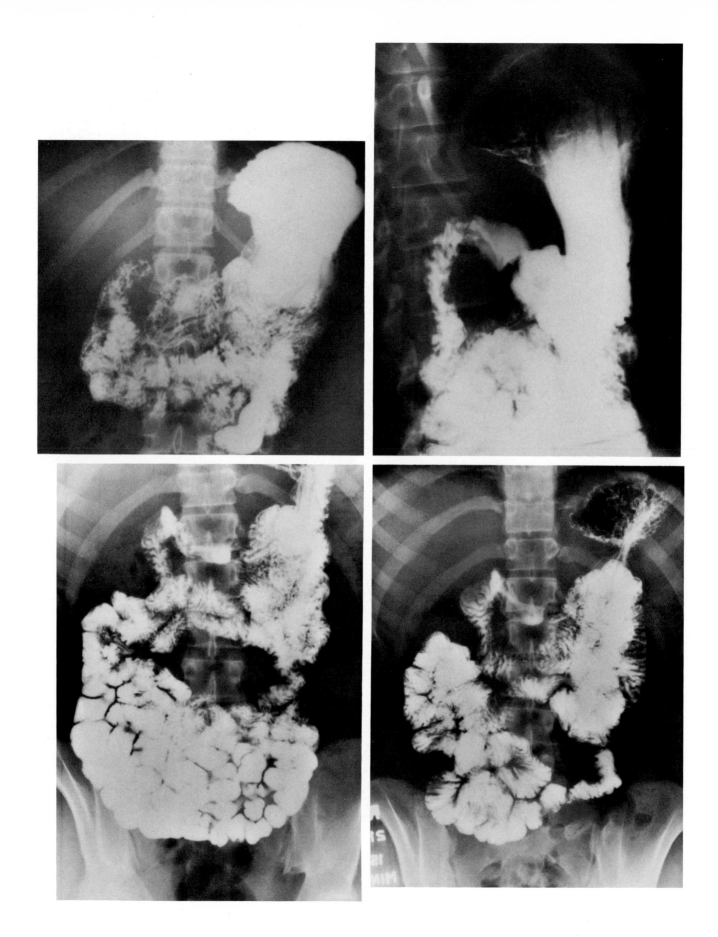

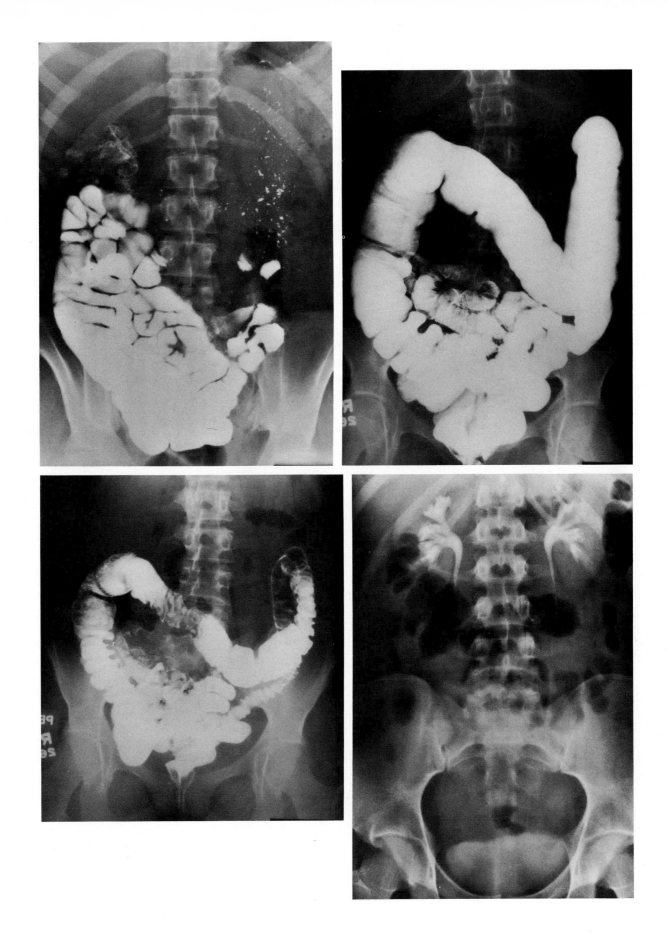

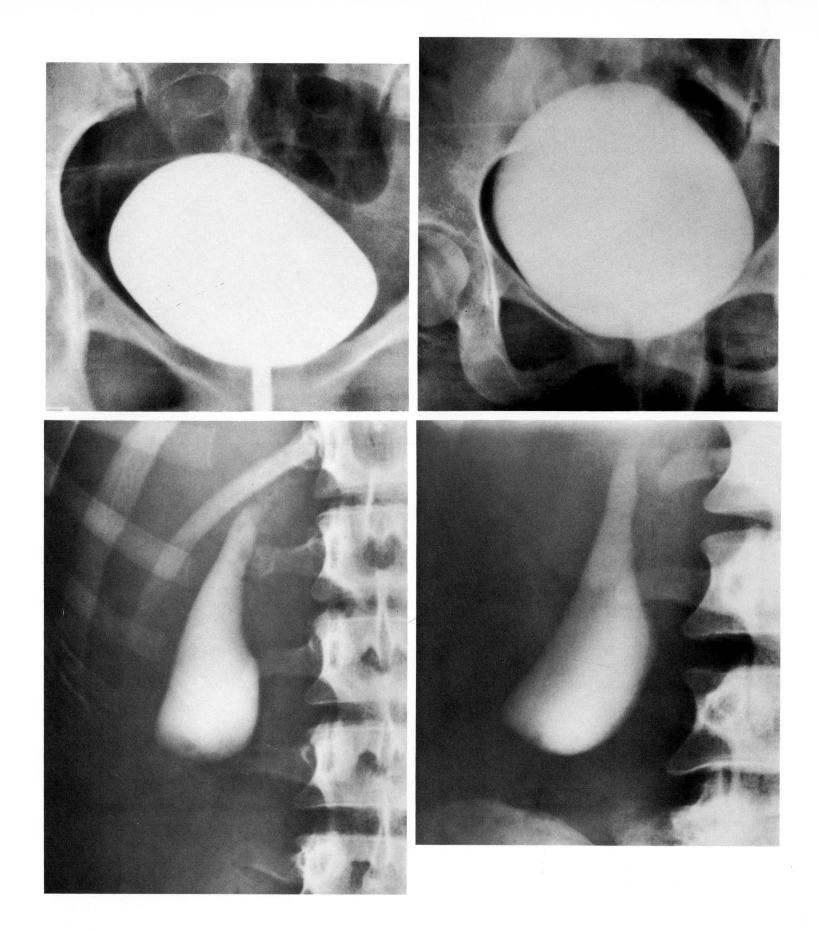